Chinese Medicine Revisited

A Western View of Chinese Medicine

Hamid Montakab

Second Edition

Homaya

ISBN: -978-2-9701039-1-2

CONTENTS

Foreword

Chinese medicine peaked in popularity in the West in the past half a century, greatly due to its integrative approach, in which the totality of the person is taken into consideration, thus making it a complete holistic medicine. This contrasts with the Western allopathic medicine, which has been consistently dividing the body into parts and specialties and separating the human body from its mind and soul.

The rift between the physical and the subtle, very typical of the modern belief system, has occurred in spite of the fact that most ancient medicines around the world understood and even emphasized body, mind, and soul unity as well as considering the human as an integral part of nature.

Today, Chinese medicine together with Hindu Ayurvedic medicine, are probably the oldest surviving medical practices in the world. Although both medicines have been traced back to 5000 BC and might have at times influenced each other, Chinese medicine spread not only to the Far East but also to Persia in medieval times and to Europe, in particular to France, as early as the 17th and 18th centuries. So much so that WHO statistics at the end of the 20th century showed that the various methods of Chinese medicine were the most utilized forms of medical practice around the world.

Over the centuries, Chinese Medicine developed a variety of healing modalities, the best known to be acupuncture and herbalism, alongside massage, bone setting, diet as well as self-cultivation energy exercises. The principles that underline Chinese medicine and the Chinese thought system are fundamentally the same. The overall world-view and understanding of cyclical and seasonal evolutions, natural life transformations and changes, as well as notions of health and disease, were reflected in all aspects of the ancient Chinese lifestyle, and maybe even found today in Chinese astrology (Ba Zhi), geomancy (Feng Shui), and a popular form of fortune telling (Yi Jing). The more scientific forms of Ba Zhi, Feng Shui, and Yi Jing have been integrated into Chinese medical practices.

Philosophical and spiritual aspects of Chinese medicine find their roots in the teachings of three contemporary masters, Laozi, Confucius and Buddha. Deep understanding of the human being and what causes disease, led the early Chinese to look at inner causative factors, emotions, and mental states. Today, any of the Chinese medical methods may be applied individually and even symptomatically without necessarily involving the mental-emotional aspects of a patient. But judging from the ancient texts and teachings, the superior doctors and healers considered the human being in his or her totality, integrating all three dimensions: physical, energetic and psychological. This may also explain the emphasis on self-transformational practices and especially the cultivation of the mind, often stressed in the older texts. Western modern theories in psychology and psychotherapy, have very definitely contributed to a better understanding of the Chinese ancient concepts, and they have the advantage of offering the Western therapist more adept tools in dealing with such problems.

Ancient Chinese medicine relied on a sophisticated diagnostic system, mostly developed to predict an imbalance in order to prevent disease. This preventative strategy in medicine was praised as being superior to actually treat a manifested disease.

In the past decades, Chinese medicine has come to be known as "TCM" (Traditional Chinese Medicine), a term coined during the early years of Communist China, to distinguish it from Western allopathic medicine. Many of the ancient theories and concepts were purged out in an attempt to make Chinese Medicine more scientific and more "medicalized". For example, in earlier TCM text-books, all references to the psyche the spirit and the shamanic backgrounds of acupuncture were filtered out, reducing acupuncture to a mere reflex therapy. On the other hand, the European tradition, which had been influenced originally by Classical Chinese Medicine (CCM), allowed for a certain preservation of the tradition. Fortunately today in China the ancient roots of Chinese medicine are being reconsidered. In the past 40 years, many of the classical Chinese medical texts have been translated and commented, thus bridging the past with the present.

In the West, the Chinese medical concepts found a common ground of comprehension in France and in Germany in Hahnemann's homeopathic theories. In the early 1900's many homeopathic doctors in France took readily to acupuncture thus creating a European brand of acupuncture. Both homeopathy and acupuncture are considered "vibrational/energy" medicines and both approach the human being in a multi-dimensional manner. As such both have been strongly opposed and contested by main-line allopathic medicine as not having a material and scientific base. Furthermore, the ancient and foreign language and concepts of Chinese medicine have made it difficult for the modern Western physician to accept and to incorporate it into the Western therapeutic arsenal. In spite of scores of scientific studies, demonstrating the effectiveness of acupuncture, the Western medical body remains skeptical.

Today we are at an exciting turning point, where nuclear physics and Western medical technologies are capable of demonstrating not only the veracity of the ancient Chinese concepts but even the physical reality of acupuncture channels and points. (Please refer to the appendix).

It is my strong belief that in the very near future, Chinese medicine will become part of integrated medical practices. The main debate should not revolve around the opposition of the Eastern and Western medical approaches, but it should rather explore the areas of the efficiency of each method and select the most appropriate, least harmful and most economic therapeutic approach for the patient.

The application of superior Western technologies can only be enriched by the deeper Oriental vision and understanding of the human nature, thus combining intelligence with wisdom, beautifully represented in the Chinese parable of the union of Fire and Water.

Preface

This book is the result of 40 years practicing and teaching Chinese medicine. It is a reflection of my own struggles caused by my previous Western materialistic medical background trying to grasp the Chinese energetic concepts. In extension, it also reflects the difficulties of Western students to grasp a totally different thought system. In the early '70s, there were very few textbooks available to the Western student, they were either technical manuals on acupuncture or herbs or else translations of ancient philosophical or spiritual texts, almost incomprehensible to a 20th-century Western mind. Teaching and answering questions on these at first alien concepts forced me to deepen my own understanding of these ideas. At times this was only made possible by integrating them into my own daily life.

I have to admit that although I have been submerged in Chinese medicine and the oriental concepts and studied and practiced many of its methods now for many years, I still feel like a beginner and I know that I will never stop learning. I am grateful to all my students for stimulating me to deepen my search and understanding, and I hope that, even in a minute way, I may contribute to help others along the same path.

The concepts presented in this text have three origins: the written ancient Chinese sources; the oral tradition as transmitted by Daoist Master J. Yuen; and the French tradition itself a heritage of their early contacts with China and Indo-China (Vietnam) as primarily transmitted through Soulié de Morant, Chamfrault and Nguyen Van Nghi.

This book addresses the Western practitioner and as such attempts to demystify and explain the oriental concepts in a language more adapted to a Western way of thinking.

It constitutes a very comprehensive text for the beginner and a solid introduction for the layperson. But it may also be an excellent reference manual for the practitioner as many theories and concepts, missing in various Eastern or Western publications, have been included and discussed.

The book is broken down into six sections:

► Part I describes the oriental vision, the notion of Qi ≈ Energy and covers all the basic Chinese dialectical systems.

► Part II: explores the physical and energetic structure of the body, the organ systems, as well as the process of energy production and energy circulation.

► Part III: studies the concept of health and disease and explores the causes of disease

► Part IV: is an in-depth study of the art of diagnosis, including the classical "Four pillars" in diagnosis, but also describes the morpho-psychological assessments.

► Part V: is an overview of all the therapeutic methods used in Chinese medicine and presented by various practitioners in their respective fields of expertise: acupuncture, other auxiliary methods, herbs and diet, Tuina massage, Qi Gong, and the cultivation of the mind.

► Part VI: explores some other methods applied in Chinese medicine: such as *Yi Jing* ≈ The Book of Changes; *Ba Zhi* and *Gan Zhi* ≈ Astrology, and *Feng Shui* ≈ Geomancy.

Additionally, the Appendix includes:

► An update on "Evidence of Acupuncture".

► A brief historical overview of Chinese medicine in China and Europe.

► A Glossary of Chinese medical terms used in this manual.

How to read this book

More often than not, the translations used in the West for Chinese medical terms are misleading or confusing. In this text, attempts have been made to address this issue. The Chinese terms have been designated in Pinyin with their most common translation as well as the Chinese ideogram.

To avoid further confusion, Chinese organ names have been capitalized to distinguish them from common Western anatomical terms, for example, "Liver" relates to the Chinese physiological concept, whereas "liver" is the Western anatomical organ. The same applies to the Chinese concepts of "Heat, Cold, Damp ..." as opposed to actual climatic heat, cold or dampness.

Acknowledgments

The incentive for writing this book was mainly initiated by colleagues and co-teachers and further supported by students who were missing many of the explanations of the Chinese medical concepts in the current literature. I express my gratitude to the co-authors, Simon Becker, Dr. Bartosz Chmielnicki, Christine Dam, Dr. Stefan Englert, Peter Firebrace, Phillip Haas, Solange Montakab, Bernhard Nessensohn and Christine Reist who contributed in the realization of this manual. Special thanks to Pia Huber for reviewing the text and to Yang Wang for correcting the Chinese terms. And above all to my wife Solange, who not only co-authored the book but also had the difficult task of being the first critic.

INTRODUCTION

Historical Background

The theoretical concepts of Chinese medicine are an integral part of Chinese history and cannot be separated from the 5000-year-old myths and legends that surround its origins. Historically speaking, no written document has been dated with certainty prior to the 12th century BC. It can be said that Chinese medicine, as we know it today, has three origins: the historical records partly lost in the mists of legend, the written tradition, and oral transmission.

On the one hand there are the legends of the three Emperors: Fu Xi, circa 2900 BC, inventor of the "Trigrams" and rudimentary writing, instigator of the rites of marriage. Followed by Shen Nong, estimated around 2800 BC, named the “Divine laborer", who instructed on the use of the plow and the hoe in agriculture, and to whom is attributed the knowledge about plants and herbal medicine. The third Emperor is Huang Di, estimated around the 26th century BC, the organizer of the state and the government, who refined writing and would be the author of the oldest medical classic the Nei Jing Su Wen (► Fig. 01).

On the other hand, there are the classical texts, the oldest being the Huang Di Nei Jing known as the Yellow Emperor’s Classic of Internal Medicine. Historians are still debating about the period of composition of the Nei Jing that could be anytime between 1000 and 200 BC. The legend has it that the Nei Jing consisted of four books: the *Su Wen* ≈ Simple Questions on general concepts of Chinese Medicine, and the *Ling Shu* ≈ Spiritual Axis, which describes the primary and secondary channels of Acupuncture. Two other books have been lost: the *Tai Shu* and the *Ming Tang*. The *Nei Jing* together with the third century BC *Nan Jing* and the first century AD *Shang Han Lun*, constitute the backbone of Chinese medical literature.

Between the two, the oral transmission passed from master to disciple, that has reached the present times, and often disputed by sinologists

To complicate matters further, as Chinese medicine evolved, and as new theories and concepts were added, out of deference for the ancients, the older concepts were not removed. As a result, the present time students and practitioners find themselves struggling with concepts that overlap, differ or sometimes even seem to contradict one another.

The Oriental vision – West versus East

When the Western scientific medicine encountered the ancient Chinese healing tradition, it had no choice but to term it "empirical", and even attributing the discovery of acupuncture and the complex channel pathways to pure chance.

I believe that between the mystical and mythical origins attributed to god-like personalities and the accidental discovery of an extremely complex system, there could be another possible explanation.

What could be the reason that would explain that the Chinese discovered and developed numerous technologies centuries before the West, for example:

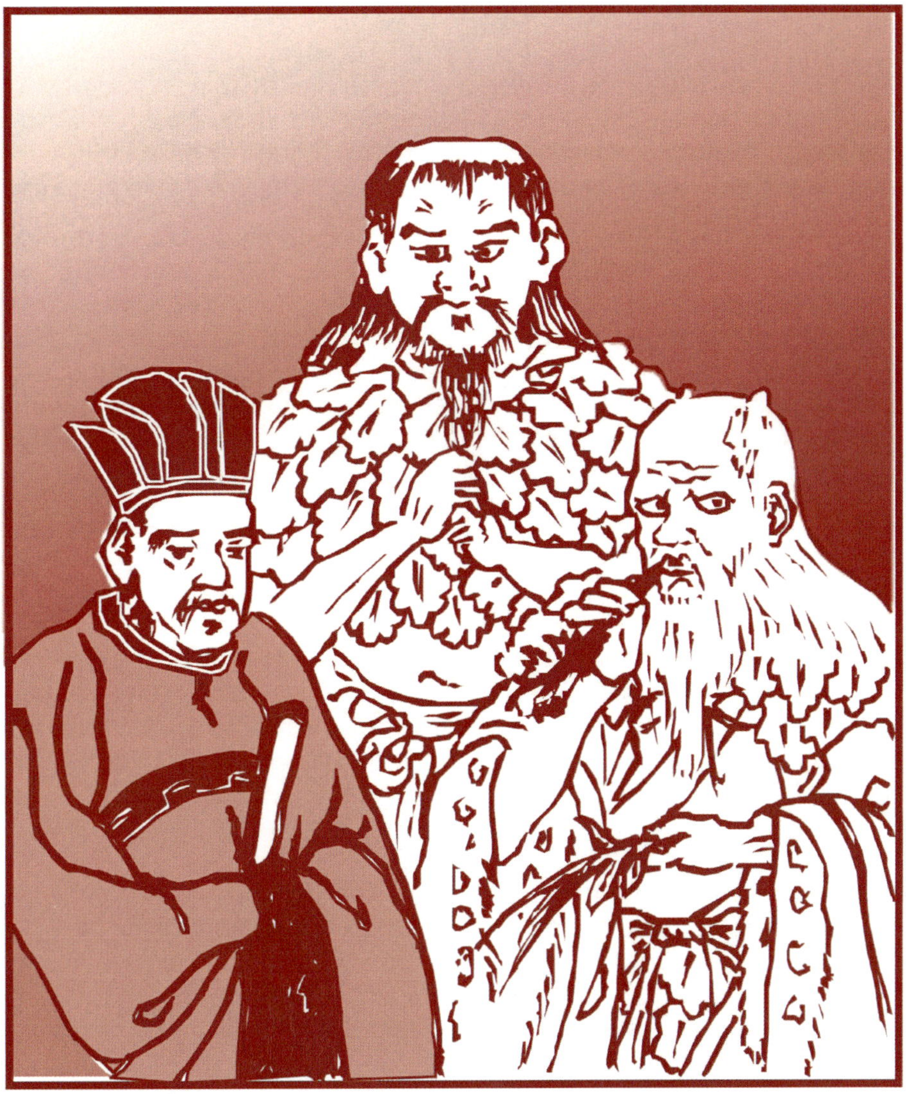

Figure 01: The three mythical emperors: Huang Di (left), Fuxi (center), Shen Nong (right)

- Agricultural technologies 2000 years before the same were applied in the West,
- The processing of iron steel, the printing press, and the compass almost 1400 years before the West,
- Discovery of the blood circulation system, 1800 years before Harvey,
- The various concepts about the human physiology and the interactions between the psyche and the soma, and the deep understanding of the origins of disease, prognosis, and treatment,
- Emphasis on prevention, with attempts at vaccination as early as 200 AD
- And most relevantly, the discovery of the binary language 27 centuries before the West invented the computer language

I truly do not believe that the above discoveries were due to supra-human qualities but rather a different way of looking at the world we live in, a totally different conception of reality.

The Oxford Dictionary defines reality as "the state of things as they actually exist", this includes everything that is, whether or not it is observable or comprehensible. On a more subjective level, private experiences and interpretation of events shape personal reality of an individual, called phenomenological reality.

Historically in the West, the reality was based on facts. A fact is an observed phenomenon in the natural world that is perceived as an elemental principle. It is rarely one that can be subject to personal interpretation. And yet facts such as "the earth is flat" or that "the sun is at the center of the universe", for centuries dominated man's perceptions and definitions of what is real. Today, the most pertinent of these facts could be said to be the "solid" nature of matter. Even though today we know that the smallest constituent of matter, the atom, is made of primarily empty space or void, our age-old conditioning does not allow us to perceive it other than solid.

The oriental and specifically the Chinese age-old vision of the human being and the world is based on a uniting and globalizing principle, with an analogical approach to phenomena, whereas the Western approach is based on separating and analyzing the phenomena situated on the same plane. The oriental approach is therefore much more intellectual and intuitive in nature, where symbols take an important place. Even the Chinese language and writing, the "ideograms", demonstrate this point. On the opposite the Western vision is much more scientific and technological, relying more on the visible rather than the occult.

It is often deeper to know why something is true
rather than to have a proof that it is true. — *A. Zee*

In quantum physics, Heisenberg's Uncertainty Principle led the nuclear physicist Amit Goswami to assume that no reality exists independently of our own consciousness as an observer. Whether this is true or not, this line of thinking brings us back to the ancient philosophical systems such as Buddhism or Daoism, which state that life, as we conceive it, is but an illusion. This illusion is created by the mind, which perceives the natural phenomena and interprets them according to the socio-cultural conditioning. This social framework gives a semblance of coherence and maintains mental sanity, but in exchange prevents one from conceiving the "impossible". In the West, great breakthroughs in science could only occur when an individual managed to break away from the established frameworks of thinking, such as with Galileo, Newton or Einstein.

Therefore to understand Chinese medicine and the ancient Chinese vision, it is imperative to adopt a global and analogical approach, where symbols take on crucial importance, and where numbers become symbols.

When the finger points to the moon, look at the moon, not at the finger! — Zen saying

Numbers have the great advantage of having a universal symbolism that goes beyond the barriers of culture and language, and as Pythagoras would put it:

Evolution is the law of life;
Numbers are the law of the universe,
Unity is the law of God.

Part I- Principles of Chinese Medical Thought

1. The vision of the universe

Microcosm-Macrocosm

In the Chinese vision, the human is a reflection of the universe. The Chinese refer to the human being as Ren人“Man or Human”.

The laws which govern the universe “macrocosm”, also govern the human “microcosm”, thus to understand humanity we can study the world that surrounds us ....as above, so below

Hermes Trismegistus

Life, as we experience it, is the result of the interaction of two opposite forces, symbolized by "Heaven and Earth" within a "Time" and "Space" framework.

The universe is a dynamic system within which all phenomena are inter-dependent.

This dynamic system, the macrocosm, is in constant change, but there is a self-regulating mechanism, which maintains equilibrium and harmony

The human in the world is like a microcosm within a macrocosm. The humans are submitted to the same constant external changes, and their self-regulating mechanisms, by constant adaptation, spontaneously maintaining a state of balance and health or "ease", the so-called "homeostasis".

A loss of this adaptation will cause "dis-balance" and "dis-ease".

We cannot study humans and their states of Health and Disease, without considering the world that surrounds them. This then is the basis of "holistic medicine".

The variations of the macrocosm, are mainly experienced as the cycles of day and night, the seasons and the climates. In humans, these variations are described as the changes in their vital activities or vital substances, called the movements of "*Qi*" (energy).

Know thyself and you will know the universe and the Gods. Socrates

The Substance of the Universe: Energy "Qi" 气/氣

The universe and its multitude of manifestations are expressions of variations and movements of a vital substance called "*Qi*" (▶ Fig. 1.1).

Between Heaven and Earth, there is Qi and the Law.

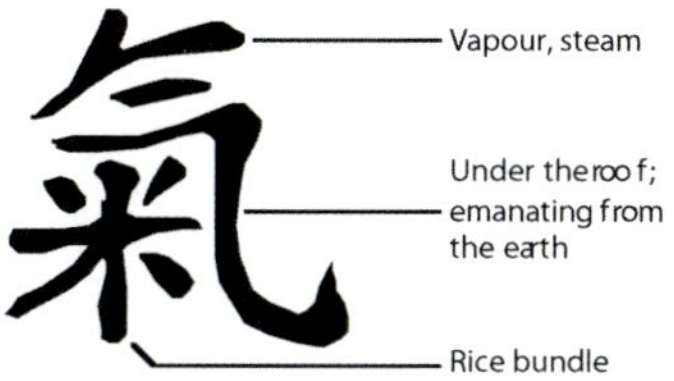

Fig. 1.1: The ideogram of Qi represents the steam that rises when rice is cooked. Evoking the idea of the transformation of visible matter into invisible vapor under the influence of fire.

All phenomena in the universe, as well as all the states in human beings, are expressions of this vital substance "*Qi*", in various degrees of movement and of concentration.

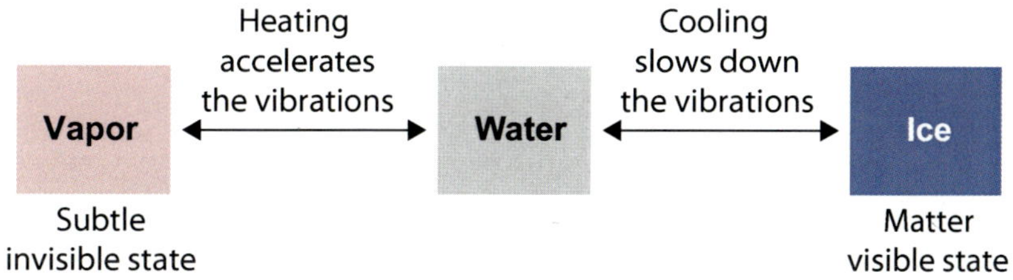

Figure 1.2: The three states of water, solid-liquid-vapor, represent the states of *Qi*

All phenomena in the universe, as well as all the states in human beings, are expressions of this vital substance "*Qi*", in various degrees of movement and of concentration.

A concentration-densification of *Qi* produces the material state, its dispersion-rarefaction produces the immaterial, the subtle or invisible state. A clear example may be observed in the various states of water, which is fluid in its normal state, becomes ice when concentrated and made dense, or vapor when it is dispersed and rarefied (▶ Fig. 1.2).

Qi has been translated as the vital force, energy, material force, vapor, emanation, fluid, life spirit, ether, etc.

In Chinese understanding, life is a materialization of *Qi* and death is a dispersion or de-materialization of *Qi*.

Humans are subject to the interaction of two opposite and complementary forces, represented by the concept of "Heaven and Earth".

Here "Heaven" symbolizes all, more subtle energies, and "Earth" represents all that is material.

We always study humans in this three-dimensional system (▶ Fig. 1.3):

- the subtle: the mind, the spirit,
- the fluid: the emotions, the energies,
- the material: the body.

These are the states of "*Qi*", in constant change, manifesting differently.

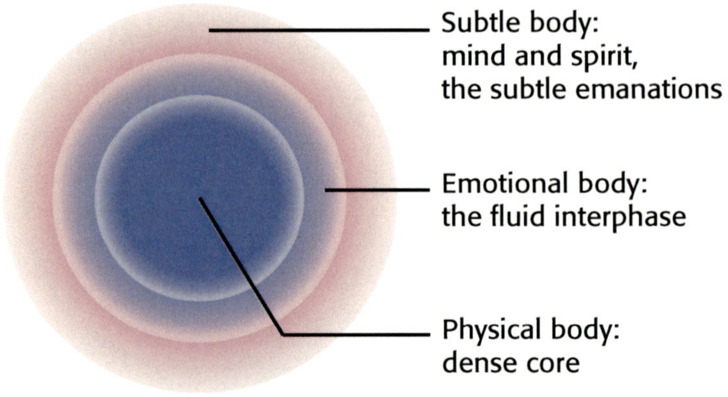

Figure 1.3: The three dimensions of the body

The matter is condensed *Qi*, the spirit is non-substantial *Qi*, in between we have the flowing *Qi* that we refer to simply as *Qi* $\approx$ Energy. The body itself is made of different degrees of density: bones, muscles, fluids and even electromagnetic fields.

On the one side there is the body, which is the condensed aspect of *Qi* and on the other side, there is the spirit that we can refer to as the mind or mental activities, resulting from neuro-hormonal impulses, hence much less condensed. Between the two extremes, there are the emotions which are much more subtle than the body, yet less subtle than the spirit-mind.

In Chinese medicine, the body, the emotions, and the mind are aspects and manifestations of the same *Qi*, and cannot be considered separately.

Qi changes its form and is given a different name, but ultimately all is a manifestation of the same "substance", the same *Qi*.

The variations of *Qi* follow certain laws. These laws are given as basic principles, in the form of dialectical systems:

- The "*Yin-Yang*" system studies the interaction of the subtle and the material.
- The "Heaven-Human-Earth" system, considers 3 states in all that exists.
- The "4 phases", are explaining the basic changes in the variation of *Qi*.
- The "5 movements", describe the 5 dynamic aspects of *Qi* in the universe and in the human being.
- The "6 energies", state all the possible variations of *Qi*: the 3 intensities of each *Yin* or *Yang* principle.

It is interesting to note that in modern nuclear physics, Einstein's theories, relating matter to energy, had already demonstrated that the state of matter changes with the speed of vibration. For decades, physicists have been attempting to reconcile quantum mechanics and general relativity and have proposed the "String theory", a mathematical model that may describe all fundamental forces and forms of matter, a concept that singularly approaches the ancient Chinese notion of "*Qi*" as the basis for all phenomena in the universe.

2. Dialectical Systems

The Dialectical Systems constitute the basis of the ancient Chinese thinking and their vision of the world. All form of arts, as well as Chinese Medicine, are established on these thought systems. We cannot truly understand the Oriental thinking if we do not grasp the symbolic meaning of the various dialectical systems.

1 (Yi 一) Creation, "The human in the image of the Dao"

The wisdom of the ancients has been passed down to us in a series of symbols.

In fact, numbers, before being used for counting and arithmetic, were universal symbols found in all ancient philosophical systems, and interestingly have the same metaphorical representations.

The Void

The concept of the Void is of capital importance in oriental and in particular in the Chinese, Daoistic principles (► chap. 21.2). It is considered the origin and the term of all form of creation, the space where *Qi* changes form and mutates.

The fullness is the appearance of a form,
It is the void of the form that gives its utility. *Lao Zi*

The void is not the absence of something, but instead, it is where the creative forces meet, it is the void at the center that gives the wheel its utility. The silent space between the notes that makes a musical harmony and the empty space between the letters that constitutes the word (► Fig. 2.1).

As was mentioned before, in nuclear physics, it is the empty space between the atomic particles that gives the form to matter, and the space between the molecules, that defines the state of matter as solid, liquid or gas.

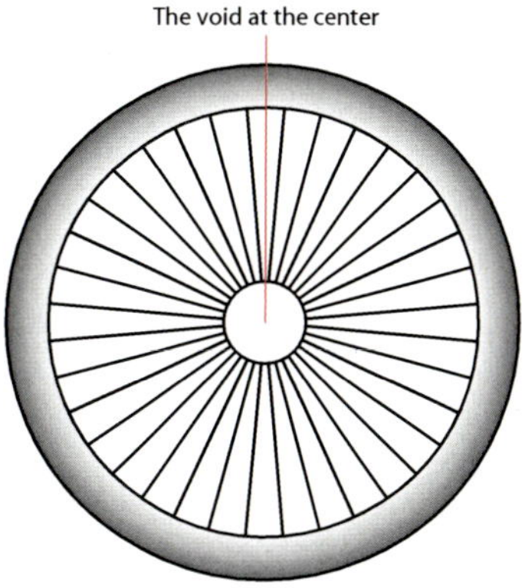

Figure 2.1: The void at the center of the wheel

Creation, Tai Ji, Dao

The Primordial Chaos ≈ *Wu Ji*無極 is the state before creation, formless, boundless and infinite; it is assimilated with the concept of Void (▶ Fig. 2.2).

The appearance of a center puts order into the disorder. Different terms refer to this center: *Zhong Ji* ≈ Central Ridge中極or polar star is the organizing center, also referred to as *Tai Ji* ≈ Supreme Ridge or Great Pole太極.

Hence the symbolism of number "one" as being the origin of creation as it contains all other numbers, and that all numbers are mere expressions of one.

This order separates above from below, light from dark, heaven from earth, or *Yang* from *Yin*.

Heaven was created by an accumulation of Yang, the element of light,
Earth was created by an accumulation of Yin, the element of darkness.

Su Wen, *chap.5*

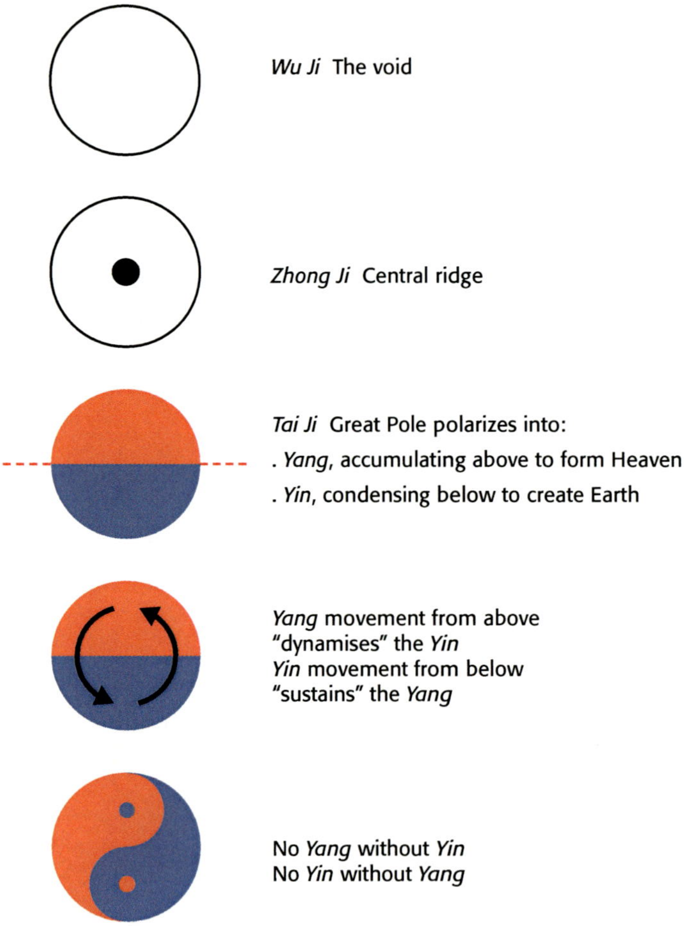

Figure 2.2: Stages of creation.

The combined movements of *Yin* and *Yang* define the basic rhythms of life, in the image of a spiral movement with the two opposite, centrifugal and centripetal movements. In the Chinese concept, life and all transformations evolve in a spiral form (▶ Fig. 2.3).

This model, also present in the West, is quite apparent in nature, having inspired the 300 BC Euclidean concept of the "Golden mean, or ratio" also called the "Divine proportion" (▶ Fig. 2.4).

It is therefore not surprising that the basic constituent of living organisms, the DNA, has a spiral structure.

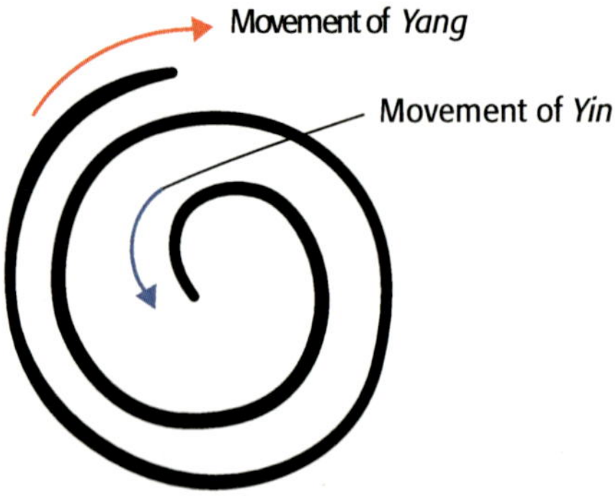

Figure 2.3: The Spiral of Life; *Yang* expands from the center, *Yin* condenses towards the center

The passage or way from the original chaos to the manifested order is known as *Dao*道 (or *Tao*) ≈ Path (▶ Fig. 2.5).

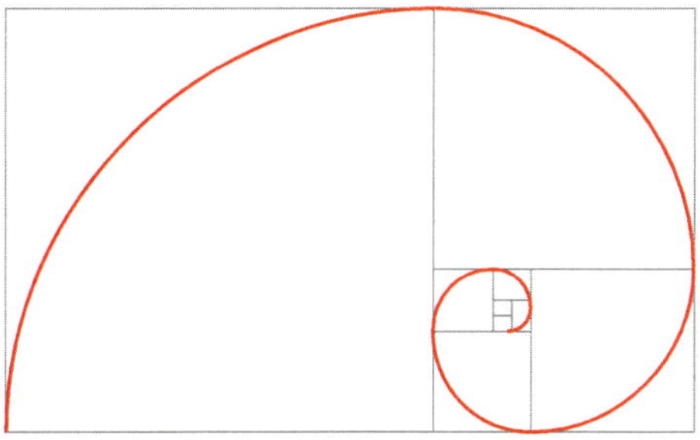

Figure 2.4: The Golden mean or Golden Ratio (Φ = 1.618...) applied to the spiral (Fibonacci spiral).

It is said that the *Dao* has no definition, the *Dao* that is defined is not the *Dao*.

Dao is pure potentiality and as Lao Zi points out in *Dao De Jing (or Taoteking)* (chap. 42);

Dao generates the One. One gives birth to Two.
Two gives birth to Three.
Three gives birth to all things

The Dao that can be told is not the eternal Dao.
The name that can be named is not the eternal name. *Lao Zi*

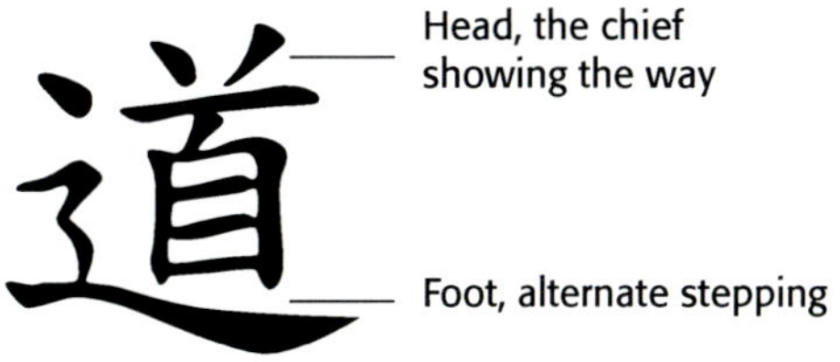

Figure 2.5: Dao, the Path as indicated by the Principle.

Humans as part of creation are subject to an order and cannot comprehend the notion of chaos. Humans as manifested beings are under the law of duality and can only have a taste of unity, but not reside in it.

With the body, Unity cannot be realized;
but without the body, the Dao may not be experienced.

Daoism is not a religion, rather a thought system. According to this philosophical concept, our origin is a mystery that we may ponder over but not fully comprehend as long as we are in this limited physical body.

The revelation that all things previously believed to be different are actually one, is an insight found in various mystical traditions such as Tantric Hinduism, Buddhism, Daoism, Zen, and Sufism, amongst others.

A very similar concept existed in the West, attributed to Aristotle, according to whom the Chaos or Prima Materia is separated into an active principle, the soul, and a passive principle, the body. The two opposites need to reunite to form the magical child in an alchemical ritual. The creation of the cosmos and the personified "Self" was said to require the intervention of a demiurge. This notion was contested by the church and replaced by the concept of an omnipotent God.

The theories about creation are equally found in the Big Bang cosmological model explaining the development of the universe.

2 (Er 二) Duality: Yin and Yang

The *Yin-Yang* theory is a symbolic and dialectical system signifying that nature and existence are dual. This concept constitutes the core of not only Chinese medicine, but also the Chinese culture and in general the oriental vision. It represents probably the most important difference between the oriental and Western way of understanding the world. In the West, the deductive logic of the early Greek philosophers, such as Plato and especially his student Aristotle, lead to opposing contrary phenomena. This analytical and therefore reductive way of thinking has dominated the Western mind ever since. The basic premise in the Chinese concept of the world is that opposites are complementary, that one could not exist without the other. In the Daoist vision, two is not the double of one but rather a distinction within the one. In other words, each aspect of duality *Yin-Yang*, not only contains the opposite but is also the originator of the opposite (see below).

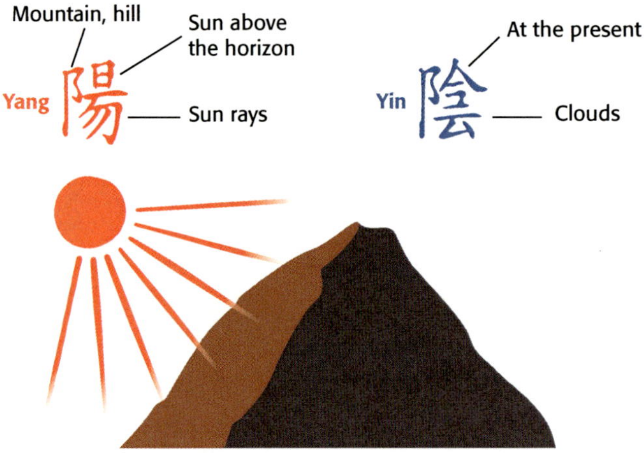

Figure 2.6: Yang, the sunny side of the mountain; Yin, the shady side.

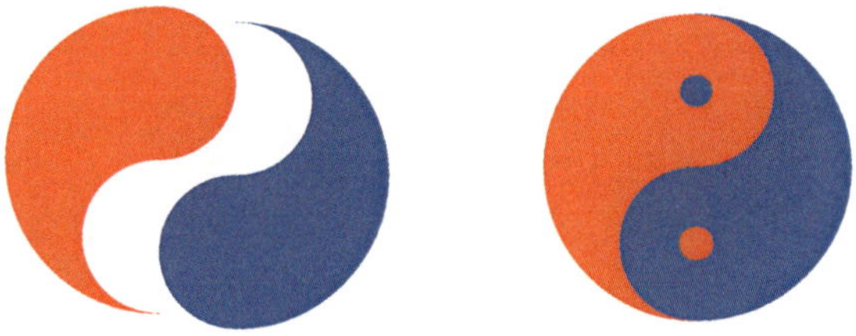

Figure 2.7: *Tai Ji*: Symbolizing the fundamental laws of *Yin* and *Yang*

Observing nature, and the cyclic changes of day and night obviously led the early thinkers to understand life and all phenomena as a permanent flow or movement between two opposite poles.

This explains the ideograms representing *Yin* and *Yang* in relation to darkness and light (▶ Fig. 2.6).

Tai Ji ≈ Supreme Ridge polarises the primordial chaos into *Yang*, the subtle and volatile, and *Yin*, the more dense and heavy.

Therefore, life is made of a dense "material" and a subtle "immaterial" energetic part.

Existence is made of two opposite, but complementary principles.

The Laws of Yin and Yang

The ancient and well-known symbol of *Tai Ji* representing a circle made up of two interwoven spirals is actually symbolizing the four basic laws of *Yin* and *Yang* (▶ Fig. 2.7). This plain image, with its harmonious beauty and elegant simplicity, conveys the most fundamental laws that govern human beings and the universe, and that constitute the very fabric of the oriental philosophical and medical thought.

- **Opposition and complementarities:** the circle is made up of two opposite principles that complement each other to create a whole, signifying that for each phenomenon there is an opposite phenomenon that is complementary to it, like the two sides of a coin. There cannot be light without darkness, activity without rest, Heaven without the Earth, or health without disease.
- **Relativity:** Nothing is absolute. The small dot in the middles of the bigger circle signifies that even a maximum of Yang contains a trace of Yin and vice versa. Also, this law signifies that Yin is defined in relation to Yang and Yang in relation to Yin. This is a very important notion, as nothing in existence is definitely Yin or definitely Yang, but phenomena appear Yin or Yang in relation to one another. For example, the sun is considered Yang in relation to the earth; the moon is also considered Yang in relation to the earth, but the moon is considered Yin in relation to the sun.
- **Interaction:** the law of inter-dependence or dynamism states that Yin produces and nourishes Yang, in return, Yang protects and moves Yin. This interaction explains that when one polarity is out of balance, it automatically will affect its opposite. For example in medicine, Blood and Qi constitute a Yin-Yang couple. It is said that Qi moves Blood and that Blood sustains or nourishes Qi. So when Blood is deficient, Qi is weak, and when Qi is deficient, Blood tends to stagnate. This dynamic inter-dependence also explains the four possible states of imbalance that are seen in pathology (► Fig. 2.8):
- When Yang is predominant: this can be due to an excess (exuberance) of Yang or a deficiency (vacuity) of Yin.
- When Yin is predominant: this can be due to an excess (exuberance) of Yin or a deficiency (vacuity) of Yang.
- **Transformation:** Each spiral starts when the opposite has reached a maximum. It is said that extreme Yin transforms into Yang and that extreme Yang transforms into Yin. For example, this law explains how an external cold (Yin) causes a fever (Yang). Transformation can only happen at a particular moment when all the conditions are met, in other words when one polarity has reached full amplitude. A good example of this would be the movements of a pendulum. In its trajectory, the pendulum starts with a slow speed, reaches maximum velocity, begins slowing down to reach maximum amplitude with zero velocity, at this point the conditions are set for the pendulum to change direction and start its opposite movement.

The *Yi Jing* (or *I Ching*) ≈ Book of changes, would be the oldest reference to the above laws, in which *Yang* is represented with a continuous line and *Yin* with a broken line. Symbolically, all possible energetic combinations in existence could be represented by various combinations of *Yin* and *Yang*. We see here the same concept that was used 27 centuries later in the West to create the first binary computer language. The *Yi Jing* describes 64 hexagrams, indicating that 64 would be the sum total of all possible phenomena between Heaven and Earth. This approach was the founding principle of the *Yin-Yang* school also known as the Naturalist school, with Zou Yan (305–240 BC) as the most prominent scholar, that J. Needham considers "The real founder of all Chinese scientific thought.."

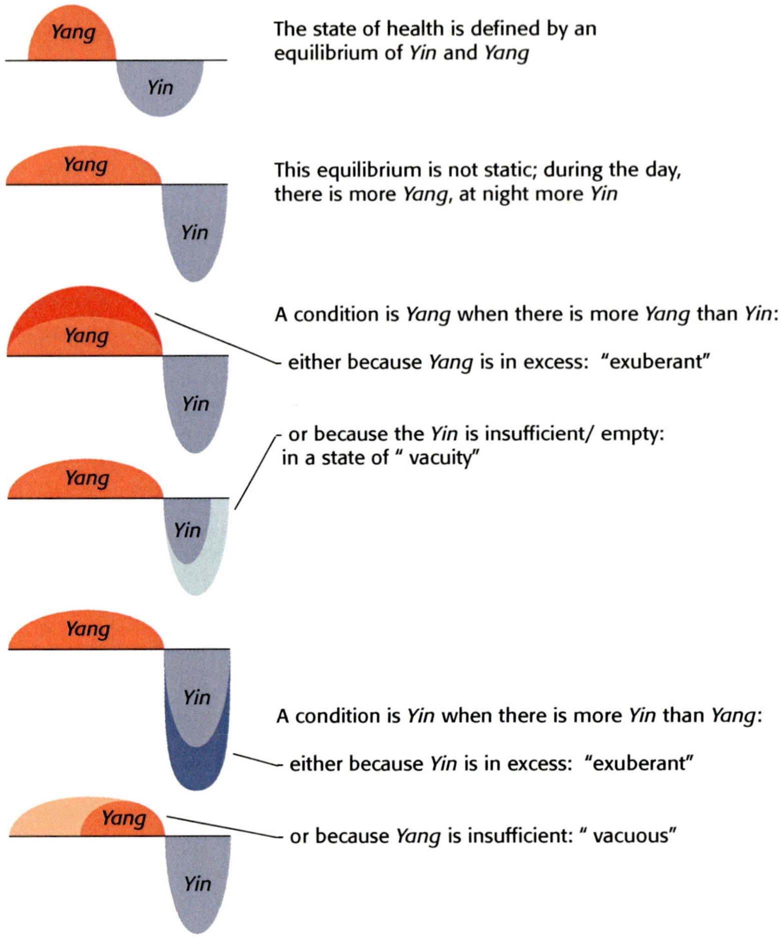

Figure 2.8: Variations of *Yin* and *Yang*: a–b) Equilibrium (state of health); c–d) *Yang* condition either from *Yang* exuberance of *Yin* vacuity; e–f) *Yin* condition either from *Yin* exuberance or *Yang* vacuity.

Classification of Yin and Yang phenomena

The *Yin* and *Yang* concept is extremely simple; nevertheless, it represents a constant challenge for the beginner and especially to the Western mind. It is often difficult to understand that although a particular phenomenon might be *Yin* in one context, it may be *Yang* in another (▶ Table 2.1)

Table 2.1 Attributes of *Yang* and *Yin*

	Yang	Yin
Yin/Yang in the cosmos	Heaven	Earth
	Sun	Moon
	Day	Night
	Fire	Water
	Hot	Cold
	Summer	Winter

Yin/Yang in general aspects	Up	Down
	Exterior	Interior
	Expansion	Contraction
	(+)	(-)
	Active	Passive
	Male	Female

	Fast	Slow
	Dry	Moist
	Young	Old
	Diffusion	Concentra-tion
	To give	To receive
Yin/Yang in the body	Back	Front
	Head	Body and limbs
	Left	Right
	Surface: *Biao*	Depth: *Li*
	Organ function(i.e. breathing)	Organ structure (i.e. lung)
	Channels	Organs
	"*Fu*" Yang organs	"*Zang*" Yin organs
	Energy: *Qi*	Blood: *Xue*
	Sympathetic	Parasym-pathetic
	Outbreath	In-breath
	Intellect	Intuition
	Extroverted	Introverted
	Excited	Calm
	Wei Qi - Defensive Energy	*Ying Qi* - Nourishing Energy
Yin/Yang in pathology	Excess/ repletion	Deficiency/ vacuity
	Acute	Chronic
	Red	Pale
	Fever	Coldness, chills
	Agitated	Depressed
	Inflammation	Oedema
	Anuria	Polyuria
	Cramps	Paralysis
	Thirst/ cool drinks	No thirst/ warm drinks
	Loud voice	Weak voice
	Course breathing	Weak breathing
	Full or fast pulse	Weak or slow pulse
	Red tongue, yellow coat	Pale tongue
Yin/Yang in relation to pain	Intense	Dull
	Localised	Diffuse
	Surface	Deep
	Intermittent	Continuous
Pain gets worse	In day-time	At night-time
	With heat	With cold
Pain gets better	At night-time	In day-time
	With cold	With heat

Another difficulty comes from value associations and judgments. Certain attributes of *Yang*, such as activity, dynamism and logical thinking, are greatly valued in the West, whereas passivity, quietness, and intuition attributed to *Yin*, are great assets in the East. 'Positive' and 'male' are attributed to *Yang*, 'negative' and 'female' are referred to as *Yin*. This often greatly irritates the Western beginners, who tend to view positive and negative in a Judeo-Christian context and not as two poles of the same movement.

Health is defined as the state of equilibrium between *Yin* and *Yang*. In general, the human being is more *Yang* during the day and more *Yin* at night. The equilibrium of *Yin* and *Yang*, therefore, is not static but dynamic in "space" and in "time".

The 8 Diagnostic Principles

This is the most important diagnostic tool in Chinese medicine and is applicable to every situation.

Every symptom has to be analyzed separately according to the 8 principles. This analysis is done by the classical Chinese diagnosis (observing, listening, smelling and touching), although not every symptom might have all of the characteristics:

- **Yin-Yang**: defines the sum total of the manifestation, and as seen above, it narrows down the investigation. The clinical manifestation, no matter how complex, can always be classified as *Yin* or *Yang*. Pathological phenomena are classified as *Yin* when there is more *Yin* than *Yang*, as is the case when there is coldness, wetness, softness, slowness, quietness, or mass. Symptoms are classified *Yang*, when *Yang* is stronger than *Yin*, manifesting with heat, redness, dryness, hardness, excitement, rapidity and expansion.

- **Biao-Li** (Surface/ Interior): situates the location of the disease, its origin, its evolution, and the prognosis. The *Biao-Li* concept is difficult to translate as it refers not quite to surface and depth which is expressed by the *Wai* and *Nei* concept, but rather to the outer layer and its lining. As for a coat that has two functions: the outer layer functions mainly as a windbreaker and water repellent, whereas the inner lining is mainly for warmth. Similarly, the *Biao* concept is referring to the outer energetic structures rich in *Wei Qi*, namely the *Pi Bou* ≈ Skin zones, and the *Jing Jin* ≈ Sinew channels. Here *Wei Qi* ≈ Defensive energy concentrates to protect against external climatic aggressions, mainly the Wind and the Cold. The *Jing* ≈ Primary channels and the blood vessels, which carry the *Ying* ≈ Nourishing energy to support the *Wei Qi*, constitute the lining "*Li*" with the exception of the *Zu Tai Yang* (Bladder) channel, which also belongs to the *Biao*. A "*Biao*" pathology, is considered acute, caused by external causes, and would be easy to treat. A pathology that has progressed to the "*Li*", could then progress to the inside "*Nei*" and affect the organs, become chronic and potentially more severe.
- **Hot-Cold**: defines mainly the nature of the disease and its clinical manifestation such as heat, acceleration, redness, dryness etc.. It is also often used to confirm the *Yin-Yang* categorization: a *Yin* condition gets better with heat and worse with cold; a *Yang* symptom gets better with cold and worse with heat.
- **Excess-Deficiency** (*Shi-Xu* ≈ Repletion-vacuity): is a very important concept in diagnosis. On the one hand, evaluating the state of a *Yin* or *Yang* condition, that is, whether a *Yang* state is due to *Yang* repletion or to *Yin* vacuity, or if a *Yin* state is due to *Yin* repletion or rather *Yang* vacuity. This assessment is of course of capital importance as it leads to a totally different therapeutic approach, to supplement (tonify) a vacuity or to reduce (disperse) repletion. On the other hand, the *Shi* ≈ Excess and *Xu* ≈ Deficient notion also explore the presence of an external pathogenic factor (excess/ repletion) and the weakness of the True energy (deficiency/ vacuity). Normally the term "Excess" should only refer to an excess of one of the "6 evils": Wind, Cold, Heat, Fire, Dampness, and Dryness, although in most literature this term is equally used for excessive conditions arising from internal causes, such as stagnations or emotions. A balanced

system does not produce excess energy, so in conditions of apparent excess such as in hyperactivity, either the controlling system is not functioning (deficiency), or the energy is not flowing freely and is accumulating in one area (stagnation). In other words "Stagnation" is the internal equivalent of "Excess".

Applying the 8 Principles to a symptom such as pain is very interesting, as a lot of information may be gathered directly; for example a *Yang*-type headache gets worse with heat or bright light; a deficiency/vacuity pain gets better with pressure, whereas an excess type pain gets worse with pressure; a stagnation gets better with movement or heat and worse with rest etc.

In certain pathological conditions such as in organic diseases, mechanical (osteopathic) dysfunctions, tumors, scar tissues or certain neurological diseases, the symptom may not give a coherent pattern according to the 8 diagnostic principles, for example, a pain getting worse with both heat and cold, or with rest and activity.

3 (San 三) Trilogy: Heaven-Human-Earth

According to this dialectical system, "Heaven" represents the *Yang* energies, "Earth" represents the *Yin* energies; and "Human" symbolizes all that is created or in other words the interaction between *Yin* and *Yang* and all of the possible combinations.

> *The pure and lucid element of light represents Heaven, the turbid element of darkness represents Earth.* *Su Wen, chap.5*
>
> *Everything in creation is covered by Heaven and supported by Earth.* *Su Wen, chap.6*

Heaven and Earth are the first *Yin* and *Yang* couple, they constitute the initial state of existence, setting forth the minimum conditions for existence defined by a "moment" in time and space (► Fig. 2.10).

Heaven represents time, the basic rhythm of life: day-night, seasons, etc.

Earth represents the space where time could be perceived: the four directions.

Heaven is symbolized by a circle, whereas Earth is oriented in relation to a center in four directions, hence the symbol of the square.

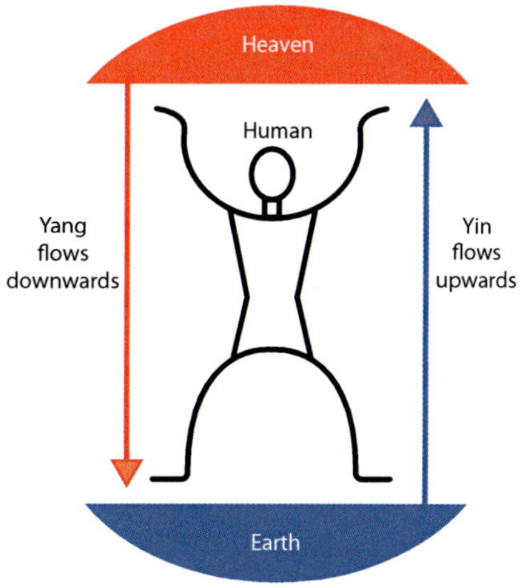

Figure 2.9: Trilogy: Heaven – Human – Earth

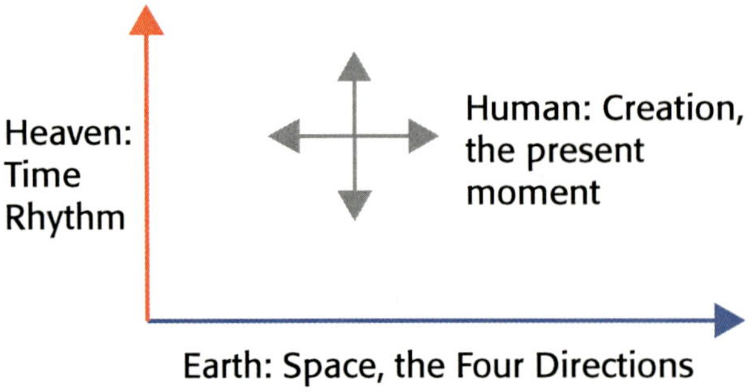

Figure 2.10: Heaven – Human – Earth : Time – Space – Creation

This analogy is to be found in all aspects of the Chinese vision and daily life even symbolized in the form of the ancient Chinese coins with a square hole in the middle (► Fig. 2.11).

Anatomically the head, which is round, represents the Heaven, and the body with its square form represents the Earth.

Heaven, the ultimate Yang principle, initiates life.
Earth, as the Yin principle, receives and nourishes life.

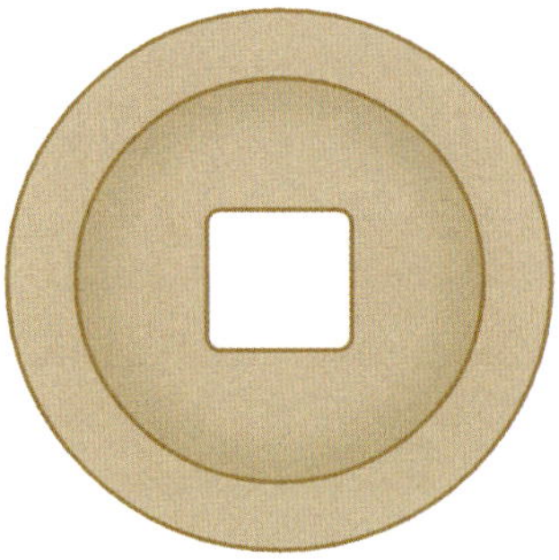

Figure 2.11: Chinese coin: Heaven-Earth

The human being, symbolizing manifested life, is defined by the interaction of time and space, of Heaven and Earth.

Human, together with Heaven and Earth represents a trinity or a trilogy called the three *Cai*才, translated as the "Active agents of the universe".

- *Tian* (天): Heaven
- *Ren* (人): Human
- *Di* (地): Earth

Where Duality represents the two poles or principles, three is the number representing actual creation or existence, as we perceive it. This concept of a trilogy can be found in many Eastern or Western traditions at the origin of creation. In the Hindu tradition, Brahma, the God of creation has two other aspects, Vishnu and Shiva. In the Egyptian mythology Atum, the creator became three by giving birth to Shu and Tefnut, to originate life. The Hebrew Qabalah places Kether at the origin materializing as Chokmah, the male principle, and Binah, the female principle. In the middle-eastern religious metaphors, the creation of humanity started with Adam and Eve having tasted the forbidden fruit, the third element and their consequent expulsion from the Garden of Eden. And again in Christianity, the concept of Trinity, at the origin, could be a reference to the same numerological symbolism.

The Dao gives birth to "One". "One" gives birth to "Two".
"Two" gives birth to "Three". "Three" gives birth to all things ("10000 beings").
Lao Zi, Dao De Jing, *chap. 42*

This is to say that humans and all beings, are the result of the interaction of the pure *Yang* of Heaven and the pure *Yin* of Earth, with which the human being is in relation through breath and food on one level and on a more subtle level through special windows and doorways: the nine portals (openings), the 10 Windows of Heaven and the 12 Doorways of the Earth.

The Heaven-Human-Earth concept is also represented in the ideogram of *Wang* ≈ Emperor 王, where a vertical line joins Heaven and Earth with a third horizontal line crossing the vertical, representing creation, and at the center of this creation, the Emperor, and envoy of heaven.

In Chinese vision and especially medicine, the symbolism of "Three" has a very important place. It is suggested that all phenomena in existence have 3 dimensions or divisions;

- 3 divisions of the body: head – body – limbs
- Each limb has three main joints (sections)
- 3 aspects or realities of human beings: physical – emotional – mental
- The 3 constituent energies: *Yuen* ≈ Source *Qi*, *Jing* ≈ Essence and *Zong* ≈ Ancestral *Qi*
- The 3 treasures: *Shen* ≈ Spirit, *Qi* ≈ Energy, and *Jing* ≈ Essence
- Triple Warmer: 3 centers: food processing, energy production, waste elimination
- The 3 energetic layers: *Wei* ≈ Defensive, *Ying* ≈ Nourishing, *Jing* ≈ Essence
- The 3 intensities of Yin and Yang (see below)
- The 3 *Dan Tian*: spiritual centers, referring to areas of alchemical transformation
- The concept of Root ≈ *Gen*, Knot ≈ *Jie*, and Branch ≈ *Zhi*, which has a very important place in Chinese physiology, diagnosis, and therapy.

Even in Western embryology, from the original cell, producing identical daughter cells, which at one point differentiates into three layers, the ectoderm, mesoderm, and endoderm, the origin of the 10 trillion of differentiated cells of the body.

In Chinese energetics, *Yin* and *Yang* also have three degrees or intensities:

- **Yang** can be:
  - *Tai Yang* (太陽): supreme *Yang* (biggest, oldest, superior, first).
  - *Shao Yang* (少陽): lesser *Yang* (young, second, little).
  - *Yang Ming* (陽明): brightness of *Yang* (clear, perfect, known)
- **Yin** can be:
  - *Tai Yin* (太陰): supreme *Yin*.
  - *Shao Yin* (少陰): lesser *Yin*
  - *Jue Yin* (厥陰): terminal *Yin* (diminished, exhausted, used up, fallen).

4 (Si 四) The Four Phases 四時 and the Five Elements (4 + 1)

Four is a further important figure relating to a division of each principle of *Yin* and *Yang*, the four territories or directions and the four seasons. Four is therefore symbolic of form, of what is material, hence the Earth (▶ Fig. 2.12)

Life is movement, and every movement has four strong moments or phases, the biphasic movements or oscillations when related to *Yin* and *Yang*, would represent a growing phase of *Yang*, a maximum expansion of *Yang*, a growing phase of *Yin* and a maximum concentration of *Yin*. The four phases are clearly represented in the *Tai Ji* model.

These four strong moments *Si Shi* 四時 are:

- In the day/night cycle: sunrise, midday, sunset and midnight.
- In the cycle of the year, they are spring, summer, fall, and winter.
- In the evolution of life, they are birth, maturity, old age, and death.

These four "moments" are represented by the first polarization of *Yin* and *Yang* into a *Shao* ≈ Lesser and *Tai* ≈ Supreme *Yin* and a *Shao* ≈ Lesser and *Tai* ≈ Supreme *Yang*.

Four is also the number representing the Earth's four directions in relation to a center. Historically, mythical animals, protectors of the four orients, represented the four directions (▶ Fig. 2.13):

- The *Qing Long* ≈ Green Dragon 青龙; the symbol of *Dong* ≈ East 东 and of benevolencee

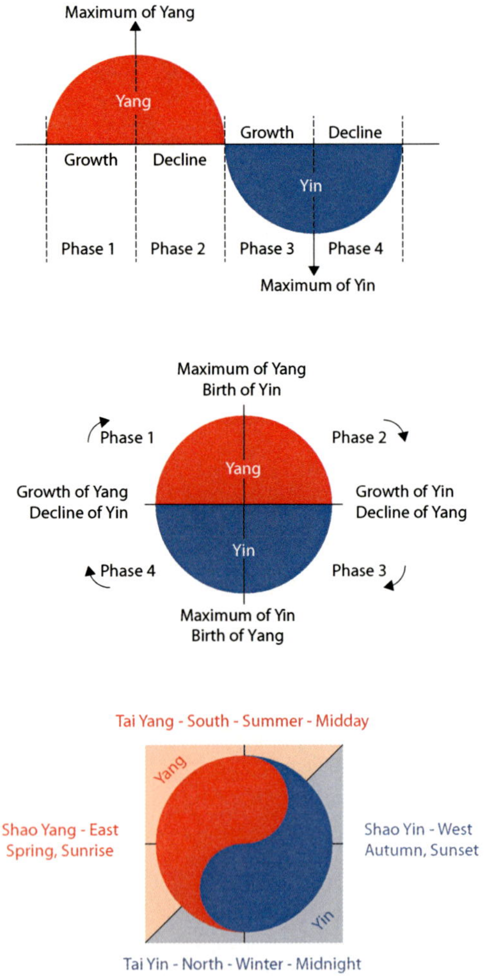

Figure 2.12: Four Phases, four Directions: *Tai Yang*/ South, *Shao Yin*/ West, *Tai Yin*/ North, *Shao Yang*/ East

- *The Zhu Qiao* ≈ Red Bird朱雀 or Phoenix, the symbol of *Nan* ≈ South 南 and of radiance and joy of life
- The *Bai Hu* ≈ White Tiger 白虎, the symbol of *Xi* ≈ West 西 and of virtue
- The *Xuan Wu* ≈ *Dark warrior* 玄武 or *Gui Xian* ≈ Black Turtle, the symbol of *Bei* ≈ North 北 and of wisdom

In the Chinese tradition, the "wise man", stands in the center facing the South, North is behind him, East and the rising sun on his left and West and the setting sun on his right. This "correct" positioning of the human body, explains the fact that the left side of the body is considered *Yang* and the right side is *Yin*. In *Feng Shui*≈ Wind and Water (Chinese Geomancy), consideration of these positions is of primary importance.

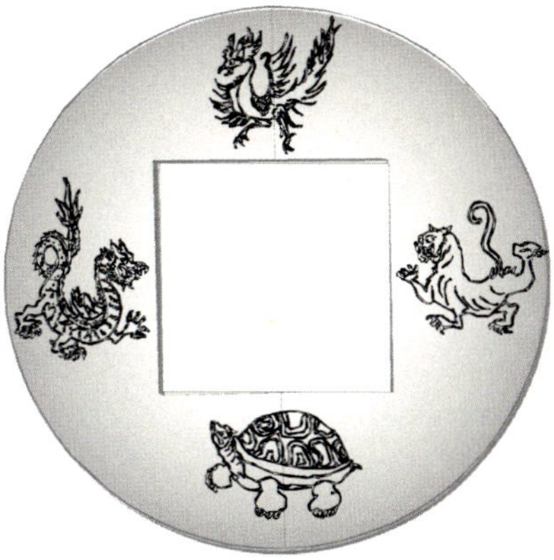

Figure 2.13: Ancient mirror with the four mythical creatures

The addition of a center to these four directions produces the five fixed positions in space and time, referred to as the Five Elements (▶ Fig. 2.14). Five is considered to be the crossing between Heaven and Earth. In this manner, all *Yang* and *Yin* phenomena gather around a center, called the "organizing center". This center is the organizer of life and of the human body.

- South, symbolized by the Fire element, represents an expansion
- North, symbolized by the Water element, represents internalization
- East, represented by the Wood element and evokes exteriorization
- West, symbolized by the Metal element, represents interiorization
- The Earth element is placed in the center, symbol of transformation

In Chinese thought, this model represents the structure of the universe and of all things. That means that any cycle, be it day and night, the seasons or life cycles, or other phenomena in the universe contain these four phases, hence the

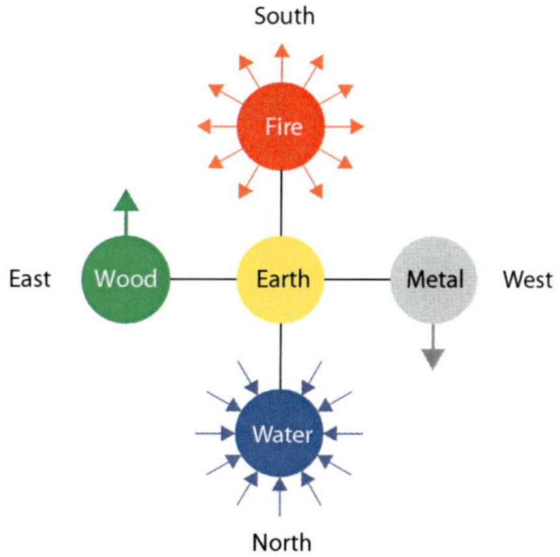

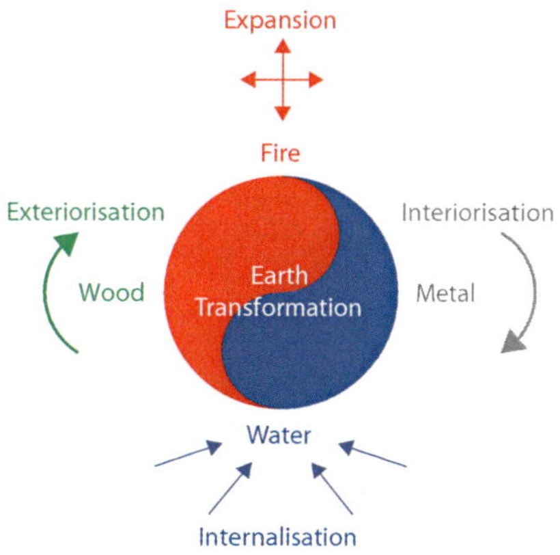

Figure 2.14: The Five Elements, the directions, and their respective movements

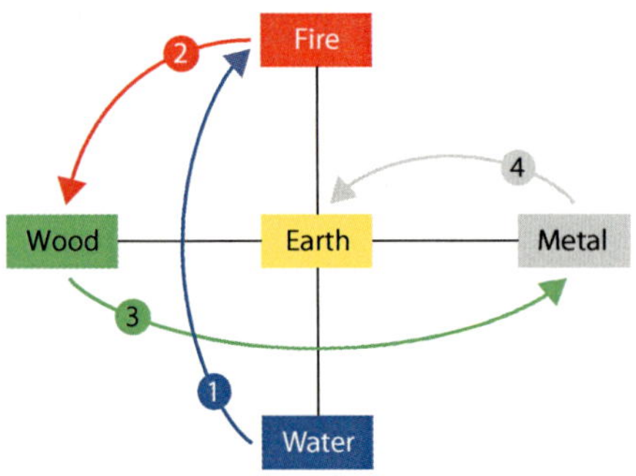

Figure 2.15: Creation order of the 5 Elements.

term of "Internal Structure" given to this model of the Five Elements.

The analogy is found in the ideogram the Chinese have used to represent their country China, or *Zhong Guo* ≈ Central Empire 中國.

The empire is structured in the model of the universe. The individual is also structured in the same way. Human-microcosm is in the image of the universe-macrocosm.

This analogy is further used to represent the order of creation, starting with Water as the base, then Fire, followed by Wood and Metal. The Earth is placed in the center. (▶ Fig. 2.15).

Here the importance of the Water element as base and source of life is underlined. This organization represents the creation and the "Internal Structure" of life and of all phenomena, the four "strong" moments and the transformation principle.

From the point of view of numerology, this "Cosmogenic" model of the Five Elements could be represented as "4+1": the four directions and the four basic movements in relation to a center.

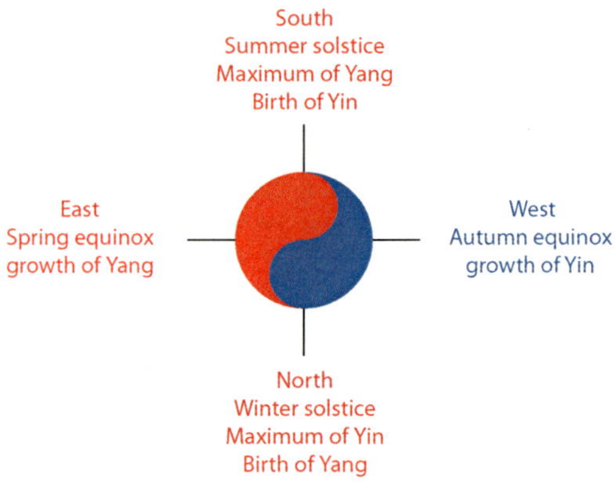

Figure 2.16: The four Directions and the Seasons.

When applied to the *Yin-Yang* and the *Taiji* model, the South and Maximum of *Yang*, the summer solstice, will also correspond to the birth of *Yin*, as the evening starts after midday, and the maximum of *Yin*, the winter solstice, is also the birth of *Yang*, as a new day starts after midnight. The equinoxes correspond to spring and autumn, where the *Yang* is growing in the former and *Yin* is growing in the latter.

These strong moments can be described dynamically as four types of movement in relation to a center. Traditionally symbolized by an element, in analogy with a season (▶ Fig. 2.16).

- **Wood-green:** symbolizes a young bamboo shoot, the manifestation of spring and the outward movement of energies. In this analogy, the bamboo shoot symbolizes the outward momentum of life as the young sprout pushes its way out of the earth in spring. The Wood element conveys an idea of coming to the surface, of bringing out and of expressing. The dynamic force is tremendous, it is directed more upwards and outwards, hence the association with birth and sunrise and is placed to the East. The childhood period corresponds to the Wood phase, with its rapid growth, great mobility and realization of potentials.

- **Fire-red:** symbolizes midday and full summer, when the dynamic forces of Yang reach their maximum expansion. The analogy of the Fire symbol, the red color, the rays of the sun at midday and the heat in summer is quite clear. The dynamism is that of expansion, of sending the rays out to the furthest points. In nature as in the body, heat dilates and expands. Fire is positioned in the South where the sunshine is greatest. In life cycles, the Fire phase corresponds to full growth and the powerful adult state, when one is in full possession of one's capacities.
- **Metal-white:** symbolizes sunset and autumn, when all movements start to slow down and gather inwards. The analogy with metal, a mineral, is that of condensation or of taking shape or of taking a looser form of matter, so all in nature with a similar dynamic will be associated with metal: sunset, when the energy moves inwards; fall and aging, when the fruits are harvested and the efforts are condensed and taking shape. The "Metal phase" is placed in the West. The white color of metal symbolizes accumulation and condensation. In the body, all inward movements correspond to Metal, such as absorbing food and the world and receptivity, which all have a similar directionality.
- **Water-black:** is the dark of the night and winter, a symbol for a gathering of energies deep inside, the consolidation of Yin. All movements come to an apparent stop. Only in appearance, because it is not a full stop but actually a preparation of the energies within to initiate the next cycle of movement. This is the moment when the pendulum has reached the maximum of its arc and marks a pause before starting its opposite movement. The movement is deep within, internalized, while the surface is still. Symbolically this moment is represented by the "Water phase" and the color black of depth, of the unknown, of the unlimited, of the potential and of wisdom. It is situated to the North. In nature, night-time, winter, and death are such moments of stillness in preparation of dawn and rebirth. It is a time for regeneration, where nothing happens on the surface, but tremendous changes are taking place internally. Water represents all movements that gather inwards, like water that seeps inwards, or as the cold that makes the heat withdraw inside. Often the original matrix of creation is represented by the Water element, from where the germ of creation grows until it can break the surface and appear as manifested life.
- **Earth-yellow**: in the middle, represents the symbol of maturity, transformation, and metamorphosis. For each strong moment to transform into another strong moment a metamorphosis is needed. Earth constitutes the axis around which the other movements may evolve. The color yellow, symbolizes the maturity of the wheat, a reminder of the rich and nourishing quality of the soil. As the agent of transformation, the Earth phase is situated in the center, it signifies that each transformation has to go through the earth. For example Earth-phase corresponds to puberty, which represents the passage between childhood-Wood to adulthood-Fire, and menopause as the moment when the adult-Fire moves to old age-Metal, and finally death, a radical change and separation of the body from the spirit, through which the body returns to the earth and the spirit is free

for a new rebirth. There is no specific season for the Earth phase, but it is customary to associate the 18 intermediary days between two seasons to the Earth element. In the West, some authors have proposed a fifth season, calling it the Indian summer to complete the Five elements. Personally, I do not adhere to this idea.

A simple image that may help visualize these four types of energy would be the watering hose (▶ Fig. 2.17):

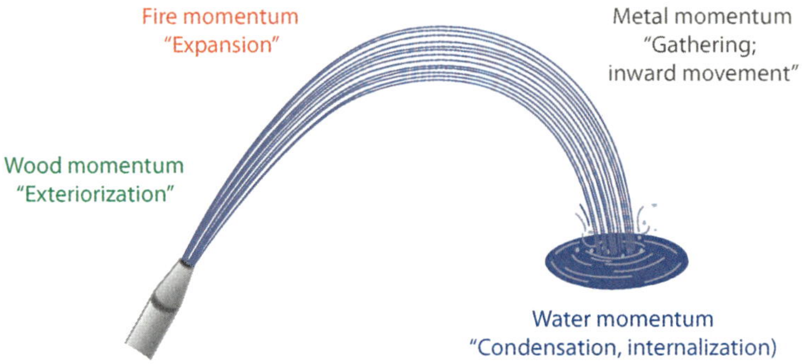

Figure 2.17: The four momentums of water reflecting the Four Phases

- Water comes out of the nozzle with force and an outward momentum, this is the Wood Phase
- Water then spreads out and up, the Fire Phase
- The water reaches a maximum height and width and starts to fall back down, represented by the Metal
- To finally gather on and seep into the ground, symbolized by the Water phase.
- In this "Cosmogenic" model each phase is balanced by another:
- The outgoing energies of Wood are countered by the inward gathering of Metal
- The expansive and centrifugal movement of Fire is limited by the condensing centripetal movement of Water.
- The Earth phase allows the transformation between each movement.

5 (Wu 五) The Five Moving Forces 五行 (3 + 2)

Wu Xing ≈ Five movements has also been translated as the five moving forces five agents, or five phases, or more commonly as the five elements.

This dialectical model represents five categories of phenomena in the world and within the human being. The phenomena in each category have in common certain structural, energetic or relational characteristics. As the human being is in the image of the universe, the internal physiological and organic functions, have energetic analogies with the external phenomena, hence the "Correspondence system", a term which is often attributed to this model.

The *Wu Xing* ≈ Five Moving forces are the most original and widely utilized system in the Chinese tradition. Already described in the *Nei Jing*, the concept was initially used in astrology and predictions and was not applied to medicine until the 11th century AD.

The *Wu Xing* categorization is based upon five types of mobile force, in permanent interaction with one another to ensure equilibrium in nature and in mankind. The *Wu Xing* ≈ Five movements should not be considered individually but as a whole with their constant interactions and relations.

Sheng ≈ Creation cycle

The Chinese describe these five movements in an order representing the creation *Sheng* cycle:

- Wood ≈ *Mu* 木
- Fire ≈ *Huo* 火
- Earth ≈ *Tu* 土 (a different concept from Earth ≈ *Di* 地 as in the pair Heaven and Earth, *Tu* represents the soil when *Di* is more the earth planet itself)
- Metal ≈ *Jin* 金
- Water ≈ *Shui* 水

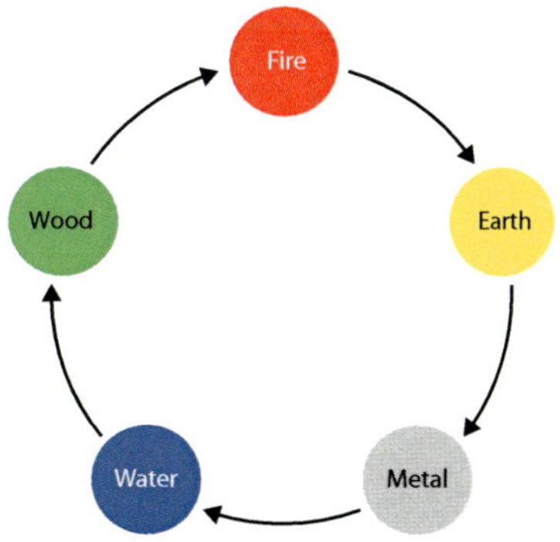

Figure 2.18: *Sheng* ≈ Creation/ nourishment cycle

This cycle is represented on a circle, a perpetual and reproductive cycle. It is said that each element is producing, engendering or nourishing the following element. Hence each element acts as the "mother" of the following element that represents the son. This relationship is called the mother-son relationship (▶ Fig. 2.18):

- Wood nourishes or engenders the Fire, Wood is the mother of Fire, Fire is the son of Wood
- Fire, in turn, engenders Earth, Fire is the mother of Earth, and Earth is the son of Fire.

In medicine, this relationship is used when supplementing an element or an organ. For example, the Metal/ Lung is supported to supplement the Water/ Kidney.

Ke ≈ Controlling cycle

Each element is in turn controlling another element, named the grandson, following a cycle represented by a pentagram (a five-pointed star) (▶ Fig. 2.19). For example, Wood is the mother of Fire and the Grandmother of Earth. Wood engenders Fire but controls Earth.

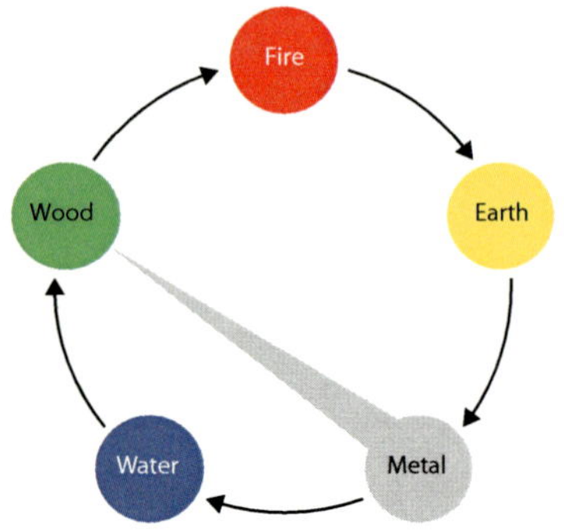

Figure 2.19: *Ke* ≈ Controlling cycle

Destruction cycle

This is the same as the *Ke* ≈ Controlling cycle, but here control is exaggerated to the point of destruction. This cycle usually implies that the controlling element, the grandmother, is not being sufficiently controlled, therefore becoming destructive to the controlled element. For example, when Wood is not checked by Metal, it becomes destructive to Earth, or in a different context, if Wood has become overactive and Metal has lost control over it, then Wood becomes destructive towards Earth (▶ Fig. 2.20). The destruction cycle may also result from the weakness of a particular element. For example, when Water is deficient, Earth may become destructive towards it.

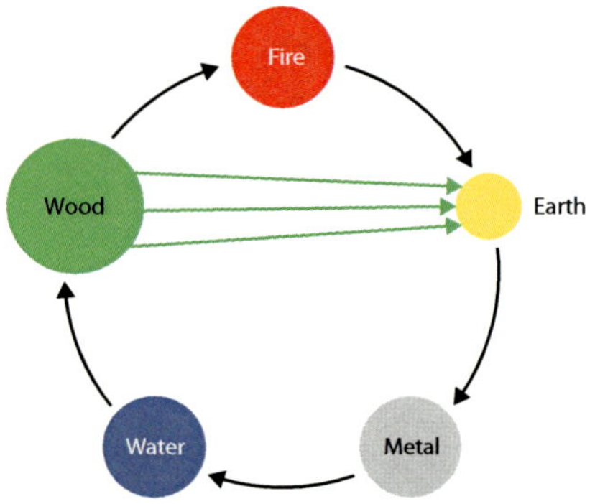

Figure 2.20: Destruction – exaggerated *Ke* ≈ Controlling cycle

Wu ≈ Insult cycle

This is, in fact, the reversal of the *Ke* ≈ Controlling cycle, when an element is rebelling against the controller (▶ Fig. 2.21). In a Confucian ordered society, the rebellion of the grandson against the grandmother is an insult and is considered a grievous act. In medicine, such a counter-action has to be rapidly rectified.

It should be understood that the *Sheng* ≈ Production/ stimulation and the *Ke* ≈ Controlling cycles are considered normal and healthy (the concept of "Homeostasis"), whereas the destruction

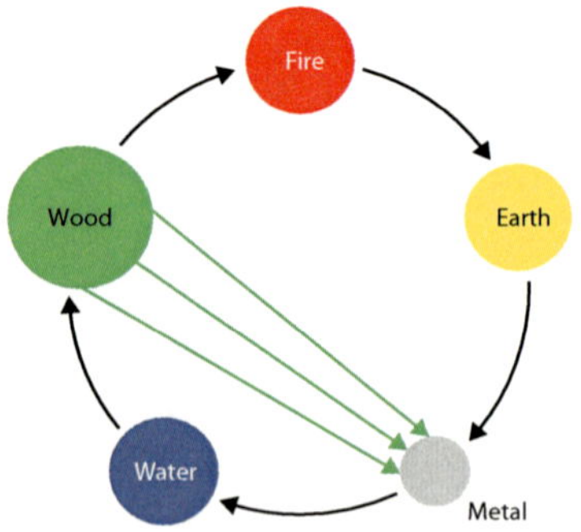

Figure 2.21: *Wu* ≈ Insult cycle (reversed *Ke* ≈ Control cycle)

and the *Wu* ≈ Insult cycles are only observed in pathological situations.

The *Sheng* and *Ke* cycles define a simultaneous inter-relation between all five movements. For example, Fire is the son of Wood, the grandson of Water, the mother of Earth, and grandmother of Metal. These perpetual relations of control and regulation allow for perfect homeostasis in the body. The same inter-relation is to be found in natural phenomena as well as in matters of state and government, hence the earlier applications of the laws of the "Five Movements" to astrology and the study of power and politics.

We see very clearly that the concept of the Five elements refers to a dynamic and mobile model and not a static and material notion as the word "element" might suggest, therefore the terms " Five Movements", "Five Moving Forces" or "Five agents" would be a more appropriate translation for *Wu Xing*.

Furthermore, the symbolic representation of the "Five Elements" with Earth in the center, as discussed in the previous chapter, is very different to the *Sheng* ≈ Creation cycle, although too often these two have been mixed up and confused with each other, presenting a very muddled picture to the beginner.

The Correspondence System

In this very original and unusual approach, all phenomena are classified into five categories, based on their energetic analogies. Similarly, in the body, the energetic movements and physiological functions with the same similarities will be classified into one of these categories.

The symbolism of each element suggest a type of movement or momentum in the *Wu Xing* ≈ Five moving forces, slightly different from the dynamics described in the previous chapter for the *Si Shi* ≈ Four Phases:

- Wood: represents mobilization in the *Wu Xing*, the capacity and agility to move quickly, flexibility and passion. In the Four Phases, it represented exteriorization, bringing out what is within, expression of feelings or artistic talents.
- Fire: represents expansion in both systems; in the Four Phases it also signifies bringing to the surface. Heat, which expands the tissues, and Joy that expands the energy from the chest, will be both attached to Fire.
- Earth: symbolizes transformation in both systems, with an added element of metamorphosis and changing of form in the Five Movement model. All transformative processes in the body, such as digestion or analysis, thinking, and memory or major life changes such as puberty and menopause are attached to the Earth Phase.
- Metal: represents condensation in the *Wu Xing*. This is the first stage of taking form, which will be completed by consolidation in the Water Phase. In the Four Phase context, Metal represents gathering and bringing inside. In the body, all processes of absorption, such as breathing or eating, as well as receptivity and empathy, but also melancholy or sadness, have the same inward movement.
- Water: is both fluid and yielding, but can also take on the form to produce consolidation and coherence. Hence not only are all the fluids of the body related

to Water but so are also the hardest structures in the body, the bones, and the teeth. Water represents the capacity to yield and the strength and willpower to resist. In the Four Phases, Water represents internalization and depth, symbolizing the potential and creative powers.

In the Five Movements, three movements are considered *Yang*: Wood-Fire and Earth, and two are classified *Yin*, Metal, and Water, hence the differentiation of 5 into "3+2", clearly referring to the Five Movements (3 *Yang* and 2 *Yin* movements), and "4+1", signify*in*g the four directions and the center as described in the Four Phases.

Certain correspondences clearly belong to the Four Phase model:

- Wood: East, sunrise, spring equinox; birth
- Fire: South, midday, summer solstice; full growth
- Metal: West, sunset, autumn equinox; decline
- Water: North, midnight, winter solstice; death
- Earth: center, change of seasons; change

On the whole, everything between Heaven and Earth could be categorized according to their affinity or analogy with one of the Five Movements. In Chinese medicine, this relation has the great advantage of explaining how external factors such as climates, colors, smells, foods, and flavors will affect the internal organs and how the internal organs are related to certain physiological functions, body parts, emotions, and mental functions. Different passages of the *Nei Jing Su Wen* have described these relationships:

> *The East engenders the Wind, which in turn engenders the Wood that produces the sour taste, which nourishes the Liver.*
> *The Liver nourishes the muscles and allows the eyes to see.*

And in another passage:

> *Green, the color of the East, penetrates the Liver and helps store it's essence, which opens at the eyes, it's taste is the sour, it belongs to the Wood phase, it has for an animal the chicken, and for cereal the wheat, the planet is Jupiter, the musical note is the Jiao, the number is 8, it presents muscular symptoms and its smell is rancid.*

For example, Wood represents exteriorization (Four Phases) and mobilization (Five Movements). In the body, expression, passion, and anger will reflect the same quality of energy and will be attached to Wood, as well as the muscular system, responsible for mobility.

In the Chinese vision, the body is made up of five layers: skin, flesh, sinews, vessels and bones, and often organic systems: five *Zang* ≈ *Yin* organs and five *Fu* ≈ *Yang* bowels. Each *Zang* and each *Fu* will correspond to one Phase, and these organic pairs constitute the core of the Five Moving forces in medicine. (▶ Fig. 2.22)

- Liver and Gallbladder belong to the Wood element,
- Heart and Small Intestine represent the Fire,
- Spleen and Stomach symbolize the Earth,
- Lung and Large Intestine are associated with Metal,
- Kidney and Bladder belong to Water.

Table 2.2 shows the most pertinent correspondence points.

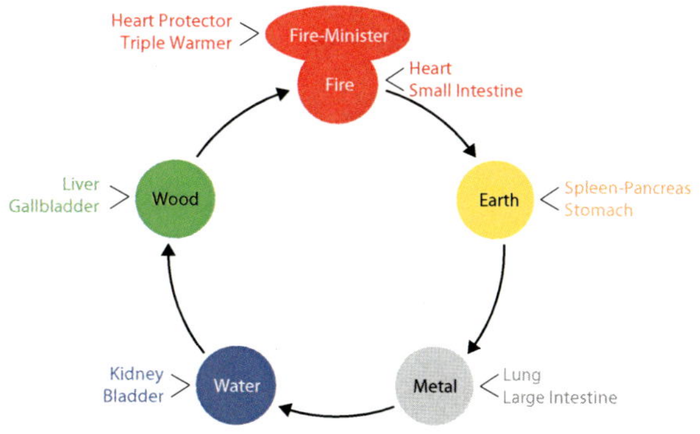

Figure 2.22: *Zang-Fu*-organs and the Five Phases.

For example, the wind, belonging to Wood, will affect the Liver, which in turn will manifest in the muscles (muscle cramps, neck tension) or in the eyes, (tearing, irritation, itching). Furthermore, Liver disharmony will produce manifestations that resemble wind, such as cramps, tremors, tics, vertigo, or emotional outbursts and anger.

Naturally, for the treatment, foods, tastes, and colors or sounds may be selected either from the Wood category or according to the inter-relation of the Five Movements, as discussed above, to supplement Wood, the Water and Kidney system may be supported. Or if the wood is overactive, the Metal and Lung system could be supplemented.

Table 2.2: The Five Phase correspondence system

Phase	Wood	Fire	Earth	Metal	Water
Correspondence to the Four phases					
Evolution	Birth	Growth	Transition	Decline	Death
Direction	East	South	Center	West	North
Season	Spring	Summer	Change of season	Autumn	Winter
Day & night	Sunrise	Midday	–	Sunset	Midnight
Correspondence to the Five Movements					
Movement	Mobilization	Expansion	Transforma-tion	Condensation	Coherence
Climate	Wind	Heat	Dampness	Dryness	Cold
Color	Green	Red	Yellow	White	Black
Smell	Rancid	Burnt	Fragrant	Acrid	Rotten
Taste	Sour	Bitter	Sweet	Spicy	Salty
Zang: Yang	Liver	Heart	Spleen	Lung	Kidney

organ					
Fu: Yin organ	Gallbladder	Small Intestine	Stomach	Large Intestine	Bladder
Sensory system	Sight	Speech	Taste	Smell	Hearing
Opening	Genitals	Tongue/ eye	Mouth	Nose	Urethra
Body layer and function	Tendons, mobility	Vessels, pulse	Flesh, muscle mass	Skin, body hair	Bones, marrow
Body part	Neck , shoulder, breast, genitals	Pulse, blood vessels	Abdomen, digestion	Mucous membranes, skin	Lumbar, knees, ankles
Manifest-ing in:	Nails	Complexion	Lips	Body hair	Hair
Voice	Shouting	Laughing	Singing	Moaning	Groaning
Fluid	Tears	Sweat	Saliva	Mucous	Urine
Quality	Friendliness flexibility	Happiness, joy, liveliness, compassion	Sympathy, caring, nourishing	Being in touch; empathy	Courage, character, will power
Emotion	Anger, rage, reactivity	Excitement, pleasure	Worry, obsession	Sadness, grief	Fear
Mental function	Imaginationl deas, dreams	Intelligence, Coherence, memory	Logic, analysis, synthesis, memory, ideas	Precision, introspection	Will, coherence, memory
Spiritual	Intuition	Enlighten-ment	Contempla-tion	Witnessing	Wisdom
Spirit	*Hun*	*Shen*	*Yi*	*Po*	*Zhi*
Musical note	*Shu or Jiao*	*Zhi*	*Gong*	*Shang*	*Yu*
Planet	Jupiter	Mars	Saturn	Venus	Mercury
Cereal	Wheat, barley	Buckwheat, red millet	Yellow millet, sticky rice	Rice, oats	Soya, Beans
Vegetable	Green peas	Turnip	Potato, pumpkin	Onion, radish	Leaks
Animal	Chicken	Lamb	Beef	Horse	Pork
Fruit	Prunes	Apricot	Melon	Peach	Dates

It is fundamental to keep in mind that life is encompassing the whole, this means the interaction of the "Five Movements" as they do not exist independently. This will further explain the fact that certain characteristics can be found under several categories. For example, memory is usually related to the Earth, but can also involve the Fire, Water or even in some cases Wood and Metal. Mental coherence depends on the coordinating aspect of Fire, but also the consolidating aspect of Water. Courage, which is an attribute of the Kidney, will also manifest in the Wood, and especially with the Gallbladder.

Another difficulty concerns the openings or portals. The portals are the openings through which the human being communicates with the outer world. The portals situated in the head are also where the sensory organs are located. The *Zang* (*Yin*) organ that is in charge of maintaining the sensory function is not the same organ system that controls the portal. For example, the Liver maintains the eyesight, whereas the eye portal is controlled by the Heart channel system.

In conclusion, the correspondence system explores the inter-relation of the macrocosm – the world, with the microcosm – the human being.

6 (Liu 六) The Six Energies: The Six Levels and the Six Layers

Qi in its transformations between Heaven and Earth goes from one extreme, *Yang*, to the other extreme, *Yin* and vice versa.

Six represents the number of resources, which maintain life. It is the number of the channels, of the *Fu* organs, of the *Liu Qi* ≈ Six forms of energy that constitute life: *Jing* ≈ Essence, *Qi* ≈ Energy, *Jin* ≈ Thin fluids, *Ye* ≈ Thick fluids, *Mai* ≈ Vessels and *Xue* ≈ Blood.

Six also represents all possible life situations as defined by the six hexagrams (described further). Even the Chinese time reflects this number, the century, is 60 years long: 6 x 10.

As we saw in section 2.3, for each polarity of *Qi*, there are three stages or three degrees:

- **Yang** is:
  - *Tai Yang* (太陽): supreme *Yang* (biggest, oldest, superior, first).
  - *Shao Yang* (少陽): lesser *Yang* (young, second, little).
  - *Yang Ming* (陽明): brightness of *Yang* (clear, perfect, known)
- **Yin** is:
  - *Tai Yin* (太陰): supreme *Yin*.
  - *Shao Yin* (少陰): lesser *Yin*
  - *Jue Yin* (厥陰): terminal *Yin* (diminished, exhausted, used up, fallen).

The terminology used for the *Yang* and the *Yin* is slightly different. The last stage of *Yin*, *Jue Yin*, designates a state of exhaustion and termination. The concept of *Yang Ming* does not apparently convey the same idea. The explanation is to be found in the symbolism for the *Yang*. The realm of reality in ancient times was the solar system, and the ultimate and supreme *Yang* would then be the sun. Hence the Chinese term for the sun, *Tai Yang*. What humans perceive of the sun on the earth therefore is but its brightness, *Yang Ming*, which in a sense represents a certain terminal phase of *Yang* (*Jue Yang*).

These six states of *Qi* resume all possible variations of *Yin* and *Yang* between Heaven and Earth. By their impact on the Five Movements, the Six Macrocosmic energies, maintain the rhythms of the universe. Six represents the natural forces from which humanity is drawing from. (► Fig. 2.23)

These six energies, at the level of the planet, manifest themselves as the six climates. It is stated in the *Su Wen* chapter 71, that:

- *Tai Yang* manifests as "Cold" to affect the Water Phase
- *Jue Yin* manifests as "Wind" to affect the Wood Phase
- *Shao Yin* and *Shao Yang* manifest respectively as "Fire" and "Heat" affecting the Fire Phase

- *Tai Yin* manifests as "Dampness" to affect the Earth phase
- *Yang Ming* manifests as "Dryness" and goes to the Metal

It is naturally difficult to understand as to why the *Tai Yang* ≈ Greater *Yang* should manifest as the Cold, we can only refer to *Su Wen's* explanation:

> *"...creation in Heaven is a mystery,*
>
> *at the level of the human being it is called the Dao".*

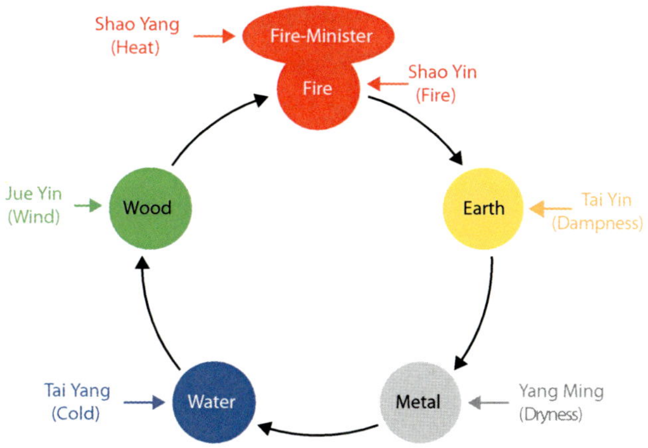

Figure 2.23: Six energies and the climates

Many attempts have been made to explain this arduous concept; none, in my opinion, are really satisfying to our Western logic. (See further comments in ▶ chap. 25 "Chinese Astrology")

To accommodate the system of Five Phases to that of the Six levels, the Fire Phase was sub-divided into Fire Emperor and Fire Minister, and two functions were added to the Fire Minister, the *Xin Bao* ≈ Heart protector also called the Pericardium, and the *San Jiao* ≈ Triple Warmer or Triple Burner.

In the body – the microcosm – these cosmic energies are received by 6 "Grand channels", having the same nomenclature as the Six energies, and each composed of 2 parts (▶ Fig. 2.24 and 2.25):

- An upper section named as *Shou* ≈ Arm
- A lower section called *Zu* ≈ Leg

This sub-division gives us the 12 Primary channels previously called the meridians of acupuncture.

- *Shou Tai Yang*- Small intestine channel

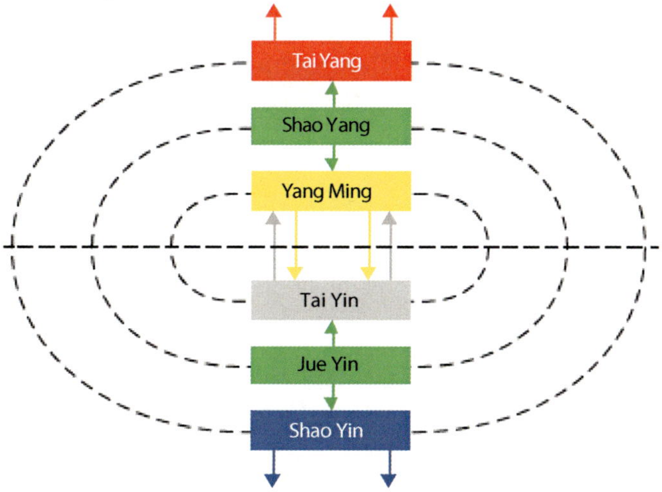

Figure 2.24 S ix levels and the Six Energetic Layers: the channel system

- *Zu Tai Yang*- Bladder channel
- *Shou Shao Yang*- Triple Warmer channel
- *Zu Shao Yang*- Gallbladder channel
- *Shou Yang Ming*- Large Intestine channel
- *Zu Yang Ming*- Stomach channel
- *Shou Tai Yin*- Lung channel
- *Zu Tai Yin*- Spleen channel
- *Shou Jue Yin*- Pericardium channel
- *Zu Jue Yin*- Liver channel
- *Shou Shao Yin*- Heart channel
- *Zu Shao Yin*- Kidney channel

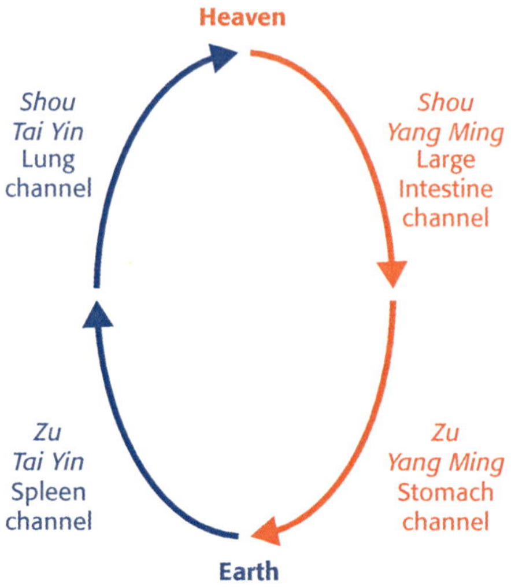

Figure 2.25: Circulation of *Yin* and *Yang* between Earth and Heaven

The channels having the same energetic nomenclature, constitute an upper and lower, Heaven and Earth, connection. For example, the *Shou* and *Zu Yang Ming*, bring the *Yang* of Heaven down and are coupled with *Zu* and *Shou Tai Yin* that bring the *Yin* of Earth upwards, completing the cycle (▶ Fig. 2.25).

Unfortunately, when Chinese medicine was introduced to the West, it was complicated for the Westerners to learn all the Chinese terms in relation to the channels, as well as the Chinese point names, so there was a simplification, for example, the *Shou Tai Yin*-Lung channel was simply called Lung channel, and the points were given numerical identifications: LU-1, LU-2 etc. The result of this unfortunate simplification is that many of the energetic characteristics of the channels as well as that of the points were lost to the Westerner.

It should be further noted that the disposition of the Six Levels, according to the intensity of *Yang* and *Yin*, is slightly different from the disposition of the channels on the body according to the energetic layers. In fact, from the surface towards the inside, the *Yang* layers keep the same disposition as in the order of their intensities. But this order changes for the *Yin* where it is: *Tai Yin – Jue Yin – Shao Yin*. In this spatial disposition, *Shao Yin* becomes the deepest layer. Here again, it is important to remember that the Six Divisions are another dialectical system and that their disposition changes according to the reference.

- In intensity: *Tai Yang- Shao Yang- Yang Ming-- Tai Yin- Shao Yin- Jue Yin*
- Spatially: *Tai Yang- Shao Yang- Yang Ming-- Tai Yin- Jue Yin- Shao Yin*
- Chronologically: *Shao Yang- Tai Yang- Yang Ming-- Shao Yin- Tai Yin- Jue Yin.*

This order signifies that all phenomena start “small” and grow “big” to reach the “end”.

All phenomena in existence could, therefore, be defined either by their dynamic similarity to one of the "Five Movements", or by their particular combination of *Yin* and *Yang* to one of the ”Six Levels”.

The combination of the three *Yin* and the three *Yang* is called a “Hexagram“ and is studied in the *Yi Jing* ≈ Book of changes易經. According to this very original text, there are only 64 possibilities of combination of the trigrams to form the hexagrams. In the binary language of the computer, the two symbols of “0” and “1”, can be combined to infinity: 01, 10 or 010, 100, 001, or 0011 etc.

The Chinese vision limits these sub-divisions to three degrees of *Yin* and *Yang* and their dual combinations, signified by the 64 hexagrams. That there are only a limited and defined number of hexagrams signifies that every moment in time and space is defined by a particular hexagram and that any given moment or any situation is a repetition of a similar moment, occurring in a different setting. This evokes the idea that time is not linear but rather spiral, as, with the passage of the seasons, there is a certain fixity and regularity, even though seemingly different from the previous cycles. The fact that time seems linear is an illusion created by our vision limited by birth and death. A given Hexagram, like any given situation, may evolve only in a limited manner, evoking a certain cause and effect relationship between the present moment and the next.

Yi Jing was and is primarily used for the purpose of divination, but may also be applied in therapy (▶ Part VI, chapter 23)

7 (Qi 七) Accomplishment

The Chinese ideogram represents the sprouting of a seed, breaking through the surface of the earth. It is the manifestation of the full strength of life, it is the number attributed to *Shao Yang*. The cycles of seven represent the accomplishment of creation, as seen in:

- The “7” days of creation
- The “7” planes of creation
- The “7” chakras
- The “7” challenges
- The “7” planets, regulating the passage of time together with the sun and the moon
- The lunar cycle: 4 X 7 = 28
- The “7” constellations of each season

In Chinese medicine:

- The “7” cervical vertebrae that link the head (Heaven) to the body (Earth)
- The “7” upper portals (openings), communication between the microcosm and the macrocosm
- The “7” passions that cause disease
- The “7” *Po* ≈ Corporeal soul, linking with the natural life force
- The human procreation cycle: 4 X 7 X 10 = 280 days
- The female number: the cycles of 7 years define the female physiology and procreative functions, based on the development of the Kidney’s reproductive capacities, referred to as Kidney-*Jing* ≈ Essence.

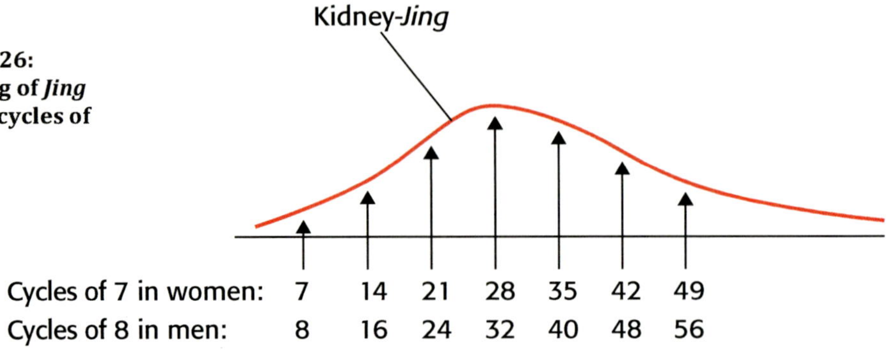

Figure 2.26: Unfolding of *Jing* through cycles of 7 and 8

The classical aging process for women is described in the *Suwen*, chapter 1, referring to the unfolding of *Jing* ≈ Essence according to defined cycles of 7 years (▶ Fig. 2.26)

- At the age of 7: the Kidney *Jing* becomes abundant, teeth change and hair grows longer;
- At 14: the *Ren* and *Chong Mai* fill up and the *Tian Gui* starts flowing (menstruation);
- At 21: the Kidney *Qi* is even and strong, wisdom teeth appear and she is fully grown;
- At 28: the muscles and bones are strong, the hair has reached its full growth, the body is flourishing and fertile, the mind is at its strongest state;
- At 35: the *Yang Ming*, weakens, the complexion withers, wrinkles appear and hair starts falling
- At 42: the upper parts of the 3 *Yang* weaken, face wrinkles and the hair turns white
- At the age of 49: the *Ren* and *Chong Mai* dry up, the *Tian Gui* stops, she is no more fertile.

A similar aging process is described for men following a cycle of 8:

- At the age of 8: the testis, which is an emanation of his Kidney *Qi*, is fully developed and teeth change;
- At the age of 16, semen is secreted and fertility is possible;
- At 24: the Kidney *Jing* is regular, muscles and bones are firm, wisdom teeth appear, and full growth is achieved;
- At 32: the muscles and bones are flourishing and the flesh is healthy;
- At 40: the testicles become smaller, hair starts falling and teeth begin to decay;
- At 48: his masculine vigor is reduced, wrinkles appear, hair turns white at the temple;
- At 56: the Liver *Qi* deteriorates and the muscles cannot function properly, vitality diminishes, semen secretion is exhausted;
- At the age of 64: teeth and hair fall out.

8 (Ba 八) Infinity: All in Existence

In numerology, the number eight is seen as 2 x 2 x 2, or again 2^3, this would symbolize duality in all its possibilities, or in other words, all that exists between Heaven and Earth. In the Chinese tradition, the number Eight has a very important symbolic significance, representing creation in all its forms.

- The "8" directions of the compass
- The "8" Winds, representing the 8 forces that maintain life
- The "8" Extraordinary vessels, responsible for the perpetuation of life and the transmission of *Jing* ≈ Essence
- The "8" Trigrams
- The "8X8" Hexagrams
- "8" is the *Shao Yin* number
- The life cycles of "8" years in men

We have seen how life evolves from the mutation of "One" into "Two", duality, *Yin-Yang*, represented by a full line "–" for *Yang* and a broken line "--" for *Yin*. A second mutation from "Two" to "Four", produces the four phases or directions, with a final mutation of "Four", into "Eight", referred to as the *Ba Gua*八卦 "☰ ☱ ☲ ☳ ☴ ☵ ☶ ☷" (▶ Fig. 2.27)

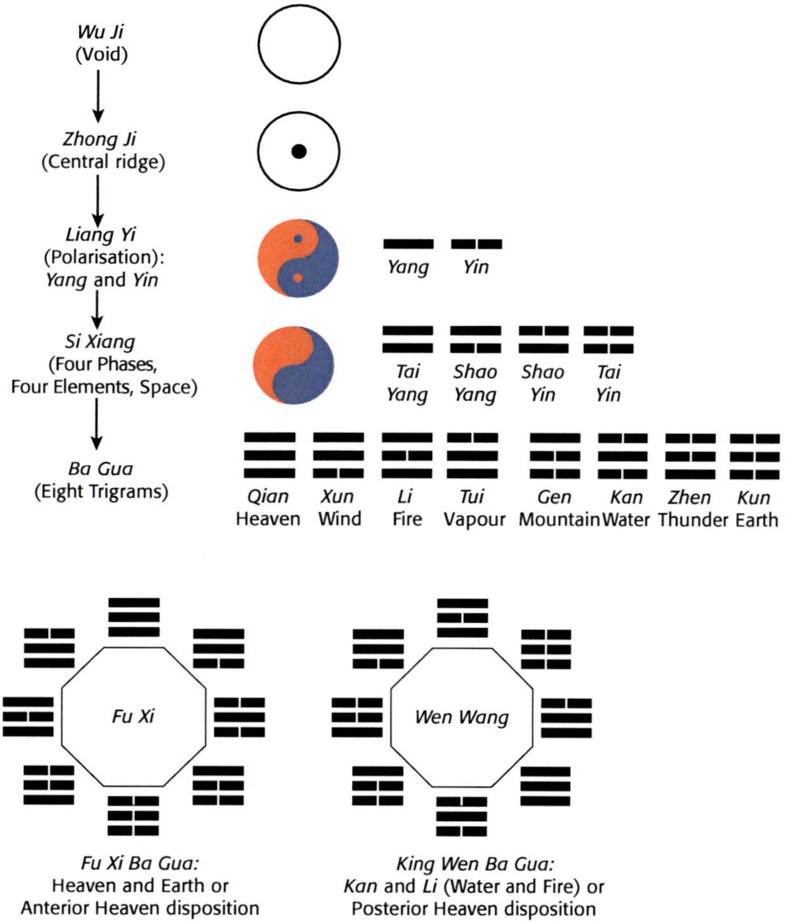

Figure 2.27 : Development of the *Ba Gua*, the Eight Trigrams

The combination of two Trigrams produces six lines called a Hexagram. The *Yi Jing* ≈ Book of changes, describes 64 Hexagrams, signifying that the totality of all possible evolutions between Heaven and Earth can be reduced to 64, and not more. This concerns not only the vital energies but also all the evolutions in nature as well as in an individual's lifespan. The *Yi Jing* represents the 64 Hexagrams in two different dispositions, a circle, representing Heaven, and a square representing Earth.

Therefore eight in its duality (8X8), represents infinity. Is it then a coincidence that the number 8, in the western numeral system, has been used to represent infinity "∞"?

In the fifties, Watson and Crick discovered the DNA structure and the genetic coding. The genetic code is the set of rules by which information encoded in genetic material, DNA, RNA, is translated into proteins by living cells. A sequence of three nucleotides, called a codon, will specify which amino acid should be synthesized for the construction of a specific protein. In order to specify the 20 naturally occurring amino acids, only four different nucleotides in combinations of three each are utilized for their coding; Adenine, Guanine, Cytosine and Thymine, the latter is replaced by Uracil in the construction of the RNA. Interestingly the combination code of 3 nucleotides could code for only a maximum of 4^3 or 64 amino acids. Again is this a coincidence?

Legend attributes the "Eight Trigrams ≈ *Ba Gua*" to Fu Xi circa 3000 BC; it is said that "with the *Ba Gua,* Fu Xi penetrated the divine spirit and by doing so classified the nature of all beings" (historical memories by Si Ma Qian).

The *Ba Gua* is placed on a circle presenting two different dispositions. The original disposition with Heaven on top and Earth below, attributed to Fu Xi, is commonly known as the "Pre or Anterior-Heaven", the second disposition with Fire on top and Water below, attributed to King Wen and is referred to as the "Later or Posterior-Heaven" (▶ Fig. 2.27).

The mating of Heaven with the Earth gave birth to everything in the world, hence the reference to the children as well as to the four primary and the four intermediary directions.

The Trigrams and Hexagrams are always read from below (▶ Table 2.3).

Table 2.3: The Anterior Heaven disposition attributed to Fu Xi

Name	Ba Gua	Nature	Season	Family	Direction	Personality
乾 Qián	☰	天 Heaven	Summer	父 Father	南 South	Creative
坤 Kūn	☷	地 Earth	Winter	母 Mother	北 North	Receptive
巽 Xùn	☴	風 Wind	Summer	長女 Eldest Daughter	西南 South -West	Gentle
坎 Kǎn	☵	水 Water	Autumn	中男 Middle Son	西 West	Abysmal
艮 Gèn	☶	山 Mountain	Autumn	少男 Youngest Son	西北 North-west	Still
震 Zhèn	☳	雷 Thunder	Winter	長男 Eldest Son	東北 North-East	Arousing

離 Lí	☲	火 Fire	Spring	中女 Middle Daughter	東 East	Clinging
兌 Duì	☱	澤 Lake	Spring	少女 Younger Daughter	東南 South-East	Joyous

The Posterior Heaven disposition attributed to King Wen; also known as the *Kan* and *Li ≈ Water and Fire Pa Gua*, here the season and direction references change (▶ Table 2.4)

Table 2.4: Posterior Heaven disposition attributed to King Wen.

Name	Nature	Season/ Element	Family	Direction	Nature
離 Lí	**火 Fire**	**Summer/ Fire**	**中女 Middle Daughter**	**南 South**	**Radiating; sun**
坤 Kūn	地 Earth	Summer/ Earth	母 Mother	西南 South-West	Receptive; yielding
兌 Duì	澤 Lake	Autumn/ Metal	少女 Youngest Daughter	西 West	Joyous or stagnating
乾 Qián	天 Heaven	Autumn/ Metal	父 Father	西北 North-West	Creative; expansive
坎 Kǎn	**水 Water**	**Winter/ Water**	**中男 Middle Son**	**北 North**	**Deep; moon**
艮 Gèn	山 Mountain	Winter/ Earth	少男 Youngest Son	東北 North-East	Still
震 Zhèn	雷 Thunder	Spring/ Wood	長男 Eldest Son	東 East	Arousing; changing
巽 Xùn	風 Wind	Spring/ Wood	長女 Eldest Daughter	東南 South-east	Gentleness, flexibility

9 (Jiu 九) Completion: End of a Cycle

The manifested existence, represented by the number "3", attains its full cycle of development on the 3 planes: Heaven-Human-Earth represented by the number "9".

In numerological symbolism, nine represents wisdom and achievement. In the tarot cards, the ninth card, called the Hermit, depicting an old man carrying a lit lantern. The Hermit, is representative of a person having completed and assimilated the lessons of life and is prepared to withdraw or to return with the new cycle, number "10", representing the new beginning: "zero", void and one. In the Chinese numerology, the number nine is attributed to Heaven.

- "9" : 3 x 3 = totality of the variations of *Qi*
- The "9" provinces
- The "9" levels of Heaven and of Death (underworld)
- The "9" Palaces
- The "9" pulses
- The "9" Heart channel points symbolizing the nine steps or stages of our life towards redemption, recovery and sovereignty:
- The "9" sections of the *Ming Tang* ≈ Hall of light (enlightenment)
- The magic square

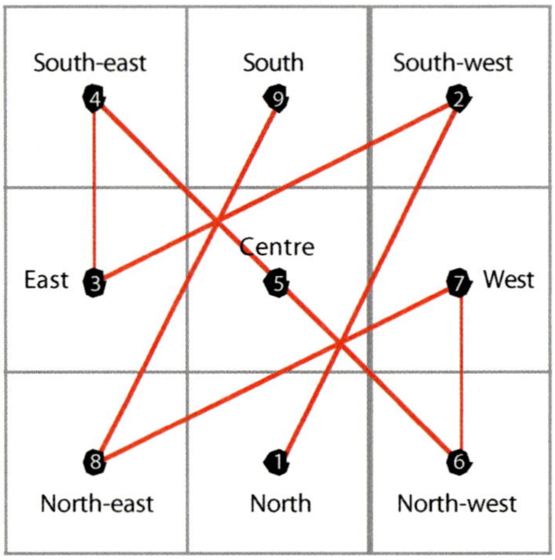

Figure 2.28: The Magic square symbolizes the *Dao*

According to legend, the disposition of the nine numbers was transmitted by the heavens to the emperor Yu the Great through the markings on the shell of a turtle that emerged from the river Luo. The special disposition of these nine numbers is considered emblematic of Heaven and is referred to as the *Lo Shu* or the "Magic square", in which the sum of the numbers in each row adds up to 15.

The Magic square symbolizes the *Dao*. In fact, *Tai Yi*, the Supreme Unity, disposes the numbers in this particular order, defining the eight directions and the center:

The Magic square is greatly used in all ancient references, such as the nine sacred mountains, the nine rivers, the nine provinces, and the nine edits or commandments that *Yu* the Great received from the Heavens to manage the earthly matters, and the nine halls of the heavenly palace.

- The 9 x 9= 81 chapters of all ancient texts are a reminder of the wisdom they imparted
- In the *Feng Shui* art of geomancy, the *Loshu* has great importance.

Table 2.5: Magic square, the sum of the numbers in each row adds up to 15

4	9	2
3	5	7
8	1	6

- In *Qi Gong* general practice, most health care exercises are performed in multiples of nine.
- In medicine, nine is also the number given to the "Portals", or human's openings to the outside, through which communication and interaction are possible:
  - 7 are *Yang* and located in the head: eyes, nose, ears, and mouth
  - 2 are *Yin* and located in the lower parts: anus, genitals

Again, these numbers are symbolic and should not be taken literally.

The symbolism of nine is clearly depicted in the ancient ideogram representing the "human", with arms stretched to receive the energies of Heaven (▶ Fig. 2.29).

- The head is represented as an open circle, signifying the communication between the human's *Shen* ≈ Spirit with the Universal *Shen*. The up-lifted arms represent the apprehension of the world by the mind, the intellect. Shen and mind, both belong to the realm of Heaven.
- The human level represents the emotions, in their dual aspect of driving force

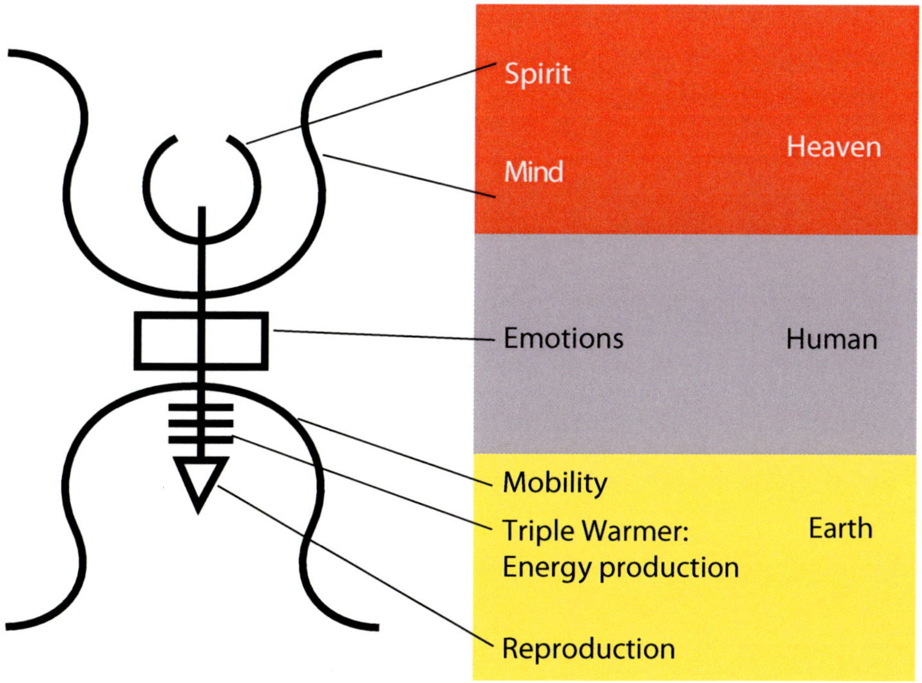

Figure 2.29: Heaven-Human-Earth and the nine levels

and pathological aspect.

- The Earth level represents what the human being has in common with animals, which is mobility, energy production, and reproduction.
- The three short lines are symbolic of the Triple Warmer system. The vertical line pointed downwards is both symbolic of gravity and of the most powerful energy in the human and animal alike, the sexual energy. In the Daoist esoteric and Tantric practices, this energy needs to be redirected upwards, through nine successive "barriers" to enable the opening of the crown center (Chakra), to allow the merging of the individual Shen with the Universal Shen.

10 (Shi 十) Perfection: Integration

With ten, a new cycle is starting.

Ten is the integration of all numbers back into one, it is the completion of human life as represented by the notion of the 7 *Po* ≈ Corporeal souls and the 3 *Hun* ≈ Ethereal souls: 7 + 3 = 10.

Ten is also the number for Heaven, 2 X 5, the 10 Heavenly stems when 12 represents the Earthly Branches.

Part II- Physical and Energetic Structure of the Body

3. The Chinese conception of the body and the organs

The ancient Chinese, similarly to most oriental and Western civilizations, had a respect for the body and would not indulge in post-mortem dissections, hence the limited and quite sketchy knowledge of physical anatomy. What little they knew was from observing the insides of animals or of humans after injury. On the other hand, they had an incredible insight into the physiological and energetic workings of the body and of the mind. The physical body was often looked at symbolically and seen as a reflection of the universal laws.

3.1 Head, Trunk, and Neck

Humans are in the image of the universe. Heaven is symbolized by a circle and Earth by a square.

The head is round and represents Heaven, the most *Yang* part of the human being. All *Yang* channels reach and meet at the head. The head is the seat of the subtlest energies, the mental and the spiritual. The heavenly palace of the envoy of heaven, *Xin*≈ Heart, the emperor, is located behind the third eye when its earthly palace is in the chest. The human being communicates with the world through its portals and sensory organs. Seven of the nine portals are located in the head, as well as all five sensory organs: sight, hearing, smell, taste, and speech.

The trunk is square, representing the Earth. All *Yin* channels converge and meet at the trunk. The trunk is the residence of all of the officials, the *Zang* organs: Heart, Lung, Spleen, Liver and Kidney, and the *Fu* organs: the Stomach, Small Intestine, Large intestine, Gallbladder, and Bladder. The trunk is where all physiological processes take place: production of the Five Substances, *Qi* ≈ Energy, *Xue* ≈ Blood, *Jinye* ≈ Body fluids, *Jing* ≈ Essence, and *Shen* ≈ Spirit/mind.

The trunk is sub-divided into three sections: the upper, middle and lower heating areas known as the Triple Warmer (or Triple Heater).

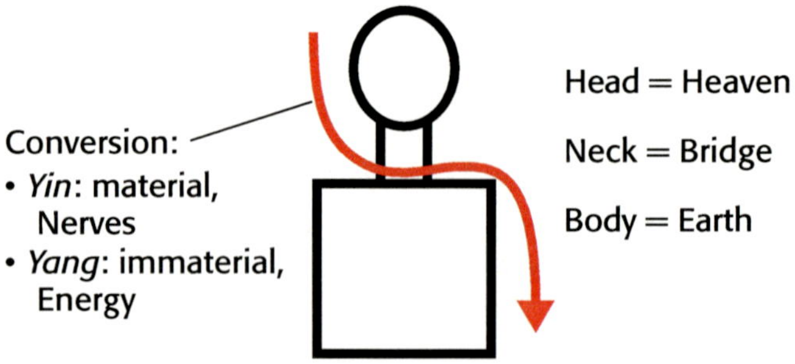

Figure 3.1: Head, Body and Neck (Conversion)

The neck is the passage between the human's Heaven, the head and the Earth, the trunk of the body, where *Yang* energies of heaven descend and the *Yin* energies of Earth ascend. There is a phenomenon of "conversion" that takes place in the area of the neck. On the material level, the cerebral nerve fibers cross over, the left brain controlling the right side of the body and vice versa. Energetically, a similar conversion occurs mainly involving the *Yang Ming* level. In fact, both the arm *Yang Ming*-Large Intestine Primary and Sinew channels, as well as the leg *Yang Ming*-Stomach *Luo* ≈ Connecting channel cross over to the opposite side. This crossing over is also observed with the leg *Shao Yang*-Gallbladder Sinew channel. Most of the "Windows of Heaven" points are located on the neck, regulating the passages of the vital substances to the head and the interaction of humans with the world.

3.2 Four Limbs

The human stands with arms raised to Heaven to receive the *Yang* energies from above. The *Yin* energies of Earth ascend through the feet. *Yin* and *Yang* channels meet and change polarities at the extremities, finger and toe tips.

Each limb is further sub-divided into three sections.

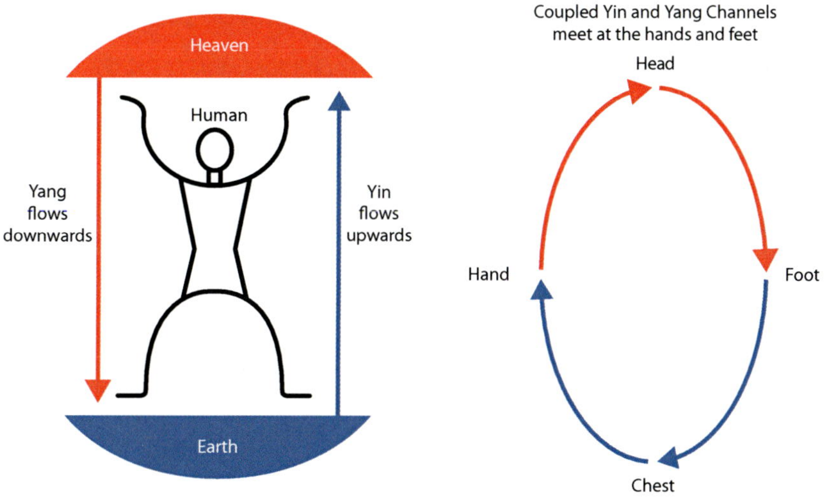

Figure 3.2: The 4 limbs and the circulation of channels

3.3 Ten Officials

The body, in the image of the state, is governed and managed by ten administrators also called officials. They are responsible for governing the body in accordance with the "universal order". These ten organs maintain life by producing the five substances, managing and adapting the energies to the outer changes, and fulfilling the human destiny. Five of the organs are considered *Yin*, *Zang*-organs and five are *Yang*, *Fu*-bowels. They constitute *Yin-Yang* couples, complementing each other in their functions.

Table 3.1: *Yin-Yang*-coupling of the ten organs

Yin, "Zang"	Yang, "Fu"
Liver	Gallbladder
Heart	Small Intestine
Spleen/ Pancreas	Stomach
Lung	Large Intestine
Kidney	Bladder

- Zang-organs are defined as being "full", not necessarily from a structural and anatomic perspective, but rather as organs that store and conserve the vital *Qi* and essences. They are *Yin*.
- The Fu-bowels are "hollow" and primarily function as a means of action, such as separation, transportation, and excretion. They are *Yang*.

Two organic functions are added to complement the physiology of the other organs (► Fig. 3.3):

- *Xin Bao* ≈ Heart Protector also named the Pericardium, as the minister to the Heart
- *San Jiao* ≈ Triple Warmer or the Triple Heater, coordinating the digestive processes involved in the production of the Five Substances.

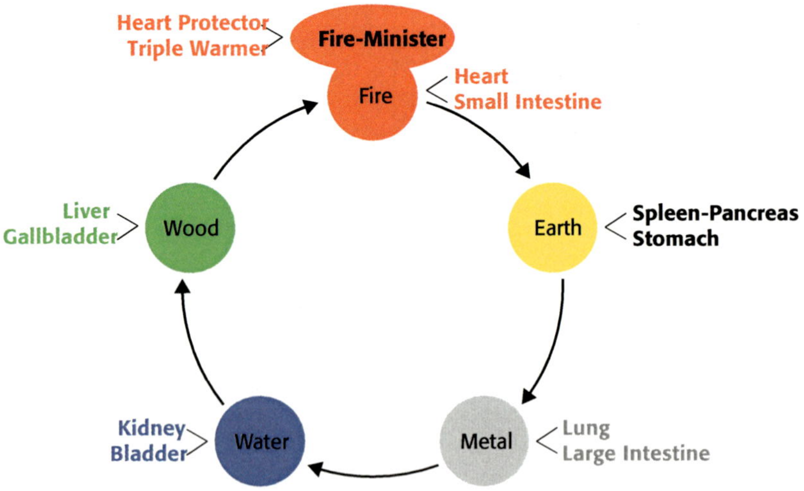

Figure 3.3: ***Zang-Fu*-organs and the Five Phases**

These six *Yin-Yang* couples are each related to one of the Five Phases, hence they will also present interactions of *Sheng* ≈ Nourishment and *Ke* ≈ Control (► chap. 2.5).

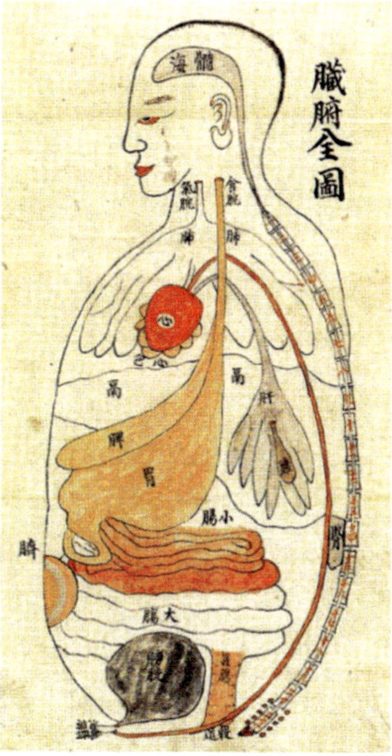

Figure 3.4: Ancient view of the internal organs

It is very important to underline that in Chinese medicine a *Zang*-organ or a *Fu*-bowel does not just designate the anatomical organ but a rather complex system including the Western anatomical organ, the specific physiological functions attached to it, the related anatomical layers and body parts, the sensory organs, the type of emotion it produces and the role it has in the mental functions. The Chinese *Zang-Fu*-organ concept is not really in contradiction with the Western notion of the organs, as many of the functional aspects are similar, nevertheless the Chinese perspective gives a much broader and richer context to the organ system, adding several dimensions to it, and describing inter-relations, which have no anatomical foundation, and can yet be observed on a daily basis.

It should be understood that the "anatomical organ" as we know it in the West, is itself a product, a materialized form, of the particular *Qi* which defines the Chinese notion of "organ system".

When an organ is removed surgically, only a small part (the physical) is removed; the other dimensions of the Chinese organ, its channel networks, its physiological, hormonal, mental and emotional functions, and manifestations all remain.

Each organ-system participates in the production of the Five Vital Substances: *Qi* ≈ Energy, *Xue* ≈ Blood, *Jin Ye* ≈ Body fluids, *Jing* ≈ Essence, and *Shen* ≈ Spirit/mind, as further described in the Triple Warmer system, but they also have other functions. Each organ has its own particular type of momentum, based on this and the physiological functions attached to the organ, they are related to one of the Five Movements. Each organ, in turn, entertains a closer relationship with one or several of the substances, for example, Heart and Liver are very dependant on *Xue* ≈ Blood, Spleen, and Kidney on *Qi* ≈ Energy, Stomach on *Jin Ye* ≈ Body fluids, etc.

Each of the five types of the momentum of each organ is considered, the "Spirit" of that organ, and is given the image of a "Spirit Residing" in that particular organ and directing its *Qi*. An analogy would be a car, representing the organ, and its driver, symbolizing the spirit. The resulting performance, the functions of an organ, is dependent both on the mechanical quality of the vehicle and the dexterity of the driver. E. Rochat, calls this spirit the "Will" of the organ.

- The Spirit of the Liver is *Hun*, its Will is to mobilize (maintain free flow).
- The Spirit of the Heart is *Shen*, its Will is to expand.
- The Spirit of the Spleen-Pancreas is *Yi*, its Will is to transform.
- The Spirit of Lung is *Po*, its Will is to condense.

- The Spirit of Kidney is *Zhi*, its Will is to consolidate.

When the will of an organ is hampered in its momentum, an emotion is produced. For example, when the Liver cannot mobilize, there will be irritability and anger; or when the Kidney cannot consolidate, there will be fear etc...

This notion of a "Spirit Residing" in an organ is not easy for the Western mind to accept and digest, which explains why there are so many different translations for the Chinese terms signifying the five spirits. Commonly they are designated by the mental attributes they represent:

- *Shen* may be referred to as "Mind".
- *Yi* is called "thought" or "Memory".
- *Zhi* is often named "Willpower".
- *Hun* is related to "Imagination".
- *Po* corresponds to "Precision".

Translations of these five Chinese terms are necessarily insufficient and misleading. For example, "*Shen*" has over 20 different meanings, in any particular context calling it simply "mind" would be extremely limiting. Personally, I prefer using the Chinese term rather than the translation.

Besides these 10 organs, there are 6 extraordinary organs that do not participate in energy production and yet store Essence and participate in various transformations (► chap. 3.4).

The organs are deep inside the body and communicate with the surface and the outside, via their channel connections and their openings "portals" and sensory organs. (► Table 2.2)

The Heart (Xin 心), Heart Protector (Xin Bao 心包)

The Heart has the function of the "emperor", the monarch that governs the nation through the state officials which are the other *Zang* and *Fu* organs and bowels.

The *Wang* ≈ emperor 王, placed at the center of creation (▶ chap. 2.3), emanating and transferring the virtues of Heaven and Earth upon humanity without any change or alteration. By the same analogy, the blood circulation system is attached to the Heart, through which the emperor communicates with the nation. (▶Fig. 3.5)

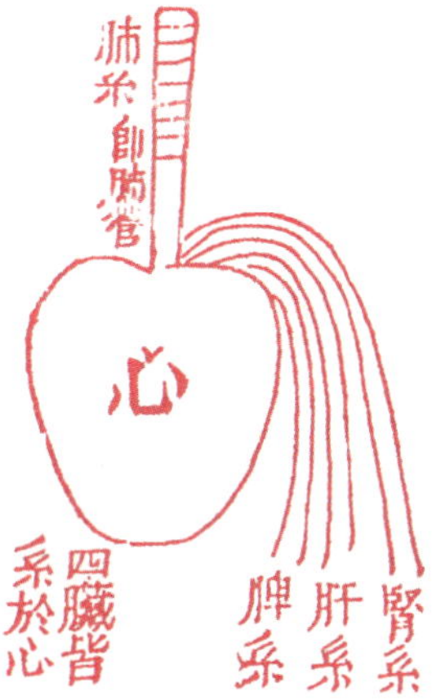

Figure 3.5: Heart (Zhen Jiu Da Cheng)

As the sun is the center of the universe so is the Heart the center of the human being, it is the inner sun, the "Source of life". (▶Fig. 3.7)

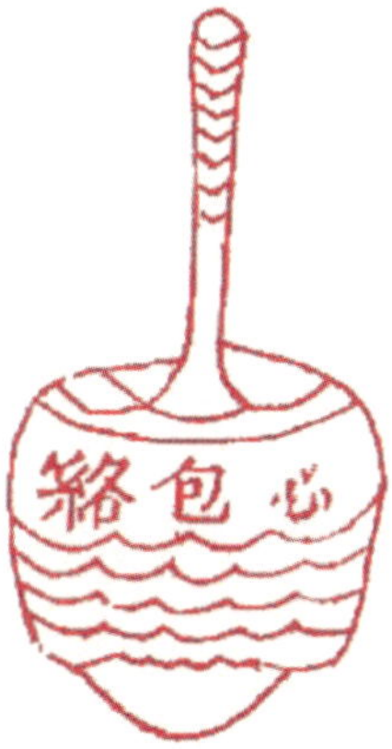

Figure 3.6: Pericardium *(Zhen Jiu Da Cheng)*

The Heart is the residence of the *Shen* representing the mind and the spirit. A clear *Shen* receives all the information and restores it without any alteration. These are attributes of a clear mind and virtues of spiritual consciousness. This can explain why the eye portal (not eyesight), is attached to the Heart, and again why speech is considered the manifestation of the *Shen*, signifying the reception and restoring of all information, expressed by the correct “word”, preceding the correct action. This concept very much joins the thinking of Aristotle (350 BC), that considered the human as “the rational animal that has language”.

The emperor governs but is not actively involved in the functions of the state. The heart pump and circulation system are actually controlled by the system called *Xin Bao* (心包), literally the heart envelope, which originally was translated as “Master of the Heart” by the French school, signifying the master of the household, referring to the Chinese term *Xin Zhu*. The English texts used the term "Heart Protector", and in some earlier Chinese manuals in English, it was even designated as “Circulation and Sex”. In the *Nei Jing*, it is referred to as *Tan Zhong* ≈ Center of *Tan*, translated as chest center, which today designates the point RM-17. Currently, in most Western literature, the term "Pericardium" or more simply

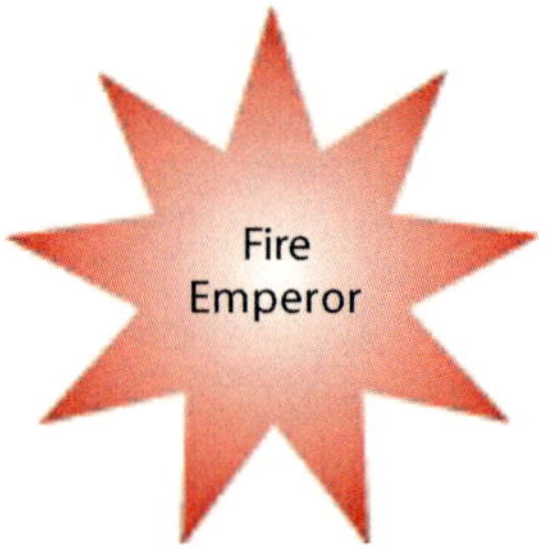

Figure 3.7: The Center, Inner Sun, Source of Life, Life principle

"Pericard" is used, which in my opinion is misleading for the Western students. To clarify this point, the Heart's main function, as the manifestation of the heavenly order, is primarily spiritual. To manifest this immaterial aspect, the Heart needs a physical, material residence, as well as certain organic functions, hence the concept of a material envelope for the Heart, the *Xin Bao*. (▶Fig. 3.6)

"*Xin Bao*" is like an ambassador, a minister carrying out the orders of the emperor. *Xin Bao* is not an organ but a function and is assimilated to the *Zang* ≈ *Yin* organs. In earlier times, the Heart channel was not even described. It was believed that the Heart, representing the Heavenly manifestation, could not be subjected to human influence, therefore all matters pertaining to the heart and circulation was treated via the *Xin Bao*.

The Heart and the Heart protector are related to the Fire phase of the Five Movements. By similarity to the life-giving property of heat, the Heart is "Source of Life" and by analogy to the expansive quality of Fire, the Heart via the *Xin Bao*, circulates blood throughout the system. The Heart is considered the "Fire emperor", whereas the Heart protector is considered the "Fire minister". The Fire minister is, in reality, an extension of Kidney-Fire, and in this manner, it links the Water to the Fire and is sometimes referred to as the envoy of the Kidney.

The functions of the Xin ≈ Heart and Xin Bao ≈ Heart Protector/ Pericardium

- Residence of *Shen:* The one and only main function of the Heart is to house the *Shen* ≈ Spirit/mind. All other functions attributed to the Heart are actually carried out by the Heart's minister, *Xin Bao. Shen* refers to the sum of mental functions: consciousness, mental faculties, and intelligence. *Shen* also refers to all the emotional as well as the spiritual phenomena; therefore the Heart is responsible for harmonious mental, emotional and spiritual evolutions. Although each mental function and each emotion pertains to its particular spirit, *Hun, Yi, Po,* and *Zhi,* in actual fact *Shen* acts as the coordinating factor giving cohesion and coherence to the mental process and harmony to the emotions. In the image of five musicians whose playing should be coordinated by a band-leader for musical coherence.

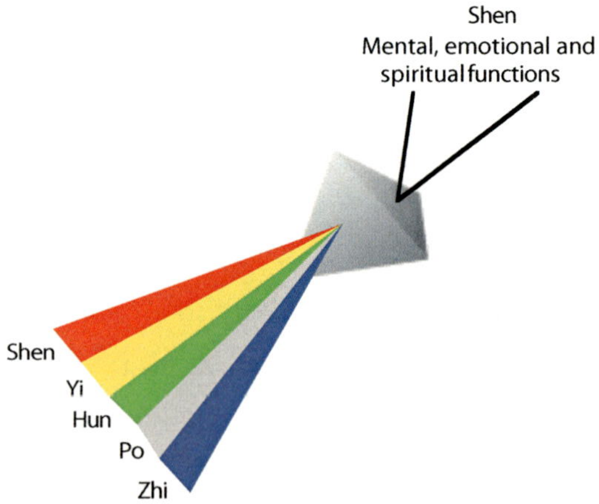

Figure 3.8: The manifested *Shen* is the sum total of *Shen, Yi, Hun, Po*, and *Zhi*

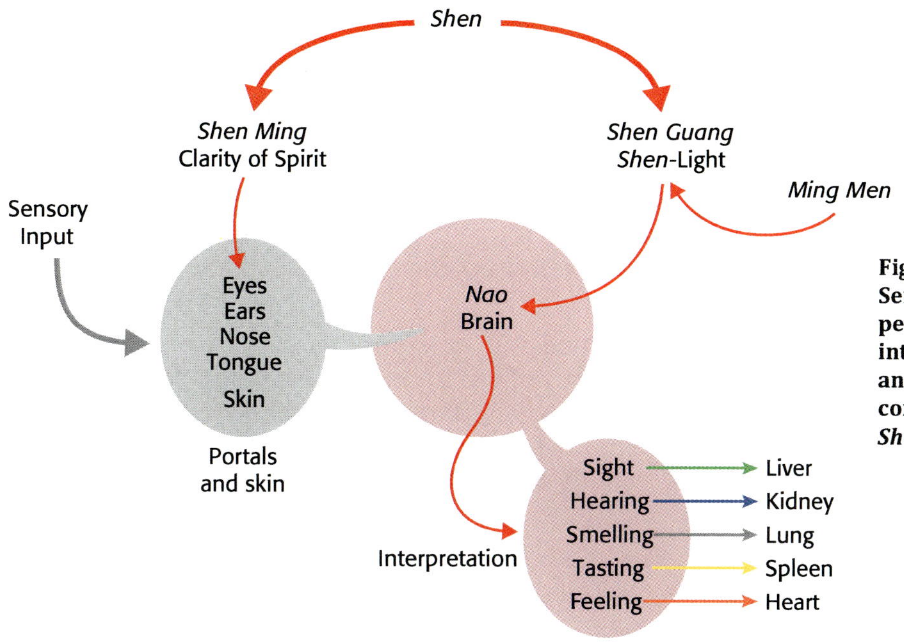

Figure 3.9 Sensory perception, interpretation and routing controlled by *Shen*

Or the image of white light that in fact is composed of all the colors of the spectrum (▶ Fig. 3.8). *Shen* is on the one hand responsible for being conscious and on the other hand for perceiving and interpreting the sensory input. *Shen* is considered disconnected in sleep, hypnosis or coma; any state in which there is no conscious awareness of one's participation. All sensory functions depend not only on the related *Zang* organ but equally rely on the acuity of the *Shen,* the "*Shen Ming*". Sensory input may be reduced, misinterpreted, or simply blocked by a dysfunctional *Shen* (▶ Fig. 3.9).

- As the Heart-emperor has the charge of the harmony within the state and the empire, Shen has the position of coordinator for the other four "Spirits", the Hun, Po, Yi, and Zhi, maintaining a coherent mental function, manifested in an appropriate connection with the inner and outer worlds, the micro and macrocosm (▶ Fig. 3.9). Shen is reflected in the eyes and manifests through a clear and coherent speech. As the emperor receives the virtues of Heaven and Earth and transmits them without alteration, on an emotional level, universal love and compassion are the attributes of the Heart. The rather earthly and human relations, love and passion as well as sexuality are the domain of the Xin Bao ≈ Heart Protector. Sexuality, in fact, is an expression of Kidney-Fire that has reached maturity, and through its connection with the Xin Bao finds an outer expression.
- It is said that the Shen-emperor has two residences, the earthly residence in the center of the chest, Tan Zhong, signifying the earthly matters that are in fact managed by the Xin Bao, such as the heart pump and circulation, as well as human relationships. The heavenly residence is in the Ming Tang, behind the third eye. In alchemical practices, this signifies that the monarch should not be concerned and distracted by earthly affairs and pleasures, but rather with spiritual awakening.

- Governing Blood: This function refers to the fact that the final transformation of food essence, body fluids, and hereditary energy into Xue ≈ Blood takes place in the Heart, although the heart does not actively participate in this process. Symbolically the blood takes on its red color from the Heart. Due to the Heart's close connection to Blood, Blood disharmony patterns such as Blood Xu-vacuity or Blood-Heat will have immediate impacts on the Shen, resulting in mental or emotional manifestations. Hence the constitutional, emotional and mental strength depends on the strength of the Heart as well as that of the Kidney essence.
- Governing the circulation: This function is delegated to the minister Xin Bao ≈ Heart Protector. The pumping action of the heart and the blood flow in the vascular system are controlled by the Xin Bao ≈ Pericardium, in practice, this signifies that all organic pathologies pertaining to the heart and the arterial system should be treated with the Pericardium channel.
- Reflects in the complexion: a pink complexion is the result of rich Blood and good circulation. In practice, a pale complexion informs more about the state of Xue ≈ Blood, rather than on the heart organ. This could be the case with Blood-vacuity affecting the heart. Excessive redness in the face, signifying excess/ repletion of Heat could express a condition of Heart-Heat or Heart-Fire, but again is not exclusively associated with the Heart.
- Opening into the tongue: The tongue is called the "bud" or offshoot" of the Heart. This refers primarily to the tongue's function of speech. A clear and coherent speech reflects the normal functioning of the mind. In Shen disturbances, speech may be disturbed, or incoherent or even become impossible which is the case either in some psychotic conditions or with loss of consciousness. The tongue is also the organ of taste, which is controlled by the Spleen-Pancreas, but like all other sensory inputs, taste is also subject to Shen. Furthermore, the color of the tongue reflects the state of Blood but not specifically the Heart-blood.
- Controlling Sweat: The specific fluid of the Heart is the sweat. Again, abnormal sweating does not only signify a Heart disharmony pattern and could be seen in a multitude of other organic imbalances.
- Modern Western physiology and in particular embryology may explain many of the ancient Chinese concepts pertaining to the Xin ≈ Heart and Xin Bao ≈ Pericardium (► table. 3.2).

Overview of Heart Functions

- Residence of Shen
- Governing Blood
- Governing the circulation
- Reflection in the complexion
- Opening into the tongue
- Controlling Sweat

Overview of Pericardium Functions

- Heart pump and Blood circulation

- Relating emotionally to the outer world: "Circulating in the world"
- Sexuality

Table 3.2: Physiology of Chinese and Western Heart (*Xin* 心) & Pericard (*Xin Bao* 心包)

Chinese Heart functions	Western physiology	Linking the two concepts
The "Emperor": seat of life	Embryology: the first organ to be formed; the cardiac conduction cells (myocytes) are issued from the "neural crest" cells, the same as the brain	Relation between the brain and the heart
Fire emperor: "Source of life"	Heartbeat: defines life	
Residence of *Shen*: mental and emotional coherence	The brain's function of consciousness, perception, coherence	Relation between emotions /psychology and heart functions (physiology)
Relating aspect: *Xin Bao* ≈ Pericardium	• Emotional heart; empathy • Social - human relating, sexuality	
Governing Blood circulation (*Xin Bao* ≈ Pericardium)	Heart pump; vascular systems; carotid sine to modify heartbeat and blood pressure	Relation between peripheral needs and blood pressure
Governing Blood: final transformation of substances into *Xue* ≈ Blood	• Right heart: pumps blood to the lungs (removes CO_2 adds O_2) • Left heart: pumps O_2-rich blood throughout the system	Relation between heart and lungs
Opening into the tongue (speech)	Coherent speech reflects the coherence of the mind	Heart- *Shen*- speech
The eyes as windows of Shen	Embryological connection between the brain, eyes and heart	Brain-eyes-heart-*Shen*
Connection with the Kidney (*Shao Yin*)	• Embryological connection between heart and kidney (retro-peritoneal space) • The aorta and the renal arteries • Atrial and brain natriuretic peptides (ANP - BNP)	Interconnection between the Heart and Kidney; *Shao Yin* axis
Xin Bao ≈ Pericard as Heart "protector"	The fibrous pericardium acting as a thick protective anatomical layer	Pericardium protects the Heart against PF (climat and emotion)

The Lung (Fei 肺) (► Fig. 3.10)

The Lung is the State Minister and chancellor, in charge of policies. It administers the harmonious exchanges with the outside by limiting excess. It is also sometimes called the judge, deciding what is appropriate or not for the system, this may result in the phenomena of rejection, as seen in allergies.

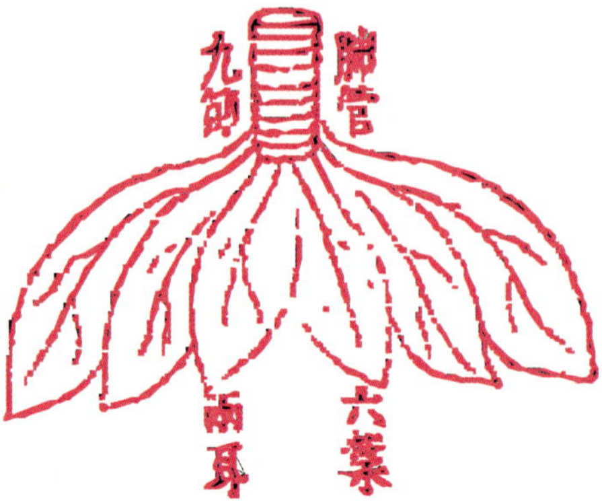

Figure 3.10: Lung *(Fei)* (*Zhen Jiu Da Cheng*)

The Lung, *Yin/ Zang*, together with its coupled *Yang/ Fu*, Large Intestine, are related to the Metal phase. Both have the role of receiving, taking in, filtering or separating and letting go of the unwanted, hence the image of a "fishing net".

The functions of the Lung

- Governing breathing by inhaling the "pure *Qi* of Heaven" (oxygen) and bringing it down to the Kidneys in the lower Triple Warmer, and by exhaling impure *Qi* (CO^2).
- Master of *Qi*: It is described that *Qi* is formed in the Lung by the mixing of the pure essence of food and fluids, with the air *Qi* before circulating throughout the body. The Lung's function is to manage the proper distribution of *Qi*, internally as well as to the surface, hence the term "Master" or "Commander" of *Qi*. This partly explains the reason that the Chinese have described the order of energy circulation in the channels by starting with the Lung channel. The Lung further protects the *Qi* stored in the chest called "*Zong Qi*" translated as "Ancestral", "Essential", "Fundamental" or "Gathering" *Qi*. The main role of *Zong Qi* is to maintain the rhythmic functions of the heart pump and breathing.

> *Zong-ancestral Qi accumulates in the center of the chest, at Shanzhong RM-17. It expresses through the throat the larynx and it links to the heart directly to the eyes. Hence liveliness and motivations, which are attributes of Jing, are conveyed through the sparkle in the eyes.*
>
> *Ling Shu, chap. 71*

- Supplying *Qi* to Blood: maintains *Qi* circulation in the Blood vessels. From a Western understanding, the Lung maintains blood pressure and may be responsible for hypotension but is not involved in hypertension.
- Controlling the diffusion of *Wei* ≈ Defensive *Qi* and *Jin Ye* ≈ Body fluids. Lung nourishes and maintains the skin, the pores, surface temperature, and skin moisture as well as all the mucous membranes; ensure the protection of the

surface against pathogenic factors. Through this function, the Lung is in charge of the first line of defense against external aggression. As it is also the highest placed *Zang*-organ, it is at times referred to as the “roof” of the *Zang-Fu*. It is the only *Zang*-organ that connects directly to the outside via the respiratory tract, the nose, and the mouth.

- Controlling the descent of *Qi* to the Kidney and the lower Triple Warmer, and in particular to the Large Intestine, its coupled *Fu*-bowel. In this manner, the Lung-*Qi* aids the urinary and intestinal functions.
- Regulating Water passages: the Lung receives the liquids coming from the Spleen-Pancreas. The lung is named the "Upper source of fluids", due to its dual action of descending and of diffusing the liquids. The Lung distributes the fluids evenly, to the skin as well as to the organs, in particular to the Kidney, which is called the "Lower source of fluids", and is in charge of the "Waterways". By this function, certain Lung pathologies are responsible for fluid accumulation and edema, urinary retention or urinary frequency.
- Governing the skin and mucous membranes and body hair: by diffusing *Wei Qi* and fluids to the surface. The thickness and smoothness of the skin depend on the quantity of *Qi* and fluids that the Lung diffuses. With Lung pathologies, the skin gets thinner and ages and wrinkles faster.
- Opening into the nose: Lung maintains the free passage of air and ensures the sense of smell.
- The fluid of the Lung is the mucous secretion.
- Housing the *Po*≈ Corporeal Soul: This is the most materialized aspect of the spirits. *Po* is the closest to the physical body and to sensations, touch, and pain. In the oriental concepts, *Po* is related to incarnation and is active during the fetal stage in the body formation. After birth it directs the inward movement of energies and maintains certain reflexes, it is also the depository of ancestral memories. *Po* represents the “instinct of protection”.

Modern Western physiology and embryology may explain many of the ancient Chinese concepts pertaining to the *Lung* (*Fei* 肺) (► table. 3.3).

Overview of Lung Functions

- Governing breathing
- Master of Qi
- Supplying *Qi* to Blood
- Controlling the diffusion of *Wei- Qi* and *Jin Ye*
- Controlling the descent of *Qi* to the Kidney
- Regulating Water passages:
- “Upper Source of Fluids”
- Governing the skin, mucous membranes, and body hair
- Opening into the nose
- In charge of mucous secretion
- Housing the *Po* ≈ Corporeal Soul

Table 3.3: Comparative Chinese and Western Physiology of the Lung (*Fei* 肺)

Chinese Lung functions	Western physiology	Linking the two concepts
The "State minister": in charge of policies	• The first independent action of the new-born • After the heart-beat, breathing defines life	"Prana"- breath links the microcosm to the macrocosm
• Governs breathing • Master of *Qi*	The alveoli allow the release of CO_2 and the absorption of O_2	The triple warmer system requires O_2 to produce *Qi* ≈ Energy
Supplying *Qi* to Blood	• In-breath allows blood to flow from the heart to the lung to be oxygenated • Out-breath pushes blood out into the heart	Breathing energizes blood and clears the toxins
Regulate the water passages: Upper source of fluids	By releasing carbolic acid, lungs also release fluids	Lung and Spleen *Tai Yin* Relation to transform Dampness
Govern the skin and the mucus membranes	• Skin complements the release of CO_2 and the absorption of O_2 • Skin releases excess fluids	Skin vitality depends on the skin's fluid content
Opens into the nose	Embryological connection between intestines, lung and the nose	Breathing starts at the nose

The Kidney or Kidneys (Shen 肾) (► Fig. 3.11)

The only pair organ in the Chinese system, not because there are two kidneys, but because they have two distinct functions: Kidney *Yin* and Kidney *Yang*.

The Kidneys are considered the "Germ of Creation" or the "Root of Life". They are in charge of the creative forces on all levels: physical, mental and spiritual. The Kidney is considered the "Counselor to the emperor". Although the Kidneys have a *Yin* and a *Yang* aspect, overall the Kidney is classified as *Zang* and *Yin* in the Chinese organ system and coupled with Bladder, its *Fu* ≈ Bowel. As the Kidney represents the fluid aspect of the body, as well as its densest structure, the skeleton, it is irelated to the Water phase symbolizing structure and coherence.

The functions of the Kidneys

The Kidneys differ from the other organs in Chinese medicine, as they present a *Yin* and *Yang* aspect as well as *Qi* function and a reservoir for *Jing*.

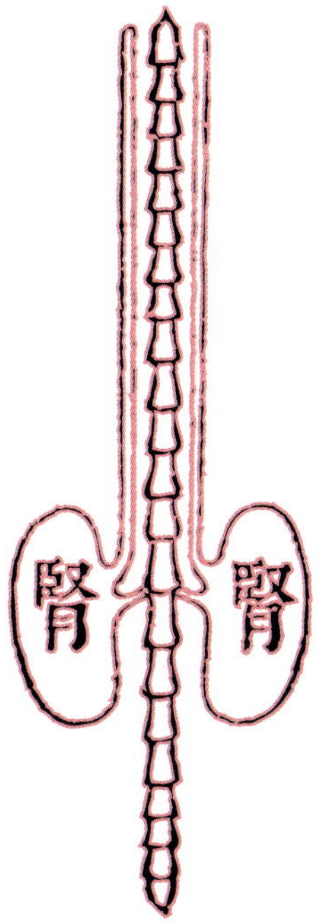

Figure 3.11: Kidneys *(Shen)*, (*Zhen Jiu Da Cheng*)

- "Root of Pre-Heaven *Qi*": The Kidneys have the charge of storing and safeguarding the pre-natal energies, the *Yuan*-Source *Qi* and the parental *Jing* ≈ Essence *Qi*. In the Chinese concept, there are three constituent or original energies: *Yuan*-Source *Qi*, *Jing* ≈ Essence and *Zong* ≈ Ancestral *Qi*, referred to as "Pre-heaven", "Anterior Heaven" or pre-natal energies.
  - *Yuan Qi* supplies the "Spark of life", it is the life principle that is going to manifest through the Heart as "Source of life" defining the desire to live, and through the Kidneys as the "Will to Live". *Yuan Qi* will constitute the *Yang* of the Kidney, Kidney Fire. Kidney Fire will later become the root of all transformative and physiological functions of the body.
  - *Jing Qi* is the parental *Jing* ≈ Essence that may be assimilated in modern times to the chromosomal inheritance, responsible for the constitution and the form. The *Jing Qi* controls growth and sexual maturation and defines the constitutional strength and vitality. At puberty, the Kidneys start producing the individual's own *Jing Qi*.
  - *Zong* ≈ Ancestral *Qi* is the cosmic *Qi* at the time of conception, which is believed to carry the destiny or mandate of the person. The notion of *Zong* ≈ Ancestral also includes transmitted character traits and habits (Ancestral) as well as the influence of the environment (Nurture). The latter joins the modern Western field of "Epigenetics".
- After birth, the combined inherited *Yuan Qi* and *Jing Qi*, are referred to as *Dong Qi* ≈ Moving *Qi* between the Kidneys and are located in the lower abdomen, an area called lower *Dan Tian*, signifying the alchemical cinnabar chamber, known as the "*Hara*" in the Japanese tradition. In

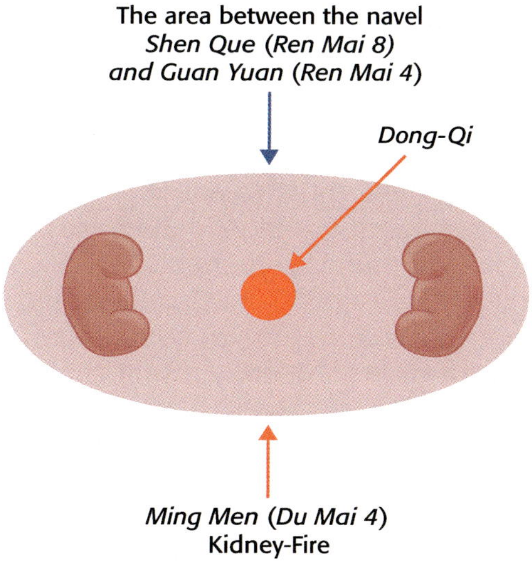

Figure 3.12: Kidneys, *Dong Qi* and *Ming Men*, Kidney-Fire

alchemical and meditative practices, this is the first area where energy is concentrated and transformed. The original *Yuan Qi* is considered the source of the "True Fire", it may be accessed by two points (▶ Fig. 3.12):

- The area between the two Kidneys called *Ming Men*, translated as Gate of Vitality, Gate of Life or Life Mandate, DM-4.
- On the lower abdomen, *Guan-Yuan*, Barrier of *Yuan Qi*, RM-4.

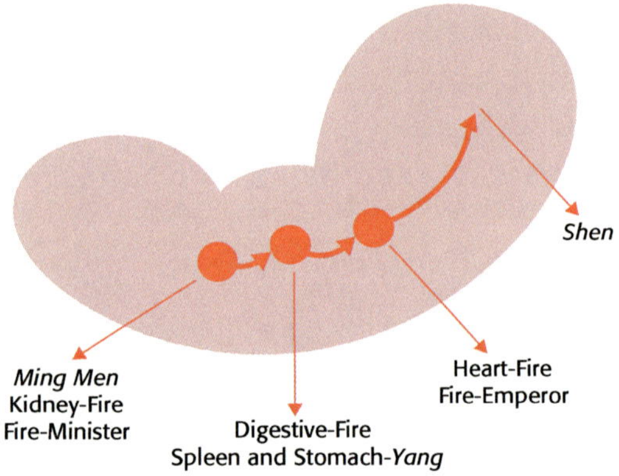

Figure 3.13: *Ming Men*, the migration of the Original Fire, -> 3 Fire centers

The Fire of *Ming Men* is the source of Fire of the whole body, it concentrates in the lower parts and is the root of Kidney *Yang*, it is referred to as "Fire Minister" (in continuity with *Xin Bao* ≈ Pericardium). This Fire migrates during the fetal phase from the lower heating center, which will later constitute the Kidney-Fire, to form the middle-heating center, the digestive Fire of Spleen and Stomach, and further to the upper heating center, to provide the Heart-Fire (▶ Fig. 3.13).

In Post-Heaven or postnatal energetics, the Kidney *Jing* is subjected to the Kidney-Fire to produce Kidney *Qi*, in the image of a candle: the wax, *Yin*, represents Kidney *Jing*, the flame, *Yang*, is Kidney-Fire, the emanating light represents Kidney *Qi*. The *Qi* thus produced in the lower parts, ascends the back via the *Du Mai* ≈ Governing channel, itself rooted in the *Dong Qi* ≈ Moving *Qi* between the Kidneys. *Du Mai* distributes this *Qi* to the *Zu Tai Yang*-Bladder channel, situated parallel and on each side of *Du Mai*. The *Qi* accumulates in certain points of the Bladder channel called Back *Shu* ≈ Transport points, from where the energy is transported to all of the *Zang* and *Fu* organs and via their respective primary channels to all the parts of the body. The dissemination of *Jing* ≈ Essence to the *various Zang-Fu* is not quite even. The body disseminates to the organs according to the pre-programmed constitution, that is, the inherited constitutional energies. For example, a Wood type constitution receives more energy at *Ganshu* BL-18,

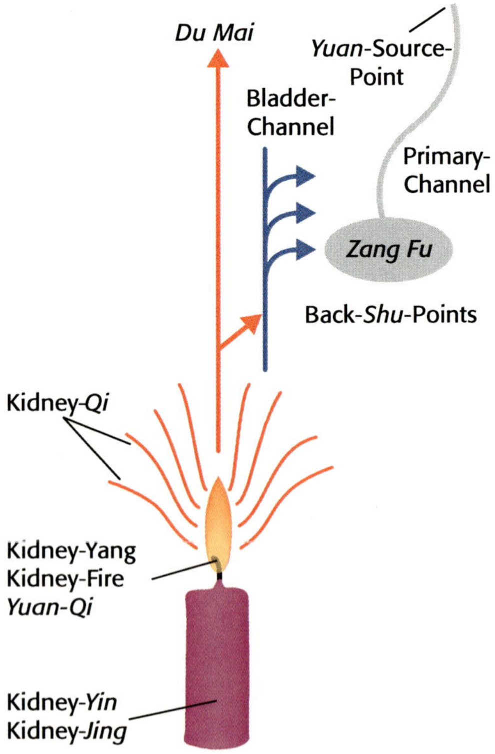

Figure 3.14: Dissemination of *Yuan Qi* from the lower Triple Warmer

the Liver Back-*Shu* point, and *Danshu* BL-19, the Gallbladder Back-*Shu*.

This process of transformation of *Jing* into *Qi* and its subsequent distribution to the *Zang-Fu* is known as the Triple Warmer process which is responsible for the production of the three substances by the Stomach and Spleen, referred to as white, grey and red substances, in the form of *Qi*, (*Ying* ≈ Nourishing and *Wei* ≈ Defensive energies), *Jin Ye* ≈ Body fluids and *Xue* ≈ Blood. (► chap. 4.4)

Jing also generates the bone via the marrow and it nourishes the brain, hence maintaining the Curious-*Fu* organs.

Furthermore, the transformation and distribution of the original *Yuan* ≈ Source *Qi* from the area of the lower *Tan Tian*, via the *Du Mai* to the Bladder channel's back *Shu* ≈ Transport points and to the various *Zang-Fu*, is reflected on the *Yuan*-Source point of the corresponding primary channels, hence their name. In fact, when stimulated, the *Yuan*-source points to direct the produced *Qi* in the Triple warmer towards the corresponding organ and channel system (► Fig. 3.14).

- "Root of *Yin* and *Yang*": The Kidneys constitute the foundation of the entire *Yin* functions and substances, and the *Yang* functions and motive forces. Besides all the fluids of the body Kidney *Yin* represents the *Jing* ≈ Essence, the structure, and the skeleton, but also the vital force and stamina. The relation between Kidney *Yin* and Heart in the *Ke* ≈ Control cycle helps to keep the Fire Phase and the Heart in check, acting as the cooling element. On the other hand, Kidney *Yang* is an extension of *Yuan Qi*, the original Fire, and sustains all of the vital functions of the body such as reproduction, digestion, blood circulation, and the mental functions. Because of their interdependent relationship: Kidney *Yin* is the material base for Kidney *Yang*, and Kidney *Yang* provides the motive force, the "Heat" for the *Yin*.
- The Kidneys are also called the origin of “Water and Fire”. This further explains the close connection between the Kidneys and the Heart.
- Storage of Essence, *Jing Qi* and sexuality: this is the *Jing Qi* produced by the Triple Warmer and stored by the Kidneys. This Essence controls the various stages of development: the growth of bones, teeth, uterus, and the stages of reproduction, sexual maturity, birth, menopause, and andropause etc. This evolution follows a cycle of 7 for women and 8 for men. Kidney Essence "*Jing Qi*" is part of the *Yin* aspect of the Kidneys, and since the *Yin* nourishes *Yang*, Kidney Essence produces Kidney *Qi* and there is thus a connection between *Jing Qi* and vitality, willpower, fertility, and sexuality.
- Production of Bones and Marrow: The production and quality of bones, marrow, and teeth depends on the strength of Kidney *Jing*. Marrow has a different significance in Chinese Medicine. It is the substance that fills up the bones, the spinal cord, and the brain; hence it contributes to mental strength, which depends on the Kidneys.
- Control of Water passages: The Kidney is in charge of controlling the separation of pure and impure fluids in the lower Triple Warmer, and the excretion of the impure by Bladder and Intestines. Hence the term of the “Lower source of fluids”.

- Control of the lower orifices: Kidney *Qi* controls the genito-urinary orifices and the anus. The *Zu Jue Yin*-Liver channel equally controls the outer genitalia.
- Reception of Lung *Qi*: Kidneys receive and hold (grasp) the pure *Qi* of air that the Lung sends down. In practice, some asthmatic conditions and breathing difficulties are due to the incapacity of the Kidney to grasp the Lung *Qi*.
- Maintain the Hair: quantity, quality, and color of hair are dependent on Kidney *Jing*. Hair quality also depends on the skin's nourishment by fluids (Lung) and Blood (Liver).
- Open into the Ears: hearing depends on the Essence "*Jing*" of the Kidneys, although external ear pathologies, such as otitis reflect on the local channels.
- Residence of "*Zhi*", which is the spirit responsible for the Creative Forces and the Will Power, and is often called the "Germ of Creation". The *Zhi* is also representing the strength of character, the will to live, courage, and sometimes called the "reservoir of desires". Where *Shen* represents intelligence, *Zhi* symbolizes wisdom, hence its title of the "Counselor to the emperor".

Modern Western physiology and in particular embryology may explain many of the ancient Chinese concepts pertaining to the Kidneys (Shen 肾) (► table. 3.4).

Overview of Kidney Functions

- The root of Inherited-Pre-Heaven Qi
- The root of Yin and Yang
- Storage of *Jing* ≈ Essence; responsible for sexuality
- Production of Bones and Marrow
- Control of Water passages: "Lower Source of Fluids"
- Controlling the lower orifices
- Reception of Lung *Qi*
- Maintain the Hair
- Opening into the ears
- Residence of *Zhi* ≈ Willpower

Table 3.4: Comparative Physiology of the Kidneys (Shen肾)

Chinese Kidney functions	Western physiology	Linking the two concepts
• The "Counselor to the Emperor" • Connection between the Heart and the Kidney (*Shao Yin*)	• Embryology heart and kidney connection (retro-peritoneal space) • Adrenal medulla issued from the "neural crest" cells (*Jing*); cortex from mesoderm • Kidneys control heartbeat and blood pressure (production of renin and aldosterone)	Relation between the kidneys, adrenals and the heart; the Kidney controlling the Heart (*Ke* cycle); *Shao Yin* axis

• Root of Yin and Yang	• Adrenaline (*Yang*): increases heart contractions; air intake (lungs) and fight-flight reflex in the brain (stress) • Cortisol (*Yin*): holds fluids, draws from reserves (muscle and bone), increases blood sugar and white blood cells	Relation between adrenaline and cortisol in response to stress or danger
• Storage of *Jing* ≈ Essence (reproductive energy)	• Embryological connection between the primitive kidneys and the ovaries and testis (*Jing*) • Production of testosterone and estrogen by the adrenal cortex	*Ming Men*: responsible for sexuality and reproduction
• Control of Water passages: "Lower Source of Fluids"	• Kidney nephrons as filtration units maintain the pH, and the fluid levels via the sodium and potassium balance • Water retention via aldosterone	Kidney adapting the fluid levels in relation to body needs
• Governing the Marrow • Controlling bones	• Production of red blood cells in the marrow via erythropoietin produced in the kidneys • Release of white blood cells via cortisol • Bone production via calcitriol (Vit. D), and calcium and phosphate metabolism	Bone density and marrow production in relation to Kidney-*Jing*
• Reception of Lung Qi • Water overflowing	• Kidneys produce renin which activates the lung's production of angiotensin • Water retention (aldosterone) causing lung edema	Relation between Kidneys and Lung; (skin vitality through the skin's fluid content)
Controlling the lower orifices	• The ureter, the bladder and urinary functions • Pelvic, vaginal and rectal connections via the testicular, ovarian and sacral arteries	Kidney Qi controls the lower sphincters
Residence of *Zhi* ≈ Willpower	• Willpower and risk-taking capacity are enhanced by dopamine mainly produced by the adrenal medulla	*Zhi* defines the strength of character
Opening in to the ears	• The bones of the ear issue from the "neural crest" cells (*Jing*)	*Jing* defines the ability to hear
Maintain hair	• The pigment cells issue from the "neural crest" cells (*Jing*)	*Jing* defines hair quality and aging

The Liver (Gan 肝)

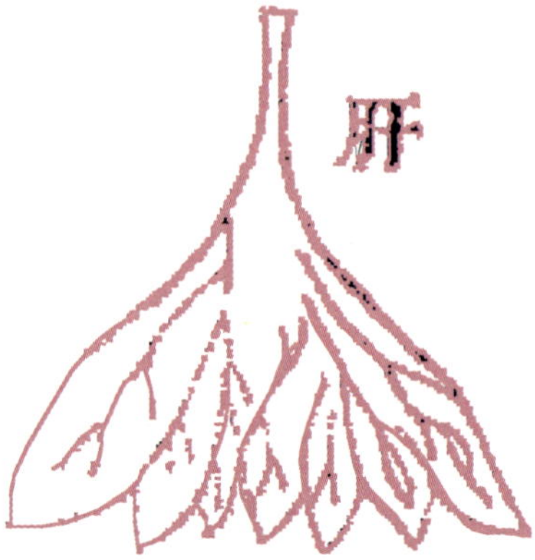

Figure 3.15: Liver *(Gan)* (*Zhen Jiu Da Cheng*)

The Liver is considered the "General of the armies" in charge of planning and strategies (▶ Fig. 3.15). The general has the role of protecting the borders, by the strategic placing of the army and thus maintaining the limits and, at the time of war, deploying the army to protect the state and the emperor. It is said that there are three kinds of generals, one that loses the war, he is usually decapitated; one that wins a battle after fighting, he has little merit, then there is the good general who wins the war without fighting a battle, he is to be praised. This analogy applied to the defensive mechanisms of the body, represented by the concept of *Wei Qi*, indicates that the Liver is in charge of managing and mobilizing *Wei Qi*. In fact many of the pathologies implicating the immune system, such as immune deficiency, autoimmunity, and hyper-reactivity (as in allergies), concern dysfunctions of the Liver. It is important to remember that the Liver only manages and mobilizes the *Wei* ≈ Defensive energy, the latter is produced by the Triple Warmer, Stomach and Spleen in particular and diffused by the Lung to the surface. It is the agility of the army that guarantees the integrity of the borders. A good general plans his strategies and is subservient to the emperor and does not rebel.

The Liver is also in charge of "becoming", one's projects and evolutions on all levels: physical (about 500 biochemical functions), psychological (resolution, prevention), and spiritual (rebirth).

By their dynamism and mobility the Liver and its *Fu* ≈ Bowel the Gallbladder are related to the Wood phase.

The functions of the Liver

- Responsible for the free flow of *Qi*: this is the most important function of the Liver. It ensures the smooth, free, relaxed and easy flow of *Qi*. Its function of mobilizing and moving out, of expanding and dispersing, affects the movements of *Qi* in all parts of the body and on all levels:
- Digestive processes and energy production: the Liver allows Stomach *Qi* to move down and aids the Spleen to move the pure energies upwards. This function is aided by the Gallbladder that stores and secretes the bile.
- The mobilization of *Wei Qi* ≈ Defensive energy: the Liver manages and moves the *Wei Qi* to where it is needed.
- The smooth expression of emotions and the management of emotional reactions also depend on the free-flowing of Liver *Qi*. Although, as discussed above, the Heart, in particular, the *Shen* is responsible for the harmony of the emotions, it is the Liver that helps in their proper expression, avoiding repression and limiting excessive outbursts. The Liver entertains with the Heart, in the Five phases, a *Sheng* ≈ Nourishing relation, "mother-son". The Liver-

Blood nourishes the Heart-Blood. As seen above, the *Shen* has an intimate connection to *Xue* ≈ Blood, further explaining the role of the Liver in emotional matters. Furthermore, the Liver and the Pericardium channels constitute the lower and upper portions of the same *Jue Yin* level. As *Xin Bao* ≈ Pericardium deals with all human interactions and emotions, the role of the Liver becomes apparent in all emotions pertaining to human relations such as passionate love, competition, anger, and jealousy as well as repression and depression.

- Storing Blood: is one of the Liver's most important function's. This concept represents two aspects: regulation and detoxification. In fact, the Liver is regulating the Blood distribution in the body; during mental activity, the brain needs more blood, during the digestive phase, the digestive and mesenteric systems have to receive blood, during muscular activity, the blood is distributed to the muscles, during rest and sleep it moves back to the Liver. When Blood is in the Liver it is "detoxified" or "cooled" down, a process by which the Liver eliminates all the excessive products such as biochemical by-products and chemical as well as emotional toxins. For this reason, the Liver is associated with the Lower Triple Warmer and in charge of elimination of toxins. The Blood cycle in women is also closely related to the smooth flow of the Liver *Qi* and its capacity to store Blood. In practice, the functions and conditions of the Liver are primarily dependent on the amount and condition of Blood, and vice versa.
- Controlling the Muscles and Sinews: this function is related to the Liver's capacity of regulating blood flow. It has to be clearly understood that the Liver is responsible only for the action (contraction) and the smooth movements of the muscles and sinews; it is the Spleen-Pancreas that maintains the "flesh" of the muscles (nourishment). Muscular agility and flexibility are expressions of the smooth flow of Liver *Qi* and the state of Liver-Blood.
- Opening into the Eyes: The Liver ensures the capacity to see "the five colors" as well as maintaining the moistening of the eyes. Eyesight and clear distinction of colors is the domain of the Liver, although many other channels also reach the eye and could be involved in a variety of eye pathologies.
- Tears are the fluid of the Liver.
- Manifesting in the Nails: nails being an extension of the sinews reflect the condition of Liver *Qi* and *Xue* ≈ Blood.
- Residence of "*Hun*": the Spirit residing in the Liver, considered the "Ethereal Soul", manages the subtler, the emotional, mental and spiritual aspects of Liver's energies: passion, anger, planning, decisions, imagination, creativity, dreams, the initiating of the new and spiritual growth. Both *Hun* and *Shen*, which are *Yang* in nature, are very dependant on the state of *Xue* ≈ Blood, *Yin*. In Liver-blood vacuity, the *Hun* becomes rootless, like a leaf in the wind, causing irritability and anger, excessive imagination, dreams and even illusions.

Modern Western physiology may explain many of the ancient Chinese concepts pertaining to the Liver (Gan 肝) (▶ table. 3.5).

Overview of Liver Functions

- Maintaining the free flow of Qi

- Storing Blood
- Controlling the Muscles and Sinews
- Opening into the Eyes
- Maintaining the tears
- Manifesting in the Nails
- Residence of *Hun* ≈ Ethereal sou

Table 3.5: Comparative Chinese and Western Physiology of the Liver (Gan 肝)

Chinese Liver functions	Western physiology	Linking the two concepts
The "General of the armies": in charge of planning, organization and strategies	• Anatomically the liver is situated in the peritoneal cavity but does not actively participate in the digestive process; it receives and transfers the nutrients and filters out toxins, metabolites, bacteria, fats and fat soluble drugs • Liver breaks down histamine (produced by mast cells, brain or certain foods)	• Liver (*Jue Yin*) protects the Heart (Emperor) • Liver is responsible for mobilising *Wei* ≈ Defensive *Qi*
Responsible for the free flow of *Qi*	• Anatomical connection with vena cava system, diaphragm, pancreas and stomach and esophagus • Seat of 500 biochemical functions: glycogen storage, protein synthesis, hormone production...	Liver dysfunctions disrupt many digestive processes, causing stagnation in the digestive tract
Stores Blood	• Liver holds 10–15% of total blood during rest • Liver filters and detoxifies blood	When needed, Liver mobilizes Blood
Controlling the Sinews	Flexibility of muscles and tendons seems to be in relation to cholesterol metabolism	Sinew function depends on Liver-Blood
Opens into the eyes, ensure sight	Management of blood flow to the head and the brain?	Liver-blood and vision
Residence of *Hun* ≈ Ethereal soul	Harmonious brain functions when the liver manages to detoxify the metabolites; otherwise there is sleeplessness and irritability in histamine accumulation	*Hun* manages planning, decisions, imagination, creativity, dreams, passion and anger

The Spleen-Pancreas (Pi 脾)

The Spleen is the "official in charge of the granaries" (▶ Fig. 3.16). Together with the Stomach, it is in charge of nourishing the body on all levels, by transforming and transporting food essence *Gu Qi*, they constitute the "Root of Post-Heaven *Qi*".

Functionally, the Pancreas and the Lymph system are also attached to the Spleen although traditionally this was never mentioned. In fact, the older images of *Pi* included both the anatomical spleen as well as the pancreas. From a Western hormonal and biochemical perspective, it becomes obvious that many of the *Pi*'s functions are those of the pancreas. For commodity, Spleen and Pancreas are now referred to as simply Spleen. The Spleen and Stomach by their central position in all transformative processes of the body are put in relation to the Earth Phase.

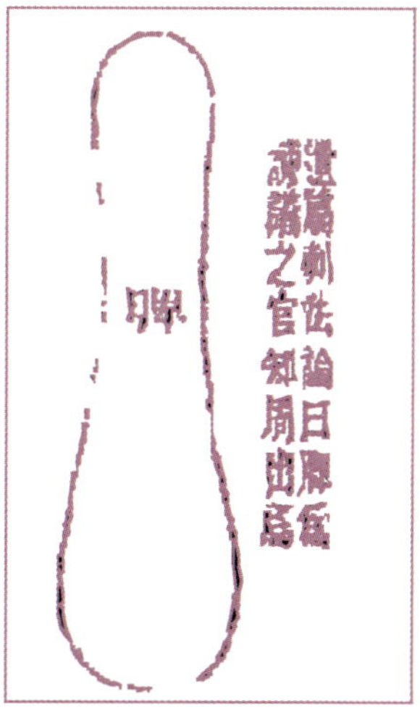

Figure 3.16: Spleen *(Pi)* (*Zhen Jiu Da Cheng*)

The functions of Spleen

- Transforming and Transporting: the Spleen is in charge of transformative processes on all levels:
- Controlling and regulating the digestive process together with the Stomach. This transformation and separation of solids and liquids into pure and impure and the transportation of the pure energy to the Lungs result in the production of *Ying* ≈ Nourishing and *Wei*≈ Defensive energy as well as Blood and Body fluids and is inseparable from the function of the Stomach.
- The mental transformative process allows for the “digestion” of concepts and information.
- Psychologically and spiritually, the Spleen presides over all mutations.
- Nourishing the Flesh and the Limbs: the Spleen maintains the strength and the volume of the muscles, while the Liver controls their contractibility. The Spleen determines the physical energy and strength of the four limbs.
- Uplifting and Holding: The upward movement of Spleen *Qi* helps to hold the abdominal organs in place. This "raising" action is attributed to the "Central *Qi*", which is an aspect of the Spleen's *Qi*, involving the Extraordinary Vessel, the *Chong Mai* ≈ Penetrating Vessel.
- Opening into the Mouth: The Spleen enables the tongue to taste the five tastes aided by the Heart.
- The saliva is the fluid of the Spleen. In fact, all salivary glands are controlled by the Spleen, except the parotid gland, which is dependent on the Kidney.
- Manifesting in the Lips: The color and condition of the lips depend on the functions of Spleen and Stomach.

- Residence of *Yi:* The spirit directing the subtler aspects of Spleen *Qi* is named *Yi* and is related to thought, the capacity to concentrate, think, analyze and memorize. Memory is a process that involves all five spirits, *Yi*'s capacity to digest, distribute and store information, *Shen*'s power of clarity and intelligence and on *Zhi*'s capacity of integration and even *Hun* and *Po* play a role (▶ Fig. 3.17). There is quite an overlap in the role of the respective spirits, *Shen, Yi,* and *Zhi*, concerning memory. The memory of past events or retained data (explicit memory), depends mainly on the *Yi* aided by *Zhi.* The memory of the performance of a particular type of action (walking, swimming, bicycling), is referred to as "procedural memory" a type of long-term memory also called implicit memory which could involve the *Shen* and the *Zhi.* In pathology loss of memory and concentration are reflected on the *Yi*, loss of short-term memory and absentmindedness on the *Shen*, and loss of long-term memory on the *Zhi*.

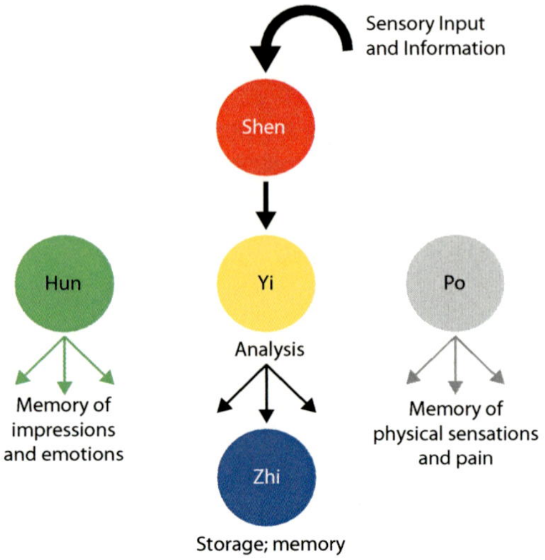

Figure 3.17: Memory process involving the Five Spirits: *Shen-Yi-Zhi, Po,* and *Hun*

- The spiritual dimension of *Yi* manifests as the capacity of contemplation and metamorphosis.

Modern Western physiology and in particular embryology may explain many of the ancient Chinese concepts pertaining to the Spleen (Pi脾) (▶ table. 3.6).

Overview of Spleen Functions

- Transforming and Transporting
- Nourishing the Flesh and Limbs
- Uplifting and Holding
- Opening into the Mouth
- Maintaining the Saliva
- Manifesting in the Lips
- Residence of *Yi* ≈ Thought/ intellect

Table 3.6: Comparative Chinese and Western Physiology of the Spleen-Pancreas (Pi 脾)

Chinese Spleen functions	Western physiology	Linking the two concepts
The "Granary official": in charge of nourishment	• Embryological common origin from the gastrointestinal tract, in particular the duodenum • Pancreas' endocrine and exocrine functions	Spleen & Stomach in charge of production of *Qi*, Blood and Fluids (3 substances)
Transformation of nutrients; transportation	• Exocrine function: enzymes to break down the food: proteases, lipase, amylase, peptidase, elastase, nuclease.... (stimulated by serotonin) • Endocrine function: glucagon (increases blood glucose), insulin (decreases blood glucose), role in sugar transport and cell uptake	Processing of food; transportation of the nutrients (mainly glucose) = *Qi* to the cells
Nourish the flesh and the limbs	• Role of insulin (cellular intake of glucose mainly in muscles and adipose tissue)	Relation between the Spleen, the flesh and body fat (connective tissue)
Producing and containing Blood in the vessels	• Spleen's role in destroying old red blood cells and recycling the hemoglobin • Spleen's role in controlling platelets (which in turn uptake the blood serotonin)	Spleen controls Blood production and prevents bleeding
Producing *Wei* ≈ Defensive *Qi*	• Role of B-lymphocytes and macrophages • Role of lymph nodes, thymus gland and bone marrow	Spleen's role in immunity
Producing & controlling Fluids	In pathology fluids accumulate in the peritoneal cavity by osmosis	Production of Dampness and Phlegm
Opens into the mouth	Salivary glands secrete enzymes to help digest nutrients: lipase, amylase, lysozyme, haptocorrin	Spleen produces saliva and allows tasting
Residence of *Yi* ≈ Thought	Relation between brain serotonin (5 hydroxytryptamine) levels and the ability to think clearly; low 5-HT levels in obsessive-compulsive disorders	In TCM Spleen disorders are responsible for worry, cogitation and obsessions

The Stomach (Wei 胃)

The Stomach and Spleen are the "officials in charge of the granaries" and the "root of Post-Heaven *Qi*" (▶ Fig. 3.18). The Stomach has a very particular position in the *Zang-Fu* organ system. Although it is a *Yang* and *Fu* organ, its function goes beyond the mere reception and transportation of nutrients. Together with its *Yin* partner, the Spleen, the Stomach represents the first stage of food transformation, hence the expression that Stomach produces three substances, white, gray and red, referring to the *Ying* ≈ Nourishing and *Wei* ≈ Defensive energies, *Jin Ye* ≈ Body fluids and *Xue* ≈ Blood (▶ Fig. 3.19). Functionally the duodenum is part of the Chinese Stomach system.

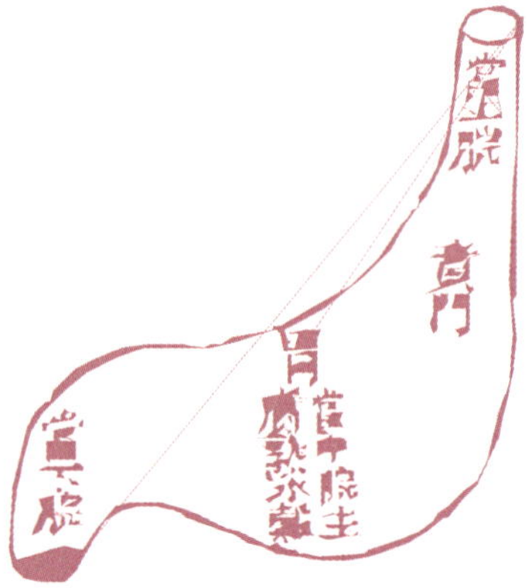

Figure 3.18: Stomach *(Wei)* (*Zhen Jiu Da Cheng*)

Stomach and Spleen are related to the central position and to the Earth phase.

The functions of the Stomach

- Reception, Fragmentation, and Ripening of food: it is said that the Stomach "Rotens and Ripens" the food, by a process of maceration and cooking; the Spleen maintains the "Transformation and Transportation ". The "Digestive Fire" represented by the Spleen *Qi* or Spleen-*Yang* supports the cooking process. This digestive Fire is an extension of the "Original Fire" or the Kidney *Yang* function. The Stomach is the most important *Fu* ≈ Bowel, and with the Spleen, they are the foundation of the body's energies. The Stomach regulates the reception of food by the sensation of "hunger".
- Transporting and Distributing Food *Qi*: again together with Spleen, the Stomach ensures the distribution of food essence *Gu Qi*, to the whole body, the organs and the limbs. Stomach *Qi* has a downward movement bringing the processed food to the Small Intestine; the Liver that maintains a free flow of *Qi* aids this action. Stomach *Qi* is evaluated in the pulse as a firm and yet gentle quality and reflected on the tongue coating as white and thin.
- Raising the "Clear *Yang*" to the head: aside from its

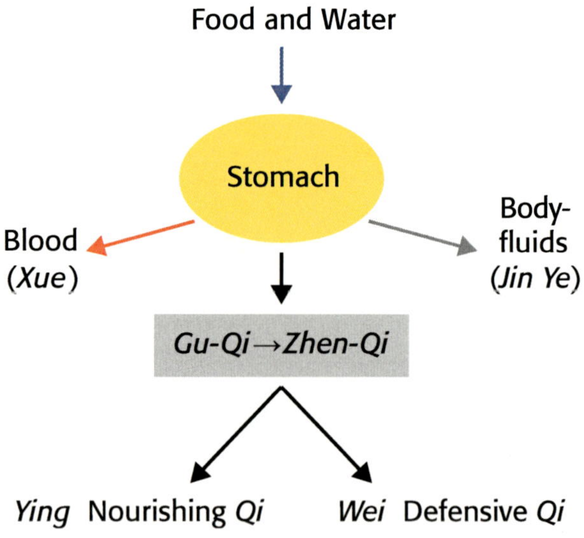

Figure 3.19: Stomach and the production of the three substances

downward movement, the Stomach channel ascends the clear *Qi* produced in the middle Triple Warmer to the head, participating in mental acuity and the sensory functions.

- The Origin of Liquids: through the sense of thirst the Stomach regulates the amount of liquids received, collaborating closely with the Kidneys in this function, hence the term: "Origin of Liquids", when the Lung is called the Upper Source of liquids" and the Kidney is named the "Lower Source of liquids".

Modern Western physiology may explain many of the ancient Chinese concepts pertaining to the Stomach (Wei 胃) (▶ table. 3.7).

Overview of Stomach Functions

- Reception, Fragmentation, and Ripening of food: production of the "Three Substances"
- Transporting and Distributing *Gu Qi* ≈ Food *Qi*
- Raising the "Clear *Yang*" to the head
- The Origin of Liquids

Table 3.7: Comparative Chinese and Western Physiology of the Stomach (Wei 胃)

Chinese Stomach functions	Western physiology	Linking the two concepts
Together with the Spleen "Officials in charge of the granaries"	Stomach represents the totality of the digestive process: breaking down of food in the mouth, blending with digestive enzymes, further processing in the stomach	Stomach is the origin of the "3 Substances": *Ying -Wei,* Blood and Fluids
Transportation and distribution of *Gu* ≈ Food *Qi*	Controlling the release of bolus (blended food, water and enzymes) into the small intestine	Control of the whole digestive process
Rotting and ripening of food	• The temperature of bolus is raised to 38° c. • Fermentation of food by the intestinal flora	Stomach likes Heat and Damp
Origin of Fluids	No relation in Western physiology to the stomach but rather the whole of the digestive tract	Fluid metabolism in the SI and LI

The Small Intestine (Xiao Chang 小腸)

The Small Intestine is the official in charge of receiving, filling up and transforming, with a notion of bringing prosperity to what is received, by separating the pure from the impure (► Fig. 3.20). By analogy, the Small Intestine separates also the pure from the impure on a psycho-emotional level, aiding the Heart to release accumulated emotions and participating in the discerning quality of the Heart.

Together with the Heart, its coupled *Zang* ≈ Organ, it is attached to the Fire phase.

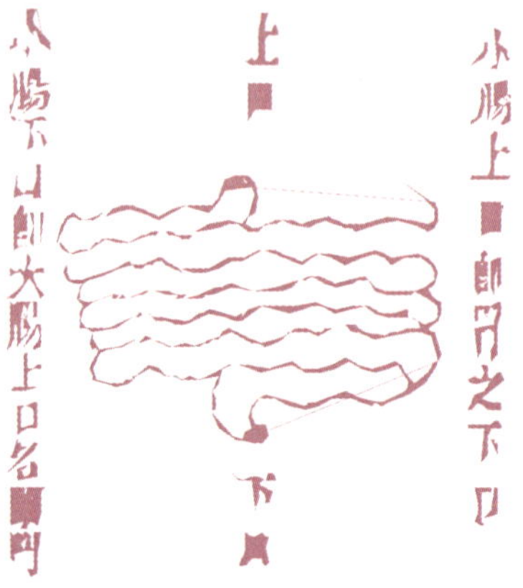

Figure 3.20 Small Intestine *(Xiao Chang)* (*Zhen Jiu Da Cheng*)

The functions of Small Intestine

- Separation of the Pure from the Impure: it receives and accomplishes the digestive processes initiated by the Stomach and Spleen. The separations of solids take place in the Small Intestine, under the control of Spleen *Qi*, the impure is transported to the Large Intestine and the Bladder.
- Separation of Liquids: takes place in the Small Intestine, presided by the Spleen *Qi*. The impure liquids are then excreted by the Bladder.

Modern Western physiology may explain many of the ancient Chinese concepts pertaining to the Small Intestine (Xiao Chang 小腸) (► table. 3.8).

Overview of Small Intestine Functions

- Separation of the Pure from the Impure
- Separation of Liquids

Table 3.8: Comparative Chinese and Western Physiology of Small Intestine (Xiao Chang 小腸)

Chinese Small Intestine functions	Western physiology	Linking the two concepts
The "Official in charge of reception and transformation"	• Importance of the duodenum in the digestive process (reception of bile and pancreatic enzymes); absorption of most nutrients: proteins, lipids and carbohydrates in the jejunum and ileum • Immunological role: Probiotic gut flora	• Separation of the pure from the impure • Site of production of Wei ≈ Defensive Qi
Separation of liquids	Absorption of water and lipids by passive diffusion	Fluid metabolism: "TW inner "duct"

The Large Intestine (Da Chang 大 腸)

The Large Intestine is in charge of receiving, transmitting and transporting, this involves the intestinal peristaltic movement and the re-absorption of fluids (▶ Fig. 3.21).

Coupled with the Lung, they are associated with the Metal phase.

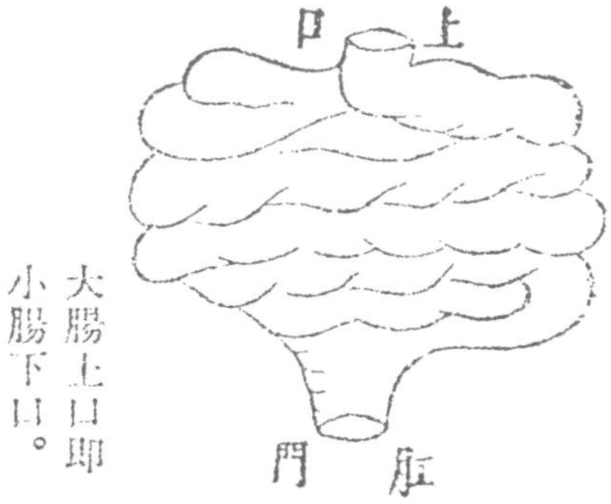

Figure 3.21: Large Intestine *(Da Chang)* (*Zhen Jiu Da Cheng*)

The functions of the Large Intestine

- The second separation of solids and liquids takes place in the Small and Large Intestine, under the control of Spleen *Qi*. Some authors believe that this second separation of solids is crucial to the production of *Wei*≈ Defensive *Qi*. This concept approaches the Western naturopathic idea of colonic irrigation. The second separation of fluids is also of major importance, as 80% of the water contained in the bowels is re-absorbed in the large intestine. French authors, namely N. Van Nghi, consider the Small and Large Intestine to be the "Inner duct" of the Triple Warmer.
- Bowel Movement: the transportation and elimination of the impure is the domain of the Large Intestine.

Modern Western physiology may explain many of the ancient Chinese concepts pertaining to the Large Intestine (Da Chang 大 腸) (▶ table. 3.9).

Overview of Large Intestine Functions

- Second Separation of Solids and Fluids
- Bowel Movement

Table 3.9: Chinese and Western Comparative Physiology of Large Intestine (*Da Chang* 大 腸)

Chinese Large Intestine functions	Western physiology	Linking the two concepts
The "Official in charge of reception, transmission and transportation"	• Completion of food digestion; absorption of Vit. K, B-12, thiamine and riboflavin (produced by the gut flora); recycling of certain nutrients (carbohydrates, fatty acids, urea) • Compaction and storage of feces; defecation • Immunological role: Probiotic gut flora	• Second separation in the TW system • Site of production of Wei ≈ Defensive *Qi*
Separation of liquids	Reclaiming water and maintaining water balance	Fluid metabolism: "TW inner duct"

The Bladder (Pang Guang 膀胱)

The Bladder is the "District official", in charge of territories and cities and water distribution (▶ Fig. 3.22).

The district official is in charge of the proper communication between the cities, symbolizing the organs, the territories, and their equilibrium by distributing the Body fluids. The concept of transporting *Qi* to the organs, produced in the lower *Dan Tian* by the transformation of Kidney *Yin* by the Kidney Fire into Kidney *Qi* was already covered under the functions of the Kidney.

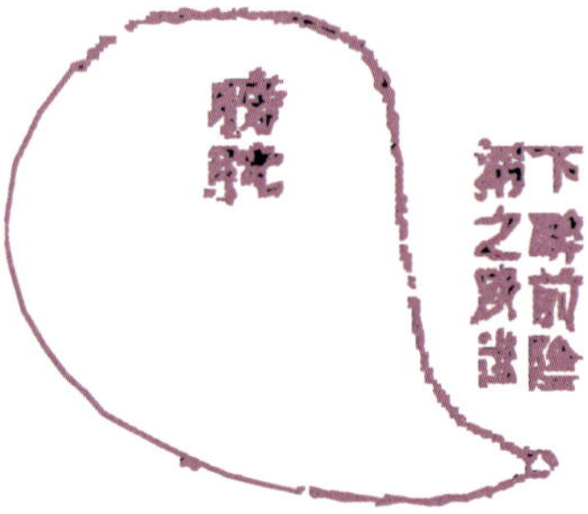

Figure 3.22: Bladder *(Pang Guang)*, (*Zhen Jiu Da Cheng*)

The Bladder, a *Fu*, *Yang*, and hollow bowel, together with its *Zang* partner, the Kidney, are attached to the Water phase.

The functions of the Bladder

- Transforming, Storing and Excreting liquids: after transforming the impure liquids into the urine, the Bladder stores and eliminates this liquid, under the control of the Kidneys.
- Distributing information: this is the territorial function of the Bladder, transporting information and coordinating the various areas of the body. This concept has an anatomical foundation in Western neurology with the principle of the dermatomes, territories irrigated by a pair of spinal nerves. This observation was probably the basis of the development of the *Jia Ji* points by *Hoa To* (2nd century AD).

Modern Western physiology and embryology may explain many of the ancient Chinese concepts pertaining to the Bladder (Pang Guang 膀胱) (▶ table. 3.10).

Overview of Bladder Functions

- Transforming, Storing and Excreting liquids
- Distributing information

Table 3.10 Comparative Chinese and Western Physiology of the Bladder (Pang Guang 膀胱)

Chinese Bladder functions	Western physiology	Linking the two concepts
The "District official in charge of territories"	Embryological relation between the neural crest cells, the back, the organs and the dermatomes	Communication of information; back *Shu* ≈ Transport points
Responsible for "Water distribution"	Storage and excretion of fluids	Kidneys control the urinary function

The Gallbladder (Dan 胆)

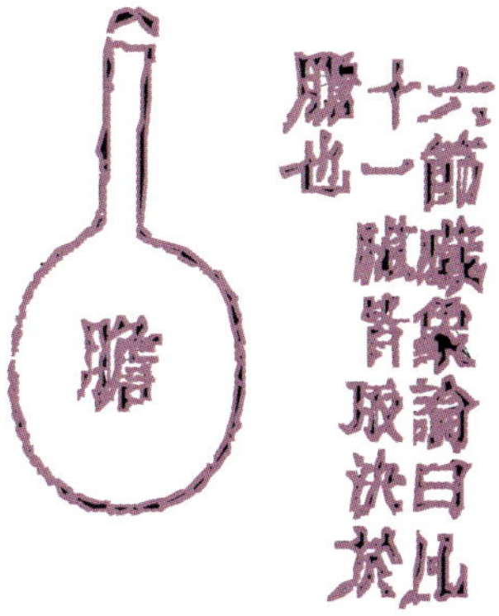

Figure 3.23: Gallbladder *(Dan)*; (*Zhen Jiu Da Cheng*)

The Gallbladder is the official in charge of *Zhong Zheng* ≈ Central Rectitude/righteousness or integrity, the just and the precise decisions and judgments (▶ Fig. 3.23). There are several mysteries surrounding the Gallbladder organ system in Chinese medicine. Central rectitude is attributed to it, this could be considered the role of the Heart-emperor; justice and the right decision could be a function of the Lung, and courage is usually attached to the Kidney. Furthermore, the Gallbladder is classified as a *Yang*, *Fu*≈ Bowel, but it does not have the transporting functions of the other *Fu* and stores pure *Qi*, the bile, similar to a *Zang* ≈ Organ. It is further classified as one of the Six Extraordinary *Fu* and is said to be the link between these six *Fu* and the ten official *Zang-Fu* organs. It would seem that the Gallbladder assimilates and integrates several of the qualities of the other organs. For example, once the Lung has passed judgment, instead of punishment, rather a rectifying action is needed. Once the Kidney has had the wisdom and fortitude to reach a decision, the courage to carry out the right action is required. In this manner, the Gallbladder can submit the precise and correct information to the emperor in order to maintain the "Central Rectitude".

Gallbladder and Liver, its coupled *Zang* ≈ Organ, belong to the Wood phase.

The functions of the Gallbladder

- Storing and Excreting Bile: the Liver produces the bile that is stored in the Gallbladder. This excretion depends on the smooth flow of Liver *Qi*. The digestive role of the Gallbladder, although mentioned in the *Nei Jing*, seems to be secondary to its other functions.
- Decision and Judgment: according to the "Central Rectitude", the Gallbladder ensures correct judgment, decisiveness and the drive and courage to move into action; the courage that comes from the Kidneys manifests through the Gallbladder.

Modern Western physiology may explain many of the ancient Chinese concepts pertaining to the Gallbladder (Dan 胆) (▶ table. 3.11).

Overview of Gall-Bladder Functions

- Storing and excreting Bile
- In charge of correct decision and judgment

Table 3.11 Comparative Chinese and Western Physiology of the Gallbladder (Dan 胆)

Chinese Gallbladder functions	Western physiology	Linking the two concepts

The "Official in charge of central rectitude": correct decisions and judgements	• Storing and excreting bile to help absorb lipids (fat) in to the lymph • Lipids (cholesterol) are essential in cell membrane structure and integrity also biosynthesis of steroid hormones, bile acids and Vit. D (bone rigidity)	Adapting bile secretion to the physiological needs and hormonal production (affecting courage and decisions)

The Triple Warmer (San Jiao 三焦)

The San Jiao, three heating centers or warmers or three hearths, is not an organ but a function and includes the combined functions of several organs involved in the processing of food, water and air, and the production of *Qi*, Blood and Body fluids(▶ Fig. 3.24).

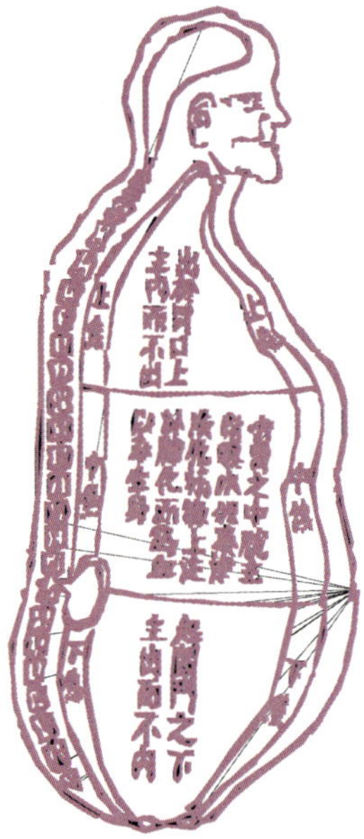

Figure 3.24 Triple Warmer *(San Jiao)* (*Zhen Jiu Da Cheng*)

The primary organs involved are the Stomach and Spleen, which have the charge of transforming and producing the 3 substances: *Ying*, *Wei Qi*, *Xue* ≈ Blood, and *Jin Ye* ≈ Body fluids. The Kidney Fire, by its transformative capacity, provides the Fire and the foundation for this cooking process. Finally, the Lung has the charge of putting the produced energy into circulation.

The arm *Shao Yang*-Triple Warmer channel, unlike all other channels that are continuations of their organ systems, does not influence the function of the Triple Warmer, except for two points (TW-4 and TW-6)

San Jiao is classified as a *Yang* and *Fu* ≈ Bowel, and is coupled with the *Xin Bao* ≈ Pericardium, and associated with the Fire phase.

Functions of the Triple Warmer

- Absorption: of food, water, and air by the upper warmer.
- Transformation: in the middle warmer and production of the "Three substances".
- Elimination: in the lower warmer, of the “impure”.
  For a detailed description see Triple Warmer-Energy production (▶ chap. 4).

Overview of Triple Warmer Functions

- Absorption: food, water, and air
- Transformation
- Elimination

3.4 Six "Extraordinary" or "Curious" Fu (Qi Heng Zhi Fu 奇恒之腑)

These organs are considered extraordinary due to their structure as well as their particular functions. On a structural level, they present the characteristics of both *Zang* and *Fu*. In fact, they are full and preserve essence as do the *Zang*, but are also hollow as a *Fu* and have the capacity to contain, but do not receive nor eliminate. On a functional level, they are extraordinary because they form the link between Pre- and Post-Heaven, and are responsible for the creation and continuation of life, and of transformation on the three levels. They do not have a *Yin-Yang* or a *Biao-Li* coupling but are in relation with the three transformational centers, the *Dan Tian* (▶ Fig. 3.25).

- The upper *Dan Tian* corresponds to the head containing the brain,
- The middle *Dan Tian*, contains the Heart,
- The lower *Dan Tian*, houses the uterus.

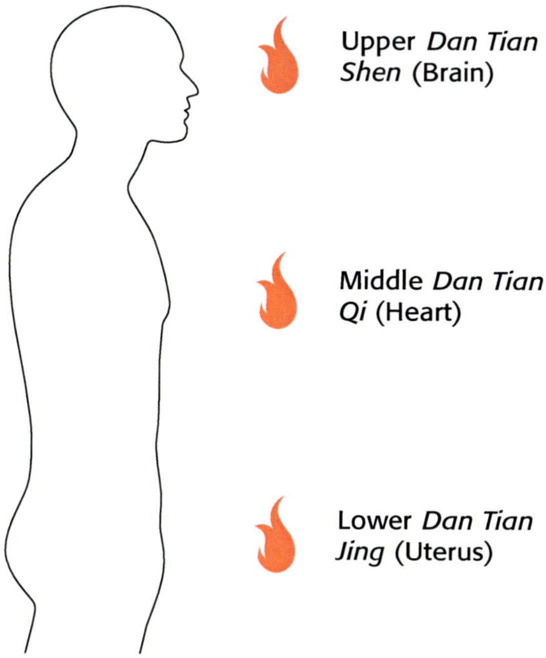

Figure 3.25: The three *Dan Tian* (Cinnabar Chambers)

In the Daoist esoteric traditions, these three areas or fields allow the transformation and refinement of the lower basic human energies into higher spiritual aspects. The term Dan Tian was translated by the French authors to "Cinnabar" a red mercury sulfide believed by the medieval alchemists to transform base metals into gold. These three centers contain the organs responsible for the human being's continuity, both on a physical as well as on a spiritual level. From the tri-partition, Heaven-Man-Earth system dialectics, these three centers conserve the "Three Treasures", *Shen, Qi,* and *Jing*, and further protected by the three bony structures, the skull, thorax, and pelvis.

The formation of these extraordinary organs precedes that of the *Zang* and the *Fu*, this was described in the following manner: from the "Vital Substances", the Brain and the Marrow are created; then the Bones form a support for the Brain and Marrow; the Vessels nourish the body and then the Gallbladder and the Uterus appear.

They are all directly or indirectly related to the Kidneys.

The Brain (Nao脑)

The Brain is produced and maintained by Kidney *Jing*, and is called the "Sea of Marrow". It is like a crossroad between the inside and the outside and is the site of integration, equilibrium, thinking, recapitulation and memory.

The Brain is considered the depository of the "Universal Law" and is the "Spiritual Matrix".

The function of the brain greatly depends on *Xue* ≈ Blood and the Heart.

The Marrow (Sui髓)

The marrow is also produced from Kidney *Jing* ≈ Essence and pertains to the spinal cord, the brain, and the bone marrow.

The function of the Marrow is to transmit central information, the "Universal Law", that is deposited in the Brain, to the whole body, via the bone marrow, Blood, and the spinal cord, the nervous system.

The Bones (Gu 骨)

The Bones are the symbol of immortality. They store the Marrow and form the material web or frame for the process of life:

- Material frame: The three bony structures, skull, thorax and pelvis, mediated by the spine. The function of the three bony structure is to protect the "Three Treasures": *Shen*, *Qi*, and *Jing*. (► Fig. 3.26).
- Immaterial web: the channel system.

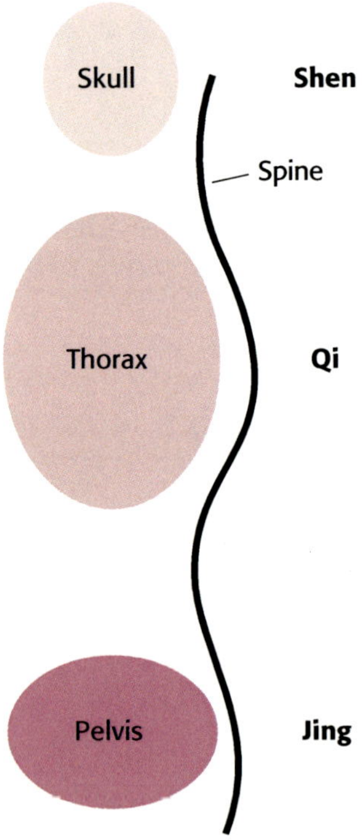

Figure 3.26: Bony structures and the Three

The Vessels (Mai 脉)

The term *Mai* refers not only to the vascular system but also seems to include the channel systems.

The blood vessels constitute a material base whereas the channels supply an immaterial framework or web in which life may develop.

The Heart controls the Blood vessels. In fact, in the embryological development of the human being, the heart is the first *Zang* ≈ Organ to develop.

In Chinese medicine, the channel system is designated by several terms, *Jing* ≈ River, *Luo* ≈ Connecting channel and *Mai* ≈ Vessel. The term *Mai* is either used for the *Luo* channels, which contain the superficial blood circulation, or for the Eight Extraordinary Vessels, that are responsible for the unfolding of life.

The Gallbladder (Dan 胆)

As discussed above, the Gallbladder is a strange *Fu* organ, storing essence and responsible for the "Central Rectitude/righteousness or integrity". It maintains authenticity and conformity in accordance with the "Universal Mandate" transmitted to "*Ming Men*" and actualized in the Uterus.

The Uterus (Nu Zi Bao 女子胞)

The Uterus is the root of life, where the entity develops on all levels:

- Physical, the fetus
- Energetic, the *Dan Tian* or *Hara*
- Spiritual, the Daoist embryo

The physical uterus is in charge of the menstrual cycle and of conception. It is closely related to the Kidneys, via the extraordinary vessels, in particular, the *Ren Mai* ≈ Conception vessel and the *Chong Mai* ≈ Penetrating vessel, and depends also on the state of Blood, which in turn is regulated primarily by the Liver, the Spleen, and the Heart.

Relation to Western physiology

In relation to Western physiology, these six organs may be assimilated to various systemic functions (► Table 3.12):

Table 3.12 The Six Extraordinary *Fu* in relation to Western physiology

Extraordinary Fu	Western anatomic and physiological function
Brain	Central nervous system
Marrow	Haematopoietic system
Bones	Electrolytic system
Vessels	Vascular system
Gallbladder	Hepato-portal system
Uterus	Genito-reproductive system

4. The Triple Warmer

4.1 Energy Production

Life is maintained by the transformation and production of energy, from air, water, and food. This process is attributed to the *San Jiao*, represented by three centers or cauldrons, called the three heating areas, the three burners or the Triple Warmer "TW".

The Triple Warmer ensures the three functions of absorption, transformation, and distribution/ elimination.

Anatomically, these functions are contained in the chest area, the upper TW, the abdomen, the middle TW, and the lower abdomen, the lower TW. (► Fig. 4.1).

Symbolically the TW is about transforming one form of energy into another form, this metamorphosis is necessitating the mediation of "Fire", hence the reference to the three Fire centers. This tri-partition is similar to the alchemical transformation symbolized by the three *Dan Tian* centers, as seen previously. It is interesting to note that the lower *Dan Tian* and the lower TW share the same Fire, the Kidney-Fire, the middle *Dan Tian* and the upper TW correspond to the Heart Fire, the upper *Dan Tian*, the seat of the *Nao* ≈ Brain and the heavenly residence of *Shen*, is not involved in energy transformation, but only with metaphysical changes.

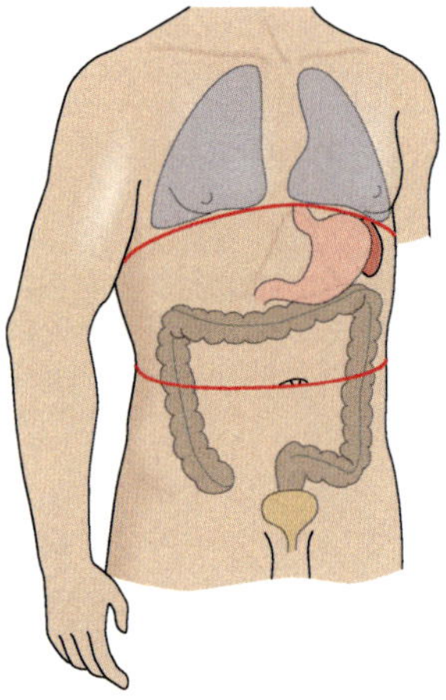

Figure 4.1: The *San-Jiao*-Triple Warmer

The energy production by the TW is a function and depends on the participation of organic systems, grouped into three sections: upper, middle and lower.

In a nutshell, the Triple Warmer is like a cooking pot in which the food and water and air are absorbed. The image of the upper TW corresponds to food and water that is placed in the pot as representing the Stomach. The air is brought down to the fuel that is located below the pot, the lower TW. The pilot light that starts the fire is the *Yuan Qi*, the "Fire of life", which stays lit from conception to death. The vapor that rises from this cooking process is symbolized by the ideogram of *Qi* ≈ Energy. (► Fig. 4.2). Chinese medicine relates the coating of the tongue to this cooking vapor, the state, and color of which is a direct reflection of the digestive function. The Triple Warmer function in general represents the transformation of solids and liquids, and is controlled by the Spleen's organic function, which includes the Pancreas and the lymphatic system. It is important to keep in mind that Spleen and Stomach are in dissociable *Zang-Fu* organs in their functioning.

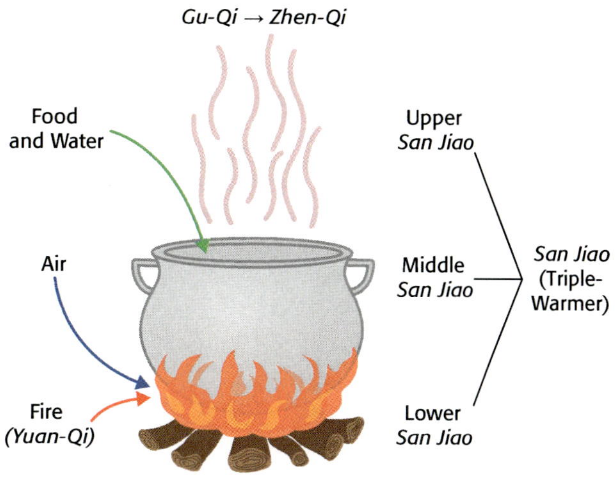

Figure 4.2 The Triple Warmer in the image of a cooking pot

Overall, when compared to the digestive process and the biochemical transformations as science has discovered today, the ancient Chinese Triple Warmer model has an uncanny similarity and accuracy, and even explains organic inter-relations and inter-functions, not apparent in modern anatomy and physiology.

4.2 Structure of the Triple Warmer, the three sections

The Upper Triple Warmer

Anatomically it extends from the nose and the mouth to the diaphragm.

The functions of the upper TW are:

- To absorb food and water and bring them to the middle TW, Stomach, and Spleen
- To direct air to the lower TW, the Kidney
- To diffuse and circulate the three substances produced by the middle TW, *Ying*≈ Nourishing and *Wei* ≈ Defensive *Qi*, *Xue* ≈ Blood *and Jin Ye* ≈ Body fluids, into the whole body.

The image of the steam rising from the cooking process evokes a vaporous state and is symbolized by the analogy to the “Mist”.

Physiologically the upper Triple Warmer corresponds to the Lung and Pericardium. The Lung, in charge of governing breath, brings the pure *Qi* of Heaven down to the Kidney in the lower TW; then in its function of "Commander of *Qi*", it receives and circulates the *Ying* and *Wei Qi*, processed in the middle TW; the Lung, further supplies *Qi* to Blood, to help it circulate. *Xin Bao* ≈ Pericardium is in charge of distributing the blood. Although the Heart is situated in the thorax, it does not actively participate in any of the functional aspects of the upper TW. In practice, the functional aspect of the upper TW is summarized by the Lung functions.

The Middle Triple Warmer

Anatomically the middle TW extends between the diaphragm and the navel.

Functions of the middle TW which represents all of the digestive physiology:

- Absorption of nutrients by the process of breaking down
- Filtering of fluids,
- Transportation and distribution of nutrition

Symbolically the image is that of “Maceration“.

Physiologically it corresponds to the functions of Spleen and Stomach. Paradoxically although the Liver is anatomically situated in this section, it is only aiding in maintaining the free flow of the *Qi*, and does not participate actively in the energy transformation of the middle TW.

The Lower Triple Warmer

Anatomically the lower TW is situated between the navel and the perineum, including the pelvic area.

Functions of the lower TW

- Separation of the pure from the impure
- Elimination of the impure by the intestines and bladder

Symbolically the image is that of a “Canal” or a “Ditch”.

Physiologically it includes the Kidneys and Bladder and the Intestines. The Liver, in its quality of filtering and purifying the blood, could also be attached to the functions of the lower TW.

4.3 Processing of nutrients by the Triple Warmer System

Transformation of Solids, production of Ying ≈ Nourishing and Wei ≈ Defensive Qi

Solid food is received by the Stomach, broken down and processed, and sent on to the intestines, for the extraction of the nutrients.

Along the Small Intestine, the processed food undergoes two separations:

- The first separation of food into pure and impure takes place mainly in the Small Intestine. Pure food, called the essence of food, or "*Gou Qi*", is absorbed and sent to the Liver, which passes it on to the Upper Triple Warmer and the Heart, to be circulated in the whole body in the form of *Ying* and *Wei Qi*, by the actions of Lung and *Xin Bao* ≈ Pericardium (▶ Fig. 4.3).
- The leftover nutrients, the impure, will undergo a second separation further down, probably in the Large Intestine. Again the pure "essence" is absorbed and sent to the Liver, the remaining matter is eliminated by the large intestine in the process of bowel movement. There is a debate, mainly in the French school, about the relation between this second separation and the specific production of *Wei* ≈ Defensive *Qi*.

The production of *Gou Qi* ≈ Food *Qi*, necessitates the heating "cooking" process, represented by the "Digestive Fire", itself an emanation of the "Kidney Fire", stored in the Lower Triple Warmer. Under the Kidney functions, we have explored the transformation of the original Fire, emanating from the pre-natal energy the *Yuan* -Source *Qi*, into Kidney *Qi*. After the original "spark of life", in the pre-natal stage, the fuel, represented by the *Jing* ≈ Essence of the Kidneys, is supplied by the essence of food and water, and transformed by the Kidneys in the post-natal period. In other words the Kidneys supply both the *Yin*, the essence for the fuel and *Yang* the Fire for the burning, necessary in this cooking process. This relation between the Kidney-Fire and the Digestive-Fire, clearly explains the digestive difficulties, encountered in old age as well as the weight gain in some cases.

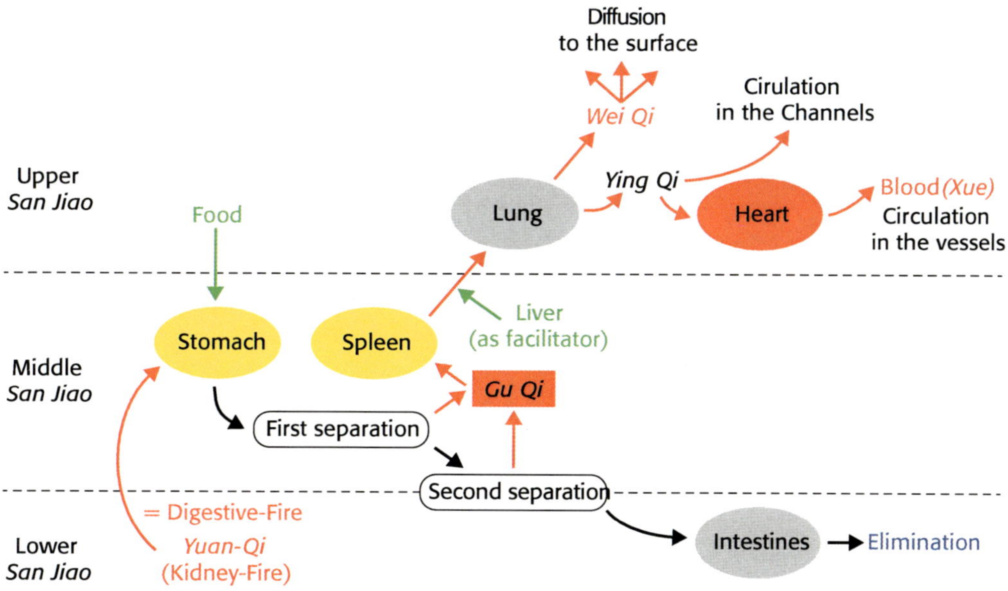

Figure 4.3: The transformation of solids and production of *Wei Qi, Ying, Qi,* and Blood

Absorption of Liquids, production of Xue ≈ Blood and Jin Ye ≈ Body fluids

The production of Body fluids is controlled by Spleen and Stomach. The action of the Stomach is primary, as it controls the intake of liquids, hence it is called the "Origin of Body Fluids".

Liquids also undergo two separations:

- First separation: the pure is sent to the Spleen, then to the Lung, the impure continues down to the intestines (▶ Fig. 4.4).
- Second separation: the pure li goes to the Kidney, then to the Spleen and up to the Lung; the impure is eliminated by the Bladder and the Large Intestine, in the urine and the stool.
- The Lung receives the fluids, diffuses them to the surface and descends excess fluids to the Kidney to be eliminated by the Bladder. The Lung is referred to as the "Upper Source of Fluids", and the Kidney as "Lower Source of Fluids".

The Body fluids contain:

- *Jin* ≈ Thin fluids or *Yang* aspect, diffused by the Lung, to lubricate the portals, the skin, and the sinews, and they accompany the diffusion of the *Wei Qi*.
- *Ye* ≈ Thick fluids or *Yin* aspect, which is distributed to the organs and to the Curious *Fu* ≈ Bowels, and will constitute the material base for *Xue* ≈ Blood.

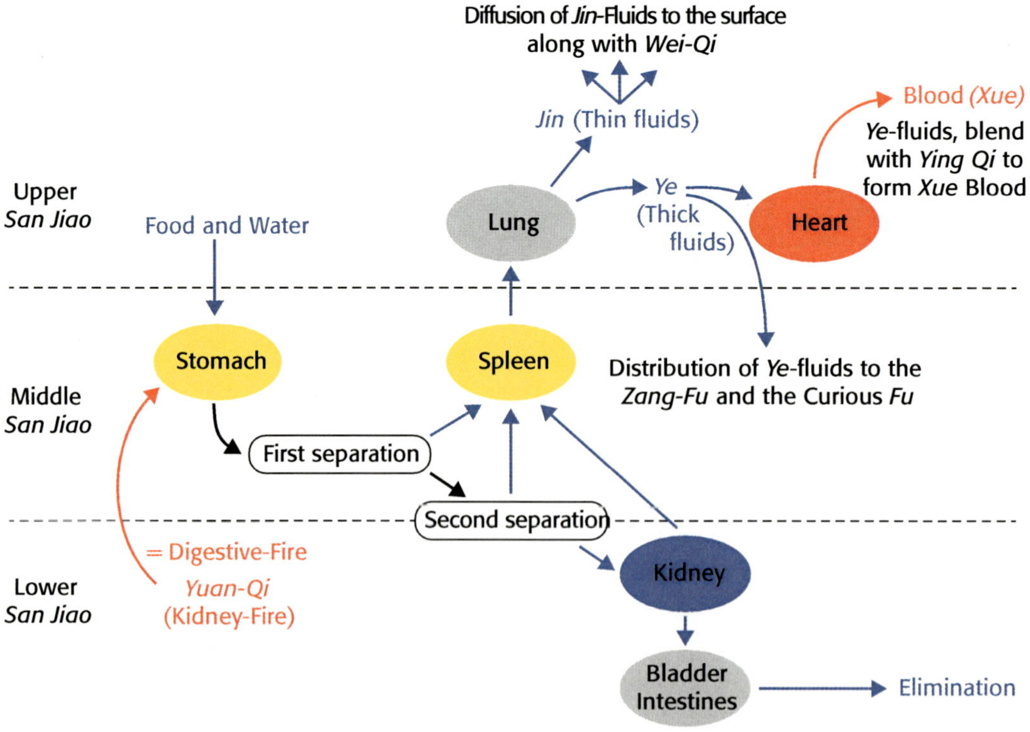

Figure 4.4 The transformation of liquids and production of *Jin Ye* body fluids and of Blood

Blood is a combination of:

- *Ying* ≈ Nourishing *Qi*, produced from the essence of food by Spleen and Stomach, carried to the Lung and transferred to the Heart
- *Ye* ≈ Fluids, produced by the Stomach and Spleen, transferred to the Lung and the Heart

The last transformation, the blending of *Ying Qi* and *Ye* ≈ Thick fluids into *Xue* ≈ Blood takes place in the Heart. It is fundamental to note that the Heart as the "Governor of Blood" does not actively participate in its production, but in turn, all the states of the Heart, will automatically affect the state of Blood and vice versa.

4.4 The Five Vital Substances

Qi in Chinese Medicine

"Qi" should be understood as that which contains, underlies, expresses and gives the dynamics to all phenomena in life.

It is the means by which *Yin* and *Yang* manifest themselves, but also the force that mobilizes them, it is the "breath of life".

Every form of manifestation is just a different vibration or shape of *Qi*. This energy circulates in the body, nourishes the physical and the subtle, maintains homeostasis and protects against pathogenic influences.

In Chinese Medicine the concept of *Qi* refers to the circulating *Qi*, in its more dense form it is called *Xue* ≈ Blood and *Jing* ≈ Essence, otherwise, the subtler aspects, the emotions, and the mind are referred to as *Shen*.

The *Qi* in the human being is partly inherited from the parents, called "Hereditary *Qi*", and partly acquired from the transformation of food, water and air, named "Acquired *Qi*".

The inherited *Qi*, as it exists before one is capable of producing one's own energy, is referred to as "Pre- or Anterior Heaven"; all the other forms of *Qi* that are produced after birth will be referred to as "Post- or Posterior Heaven".

"Anterior Heaven" or "Pre-Heaven" (Xian Tian 先天)

The "Inherited *Qi*" or pre-natal *Qi* contains three different origins:

- **Yuan Qi ≈ Source/ original 元/ 原气:** Considered the life principle, it joins all life forms to the source, "*Tai Yi*". *Yuan Qi* is the source of the body's "Fire", necessary for the transformative processes in life, in particular, the production of the "Vital Substances", through a process called the Triple Warmer "*San Jiao*". As seen previously, the *Yuan Qi* irrigates the organs and emerges at the *Yuan*-Source points of the channels. It is believed that the quantity of *Yuan Qi* is fixed at the moment of conception and defines the length of life. The *Yuan Qi* is stored in an area behind the navel and in front of the Kidneys, the *Dan Tian*, and is protected by the Kidney's *Qi*.

- **Jing Qi ≈ Essence 精气:** This is the essence of the parents, which is concentrated in the father's sperm and the mother's ova, and may be assimilated to the genetic code. *Jing Qi* is in part responsible for the development of the physical body of the child. After birth one produces one's own *Jing Qi*, which is stored in the five Zang-organs. After puberty, the Kidneys produce the sexual *Jing*, stored in the gonads.
- **Zong ≈ Ancestral Qi 宗气:** Also translated as "Essential", "Fundamental" or "Gathering" *Qi*, it is responsible for transmitting the ancestral characteristics. *Zong Qi*, is partly influenced by the surrounding, hence the denomination of "Cosmic *Qi*", it is believed to carry the destiny of the future being; and in part it is the parental *Zong* at the moment of conception. In other words, where the parents lived, what they ate, how they felt at the time of conception, and most of all the mother's lifestyle during the time of pregnancy, these are all influencing factors in the quality of *Zong Qi* passed onto the child. The *Zong Qi* is stored in the chest "*Shan Zhong*", and regulates the vital rhythmic movements of lung and heart. In the post-natal phase, it is produced and maintained by food, breathing and sunlight.

"Posterior Heaven" or "Post-Heaven" (Hou Tian 后天)

The post-natal or acquired *Qi*, is the energy which one uses daily to live, to adapt to change, to fight off disease, to think and to transform oneself.

The post-natal energies circulate in the body in two forms:

- Subtle, non-material: *Ying* ≈ Nourishing, *Wei* ≈ Defensive *Qi* and *Shen* ≈ Spirit
- Material: *Xue* ≈ Blood, *Jin Ye* ≈ Body fluids and *Jing* ≈ Essence

These energies are all derived from the absorbed food, water, and air. It is therefore logical that the quality of the produced substances greatly depends on the quantity and quality of the air, food, and water and the quality of the digestive Fire.

The *San Jiao* ≈ Triple Warmer model explores this transformative process and the production and the subsequent circulation of this *Qi*.

The numerous forms of *Qi*, have been given names and characteristics in Chinese medicine, this has at times confused the Western adept. For the sake of thoroughness, a list is given below. However, in daily practice, the *Ying*, *Wei*, and *Zong Qi* remain the main references.

Zheng ≈ Upright Qi (正气) and Zhen ≈ True or Authentic Qi (真气)

Zhen Qi or "True" energy is the sum of all the energies circulating in the human being and is synonymous to *Zheng Qi* the "Upright" energy. The term *Zheng* is used in opposition to *Xie Qi*邪气the pathogenic energy, in this context signifying a state of health as opposed to a condition of disease. *Xie Qi* usually refers to external causes, mainly the climates that have become pathogenic for the system, hence the concept of evil, vicious, nefarious, aggressive, wicked or perverse that is associated to it. In a broader sense, internal causes, such as emotions could also become pathogenic as opposed to the upright and healthy energy.

Zhen Qi is simply referred to as "*Qi*".

Qi is subject to the rhythmic internal variation of the four phases and synchronized by the macrocosmic movements as analyzed by the five moving forces.

Zheng Qi or *Zhen Qi* is the product of the transformative processes of the Triple Warmer. The part of the *Zhen* ≈ True energy that circulates in the channels and nourishes the system is called *Ying Qi*. The part circulating mainly outside the channels and on the surface and protecting the system is named *Wei Qi*.

Ying ≈ Nourishing/constructive Qi (營气)

Two ideograms represent this concept of nourishment:

- *Ying* 營: fire; rising sap
- *Yong* 禜: encampment; fire; cooking

This concept clearly denotes the fires used for cooking food for the army, a reference to the defensive energies of the body. Currently, the term *Ying* is the most utilized.

Functions of Ying Qi

Ying Qi is deep energy, extracted from food, water, and air by the Triple Warmer process, under the influence of *Yuan Qi*.

Ying Qi circulates in the channels and nourishes the immaterial, energetic body.

It also participates with the body fluids in the elaboration of Blood and thus nourishes the material body.

Each organ system receives, stores and transforms this *Ying Qi* into a specific function: physical, sensory, emotional, mental, etc.

Production of Ying Qi

The elaboration of *Ying Qi* takes place mainly in the middle Triple Warmer, under the control of Spleen and Stomach's digestive Fire, from the first separation of food. The Kidneys supply the *Yuan Qi*. (▶ chap. 4.3)

Once produced, the *Ying Qi* ascends to the chest to be circulated in the whole system by the Lung named the "commander of *Qi*".

Circulation of Ying Qi

This circulation follows a 24 hour determined rhythm, with a maximum tide of 2 hours in each channel system. This "nyctemeral" circulation is referred to as the "Midday-midnight" flow. (▶ Fig. 4.5)

From the Liver channel, the *Ying Qi* passes to *Du Mai* ≈ Governing vessel at *Bai Hui* DM 20, then to *Ren Mai* ≈ Conception vessel up to *Tian Tu* RM-22, from where the *Qi* passes back to the Lung channel.

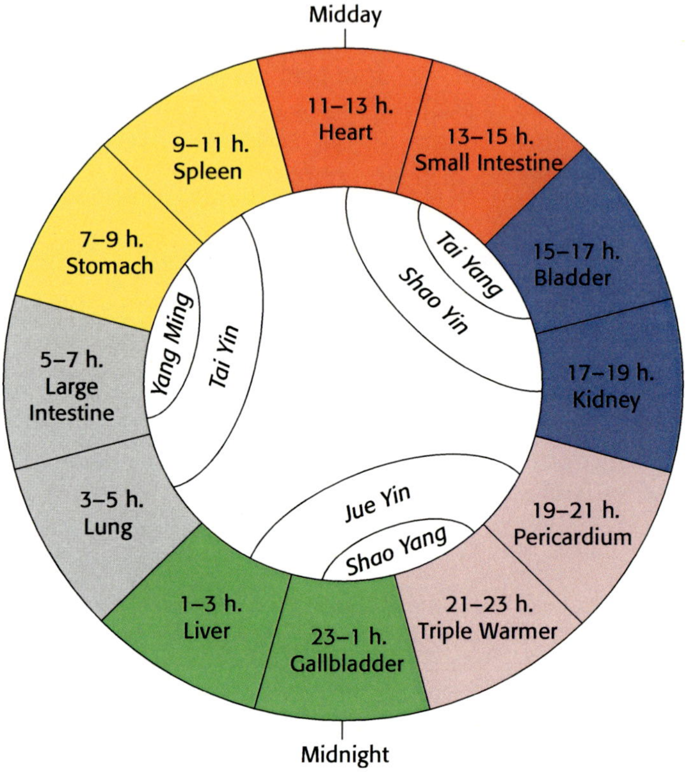

Figure 4.5: Nyctemeral circulation of *Ying Qi* in the primary channels

Wei ≈ Defensive Qi (卫气)

The functions of Wei Qi

Wei Qi's main function is protection and adaptation; it especially concentrates where there is more need of defence, such as on the surface, in the upper parts and in the superficial sinews or tendino-muscular zones.

It also maintains the surface heat and controls the opening of the pores and the moisture of the skin.

Production of Wei Qi

Wei Qi is also extracted from food, water and air in the middle as well as the lower Triple Warmer, under the control of Spleen and Stomach, from the second separation of food. This second separation takes place in the end parts of the small intestine and the large intestine, the latter seems to play an important role in the elaboration of *Wei Qi*. The Kidney-Fire supplies the *Yuan Qi*, necessary for the digestive process. (▶ chap. 4.3)

The Lung diffuses *Wei Qi* from the chest to the surface.

Circulation of Wei Qi

Wei Qi is also distributed from the chest by the Lung, but circulates freely everywhere, inside and outside of the channels.

During the day, *Wei Qi* emerges at the corner of the eye *Ying Ming* BL-1, and circulates along the 6 skin zones or *Pi Bu*, up and down 25 times. At night, *Wei Qi* penetrates into the depth, at the ankle, and circulates amongst the *Zang-Fu* 25 times, following the *Ke* ≈ Control cycle of the five phases (▶ Fig. 4.6).

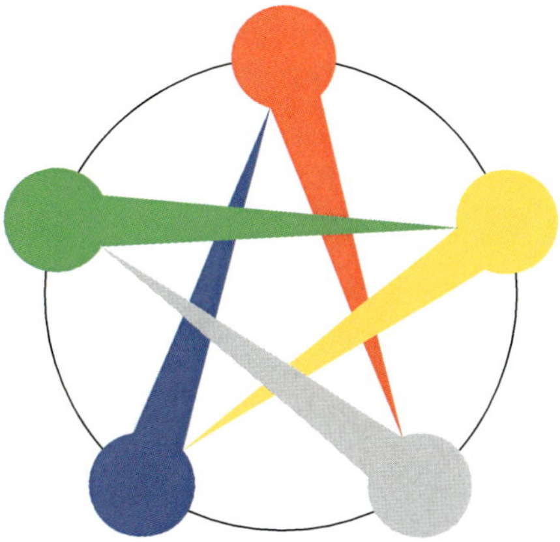

Figure 4.6: Nocturnal circulation of *Wei Qi* in the *Zang-Fu*

Zong ≈ Ancestral Qi (宗气)

Although *Zong Qi* is one of the constituents of pre-natal inherited energies, after birth and the taking in of the first breath, the Triple Warmer starts functioning and producing *Qi*, a part of which is stored in the chest centre *Shan Zhong* 膻中 an area also called *Shang Qi Hai* ≈ Upper Sea of Energy and protected by the Lung. The *Zong Qi* maintains and regulates the vital rhythmic movements of lung and heart, and manifests in the strength of the voice.

Xue ≈ Blood (血)

Blood is the material aspect of *Ying Qi*. They both have the same origin and are produced in the TW. Blood nourishes the material body and flows in the blood vessels, whereas *Ying Qi* nourishes the immaterial body and circulates in the channels.

Production and circulation of Blood

- Spleen and Stomach produce Blood in the middle Triple Warmer, from the essence of food and the pure body fluids. The digestive-Fire is provided by the Kidney-Fire, itself an expression of *Yuan Qi*. All these elements are integrated into the Heart to form the Blood. The Heart only governs Blood but has no direct action in its production. (▶ chap. 4.3)

- The Spleen is also responsible for maintaining Blood in the vessels. A Spleen *Qi*-vacuity may cause vascular fragility or coagulation problems.
- Liver stores Blood. During an activity, Blood is distributed to the muscles, but during rest and sleep, Blood is stored in the Liver, where it is regenerated and detoxified. Good quality of sleep is important in this process.
- Liver Blood nourishes muscles and tendons and lubricates the eyes and supports the vision. It also maintains the Blood cycle of the uterus.
- Kidneys contribute to Blood production by containing the *Yuan Qi*, by maintaining the body fluids and by nourishing the marrow, where the red and white blood cells are produced.
- Lung receives food essence and fluids, extracts the pure *Qi* of the air and passes them to the Heart, in this manner it "oxygenates" Blood. Also being the commander of *Qi*, Lung integrates the *Qi* necessary for the dynamism of Blood.
- Heart Protector (Pericardium): controls the circulation system: the heart pump.

The functions of Blood

- Nourish the material body and humidify the tissues:
  - The inside: *Zang-Fu* and their related body parts; the Curious *Fu*
  - The surface: nourish and lubricate the skin and mucous membranes, hair eyes, muscles and sinews
- Residence for the *Shen*: it is the material base for the mind
- Responsible for the menstrual cycle and milk production in women and sperm production in men. Blood maintains the fetus during pregnancy.
- Blood entertains a *Yin-Yang* relation with *Qi* (interdependence/ interaction); in this manner, Blood nourishes *Qi*, in turn, *Qi* moves and protects (holds) Blood. It is commonly said that *Qi* is the "commander" of Blood, and that Blood is the "mother of *Qi*". This relationship defines the energetic quality of Blood. The Chinese pulse diagnosis studies this relationship: the volume of the pulse reflects the amount of Blood, whereas the strength of the pulse is related to the *Qi*. This interaction could be compared to a balloon in which the ascending force, the hot air is similar to the action of *Qi*, and the descending factor is equivalent to the containing quality of Blood (▶ Fig. 4.7).

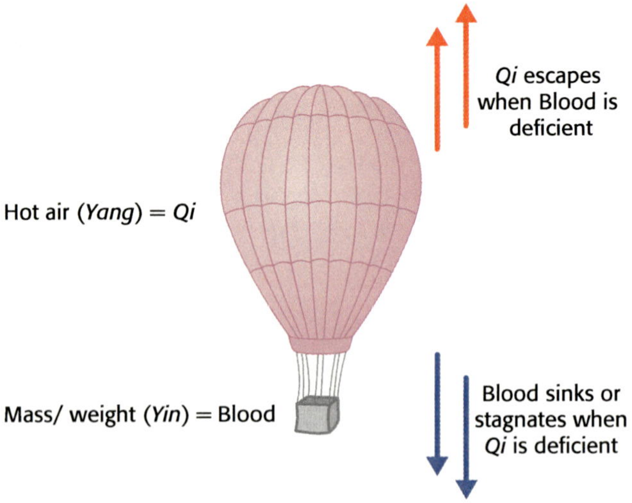

Figure 4.7: Interdependence of Blood and *Qi* in the image of a balloon

Blood is also often related to *Jing*, according to the expression "Essence and Blood are of the same source", which could be a reference to the role of the bone marrow in the production of blood and its relation to Kidney-*Jing*. This relation is further confirmed by the notion that one drop of *Jing* is equivalent to 100 drops of Blood.

Blood distribution is not equal to all the parts of the body. In fact, the Chinese have defined the ratio of Blood and *Qi* for each surface territory:

- *Tai Yang* territories contain more Blood than *Qi*
- *Shao Yang* territories contain more *Qi* than Blood
- *Yang Ming* areas contain equal amounts of *Qi* and Blood
- *Tai Yin* zones contain more *Qi* than Blood
- *Jue Yin* territories contain more Blood than *Qi*
- *Shao Yin* territories contain more *Qi* than Blood

This ratio explains certain physiological particularities, for example, the *Yang Ming* territory, containing abundant *Qi* and Blood, is where more body hair is to be found. It also has some importance in the choice of channels when treating certain pathologies, for example in treating a *Yin*-type pathology, a channel containing more Blood would be selected over one that has more *Qi*. In the older days, bleeding methods were indicated for channels containing more blood, whereas needling was preferred for channels having more *Qi*.

Jin Ye ≈ Body fluids (津液)

Refers to all the liquid elements of the body. They consist of two parts, *Jin* ≈ Liquid, and *Ye* ≈ Humour, and have slightly different functions.

Production of Body fluids

- *Jin Ye* are produced or rather extracted in the Triple Warmer, from the absorbed liquids, under the control of Spleen and Stomach.
- The Stomach is considered the "Origin of the Body fluids". This extraction takes place in the Small and Large Intestines.
- The Lung receives and diffuses the fluids from the chest to the surface, accompanied by the *Wei Qi*. The lung is called the "Upper source of Fluids".
- The Kidneys control the elimination of liquids received from the Lung. The Kidneys are the "Lower source of Fluids". (▶ chap. 4.3)

The functions of Body fluids

- *Jin* 津 ≈Thin fluids/ liquids are the clear and light part of the Body fluids. They are *Yang* in relation to *Ye* and are diffused outward by the Lung and circulate on the surface. The *Jin* ≈ Liquids are again sub-divided into:

- Pure (*Yang*): and have for a function to lubricate the portals in the form of tears, sweat, saliva, mucous, parotid secretion
- Turbid (*Yin*): they circulate with *Wei Qi* and moisten the skin, mucous membranes, and muscles.

- *Ye* 液 ≈ Thick fluids or humours are the heavy and dense *Yin* part of the Body fluids. They stay and circulate within the system together with *Ying Qi* and participate in the formation of Blood. The *Ye* fluids are also sub-divided in to
  - Pure and *Yang*, the part that permeates the *Zang-Fu*
  - Turbid and *Yin*, which lubricates the curious *Fu*≈ Bowels, the joints, the brain, the spinal cord, and the intestines.

Jing Qi ≈ Essence (精气)

Jing refers to *Qi* in its purest form, the essence. It has several meanings:

- The essence of food is called the *Jing* of food ≈ *Gou Qi* 谷气.
- The energy that is stored in each *Zang*-organ is referred to as the *Jing* of that organ.
- But most often *Jing Qi* refers to the essence of the Kidneys. This *Jing* has two origins, on the one hand, it is the inherited *Jing* of the parents, which can be considered as the chromosome lineage of the person. On the other hand, after puberty when the Kidneys have reached their maturity, the individual starts producing their own *Jing*. Therefore it can be said that the *Qi* that is stored in the Kidney is the Kidney-*Jing*. Obviously, the post-natal *Jing* not only reflects the inherited *Jing* but also the quality of food and water and lifestyle in general. This *Jing* represents the individual's life force, reproductive capacity as well as resistance to disease. There is a direct relation between Kidney-*Qi* and Kidney-*Jing*. The image of the candle is appropriate in demonstrating the transformation of Kidney-*Jing* into Kidney *Qi*, under the action of Kidney Fire (► Fig. 4.8).
- This transformative process is the foundation of all physiological functions in the body, in particular the life-sustaining "Triple Warmer".

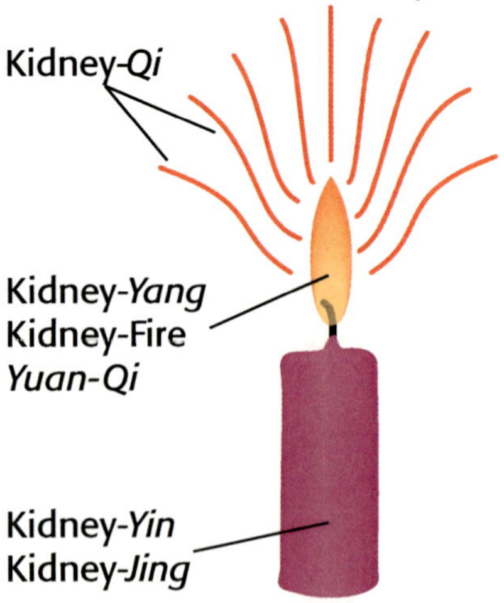

Figure 4.8: Relation between Kidney-*Jing*, Kidney-Fire, and Kidney-*Qi*

Functions of Jing

- Growth: the development of the body from the original cell to its full maturity follows a sequence partially determined by the strength of the inherited *Jing* and carried out by the eight Extraordinary Vessels.
- Development: the predetermined order of growth, following cycles of 7 and 8

which determine the various stages of maturation of Kidney *Jing*, as seen in chapter 2.7, figure 2.26, explore the development, strength, and flexibility of the bones and sinews, teeth and hair.

- Reproduction: Kidneys receive *Ying* ≈ Nutritive energy that has been produced in the TW and utilize this *Qi* for the development and maintenance of the sexual organs, and of sexual energy, and integrate it into the sperm and the ova. At puberty, the sexual organs are mature enough for reproduction. In general, *Jing Qi* represents the sexual energy. In ancient times it was believed that *Jing Qi* being strong and abundant in a young person but in turn containing valuable life experiences and wisdom in an older one, that the ideal combination to provide the best *Jing* for the child would be for old men to have very young wives!

Shen ≈ Spirit (神)

Shen signifies consciousness, intelligence, soul, spirit and life force.

Shen is the life principle; in the Chinese belief, *Shen* appears shortly after conception and leaves the body after death. It is even presumed that the *Shen* chooses the physical body that it will inhabit.

The individual *Shen* is part of the "Universal *Shen*", it is further believed that after death, the *Shen* leaving the body joins this global spirit. One of the fundamental premises of oriental spiritual thinking is that the human being, in this separate and dual body, has the opportunity to discover its oneness with existence, with the whole.

During one's life, *Shen* represents the consciousness, as well as the emotional and the mental functions, all deriving their energies from the Triple Warmer.

The three "Hereditary" energies of the human being define the body-shape, the constitution, and the temperament, whereas *Shen* defines the destiny of this form.

The image is that of each of the five organ-energy systems having a "driving spirit" directing the specific energies of that organ, producing a specific emotion and a mental or spiritual activity. These spirits are subject to the emperor, the Fire spirit, *Shen*. (▶ Fig. 4.9).

Shen could be compared to daylight, its white color being, in fact, a blending of all the other colors (▶ chap. 3.3, Fig. 3.8).

The total manifestation and mental-emotional balance of a person are referred to as their *Shen*.

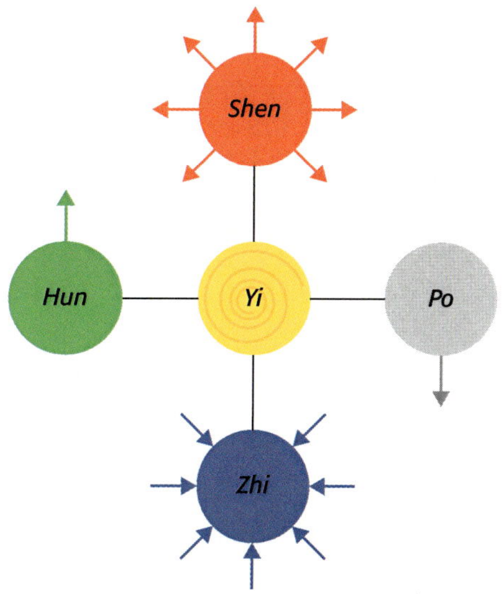

Figure 4.9: Shen-Emperor controlling *Yi, Zhi, Hun* and *Po*

The closest Western analogy for the concept of the various facets of the *Shen* and its constituents could be found in the Jungian stratification of the human psyche (▶ Fig. 4.10):

- Consciousness and the concept of the "Self": related to *Shen*
- Ego, Persona, and self-image: related to *Yi*, possibly *Po*
- Personal unconscious/ subconscious: represented by *Hun* and *Po*
- The collective unconscious, ethnical, racial, familial; anima, animus; archetypes: *Hun, Po,* and *Zhi*

The latter concept actually seems to correspond to the Chinese notion of *Zong* ≈ Ancestral *Qi*.

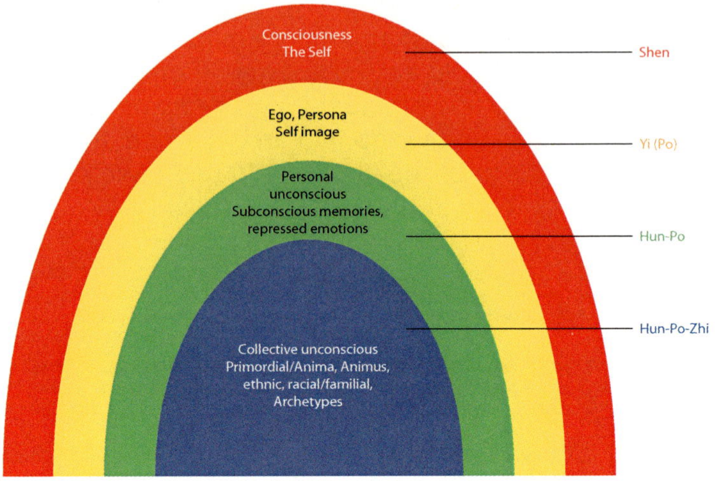

Figure 4.10: Jungian image of the stratified human psyche and it's parallel with the Chinese concepts of the *Shen* ≈ Spirit/mind

The Functions of Shen

- Consciousness: understood as awareness, cognition, and insight
- Thinking: logic, intelligence, memory, ideas, coherence, and wisdom
- Sleep, in fact, the sleep quality depends on the quietness of the mind
- Integration and comprehension of the five sensory inputs, independent of the sensory organs, the mind has to interpret the information that is received in a coherent manner (▶ chap. 3, Fig. 3.9)
- Spirituality: the capacity to live one's destiny, to comprehend the challenges and lessons, to realize the impermanence of all phenomena, and to accept the illusion of one's separateness from the whole are attributes of *Shen*. In fact, the names of the nine points of the Heart channel, symbolize the nine steps of each person towards redemption.
- Mental activity in its capacity of coherence and coordination is an attribute of *Shen* and the Heart, but it also depends on two other organs, for its functioning on Spleen-*Qi*, and for the production and the maintenance of the brain matter, on the Kidney-*Jing* (▶ Fig. 4.11).

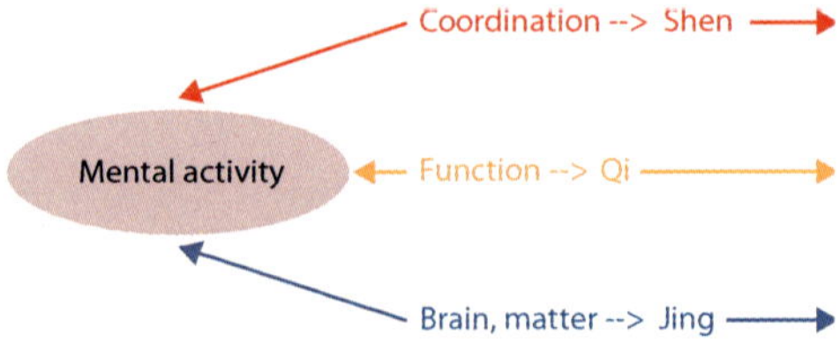

Figure 4.11: Mental activity and the Three Treasures: *Shen, Qi, Jing*

The Three Treasures (San Bao三宝)

In the Chinese art of health maintenance, transformation and search for harmony, the emphasis is put on the "Three Treasures": *Shen* - *Qi* - *Jing* (▶Fig. 4.12).

- *Jing* is produced and protected by the Kidneys and is responsible for strength, vitality and the continuation of the species. *Jing*, in turn, depends on the quality "*Jing*" of the air, water and food, and the preservation of the sexual energy.

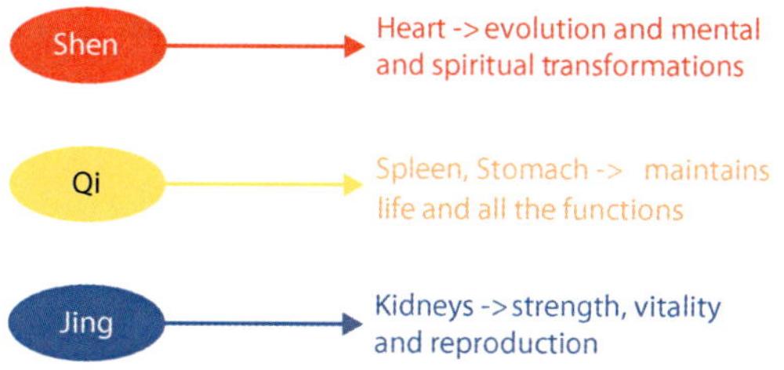

Figure 4.12: The Three Treasures: *Shen, Qi, Jing*

- *Qi* (refers to True ≈ *Zhen Qi*) is produced by the Spleen and Stomach and maintains life, it clearly depends on the quality of food and water, and the correct lifestyle and the circulation of this *Qi* through appropriate exercises "*Qi Gong*".
- *Shen* is residing in the Heart and enables the evolution and transformation of the human being, mentally as well as spiritually. *Shen* is developed by correct discipline and the cultivation of the mind and the spirit through meditative practices.

Overview of all the energies in the human being

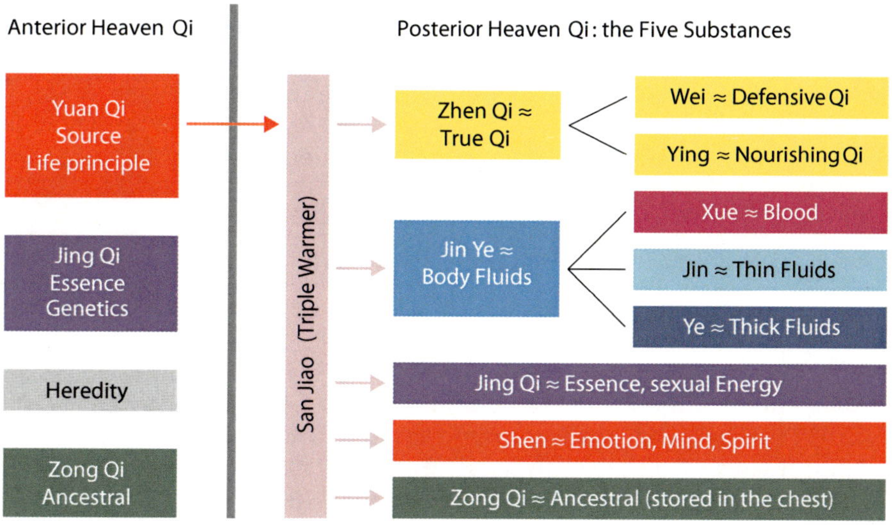

Figure 4.13: Pre- & Post-Heaven *Qi*, production of the Five substances (*Qi*, Blood, Fluids, *Jing*, *Shen*). *Yuan* ≈ Source *Qi* is the source of the Digestive Fire and the foundation of the Triple Warmer. *Jing* and *Zong Qi* influence the constitution

4.5 Circulation of Qi: Jing Luo, the Channel system

Qi circulates everywhere and maintains and mobilizes the physical body. It protects and adapts to external changes. Through the action of each specific organ system, *Qi* manifests in a multitude of functions, emotions and mental activities.

The channels of acupuncture surround and contain the body like a net or a web.

The most appropriate image is the weaving loom, with threads, which are stretched vertically and tightly, the warp, which gives the material its main shape and strength. The lighter threads, the woof, which is woven horizontally from left to right and right to left, complete and give substance to the fabric (▶Fig. 4.14).

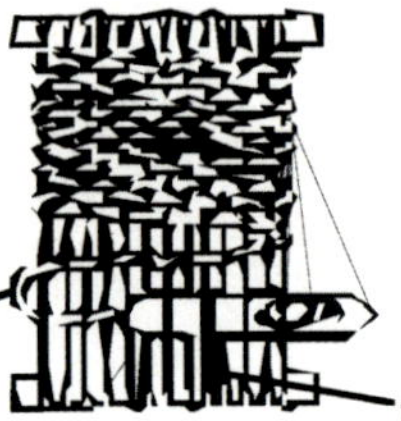

Figure 4.14: Channels in the image of a weaving loom

The Chinese expression for the channels "*Jing Luo*" evokes precisely this image.

Channels are defined as conveyers of *Qi* ≈ Energy and of *Xue* ≈ Blood, hence the image of rivers and canals. They link and connect all the body parts, the depth and the surface, the interior and the exterior, hence the image of a web.

The channels of acupuncture are intimately connected to other anatomical structures: the vascular system, lymphatic circulation, peripheral nervous system, muscles, and the fascia. As conductors of energy, the channels do not have a material base.

Skin	Related to the *Pi Bu* ≈ Skin zones
Muscles	Related to the *Jing Jin* ≈ Sinew channels
Blood vessels	Related to the *Luo* ≈ Connecting vessels
Flesh	Related to the *Zheng* ≈ Primary channels
Bones	Related to the *Jing Bie* ≈ Divergent channels
Marrow	Related to the *Qi Jing Ba Mai* ≈ Extraordinary vessels

The anatomical reality of the Chinese channel system has only recently been demonstrated by CT scans and amperometric oxygen microsensors, explaining the initial translation by the French authors of the term "*Jing-Luo*" as "Meridian". Meridians are imaginary lines traced from north to south, referred to as longitudes. The term "Meridian", although conveying certain aspects of the notion of "*Jing*", is nevertheless quite restrictive and is now being replaced by the more common expression of "Channel". A recent and very interesting explanation for the channel theory has been proposed by Dr. D. Keown to explain the anatomical basis for the acupuncture channels. According to this theory, the channels would be the space of least resistance for the electrical impulses originating in the organs and traveling to the extremities. These spaces seem to correspond to the fascia, whose embryological development would further explain the inner connections between various organs and body parts (► Appendix). It is very important not to see the channels as simple vessels or pipes carrying energy back and forth, but rather as lines of resonance, responding to all internal and external impulses. They can be compared to the strings of a musical instrument. Each string has its own tension (potential) and will resonate with a specific vibration. This vibration may be transmitted from the inside, as is the case in organic and emotional functions, similar to a finger plucking the strings of the instrument. Or the vibration may be the result of resonance with an outside source. In both cases, the string of the instrument will convey this vibration along its length as well as into the surrounding space.

A very modern and appropriate image of the channel would be the World Wide Web which, although it does not possess a physical reality, links all the points of the globe together.

Historically, the earlier descriptions of the channels presented them with the notion of *Gen* ≈ Root and *Jie* ≈ Termination. All channels supposedly started at the extremities to end on the trunk or the head. The present notion of "Root, Knot, and Branch" relates to this ancient system.

The oldest texts dealing with channels are the *Nei Jing* texts. Written or compiled approximately around 200 BC, the *Nei Jing* consisted of 4 books: the *Su Wen* and *Ling Shu*, mainly on acupuncture, and according to oral transmission, 2 lost books: *Tai Shu*, treating *Mu* ≈ Alarm and *Xi* ≈ Cleft points, and the *Ming Tang*, on the location of Acu-points. A later treatise the *Nan Jing* ≈ Classic of difficulties, further comments and analyses the *Ling Shu*.

The *Nei Jing* establishes the channel system as a continuum of a defined sequence.

Although the channels do correspond to the *Zang/ Fu* through their deeper pathways, on the surface they also establish an independent continuum through which other aspects of physiology or pathology may be explained.

Classification of the Channels

Roughly classified into "Primary" and "Secondary" channels (►Fig. 4.15).

- Primary Channels are the 12 *Zheng Jing*. They have a defined axis and direction from top to bottom or from below to above.
- Secondary Channels which include:
  - 12 *Jing Jin* ≈ Sinew or Tendino-muscular channels
  - 12 *Jing Bie* ≈ Divergent or Distinct channels

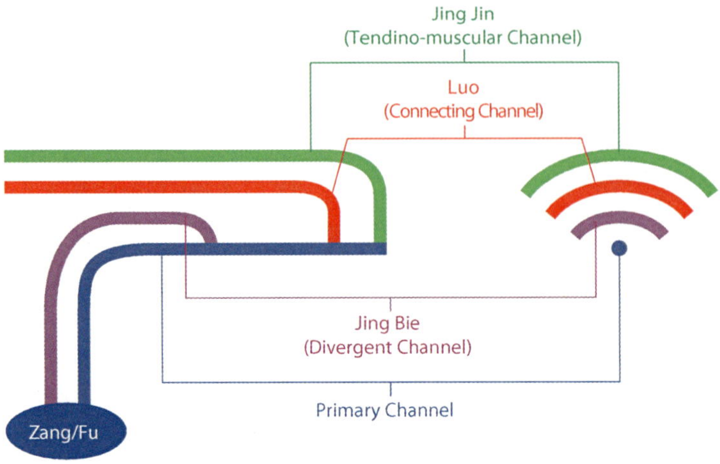

Figure 4.15: Channel stratification: each Primary channel has a network of secondary channels to complement its functions and for protection

- *Luo Mai* ≈ Connecting or Network vessels, further subdivided in to:
  - Minute *Luo*: *Sun Luo, Fu Luo*, and *Xue Luo*
  - 12 Connecting or Transversal* *Luo*
  - 16 *Luo Bie*/ Diverging or Longitudinal[1] *Luo*
- 12 Pi Bu or cutaneous zones are not really channels but territories attached to a primary channel.

- 8 *Qi Jing* ≈ Extraordinary vessels

Amongst the secondary channels, all except the 8 Extraordinary and the minute *Luo* are referred to by the name of the primary channel they are related to.

The Primary Channels describe the fundamental energetic structure, the framework of the body, on which all phenomena, be it internal or external, resonate. The Secondary channels supplement and further specify the functions of the primary channels. It can be said that secondary channels are the externalization of the primary channels. In this manner, each group, the primary with its secondary channels, has its own preferential roles and functions.

The primary channels connect the *Zang-Fu* to the head and the outside. The secondary channels complement the Primary and protect them.

The Domain of the Channels

The Channels as conveyers of *Qi* ≈ Energy and of *Xue* ≈ Blood link not only the depth and the surface, the *Zang-Fu* organs with the anatomical structures, but also the inner with the outer world as well as the post-natal "Posterior Heaven" with the pre-natal "Anterior Heaven".

The three energies: *Wei*-Defensive, *Ying* ≈ Nourishing, and *Jing* ≈ Essence, define the three energetic levels of the human being:

[1] This Terminology was given by the French-Vietnamese school.

- The *Wei Qi*, abundant on the surface, deals with contact with the outer world and helps adapt to the external changes. The *Jing Jin* ≈ Sinew channels are the main vehicles for the *Wei Qi*, and as the most superficial organized channel system, deal with the outer world, acting as a defensive layer against external influences and climatic changes. As they are also controlling the muscles and sinews, the *Jing Jin* are responsible for the physical appearance, the morphology.
- The *Ying Qi*, is responsible for the inner nourishment and is mainly carried via *Xue*≈ Blood as well as via the primary channels to the physical structures. As the *Luo*-network channels are intimately connected to Blood and the capillary system, they appear to help the processing of the outer influences, acting as a buffer system and dealing more specifically with the emotional responses. The primary channels constitute the bridge between the outer changes and the inherited energies.
- The *Jing Qi*, or constitutional energy, genetic inheritance, which according to the Daoist belief also defines, our fate and destiny, is managed and carried by the Eight Extraordinary Vessels. Additionally, the *Jing Bie* ≈ Divergent channels constitute the buffer system for the *Jing*, and act as a link between the inherited (pre-heaven) and produced (post-heaven) energies.

According to Master Yuen, the energetic anatomy of the body can be summarized as:

- The exterior or the *Wei Qi* layer as the instinctual, autonomic, involuntary and natural aspect, responding to the climate and to external influences;
- The interior *Ying Qi* layer is responsible for cognitive choices, emotions, desires, nutrition (choice of foods), moral choices (obligations) and beliefs;
- The constitutional *Jing Qi* level: represents the inherited energies and concerns survival as well as gender and ethnic issues. The Extraordinary vessels oversee the transmission of the inherited energies and thus the unfolding of the predefined destiny.
- The Primary channels, linking the surface and the interior, manifest the original *Yin* and *Yang* as post-natal *Qi* and Blood and are considered the "Path of Life", in other words how the inherited energies are actually manifested in life.

The Channels reflect the physiology (natural state of human existence) and convey movement.

Pathology is the normal physiology gone astray, a dysfunction of the movement of *Qi*. In this manner, a repletion (excess) of a channel represents a path that is often threaded, what one is attracted to, desires and propensities, whereas a vacuity (deficiency), would represent an area which is repeatedly avoided.

Anatomically the channel system relates to various layers (▶Table. 4.1):

Table 4.1: The anatomical connections of the Chinese Channel system

The Exterior: Yang aspect	Channel	Zang-Fu / Inside: Yin aspect

Pi ≈ Skin	*Pi Bu* ≈ *Skin* zones	None
Jin ≈ Sinews	*Jing Jin* ≈ *Sinew channels*	None
Mai ≈ Vessels	*Luo* ≈ Connecting vessels	None directly
Ji ≈ Flesh	*Zheng Jing* ≈ Primary channels	*Zang-Fu*
Gu ≈ Bone	*Jing Bie* ≈ Divergent channels	*Zang-Fu*
Sui ≈ Marrow	*Qi Jing Ba Mai* ≈ Extraordinary vessels	*Qi Fu* ≈ Curious *Fu*

Only the Primary and Divergent channels connect with the *Zang-Fu* with the exception of the Heart and Pericardium *Luo* vessels.

The terminology of the Primary Channels

The Primary channels are classified into three *Yin* and three *Yang* intensities or degrees, as described in chapter 2.3.

Tai	太	Great, greatest, supreme, the first, the most ancient, respectable
Shao	少	Little, small, lesser, young, insufficient, the second ...
Jue	厥	Fallen, diminished, exhausted, used up, terminal ...
Ming	明	Brightness, daylight, manifested, clarity, lucidity, vision, next ...

This defines 6 vibratory axes, 3 intensities of *Yin* and 3 intensities of *Yang*, referred to as the Six "Grand Meridians/Channels":

Tai Yang	*Shao Yang*	*Yang Ming*
Tai Yin	*Shao Yin*	*Jue Yin*

It is fundamental to underline the importance of the notion of the 6 axis or vectors, as all phenomena between Heaven and Earth, will naturally resonate with one of them, this, of course, includes all physiological functions.

Each axis has two poles: Heaven/ *Yang* and Earth/ *Yin*.

- The part of each axis is related to the upper limbs "*Shou*" 手 hand.
- The *Yin* part joins the lower limbs "*Zu*" 足 foot.

This gives us the 12 expressions defining the 12 Primary Channels:

Shou (Hand) *Tai Yang*- Small Intestine (SI)	with *Zu* (Foot) *Tai Yang*- Bladder (BL)
Shou (Hand) *Shao Yang*-Triple Warmer (TW)	with *Zu* (Foot) *Shao Yang*- Gallbladder (GB)
Shou (Hand) *Yang Ming*-Large Intestine	with *Zu* (Foot) *Yang Ming*- Stomach (ST)

(LI)	
Shou (Hand) *Tai Yin*- Lung (LU)	with *Zu* (Foot) *Tai Yin*- Spleen/Pancreas (SP)
Shou (Hand) *Shao Yin*- Heart (HE)	with *Zu* (Foot) *Shao Yin*- Kidney (KI)
Shou (Hand) *Jue Yin*- Pericardium (PE)	with *Zu* (Foot) *Jue Yin*- Liver (LR)

Again it is essential to stress the importance of naming the primary channels according to their energetic classifications rather than the simplified Westernized manner of naming them according to their *Zang-Fu* connections. Hence *Zu Tai Yang* channel, informs us about its polarity: *Yang*; its intensity: *Tai*; its connection to the lower limbs: *Zu*. Furthermore, it informs about its position on the body, the most *Yang* regions, that it is connected to *Shou Tai Yang* and that all *Tai Yang* phenomena will resonate on it etc. Instead, all of this information is lost when we call it the Bladder channel, retaining only its connection to the related *Fu* ≈ Bowel the Bladder.

The channels are first defined by their connection to the hand or the foot, then their energetic level or axis /intensity. Hence Small Intestine would be *Shou Tai Yang* ≈ Hand, Greater *Yang*.

Hand ≈ Shou	**Level/ Intensitiy**	**Foot ≈ Zu**
Small Intestine (SI)	**Tai Yang**	Bladder (BL)
Triple Warmer (TW)	**Shao Yang**	Gallbladder (GB)
Large Intestine (LI)	**Yang Ming**	Stomach (ST)
Lung (LU)	**Tai Yin**	Spleen/Pancreas (SP)
Heart (HE)	**Shao Yin**	Kidney (KI)
Pericardium (PE)	**Jue Yin**	Liver (LR)

The "six energy levels" describe the intensity of *Yang* from greater to weaker *Yang* and from greater to weaker *Yin*. In reality, the channels on the body have been described with a slight difference. The *Shao Yin* level has been placed at the deepest level. The *Shao Yin* being the vital axis of the body, it makes sense that it should also be the most protected.

Hence the disposition of the 6 energy vectors as related to the body, from the surface towards the depth, could be termed as the "Six Energy Layers":

- *Tai Yang*
- *Shao Yang*
- *Yang Ming*
- *Tai Yin*
- *Jue Yin*
- *Shao Yin*

Organization and circulation of the channels

The sequence of descriptions of the primary and secondary channels in the classical texts differs from one channel group to another. The order in which each channel system is described is signifying and emphasizing its main functions.

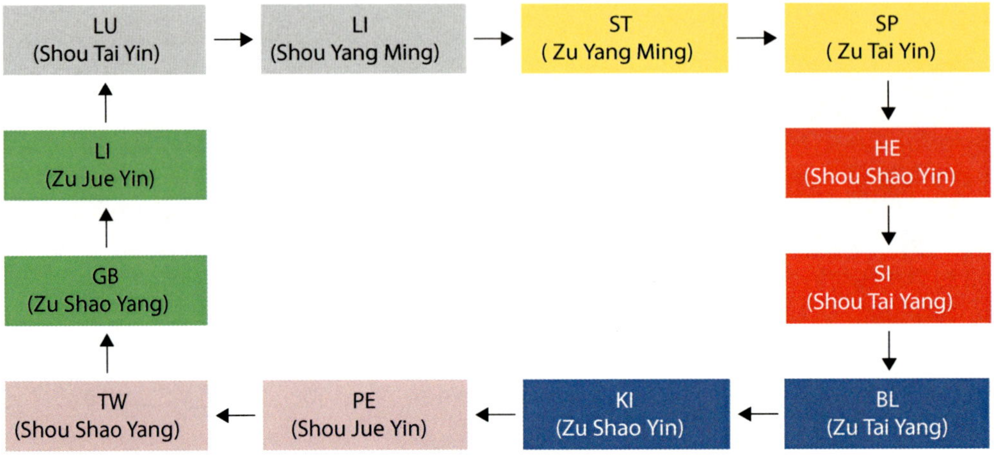

Figure 4.16 : The circulation order in the Primary Channels

The Primary Channels (正经 Zheng Jing)

They are described as a continuum in the following order (▶Fig. 4.16):

LU (*Shou Tai Yin*) Metal → LI (*Shou Yang Ming*) Metal → ST (*Zu Yang Ming*) Earth → SP (*Zu Tai Yin*) Earth → HE (*Shou Shao Yin*) Fire → SI (*Shou Tai Yang*) Fire → BL (*Zu Tai Yang*) Water → KI (*Zu Shao Yin*) Water → PE (*Shou Jue Yin*) Fire minister → TW (*Shou Shao Yang*) Fire minister → GB (*Zu Shao Yang*) Wood → LR (*Zu Jue Yin*) Wood.

All *Yang* channels flow from Heaven to Earth, descending from top to bottom. Considering a man with arms raised upwards(▶Fig. 4.17):

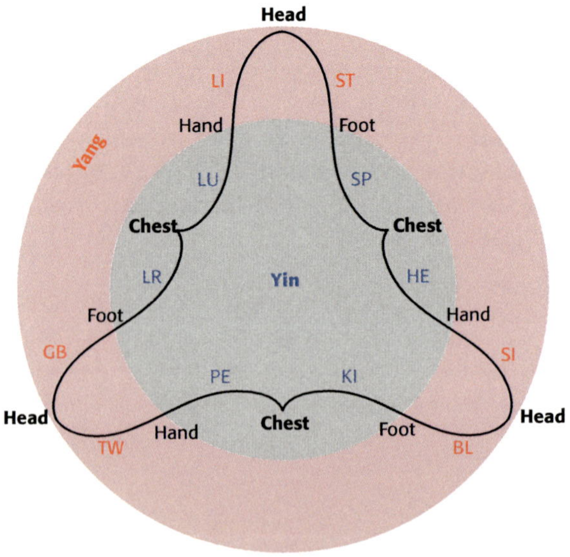

Figure 4.17: *Yang* Channels flow down: hand to head to foot; *Yin* Channels flow up: foot to chest to hand

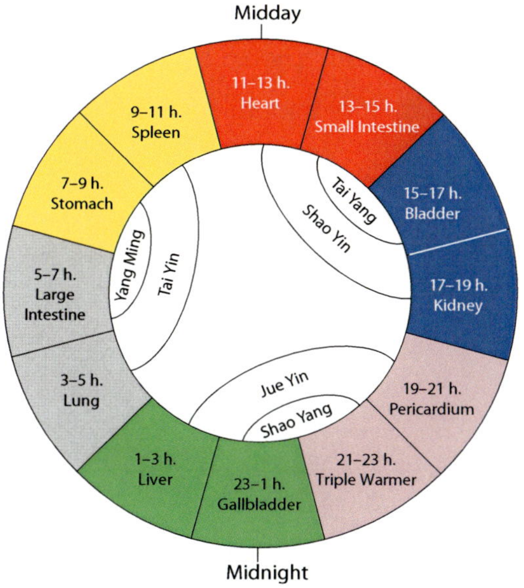

Figure 4.18: Midday-midnight relation: the high tide in a channel system corresponds to the low tide in the channel diametrically opposite to it

- *Shou Yang Ming*- LI flows from the hand to the head
- *Zu Yang Ming*- ST continues from the head to the foot, completing the first unit.
- *Shou Tai Yang*- SI flows from the hand to the head,
- *Zu Tai Yang*- BL continues from the head to the foot, completing the second unit.
- *Shou Shao Yang*- TW flows from the hand to the head,
- *Zu Shao Yang*- GB continues from the head to the foot, completing the third unit.
- All the *Yin* channels ascend, flowing from Earth to Heaven:
- *Zu Tai Yin*- SP ascends from the foot to the trunk,
- *Shou Tai Yin*- LU ascends from the trunk to the hand, completing the 1st unit.
- *Zu Shao Yin*- KI ascends from the foot to the trunk,
- *Shou Shao Yin*- HE ascends from the trunk to the hand, completing the second unit.
- *Zu Jue Yin*- LR ascends from the foot to the trunk,
- *Shou Jue Yin*- PE ascends from the trunk to the hand, completing the third unit.

The sequential flow of *Qi* starts with the Lung channel and relates to 24 hour *Qi* circulation. Each channel presents a high tide of energy for 2 hours; consequently 12 hours later it will have a period of low energy. This point is of importance in diagnosis and treatment. Repletion (excess) in a channel and its associated organ will manifest more easily at the times of maximum energy; i.e. classical asthma attacks occur between 3 and 5 in the morning. Whereas a vacuity (deficiency) will manifest commonly at the lowest energy times; i.e. lumbar pains in the early morning, 5-7 am (lowest time for the Kidney *Qi*). It becomes apparent that any given time corresponds to a maximum activity in one channel and a minimum activity in another channel. This 24-hour relationship is referred to as the Midday-Midnight system (▶Fig. 4.18). The 12 sections of time correspond to the 12 earthly branches (Chinese astrology).

In therapy, the best time to supplement a channel would be when the *Qi* starts rising, and the best time to reduce it would be when the *Qi* is waning.

It is very important to underline that the hourly slots correspond to the sun-time in a given time zone, and not to the clock time, which is often changed artificially for daylight saving purposes. In particular, in Europe, the real sun time is actually the Greenwich mean-time. For example in considering the Horary system, the LU time in England would be 3-5 a.m., whereas in France it would be 4-6 a.m. And during the daylight saving seasons, even another hour should be added.

The relation between the channel receiving the tide of *Qi* and the channel having the lowest *Qi* level is referred to as the Midday-Midnight relation. In therapy, this relation can be utilized to treat an external pathogenic repletion in a channel by using the *Luo*-network point of the channel diametrically opposite to it. For example, an external pathology of the Lung may be treated with the *Luo* of the Bladder channel, preferably between 3 and 5 p.m.

The relationship between the channels

Besides the obvious connection between each channel and its corresponding *Zang* or *Fu* organ, each channel further has two privileged relations:

- One of opposite polarity, *Yin-Yang*, but in the same section of the body, *Shou* ≈ Hand or *Zu* ≈ Foot, belonging to the same element. This constitutes the basic coupling system, joining the inside and the outside, the *Biao* and the *Li*, the *Yin* the *Yang* and is the main means for maintaining the harmony of the microcosm and the macrocosm. For example the *Shou Tai Yin*-LU and *Shou Yang Ming*-LI, or the *Zu Shao Yin*-KI and the *Zu Tai Yang*-BL.
- One of the same polarity but in the opposite section of the body. This allows for the communication of the above and the below, heaven and earth and of two different elements. This constitutes the 6 grand channels or energy axis, explaining the energetic stratification of the body. For example *Shou* and *Zu Tai Yang*, SI-BL channels.

Channel pathways

Basically, two pathways are considered:

- External pathway where the channel is more superficial and accessible to stimulation by needles or pressure or heat. On this superficial section of the channel are situated the Acupuncture Points, acting as small wells of *Qi*, through which the flow of *Qi* may be manipulated by the action of needles, pressure, heat etc.
- The deep or internal pathway is of great physiological importance because it explains the connection between the related organ and the channel as well as the internal connection between various organs and anatomical spaces. The internal pathways also explain the physiology, the pathology and many of the symptoms observed in channel disharmonies. These connections also explain some classical relations, i.e. Lung and Stomach; Spleen with the Heart; Kidney with the Liver, Lung or Heart; Liver to Lung; Small Intestine to Stomach; the Brain with *Zu Tai Yang*-BL, *Zu Shao Yang*-GB, *Zu Jue Yin*-LR, and possibly *Shou Shao Yin*-HE channels.

The preferential roles and functions of the channels

Primary channels ≈ *Zheng Jing*

The *Zheng Jing* ≈ Primary channels are the axis of the body, conveying *Qi* and Blood and defining the "Postnatal" existence. All phenomena, both external and internal resonate on the Primary channels, hence they reflect the natural order of human existence and physiology, and like their name, *Jing* ≈ River/ Pathway indicates, they convey movement. In Daoist symbolism, the Primary channels represent the “Path of life “ which leads us to our destiny.

The sequencing of the primary channels conveys physiology, which can be simplified as the three pre-requisites of life:

- Survival: as defined by air, food, and water. Survival is defined by the first cycle of circulation: LU → LI → ST → SP called the “First Unit”;
- Continuation of life and a sense of purpose: defined by the “Second Unit”: HE → SI → BL → KI;
- Mobility, choice, interaction and the sense of protection: defined by the “Third Unit”: PE → TW → GB → LR.

Sinew channels ≈ *Jing Jin*

The *Jing Jin* are in charge of the exterior/surface of the body, energetically related to *Wei*≈ Defensive *Qi* and the protection of the surface. Anatomically they relate to the muscles, the fascia and the physical appearance, the morphology.

Network/Connecting channels ≈ *Luo Mai*

The *Luo*, by their connection to *Xue* ≈ Blood and to *Shen* ≈ Spirit, are in charge of processing of the world. On the one hand, they constitute a buffer for pathogenic factors, by containing them in the superficial blood capillaries. These are the Longitudinal *Luo* establishing contact to the outer world. On the other hand, they maintain the harmony of the *Biao-Li* ≈ Surface and Lining/inside. These are the Transversal *Luo,* which also ensures and maintain the rhythmicity of the microcosm with the macrocosm in the 5 phases. In other words, they help the inner organs adapt and respond accordingly to outer changes of seasons, climates, colors, sounds etc. Energetically they are related to the *Ying*≈ Nourishing level. From a Daoist perspective, they define the emotional behavior, the temperament, and allow for life choices and beliefs.

Extraordinary vessels ≈ *Qi Jing Ba Mai*

The Extraordinary vessels transmit the constitutional energies. They define our genetic make-up and are rooted in pre-heaven (pre-natal) energies. They ensure the perpetuation of the species. The extraordinary channels are all rooted in the *Dong Qi* ≈ Moving *Qi* between the kidneys, reflected in the *Ming Men* ≈ Gate of destiny. From a Daoist point of view, they define our fate and destiny.

According to Master J. Yuen, constitutional energies are defined by the *Yuan* - Source *Qi*, which is reflected by its two components:

- Morphology, the genetic makeup, defined by the parental *Jing* ≈ Essence
- Destiny[2]*, defined by *Dai* or *Zong* ≈ Cosmic *Qi* at the time of conception

Divergent channels ≈ *Jing Bie*

The *Jing Bie* are in charge of communicating with the depth, the *Zang-Fu*, and their protection via the *Gao Huang* ≈ Membranes. They act as buffers for pathogenic factors, diverting them from the *Zang-Fu* and into major articulations. The *Jing Bie* pairs maintain the communication between the trunk and the head and maintain the flow of *Qi*, Blood, and Fluids to and from the head. As they are in contact with the Essence, with *Qi*, and with Blood, they constitute a bridge between the pre-heaven/ constitution and the post-heaven energies.

---

[2] Also referred to as Astrology.

Part III- Health and Disease in Chinese Medicine

5. Origins of disease

The first documented concern about illness appeared around 1600 BC and was attributed to the spirit of ancestors exacting punishment on the descendants. Later this notion was extended to include "Winds" symbolizing the higher powers causing disease. The notion of "Evil spirits" or *Gui*- a harming spirit, causing disease appeared around 1000 BC and still remains in the causative factors of disease nemesis. Therapy consisted therefore of rituals of dancing, chanting and amulets and involved shamans, *Shi,* and sorcerers, *Wu*. By the 2nd century BC, the importance of spirits was lessened and replaced by more scientific explanations and natural causes, as well as the concept of *Wei* ≈ Defensive versus *Xie* ≈ Aggressive energy. One of the oldest texts, *Shang Han Lun*, "Treatise on Cold-induced diseases" by *Zhang Zhong Jing* (142–220 AD), clearly demonstrates a systematic, diagnostic and therapeutic approach to disease. By the 6th century the origins of disease were discussed by *Chao Yuan Fang,* and by the Song dynasty, the causative factors were classified into three categories, which still remain current today.

Health is defined as a state of harmony between *Yin* and *Yang*. This equilibrium is relative to each individual.

A loss of equilibrium between *Yin* and *Yang* causes a state of disease. The loss of balance depends on:

- The strength of the vital energy of the person, the Upright "*Zheng* Qi"
- The strength of the pathogenic agent, the aggressive "*Xie Qi*"

Previously, we have explored the various constituents of the Vital Substances that make up the *Zhen* ≈ True and *Zheng* ≈ Upright energy of a person. In summery the strength of the vital energy depends on:

- The constitution of the individual
- Lifestyle: diet, exercise sexual activity and habits
- The environment
- Behaviour, represented by the mental and emotional equilibrium

In a nutshell, “Health” can be defined as the capacity for each person to adapt to external changes, such as the climate, food, pollution, life cycles, emotional and mental demands, etc.

These external influences, unless they are extreme, would not provoke disease unless the inner milieu, the microcosm, is weak and has lost its capacity to adapt. Schematically there are three levels of adaptation:

- Macrocosmic: climates, seasons, as well as cosmic influences
- Environmental: mainly involve the socio-affective relations

- Personal: including individual needs and desires, dietary and sexual as well as physiological changes and aging

It becomes therefore apparent as to why in the analysis of a pathological process and in particular in Chinese Diagnosis, the aim is to not only to analyze the manifestation, but also to define the causative factor as well as the deeper condition having permitted the appearance of a disease. Classically this approach had been referred to as the Root, Knot and Branch concept in the image of a tree in which the leaves are apparent, but the roots are hidden (▶Fig. 5.1):

- The "Site": where the pathological process is manifesting, such as a channel, a body layer, *Zang-Fu* organ system
- The “Cause”: the factors causing the manifestation: traditionally there are 3 categories:
- External causes: the six climatic energies (wind, heat, fire, cold, dry, damp)
- Internal causes: emotions
- Other causes: diet, exercise, sexual activity, parasites, trauma etc.
- The “Condition”: what was initially the reason for the causative factor to be able to produce an imbalance.
- The condition is the internal origin of the disease. Finding out in which period the disease has begun can help define its origin:
- The prenatal period: Pre-Heaven energies define the constitution. This does not only imply the heredity but also the state of health of the parents at the moment of conception, and of the mother throughout the pregnancy.
- The childhood period depends on the constitution and mostly on the diet (to note that a lack of maternal care at this stage would usually only manifest later in life).
- The adult period: is mainly influenced by the mental-emotional behavior, and secondarily by all the other causes.

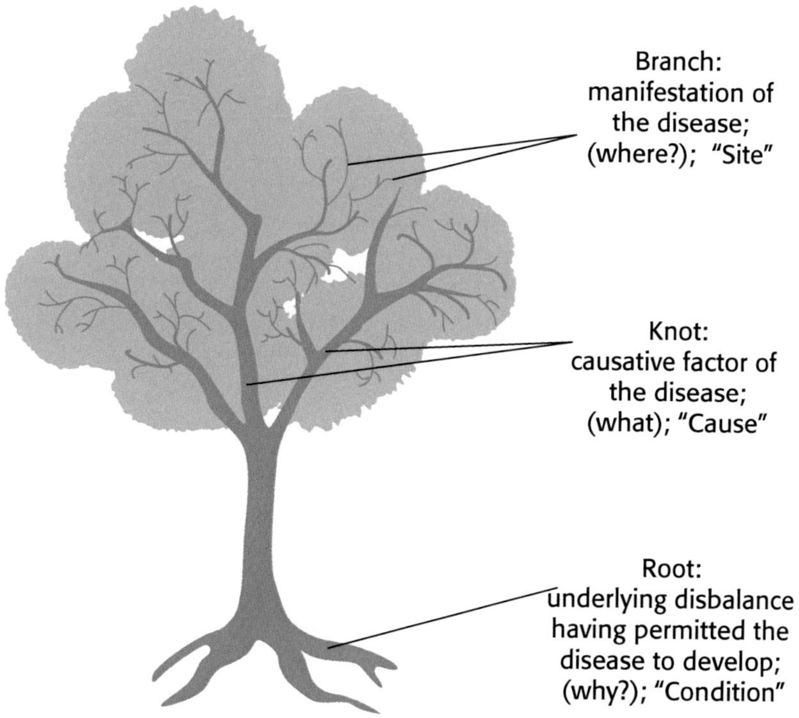

Figure 5.1: Branch-knot-root or Site-cause-condition of a disease and the aim of diagnosis

6. External Causes of Disease

The external factors causing disease are the climates, the seasonal energies, and the cosmic rhythms. In general, today mostly the climatic causes are discussed in Chinese medicine, the seasonal and cosmic influences are studied more under the topic of "Stems and Branches".

The "*Liu Yin*"- six excesses are the normal climatic energies turned aggressive "*Xie*"- perverted or pathogenic.

The normal climatic variations are:

- Wind ≈ *Feng*
- Heat ≈ *Re*, and Fire ≈ *Huo*
- Dampness ≈ *Shi*
- Dryness ≈ *Zao*
- Cold ≈ *Han*

They can become aggressive for the individual system for 3 reasons:

- They are too intense
- They are out of season
- The defensive energies of the person are deficient

In these cases, the six climates become incorrect, vicious, perverted or pathogenic and are termed "*Xie Qi*" that has aggressed or penetrated the body, in the image of the enemy that has broken through the defenses of the country.

The six *Xie* ≈ Pathogenic Factors (PF) can act singly or in combination.

Each climatic factor predominates during its corresponding season, such as cold in winter, wind in spring, heat in summer, etc. It will cause a set of symptoms only if there is a pre-existing weakness in the corresponding organ systems. For example, Wind will cause symptoms in spring if the Liver and Gallbladder are out of harmony, manifesting with Wind type patterns, such as hay fever or conjunctivitis. When this pernicious energy "*Xie Qi*" has been victorious and is said to have penetrated inside, the symptoms are classified as "*Shi*" evoking a state of excess or repletion. According to the symptoms, the type of pathogenic factor may be identified and classified as "External" Heat or Cold and referred to as "Excess or replete" Heat, Cold, Wind, Dampness or Dryness.

Similar symptoms may arise not from outside but from internal *Zang-Fu* disharmony; for example, an internal *Yang* vacuity can give rise to symptoms of internal Cold; this condition is referred to as "Internal Cold" or "Deficiency Cold or Vacuity Cold", which signifies a cold resulting from a *Yang* weakness.

The contraction "penetration" of the *Xie Qi*, into the body occurs either through

- The skin, specifically the six skin zones and mucous membranes especially of the nose and the mouth;
- The muscles, via the sinew channels;
- The Divergent or the Primary channels;
- *Xie Qi* may also penetrate some organs directly, such as Lung or Stomach
- Or direct infestation of the Blood, as in insect bites or surgical acts.

In general, the energetic stratification of the body prevents the direct penetration of *Xie* ≈ Pathogenic energy into the organs and to the Blood-level. The *Wei* ≈ Defensive energy is quite abundant on the surface and tends to stop the pathogenic factors by adapting to the outer changes via the surface body temperature and the opening and closing of the pores. One of the main functions of the secondary channel systems of each primary channel is to protect it against a PF invasion, especially to protect the organ by maintaining the PF on the surface. As long as the symptoms are in the external layers of the body, such as the skin zones, the secondary channels, and the *Tai Yang* territories, the disease is considered "*Biao*"-exterior in the image of an outer garment.

When *Xie Qi* penetrates deeper into the Primary channels or into the organs it is considered *Li* ≈ Interior, representing the lining of a coat (▶ Fig. 6.1). Once inside, one type of *Xie Qi* may transform into another: Cold into Heat; Heat into Dryness; Dampness into Heat, and Fire into Wind. Most external pathogenic factors tend to transform ultimately into Heat once inside the body, which explains the feverish episode that is typical in the externally contracted diseases.

When two or more pathogenic factors combine, their impact becomes much stronger, for example, cold-wind, or cold-damp-wind is known to be more aggressive than simple wind or a simple cold.

A particular *Xie Qi* is not only depending on the season but also on the condition; for example, Heat may cause disease not only in summer but in any season.

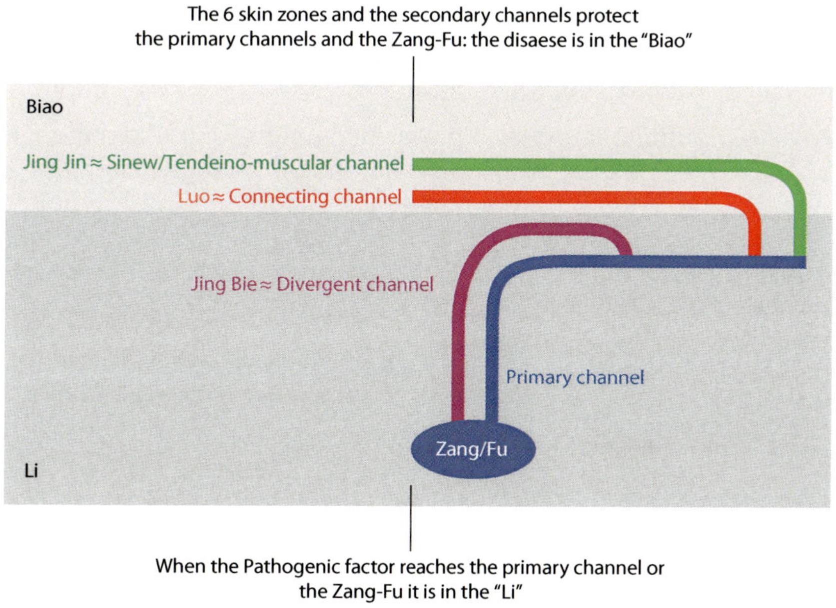

Figure 6.1 : *Biao-Li*; the protective layers of the body

Infections in Chinese Medicine

It is important here to discuss the concept of infectious diseases, as we understand them in the West. Every bacteria, fungus or virus, needs a particular milieu to grow and develop:

- Bacteria need a warm and humid milieu
- Viruses need either a warm and moist or a cold and moist atmosphere
- Fungi need a warm and moist surrounding

An "infection" does not occur only because there is the presence of a germ, but because there is a particular condition, for example, Damp-Heat, which is favorable to the growth of that particular microbe. Not every person exposed to a certain germ is going to be infected, only the ones that present the right conditions at the moment of contamination. If this condition is caused by the climate it is called "External", if it is due to a *Zang/Fu* disharmony it is classified as "Internal". This clearly demonstrates the limited action of antibiotics that only treat the incidental germ factor but not the real cause. Of course, when the infectious agent has penetrated into the Blood level directly, as is the case with AIDS or Hepatitis C or Borreliosis, the outer defenses are by-passed, and only the inherent strength of *Wei Qi* can make the difference.

It is not the bacteria causing a disease, but the disease that allows the pathogenic agent to inoculate.

In most cases, except for Wind, the manifestations of an externally or internally caused condition are quite similar; the differences reside in the evolution, the prognosis, and the treatment.

6.1 Feng ≈ Wind 风

Wind is the most mobile and erratic of the climatic forces, it is *Yang* in nature and mostly attacks the upper parts of the body, head, and neck, the eyes, and the nose.

Its mobility explains the acute onset and the erratic nature of the symptoms, such as moving pains, tics, and spasms, also quick emotional changes such as stress, irritability, and anger. Being *Yang* it harms mostly the Blood and the *Yin* of the body causing pruritis, dryness, and stiffness. Wind can associate with any of the other climatic factors, making them more mobile and more aggressive; it has been given the label of "Spearhead of *Xie Qi*" (► Fig. 6.2).

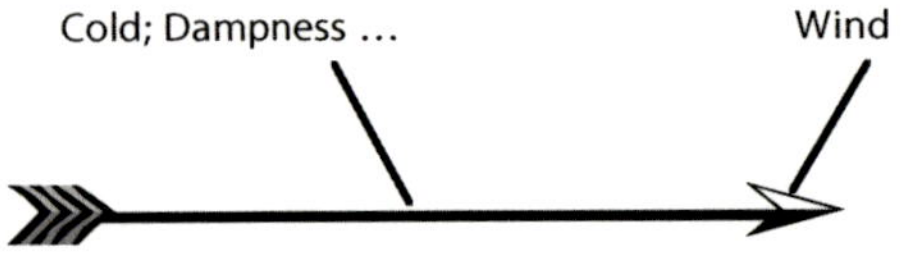

Figure 6.2: Wind facilitates the penetration of other Pathogenic factors

Wind is attached to the Wood phase and in general sensitivity to wind implies a Liver dysfunction.

Symptoms of External Wind

- Acute onset; dislike of wind or of cold
- Sneezing, rhinorrhea, stuffed nose, cough
- Itchy or a sore throat
- Headaches, neck and shoulder tensions
- Erratic joint pains as in acute rheumatoid arthritis
- Facial palsy
- Symptoms change according to PF combinations: Wind-Cold / Wind-Heat / Wind-Damp

Symptoms of Internal Wind

Internal Wind is very different in its manifestation, but has the suddenness and the mobility factor as with external wind:

- Trembling, spasms, tics, tinnitus, vertigo, convulsions,
- Itching,
- Visual spots,
- Paresthesia, loss of consciousness, stroke, hemiplegia.

In nature, the rising of warmer air currents produces wind, and depending on the suddenness and intensity of this air movement the wind may present as a breeze, strong wind, or even a hurricane or tornado. In the body, similarly, the rising of *Yang* towards the head produces Internal Wind, manifesting with mild tics or dizziness or more severe vertigo or even stroke.

Internal Wind always involves a Liver dysfunction. Liver Excess patterns (Liver-Fire, Liver-Heat, or Liver Qi stagnation), tend to produce Liver-Yang-rising and may result in Internal Wind. Liver Deficient patterns (Liver-Blood vacuity or Liver-Yin vacuity) may also produce a condition of Yang-rising and cause Internal Wind, although usually with less severe symptoms (▶ Fig. 6.3).

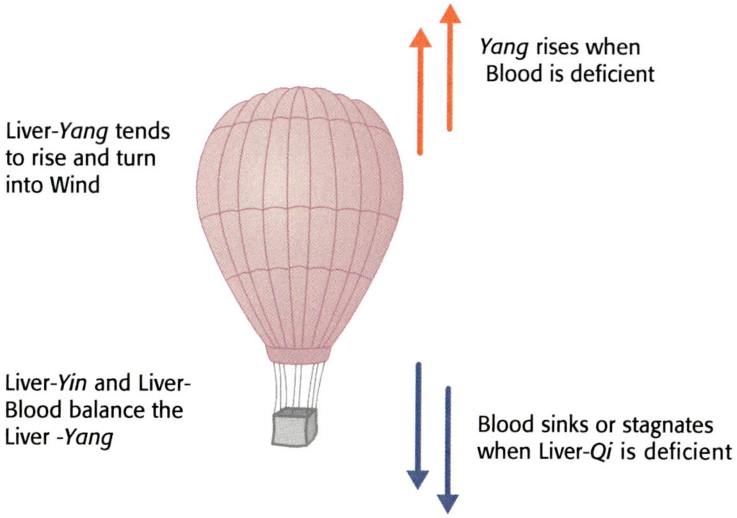

Figure 6.3: Internal Wind always involves a Liver dysfunction

6.2 Re ≈ Heat 热

Heat is *Yang* in nature, therefore, injures the *Yin*, in particular, the *Jin Ye* ≈ Body fluids and Blood. Heat accelerates all functions and tends to move upwards to the face and head and to disturb the *Shen* ≈ Spirit/mind. Heat corresponds to the Fire phase. Generally, the Heart and the Liver are most susceptible to Heat.

Symptoms of Heat

- Dislike of Heat, fever with perspiration,
- Headaches, mental agitation, insomnia,
- Dry and painful throat, dry mouth with intense thirst,
- Small amounts of dark urine
- Fast pulse

The sensitivity to external heat depends on the strength of the body's *Yin*.

Internal Heat is similar in manifestation and comes from the *Yin*-vacuity (deficiency) of the *Zang-Fu*; this condition is called "Empty-Heat", signifying that Heat is resulting from a deficient condition.

Organs that have plenty of *Yang-Qi* are more susceptible to produce Heat, for example, Liver, Heart, and Stomach.

6.3 Huo ≈ Fire 火

In Chinese medicine, Heat conditions that are more severe are classified as Fire. Heat warms whereas Fire burns and in particular damages the *Jin Ye ≈ Body* fluids and causes extreme dryness. Fire is also attached to the Fire phase.

Symptoms of Fire

Two symptoms differentiate Fire from Heat:

- Blood agitation: causing bleeding, or skin rashes
- Shen disturbance: insomnia, agitation, madness
- Other symptoms are more severe Heat signs, such as intense thirst, dry stools, various infections, and mouth ulcers

Fire results most often from the transformation of other external PF or from the aggravation of internal Heat.

6.4 Shi ≈ Dampness 湿/ Tan ≈ Phlegm 痰

Is *Yin* in nature and disturbs the *Yang* functions, especially Spleen-*Yang*. Its heavy and sticky nature makes it infiltrate and cause stagnation and slowing down. Dampness affects mostly the lower parts. Most diseases caused by Dampness become easily chronic. Dampness may be due to external climatic humidity or due to internal organic dysfunctions, mainly of the Spleen. Dampness is the climatic energy attached to the Earth phase.

Symptoms of Dampness

- Heavy head, cotton-like feeling in the head
- Heavy and achy limbs, numbness and rheumatism, edema, cellulitis;
- Body aches, fixed joint pains
- Chest oppression, excessive production of mucous and phlegm
- Abdominal fullness; bloating, knots in the stomach
- Vaginal discharge; turbid urine, soft stools
- Cysts, nodules, and tumors; wet type eczema
- Combined with Heat it provokes all kinds of infections.

Symptoms of Internal Dampness

Is due to the Spleen not transforming the fluids, the symptoms are quite similar to the above with the addition of:

- Sticky taste in the mouth, with no desire to drink
- A dull yellow complexion

Tan ≈ Phlegm/ Sputum 痰

Phlegm has the same nature as Dampness but is due only to internal causes, mainly the Kidney-*Yang* vacuity. Phlegm could also come from long-standing conditions of Dampness, or when Heat has injured the Body fluids. It is reputed that all complicated diseases involve Phlegm and that these conditions are very difficult to treat.

Phlegm is classified as:

- Visible Phlegm including all types of discharge; from the nose, the lungs, genitals, or the presence of mucous in the stool.
- Invisible Phlegm, which refers to most tumors and cysts, plum-pit feeling in the throat, arterial plaque (atheroma), joint calcifications or deformations; and a particular condition termed "Phlegm misting the Heart orifices", which includes a variety of sensory organ dysfunctions, mental disorientation, psychosis, and even coma.

6.5 Zao ≈ Dryness 燥

Dryness is *Yang* in nature and disturbs the *Yin*, in particular, the *Jin Ye* ≈ Body fluids and Blood. The Upper and Lower Source of fluids, the Lung and Kidney organs are the most sensitive to climatic Dryness, and to a lesser degree the Stomach that reacts to dietary dryness. External Dryness penetrates through the nose and the skin, whereas internal Dryness is due to the deficiency-vacuity of the *Jin Ye* ≈ Body fluids. Dryness is attached to the Metal phase.

Symptoms of Dryness

- Fever and thirst,
- A dry cough, maybe with bloody sputum, painful chest
- Anxiety
- A headache

Symptoms of Internal Dryness

- Dry skin and hair
- Reduced urine, constipation
- Emaciation

6.6 Han ≈ Cold 寒

Is *Yin* in nature and disturbs all the *Yang* functions, in particular, the Kidney-*Yang*. It slows down all functions and causes obstruction in the image of the rivers that freeze in wintertime. Internal Cold is due to a vacuity of *Yang*, in particular, Kidney-*Yang*. Cold is attached to the Water phase. Besides the Kidney-*Yang*, the Lung is quite susceptible to external Cold.

Symptoms of Cold

- Aversion to cold, chills that are not improved by heat
- In case of fever, there is no sweating and no thirst
- Clear and abundant mucous and urine,
- Diarrhea
- Intense joint pains
- Slow pulses

Symptoms of Internal Cold

- The symptoms are the same as for external Cold
- Except that the chills are improved by heat

7. Internal Causes of Disease

The internal causes of disease are the five Emotions "*Wu Zhi*" 五志and the seven Passions "*Qi Qing*"七情.

One of the originalities of Chinese medicine resides in its holistic understanding of the human being. By indicating the emotions as the only internal cause, an important emphasis is being put on two points:

- Emotions are internal and do not come from the outside, as one often tends to wrongly presume
- Emotional disturbances are the internal root of all disease and suffering

Physical and Psychological Health are interdependent

Certainly, these points were reinforced by the advent of Buddhist teachings, in which the source of human suffering is explained to be the ignorance of the four truths and inclination to the passions, in other words, one's attachments and emotional reactions to the world and to the outer changes.

In the Chinese concept, the *Zang-Fu* system, as a functional unit has three spheres of action: physical, energetic and emotional- mental. This is represented by the notion of the "3 Treasures": *Jing* ≈ Essence, *Qi* ≈ Energy and *Shen* ≈ Spirit/mind.

The *Jing* ≈ Essence of each organ is the base of, not only its physical form but also of its energetic, emotional and mental expressions.

The basic program of the body is the "Will to live" in order to fulfill ones "*Ming*" ≈ Mandate of life. The specific movement of *Qi* in each *Zang* ≈ Organ is the expression of its "Will". When this strength is used to satisfy the desires (passions) then it becomes an emotion. For example, the ability to move forward is the modality of Liver-*Qi*

- When it is balanced = there is no emotion
- When excessive = there is "Anger"; this could be explained by the Liver's potential, to be diverted into passions, irritability, and anger instead of being expressed through movement and creativity.

Emotions are the modifications of the Spirit in reaction to changes in the environment. They are necessary for the normal functioning of the organism, thus they are named the "Five emotions" in continuity with the "Five Moving forces". Emotion is considered the driving force behind motivation. When a particular emotion becomes harmful then it is classified as a "passion". Although Western psychology enumerates numerous types of emotion, the ancient Chinese symbolically classified the harmful emotions as the "Seven passions". The number seven is the symbolic number for the aging process and for destruction. Modern science is exploring the neuro-humoral factors involved in emotions. Although it is still not clear if a particular chemistry produces an emotion or vice versa, the physiological effects of emotions and their impact on health and disease are indisputable today. On this point, the ancient Chinese had a very deep understanding by delegating the inner causes of disease to emotional factors and by analyzing the physiological impact of each emotion.

In Classical Chinese medicine (CCM), emotions are believed to cause disease if they are not adapted to external changes:

- Excessive emotion
- Repressed emotion
- Unadapted emotion

Each emotion relates to one of the "5 moving forces", and is the non-physical manifestation of the corresponding organ. They are considered *Yang* as opposed to other organic functions. But in relation to one another, some emotions are classified as *Yang*, such as anger or elation, as opposed to sadness and fear, which are considered *Yin*.

- An excessive emotion harms the corresponding organ and may transform into Fire.
- Disharmony of the *Zang-Fu* may produce an emotional disturbance (excess or insufficient). This emotional disturbance may further aggravate the organ disharmony, thus producing a vicious circle.
- **All emotions ultimately affect the Heart-emperor, residence of *Shen***
- In general *Yang* type emotions manifest more easily in *Yang* conditions:
- *Yang* Excess/ repletion
- *Qi* or *Yang* stagnation
- *Yin*, Blood or *Jin Ye* deficiency/ vacuity
- *Yin*-type emotions appear more easily in *Yin* conditions:
- *Qi* or *Yang* deficiency/ vacuity
- *Yin* Excess/ repletion
- Sometimes in *Qi* stagnation
- In practice three organs are most affected by emotions:
- The Heart governs the Spirit "*Shen*", and thus regulates all the other emotions.
- The Liver is in charge of defence and of immediate adaptability, but also draining and de-congesting, in other words releasing the emotional accumulations.
- The Spleen is in charge of transforming the essence of food, but also of the processing “digesting” of the emotions and thoughts.

7.1 Anger ≈ Nu 怒

The liver produces anger that should be understood as reactivity, or a defensive mechanism, which also happens to be the mobile force behind enthusiasm, passion, competition, and decisiveness.

Pathologically, anger includes a variety of manifestations: rage, irritability, frustration, repressed anger, hate, bitterness etc.

Liver disharmonies produce anger:

- Liver-*Qi* stagnation or Liver-*Yang* rising or Liver-Fire produce an explosive anger
- Liver-Blood vacuity produces irritability and frustration
- Liver-*Qi* stagnation causes repressed anger
- On the other hand, excessive anger harms the Liver, producing:
- Liver-*Qi* stagnation or Liver-Blood stagnation;
- Liver-*Yang* rising or Liver-Fire.

Effects of Anger

Anger is extremely *Yang* in nature, and similarly to Wind, causes *Qi* to rise to the head, producing Heat and Fire symptoms:

- Dizziness, vertigo, tinnitus, which are manifestations of Wind
- Headaches, red face and neck, bitter taste and red tongue, signs of Heat
- Nosebleeds, agitation of the spirit, signifying the transformation into Fire
- Also produces a greenish complexion, a wiry pulse, and red tongue sides

Liver *Qi* stagnation very often over-controls the Earth (*Ke* ≈ Control cycle) and harms the Spleen and Stomach causing gastritis, and fatigue.

It may also insult Metal (*Wu* ≈ Insult cycle), causing Lung counter-flow *Qi* with asthma and wheezing.

Repressed anger may even manifest as an apparent chronic depression with a red and dry tongue and a tight pulse, versus real depression due to the Lung where the pulse would be weak.

7.2 Joy/ Elation ≈ Lè/ Xĭ Lè乐/ 喜乐

The Heart produces Joy and contentment. Joy is a reflection of a harmonious state of *Qi*, it calms *Shen* and *Qi*, dilates the vessels, improving the circulation in the brain helping memory and easing the communication with the world. Joy further harmonizes *Ying* and *Wei Qi* and protects against illness. Joy is *Yang* in nature and attached to the expansive movement of the Fire phase.

Effects of Joy:

Pathologically too much excitement or pleasure, harms the Heart and disperses the *Qi* outwards, causing excessive communication (talkativeness), and may produce:

- Heart-Fire or Pericardium-Fire
- Heart-*Yin* or Heart-Blood vacuity

A Heart disharmony can produce excessive or insufficient excitement:

- Heart-Fire produces over excitement: hysterical laughter
- Heart-*Qi* or Heart-*Yang* vacuity produces sadness and crying

Excessive craving or desire produces PE-Fire and vice versa.

7.3 Worry/pensiveness ≈ Si 思

The Spleen is responsible for planning and caring, and provides the Heart with accurate information "*Yi* ≈ Thought"

A Spleen disharmony produces worry:

- Spleen-*Qi* vacuity produces mental asthenia with memory and concentration problems.
- A chronic stagnation of Spleen-*Qi* gives rise to obsessions, worrying and fixed ideas.

Effects of Worry and obsession

Excessive thinking and worrying harm the Spleen by knotting and depleting its *Qi*, harming the Lung and the Heart

- *Qi* stagnation in the chest and the breasts
- Spleen-*Qi* stasis, food stasis, Stomach-Heat (ulcers)
- Yellowish-grey color; slippery or tight pulse
- Worry about the future, also affects the Lung *Qi*

7.4 Sadness/ sorrow ≈ Bei 悲/ Ai哀

The Lung produces sadness, which could be broadened to include sensitivity, perception, being in touch and the capacity for introspection. Sadness gathers *Qi* inwards, is *Yin* in nature and attached to the Metal phase.

Lung-*Qi* vacuity produces sadness, melancholy or future worry and a sense of anxiety. Prolonged sadness produces grief.

Effects of Sadness

Excessive or prolonged sadness harms the Lung, preventing its *Qi* from descending, as well as the Heart, causing loss of communication and joy. Sadness blocks the upper Triple Warmer and the circulation of *Ying* ≈ Nourishing and *Wei* ≈ Defensive *Qi*. The Lung in its function of "Master of *Qi*", is affected by sadness producing:

- Depression
- Fatigue
- Shortness of breath
- Short and weak pulse in both distal "*Cun*" positions
- In women, sadness may cause Liver- Blood-*Xu*≈ Vacuity
- Unexpressed sadness (loss of joy) may affect the Kidneys, causing a loss of will to live with suicidal tendencies.

7.5 Oppression ≈ You 憂/ Chou You 愁憂

Oppression is linked to grief and represents a condition of lack of circulation, of contraction and immobilization, causing weakness of Blood and *Qi* and ultimately producing a *Yang-Qi* vacuity.

Effects of Oppression

- Oppression is usually related to the Lung, in particular, LU-*Qi Xu* with shortness of breath and a weak cough.
- It may affect the Heart causing HE-*Qi Xu* or HE-*Yin Xu*, with mental tiredness, palpitations, agitation, insomnia, and amnesia.
- When it affects the Spleen and Stomach, it disrupts transformation and transportation, causing reduced appetite, bloating, weakness of the four limbs and injury to *Yi*≈ Thought.
- It can even affect the Liver causing Liver-*Qi* stasis

7.6 Fear ≈ Kong 恐/ Kong Ju 恐懼 (惧)

The Kidneys produce fear, anxiety, and apprehension, allowing for the spirit to adjust the true capacities of the person to the willpower and drive.

Kidney disharmonies often produce fear:

- Kidney-*Qi* vacuity produces fearfulness and indecision
- Kidney-*Yin* vacuity causes an apparent Kidney-*Yang* repletion with manifestations of temerity and authoritativeness.

Effects of Fear

Fear and chronic anxiety damage the Kidneys:

- Excessive or sudden fear produce a Kidney-*Qi Xu* and separate the *Qi* from the *Jing*, causing the *Jing* to descend to the lower TW, with the weakness of the lower orifices; and the *Qi* to rise to the upper TW producing palpitations and panic attacks
- Chronic anxiety depletes the Kidney-*Yin* resulting in *Yang* rising causing hot flushes, tinnitus, vertigo, night sweating, palpitations, and a malar flush.

7.7 Shock/Fright ≈ Jing 驚

Shock can be excessive or sudden fear or even sudden joy.

A chronic deficiency of Kidney and Heart-*Yin* may produce a propensity to be easily startled.

Effects of Shock

Emotional or mental shock can scatter the *Qi*, causing a sudden depletion of Kidney essence and of Heart *Qi*:

- Palpitations
- Insomnia
- Other “Empty-Heat” symptoms
- Fast and moving pulse
- A white face; or in children, a bluish tinged forehead, or the chin if the shock has been pre-natal.

7.8 Other Emotions

- Hatred is like anger but also affects the Heart
- Jealousy and desire, as well as obsessive and possessive love, affect the Heart and Pericardium.
- Guilt, like sadness or repressed anger, affects the Heart and Kidney, causing *Qi* to stagnate or to sink.

8. Other Causes of Disease (Half internal – half external)

8.1 Constitution

The importance of the impact of constitution on the capacity to adapt to the external changes and to resist pathogenic factors seems obvious.

Constitution depends on the Pre-Heaven energies:

- *Yuan* ≈ Source *Qi* together with the inherited *Jing* ≈ Essence defines the life expectancy,
- *Jing* ≈ Essence of the parents at the moment of conception has a very important impact on the constitution. The ancient Chinese concept of *Jing* may be equated to the modern science of genetics and the chromosomic transmission.
- *Zong* ≈ Ancestral *Qi* of the mother during the pregnancy has an important influence on the *Zong Qi* of the child. The notion of *Zong Qi* is not easily explained from a Western point of view, although the recent understanding about epigenetics seem to coincide quite well with the ancient Chinese concepts.

These points explain why in ancient times in China, great emphasis was put on the parents' health and lifestyle, in order to provide the best *Jing* and *Zong* for the child. The combination of these factors defines the constitution and may be calculated from the birth time and date.

Although each constitution seems to be quite pre-determined and fixed, it may nevertheless be maintained or even improved by a moderate lifestyle and exercise, or on the contrary harmed by an inappropriate lifestyle, by accidents or by repeated shocks. Two constitutional types are more often exposed to weakness, with many childhood diseases:

- Metal constitution: with Lung *Qi* deficiency, tuberculosis and whooping cough in the family; often presenting thoracic deformity, scoliosis, displaced front pulse and cracks on the font area of the tongue.
- Kidney constitution: with a tendency to numerous diseases and infections; often presenting small ears and various growth problems.

Again it is fundamental to underline that it is not the strength of the constitution, the genetic structure or "genotype", that guarantees a long and healthy life, but rather the correct lifestyle. How the gene will manifest itself throughout its lifetime, what is known as "phenotype" depends entirely on other factors.

According to the recent "epigenetic" research, there are certain factors that will either block or enhance the "expression" of a particular gene. These factors are not entirely inherited and may be greatly influenced by environmental and personal inputs. Lifestyle, diet, the environment, and in particular belief systems and thoughts and emotions, seem to play a crucial role in the behavior of a particular gene. The mechanism by which a particular gene will be activated or not, is transmitted equally and coded in the terminal sections of the DNA helix, a section that had previously been considered to have no importance as it did not carry the genetic information. The Chinese notion of Ancestral energy, is referring to a from of transmitted information from the ancestors, but which is greatly dependent on external as well as personal influences.

This is the concept of "Nature" versus "Nurture".

8.2 Diet

Diet is a fundamental element of health. The circulating *Qi*, in particular, the *Ying* ≈ Nourishing and *Wei* ≈ Defensive *Qi*, greatly depend on the quality of food, water, and air. The *Gu Qi* ≈ Food essence is a reflection of the *Jing* ≈ Essence of each food product. The more a food product is processed or altered, the less *Jing* it has. As a general rule, any food product that can reproduce life, such as whole grain seeds, sprouts or eggs, are richer in *Jing*, than foods that are inert. On the other hand, the richer *Jing* requires more work for the system to digest.

Diet can be a cause of disease:

- Insufficient nutrition leads to malnutrition, resulting in a deficiency of *Qi*, Blood, Stomach, and Spleen;
- Excessive eating harms the Stomach and Intestines causing food stasis, and depletes Spleen-*Qi*;
- Excess of raw or cold foods causes Spleen-*Yang* vacuity;
- Excess of fats or sweets harms the Spleen and causes Dampness or Damp-Heat;
- Excess of spices causes Stomach-Heat or Liver-Heat;
- Excess of one of the Five Tastes harms the *Qi* of the corresponding *Zang* ≈ Organ;
- Irregular eating, or eating too fast or under stress, or eating while doing something else, cause Stomach-*Yin* vacuity.

8.3 Fatigue

Health depends on a balance between activity and rest.

The normal activity uses the Post-Heaven *Qi* produced by Spleen and Stomach, in particular, the *Ying Qi*. In the case of over-exertion, energy is drawn from the reserves of *Jing Qi*. Lack of sufficient rest and sleep or poor quality of sleep put the system in a condition of *Yin* deficiency, resulting in the well-known modern-day condition of "burn out".

Sleep is as necessary to life as air, food, and water.

Sleep difficulty, in particular, insomnia, is a rapidly increasing modern day problem, affecting almost 40% of the population of industrialized societies.

- Excessive physical fatigue: depletes the Spleen *Qi*
- Excessive mental fatigue: depletes the Spleen and Stomach and then the Kidneys.
- Repetitive movements cause stagnation of *Qi* in the corresponding area leading to tendinitis, or organ taxation (*Wu Lao* ≈ Five Taxations五勞):
  - An excessive lifting of heavy weights or excessive standing taxes the Kidneys;
  - Excessive exercise taxes the Liver and harms the muscles;
  - Overuse of the eyes taxes the Heart Blood;
  - Too much lying down weakens the Lung *Qi*;
  - Too much sitting taxes the Spleen;

However insufficient exercise also causes disease by producing stagnation of *Qi* and increasing the risk of the accumulation of Dampness and Phlegm.

8.4 Sexual Activity

In chapter 1 of the *Nei Jing*, many of the wrong ways of living and eating as well as sexual activity are mentioned. Most of the older Chinese texts underline excessive sexual activity and the loss of *Jing* as a major causative factor for a disease. I do not believe this to be true in the modern world, although inappropriate sexual activity is still of actuality.

Sexual energy depends primarily on the Kidney *Qi*, but all the other organs also participate by contributing the appropriate emotional energy involved in satisfactory intercourse.

Sexual desire depends on Kidney-*Qi* and Kidney-*Yang*, The sexual act depends on the balance of the *Yin* and *Yang* of the Kidneys. Erection also is dependent on Liver-Blood.

Orgasm depends on Kidney-*Jing*, in women it also depends on Blood. Men lose an important amount of Kidney *Jing* through ejaculation, whereas women lose it to a lesser degree through menstruation but much more through multiple pregnancies and childbirths. So it is not sexual activity per se, but the rather excessive loss of *Jing*, in the form of sperm in men, which is taxing and may cause disease. Still, this has entirely to do with the constitution of the person and has to be adapted to age and to the season. Roughly the frequency of ejaculation in men is calculated by dividing the age of the person by 5 (i.e. a 50-year old man should not ejaculate more than once every 10 days). This frequency is of course very dependent on the individual constitution.

In women, sexual activity and orgasm do not have the same taxing effect.

The saying goes that one-drop of sperm equals a hundred drops of Blood.

Excessive loss of *Jing* weakens Kidney-*Qi* and especially Kidney-*Yin*, producing lumbar aches, frequent urination, fatigue, dizziness etc.

In modern times the inopportune hormonal stimulations for infertility are also causing a weakening of *Jing*.

All Kidney disharmony patterns may produce sexual problems:

- Lack of desire,
- Impotence and erectile problems, frigidity,
- Premature ejaculation, spermatorrhoea

Insufficient sexual activity and abstinence, especially if the sexual energy is not adequately transformed, may cause stagnation of *Jing*.

Unsatisfactory sex, when there is an absence of tenderness or orgasm, may also be a source of imbalance and disease.

8.5 Trauma

Wounds, fractures, dislocations, sprains, and contusions cause stagnation of *Qi* and of Blood in the afflicted area, manifesting with:

- Pain
- Swelling
- Ecchymosis (Haematoma/bruising)

In severe cases, Blood loss might lead to Blood vacuity.

The consequences are immediate and local, but can also be more secondary and may have implications in the future.

The degree of damage has to do not only with the strength of the impact but also with the training and resistance of the person and the amount of *Wei Qi* concentrated on the surface. In many forms of martial arts, the adept trains to increase the flow of *Wei Qi* to the sinews and to the surface.

Two of the Spleen's functions are to nourish the flesh and to maintain Blood in the blood vessels. Thus in Spleen-*Qi* vacuity, there is a propensity to vascular fragility and easy bruising.

8.6 Parasites and Germs

Parasites are dependent on dietary hygiene and equilibrium.

For example, an excess of oily and sweet foods produces Damp-Heat and is favorable for the development of intestinal worms.

Infections due to fungus and protozoa, also need predisposing conditions such as Damp-Heat.

The modern day concept of bacterial, viral and fungal infections can be easily attached to the ancient category of parasites in general.

As discussed in the "External Causes", all germs and parasites need a specific milieu for developing. Bacteria need a Hot and Damp condition to cause infectious diseases, whereas viruses may require more often a Cold and Damp condition, as in certain seasonal flu epidemics.

8.7 Poisons

The significance of "poison" has changed since the ancient times, nowadays actual poisoning is rare, but accidental poisoning more and more common, including chemical additives, pesticides, heavy metals, toxic fumes, industrial by-products, etc.

8.8 Radiation

Not known to the ancients, radiation has become a modern world problem. Mankind has to learn to adapt to a world exposed to all kinds of radiation: nuclear, solar (ultraviolet), medical (gamma rays), laser rays, domestic exposures to quartz batteries, cathodic tubes, microwaves, electromagnetic waves and so on. Radiations, even when weak in intensity, have known cumulative effects and should be taken into consideration.

The Liver has the charge of detoxifying the system, and the accumulated toxins will produce Liver-Heat.

The strongest impact of most types of radiations, is on the Kidney-*Jing*, affecting the brain and the marrow, and causing infertility but also possibly affecting the brain matter.

8.9 Telluric Forces

Well known to the Chinese, these influences are considered an important cause of health or disease, success, and fortune etc. The study of the earth's geomagnetic currents are not really classified as a cause of disease but part of a specialty called "Feng Shui" ≈ Wind and Water (►chap. 26). These factors are more and more recognized and known in our days and should be considered in medical practice. Although there is no actual treatment for them, there are many methods of correction that can be recommended.

8.10 Iatrogenic Factors

As early as the 2nd century AD, beginning with the *Shang Han Lun*, diagnostic and therapeutic errors and their consequences had been discussed, and therapeutic mistakes were included in the analysis of the causes of disease, especially concerning wrong herbal treatments.

It is very unfortunate that today, in the most advanced societies the cause of mortality by iatrogenic factors has rapidly taken the third or even the second position.

These factors include the adverse effect of drugs, therapeutic complications, drug interactions, medical errors or negligence; to which can be added the propensity to "over-treat", a tendency that already Hippocrates was cautioning against in the 4th century BC. In fact, recent investigations have revealed that a great number of elderly patients in hospice care have been prescribed up to 12 to 15 different drugs at one time. I do not believe that any professor of pharmacology could predict the combined effects of such a chemical cocktail on a person's physiology.

The effects of Western medicines, which are mostly synthetic molecules, may be energetically evaluated as producing Liver-Heat through their accumulation in the Liver, and subsequently Blood-Heat. But then each drug has its own energetic nature and has to be individually taken into consideration; for example:

- Antibiotics are Cold in nature and produce Cold in the Spleen, Blood-Xu and internal Wind, Liver-*Yang* rising or Stomach-*Yin* vacuity;
- Contraceptives produce Liver-*Qi* stagnation, Liver-*Yang* rising, Blood stagnation, Blood-vacuity, and Blood-Heat;
- Steroids are *Yang* in nature and produce *Yin* deficiency of Stomach and Lungs, Blood-vacuity and depletion of Kidney-*Jing*;
- Tranquilizers: depress the *Yang*, harm Spleen-*Qi*, affect the *Yi* ≈Thought/ intellect and disrupt Liver-*Qi*.

8.11 Harmful Spirits (Gui 鬼)

The concept of *Gui* was probably a leftover of the earlier beliefs that all disease was due to harmful spirits. The Chinese notion of *Gui* ≈ Ghost refers to apparently unexplained or inappropriate reactions to outer stimuli without a coherent explanation. Today this could be extended to include any unconscious conditioning, hypnosis, phobias, behavioral neurosis, many so-called psychosomatic diseases, and of course in most psychotic manifestations. An appropriate term for *Gui* could be an "un-named energy mass", due to unresolved issues causing an energetic disturbance.

Both *Hun* ≈ Ethereal soul and *Po* ≈ Corporeal soul contain the radical *Gui* in their ideograms:

The mechanism of Gui

Normally mental activity depends on the consciousness of Shen ≈ Spirit/ mind, integrating all inputs, which are then analyzed and classified by *Yi* ≈ Thought/ intellect to be stored by *Zhi*. When *Shen* is disconnected, as is the case in sleep, hypnosis, coma, or in certain intense traumatic conditions or high fevers, *Hun* ≈ Ethereal soul and *Po* ≈ Corporeal soul take over and store the memories. Therefore Yi-intellect does not analyze the sensory input anymore.

As *Hun* ≈ Ethereal soul and *Po* ≈ Corporeal soul do not analyze the experience, the memory is stored in its integrity, and when recalled or re-activated, the person will experience the whole event as though it was occurring right then and there. These unexplained and apparently illogical responses are referred to as *Gui* ≈ Ghost in Chinese medicine (► Fig. 8.1).

- *Hun* stores impressions and emotions, producing "Behavioural *Gui*"
- *Po* stores physical sensations and pain, the cause of "Somatic *Gui*"

There are two categories of *Gui*:

- Individual *Gui* due to personal un-resolved issues
- Collective *Gui*, due to social, ethnic or racial conditioning

During dreaming process, the Liver through the offices of *Hun* attempts to release many of the unresolved issues.

More serious conditions may be treated with acupuncture, although needles alone without proper psychotherapeutic support seem quite often insufficient.

The Modern significance of "Gui"

The role of the Heart as the residence of *Shen* was covered in Part II, chapter 3.3. The concept of *Shen* itself was described in Chapter 4.4, in particular the breakdown of the Psyche according to the Jungian model in relation to the "Five Spirits": *Shen, Yi, Zhi, Hun* and *Po* are demonstrated in Figure 4.10.

The human "Psyche" is made of a conscious part, that we can refer to as the *Shen* aspect of the whole mind, and

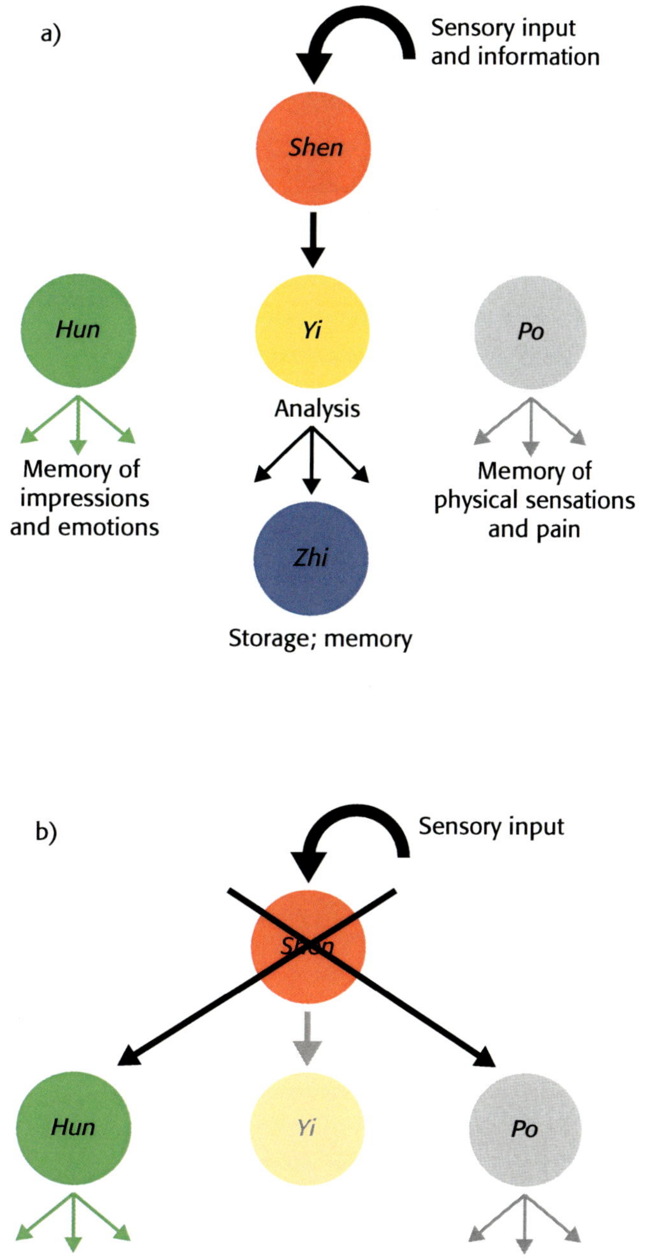

Figure 8.1 ***Shen, Yi*** **and** ***Zhi*** **deal with analysis and memory processing of all input. In the absence of** ***Shen, Hun*** **and** ***Po*** **store emotions, sensations and pain.**

an unconscious part, including the sub-conscious. The unconscious functions of the mind represent 9/10ths of the total workings of the mind. This includes the neuro-humoral functions, primarily but not exclusively represented by the sympathetic and parasympathetic nervous systems. Thoughts, feelings and emotions which modulate these systems are the results of constitution, temperament, conditioning and belief systems (▶Chapters 10.3 and 10.4). For example, an encounter with a wild animal or a reptile, often provokes an ancestral reaction of fear and a fight or flight response (sympathetic and adrenergic response), unless the person was born and raised in a tropical jungle with a daily exposure to these hasards. When a similar adrenergic reaction is manifested towards an inoucuous animal or object, it is termed a phobic reaction, and in the Chinese medical concepts a "*Gui*". In general any inappropriate, response to an outer situation may be considered a *Gui.*

Medically speaking the *Gui* can include many neurotic or psychotic conditions and even certain allergies. The concept may be extended to the following pathologies:

- Rejections
- Phobias
- Psychosomatic diseases
- Obsessive-compulsive disorders (OCD) including the OCD personality disorder
- Post Traumatic Stress Disorders (PTSD)
- Bipolar and Scizophrenic conditions
- More severe psychotic conditions

Classical Chinese Medicine has proposed a number of treatment strategies to deal with *Gui.* Although for the more serious conditions acupuncture alone, without an appropriate psychotherapeutic support, is quite insufficient

Part IV- Diagnosis in Chinese Medicine

9. Aim and purpose of Chinese Diagnosis

The central axis of Chinese medical practice is the diagnostic concept. Chinese diagnosis is in many ways similar to the Western approach of critical analysis and logical reasoning leading to a grouping of signs and symptoms into a specific disease context. The main difference resides in the approach modality. The Western diagnosis relies on internal investigations, laboratory and X-ray or EMR findings, or even some more invasive methods, whereas Chinese diagnosis emanates from the same concept of microcosm being in the image of the macrocosm, and that external signs and symptoms are reflective of internal, organic dysfunctions.

[...] all which is within, manifests without,
to know the within, observe the without. *Zhu Zheng Hen*

9.1 "Four Pillars" of Diagnosis

In order to gather the necessary information and reach a diagnosis, classically four diagnostic stages are described, known as the "Four Pillars" of diagnosis:

- **To observe:** includes the analysis of the morphology and movements, face, hands, colours, and the tongue
- **To smell:** the body's smells and eliminations
- **To listen:** to the voice and the sounds of breathing as well as asking questions and conducting a full anamnesis
- **To touch:** the taking of the pulses, palpation of various body zones and acupuncture points

It was classically agreed that a "superior" doctor needed only to observe in order to recognize the disease, an "average" physician, needed to listen as well, whereas an "inferior" physician also had to touch the patient to arrive at a diagnosis. This statement reflects a period in which examination of the body, especially that of women was considered a taboo, hence the emergence of numerous diagnostic modalities based on observation. Palpation methods of diagnosis, except for pulse taking, were not extremely popular in China, although they became quite developed in Japan.

It is the synthesis of the four stages that constitute the Chinese diagnosis and not isolated signs or symptoms.

The aim of diagnosis is to define three points:

- The "site" of the disease, that is the channel, body layer or system that has been affected;

- The "causative" factor, either external, wind-heat-cold..., or internal emotions or mixed causes such as constitutional weakness, life-style errors or dietary excess...;
- To establish the general "condition" of the person, which would elucidate the dysfunction of the system that has permitted the causative factor to produce a disease; for example, an internal weakness of *Yang*, causing a susceptibility to external cold, leading to the contraction of cold in Winter-time; or an emotional repression, causing Liver-*Qi* stasis, producing migraine headaches.

This diagnostic approach was commonly referred to as "Branch-Knot and Root", in the image of a tree, where the visible leaves and branches are compared to where the disease manifests and where the symptoms are apparent (▶ chap. 5, Fig. 5.1). The Knot is the area the branches come together, representing the causative factor. The Root, often hidden, is the true condition or the underlying internal cause of the disease.

In modern TCM, with the ascendance of herbal medicine over acupuncture, the identification of organ patterns has taken fundamental importance, whereas the more ancient, classical medical approach was primarily channel oriented.

With the further development and integration of the "correspondence system" of the "five phases" in medicine, signs, and symptoms gathered by the four diagnostic stages, colors, smells and sounds, could be attached to a specific phase and organ system. Furthermore, as each part of the body reflects the whole, special diagnostic methods were developed over the years, such as pulse, tongue, face, iris, ear, and abdominal diagnosis.

9.2 Three levels of Diagnosis, Three Levels of Treatment

The concept of Branch, Knot, and Root automatically leads to three therapeutic strategies.

Treating the "Branch" or symptom for which the patient is consulting, is very similar to prescribing a painkiller for a headache, an antibiotic for an infection or a sleeping pill for insomnia. The ancient Chinese would consider this as inferior medical practice.

Treating the causative factor, the "Knot", is already a step in the right direction.

But understanding and treating the "Root" of a disease is the domain of a superior physician and constitutes the true art of Chinese medicine and all other "Holistic" practices (▶ Fig. 9.1).

In the West, disease, and death are considered number one enemies of the doctor, whereas the Daoists understood the disease nemesis to actually be a call for health. The hidden root of a disease is the key for true healing. It is always important to keep in mind that a superior physician treats a patient and not the disease. What the disease represents for the patient is an individual process, and for profound healing to occur, the patient has to understand and connect to the deeper ramifications. The Daoist would say that in order to treat a disease one has to first name it, then own it, and only after that can it be treated. This means that a patient has first to put the correct label on their suffering, i.e. to state that there is angina caused by a staph infection, is only to define the site and the cause of the problem. The root of the disease resides in the person who is suffering. It is not for the physician to give the label, for example stating: "... you have an issue with your job, family, etc.", it is for the patient to discover the link, and only then deep healing can take place.

The art of Chinese diagnosis lies in discovering these hidden roots, and the true art of a healer is to shed light on these deep recesses and gently bring the patient to hear their inner call for help and to empower the person in making the changes that are necessary for them to heal.

Please refer to the end of part IV, chapter 15 for an overview and discussion on a comprehensive approach to diagnosis.

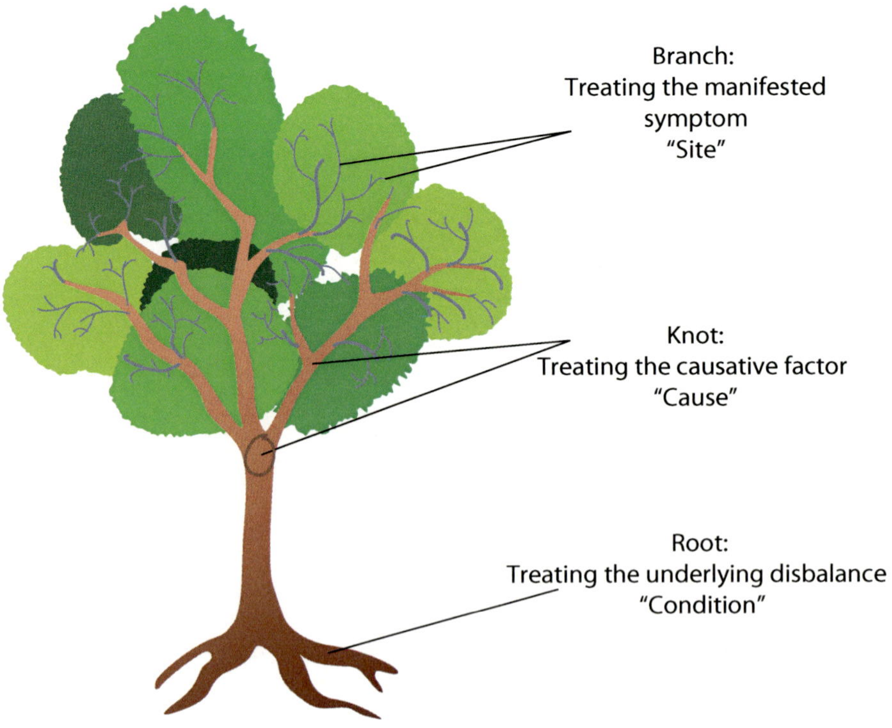

Figure 9.1: Treating the Site, Cause and Condition

10. Observation

[...] Through the outer reflection is recognized the inner organ,
and thus is known the disease. *Ling Shu, chap.47*

10.1 General Observation

Facial Expression, Shen

The "*Shen*" is the outer manifestation of the vital activity of the body as well as the mental state of the person.

It is in the eyes that is concentrated the *Jing Qi* of the organs, the eyes are the "outer orifice" of the Liver, and the "envoy" of the Heart and they communicate with the brain.

The *Shen* is conserved in the Heart and thus it is reflected in the eyes. The brightness of the eyes "*Yan Shen*" will inform on the vital activity, mental state, co-ordination capacity of the person, therefore constituting a good means of evaluating the overall strength of the patient and the intensity of the disease.

3 situations are possible:

- **Strong Shen:**
  - Eyes are lively and bright or sparkling
  - General health is good, the state of consciousness and speech are clear
  - Breathing and movements are regular
  - Facial color is bright

A strong *Shen* denotes a strong *Jing Qi*, and even if the disease is serious the prognosis is usually good.

It is interesting to note that the liveliness and brightness observed in children is a sign of the child's strong vital energy, the same brilliance in an older patient is more a reflection of the strength of their spirit.

- **Loss of Shen:**
  - The eyes are dull with a fixed look
  - There is general apathy with slow reactions or abnormal movements
  - Breathing is irregular
  - Facial color is dull

The lack of *Shen* denotes a loss of *Zheng* ≈ Upright *Qi*, in this case, the prognosis is usually not good.

- **False Shen:**
  - Observed in chronic and severe diseases: the eyes, facial color, voice, and physical and mental conditions all suddenly improve. This is often announcing the improvement before the end.
  - False *Shen* could also be observed in mentally deranged patients: the eyes have an almost abnormal brilliance. The gaze could be fixed, almost threatening, or uncontrolled and darting movement of the eyes, which is considered even more severe, especially if the white of the eye is showing on the four sides (▶ Fig. 10.13.d).

The Eye's gaze "*Jing Ming*": reflects also the constitution

- Direct gaze: Wood constitution
- Sparkling: Fire constitution
- Warm, supportive: Earth constitution
- Dreamy, hopeless: Metal constitution
- Mysterious, seductive: Water constitution

Shape and color of the face

In diagnosis, the face can reveal on the one hand the inherited strengths and weaknesses as well as the characteristics of a person and on the other hand organ dysfunctions.

In general, the facial form is a reflection of the constitution and will usually correspond to the dominant element. To determine the constitutional morphotype of a person, it is necessary to consider not only the shape of the face but also the body form and the shape of the hands. Chinese astrologers would analyze the time of birth to determine the influence of *Tian* ≈ Heaven on a person. In general, the year would inform on the predominant Extraordinary vessel, the month on the *Luo* ≈ Connecting channel, when day and time would inform on the Primary channels. In this manner, the strengths and weaknesses of a person are established. The *Ming* ≈ Destiny of the person is further analyzed by studying the lines of the hands and particularly the shape of the face and that of the ears. The presence of moles and lines are important indicators.

Analysis according to the facial form

During the fetal stage, it is believed that the *Ling Po* ≈ Corporeal Soul, *Ling Hun* ≈ Ethereal Soul – and the Individual Spirit – Little *Shen*, descend via the fontanel and DM-20 and influence the development of the facial anatomy, thus sculpting the face. In this manner, the Wood influence would manifest itself in the area of the forehead, the Fire would develop the cheekbones, the Earth would influence the chin area and the Metal energy would concentrate in the nose. The Water action would be seen in the ears. The final facial shape is the interaction and combination of these pre-natal energies.

Please note that this “Pre-Heaven” elemental influence is very different from the Five Element and organ correspondence (▶ Fig. 10.4) as described in the *Su Wen* and currently used in diagnosis.

Therefore the face is first analyzed according to its basic shape in relation to the Five Elements. For the description of the basic Five constitution types see chapter 10.2.

Most often people will present variations and combinations of these forms. In “Chinese Face Reading” the character of a person is reflected in the face(▶ Fig. 10.1, and Table 10.2).

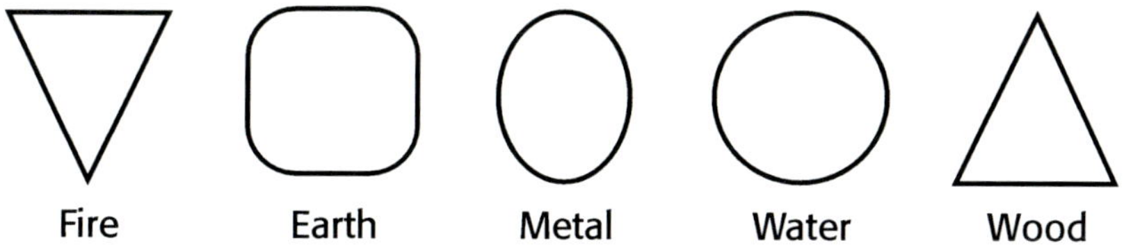

Figure 10.1 : Face shapes in relation to the Five Elements

Table 10.1 Examples of "Chinese Face Reading"

For example the trapezoid shape would combine qualities of Fire and Earth, giving the Fire more practical and realistic tendencies. L. Bridges associates this form with performers and inventors.	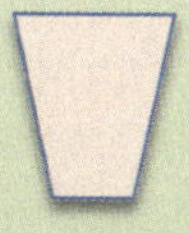
The inverted trapezoid combines qualities of Wood and Earth, and would confer to the fixity of Earth, the competitive and aggressive qualities of Wood, making the personality goal oriented and domineering. L. Bridges defines this shape as the dictator and hedonist.	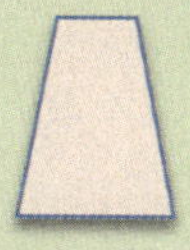
The rectangular face, combines the qualities of Earth and Metal, practical, non-emotional and secondary, thinking before they act; often found in aristocratic people, they make good politicians, teachers or physicians.	
The Diamond shape combines the nature of Fire and Wood, conferring a versatile and temperamental character to the person with tendency to be authoritative and demanding at the same time as being seductive and charming.	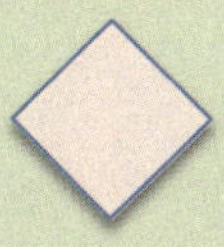

The face shape may also be modified with time and weight changes, but although the basic structure remains, certain characteristics may get enhanced or attenuated.

Analysis based on Yin and Yang

In general, a bony face is considered *Yang*, whereas a fleshy face is *Yin*.

But in addition, the overall shape of the face is divided into two halves, the right side, *Yin* and the left side, *Yang*. The right side is considered the "Public" side, the face one presents to the world, it is reflecting the left-brain's analytical, logical and linear activity (the *Yin* reflecting the *Yang)* (▶ Fig. 10.2). The left side is the "Private" side and reflects the person's true feelings. The left side of the face is controlled by the right brain, which is associated with the emotional, intuitive and creative tendencies; it is the emotional and holistic brain (the *Yang* reflecting the *Yin)*.

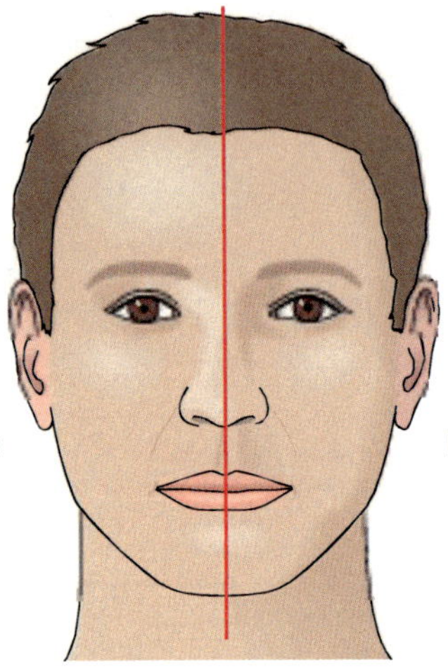

Figure 10.2 *Yin* and *Yang* halves of the face

The analysis of the two halves of the face in babies is of great interest. The side of the face showing more markings and expressions would reflect the dominant (opposite) brain side and consequently the inherent facilities. For example, a child with predominant right facial features will have greater facilities in academic pursuits and should not be forced to take art or piano lessons, and vice versa.

In adults an interesting exercise consists of cutting a frontal facial photo in half, and then recreating two new photos of the person, once using the right side of the face and its mirror copy, and once the left side with its mirror copy. This photomontage is very easy to realize with any photo software on the computer. The resulting twins will present sometimes totally different characters. The right face may be severe and sad, showing the face which the person shows to the outside world, while the left face may be a joyful and carefree reflecting the person's true nature.

Analysis based on the three regions ≈ San Bu 三部

The division into three regions (▶ Fig. 10.3):

- Upper region: extending from the hairline to above the eyebrows. Corresponding to Heaven, it reflects the mental development of the

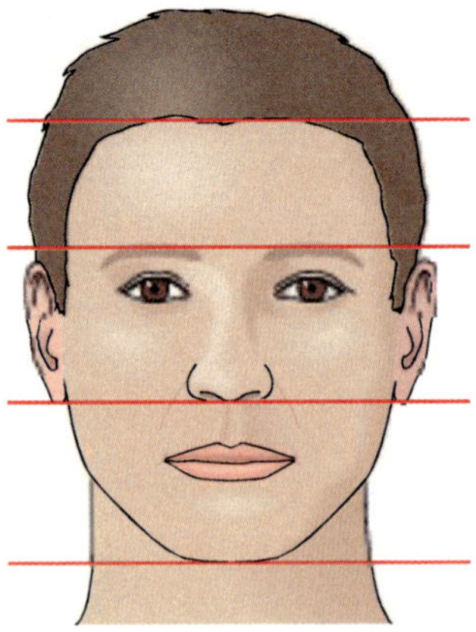

Figure 10.3: Three Regions *(San Bu)*: Heaven, Man, Earth

person. This area also represents the inherited energies and the *Ming* ≈ Destiny. A long and large forehead denotes a mental type character.

- Middle region: from the eyebrows to below the tip of the nose. The "Human" zone corresponds to the ability to construct and create. A Person with a long and prominent nose would manifest a practical nature.
- Lower region: from the tip of the nose to below the chin, this corresponds to the Earth and reflects the support from society. A long and prominent chin would often signify an emotional and instinctual character.

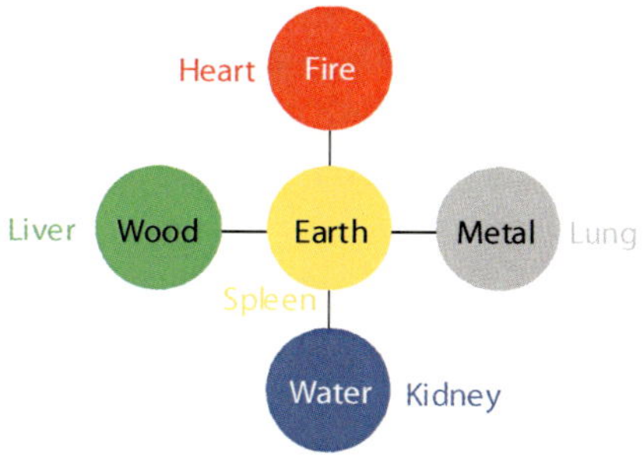

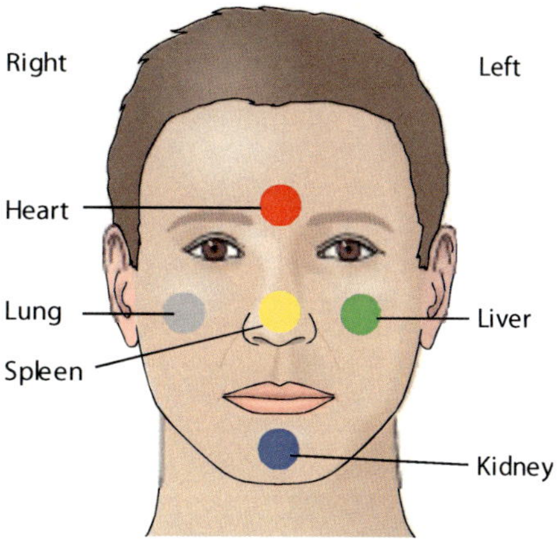

ure 10.4: Face areas in relation to Five Elements (*Su Wen*, chap. 32)

Analysis based on the Five Elements: The Facial areas

There are several facial maps reflecting the internal organs. The most commonly used is the simpler version described in the *Su Wen* chapter 32 relating the five areas of the face to the five phases and the corresponding organs. In general, the appearance of redness in these areas denotes the presence of a Heat disease in that particular organ (▶ Fig. 10.4).

Analysis based on Body parts and organs

Another facial mapping is described in the *Ling Shu* (chapter 49), in which the function of the internal organs would reflect on the face in the form of color change, the presence of pimples, boils, recurrent skin conditions, dryness or abnormal secretions (▶ Fig. 10.5).

Another facial map represents the projection of body parts on the face (▶ Fig. 10.6).

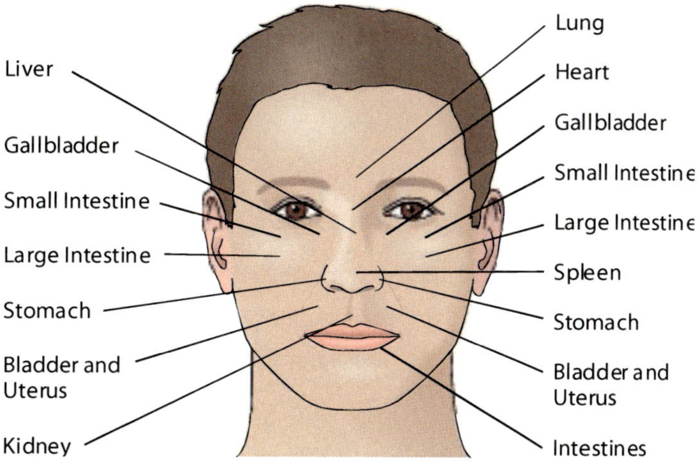

Figure 10.5: Projection of the internal organs on the face (*Ling Shu*, chap. 49)

In practice, none of these systems should be considered separately, as a particular marking could represent either a constitutional trait, or a current organic problem, or even an emotional issue. It is best to analyze different areas when evaluating a particular organ:

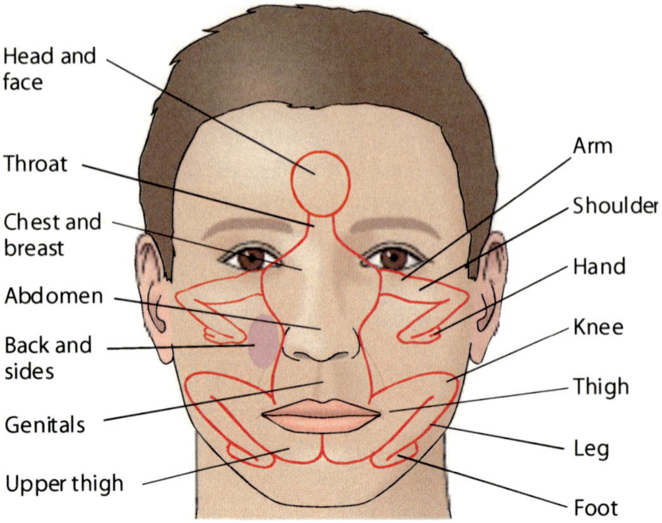

Figure 10.6: Projection of body parts on the face

Kidneys

The following areas reflect the psycho-energetic aspect of the Kidneys:

Ears	Strength of inherited *Jing*
Below the eyes	Function of Kidney *Qi, Yin* and *Yang*
Lower lid	Kidney *Yang*, Adrenals
Philtrum	Fertility, genital functions
Chin	Will power
Hair	Strength of Kidney and *Jing*

Liver and Gallbladder

Liver functions may be evaluated in the following areas:

Eyebrows	Thickness and length indicate the strength of the Liver and the Liver-Qi
Brow bone	Power and leadership
Between the eyes	The emotional expression of Wood; anger
Dark around the eyes	Liver-Qi Xu
Temple	Desire for altered states
Jaw	Strength of beliefs and will
Sclera	Liver-Heat
Tremors	Uncontrolled movements of the eyes, tics, tremors, shaking of the head: Liver-Wind

Heart

The conditions of the Heart and of the *Shen* may be assessed in the following areas:

Eyes	Strength and state of Shen
Eye corners	Emotions: joy lines or sadness lines
Complexion	Facial color: Heart's function
Nose Tip	Shape and color reflects on Heart's function
Eye canthus	Inner and outer canthus
Tongue tip	Emotional state
Speech	Clarity or difficulty: aphasia or stuttering

Spleen and Stomach

Spleen and Stomach functions are reflected on the face:

Mouth and lips	Thickness and length indicate the strength and functions of Stomach and Spleen
Above the lip	Stomach functions
Nose bridge	Emotions: worry
Moneybags	(Fleshy area below the cheeks and above the jaw): state of Spleen-Qi
Mouth ulcers	Stomach-Heat
Teeth dry yellow	Stomach-Heat

Lung

The state of the Lung and its functions are reflected in these areas:

Nose	Length and shape: strength and state of Lung-Qi
Nostrils	Color reflects the state of Lung-Qi and the type of Pathogenic factor
Cheeks	(Below cheekbones), color and fullness: state of Lung-Qi
Eye corners	Sadness or grief lines
Nasal discharge	Type of Pathogenic factor

Intestines

The state of the intestines and bowel movement, in general, may be evaluated by the following:

Lip corners	Reflect on the Duodenum
Below the lips	Coloring is in relation with the Large Intestine
Side of face	Line from corner of the eye to the cheek: chronic constipation; poor assimilation of food

Analysis based on the Mountains and Rivers

The tradition has it that Heaven sculpts the face into mountains and rivers. The mountains form the prominent areas, forehead, nose, chin, and the cheeks. The rivers are the mouth, ears, and eyes (▶ Fig. 10.7).

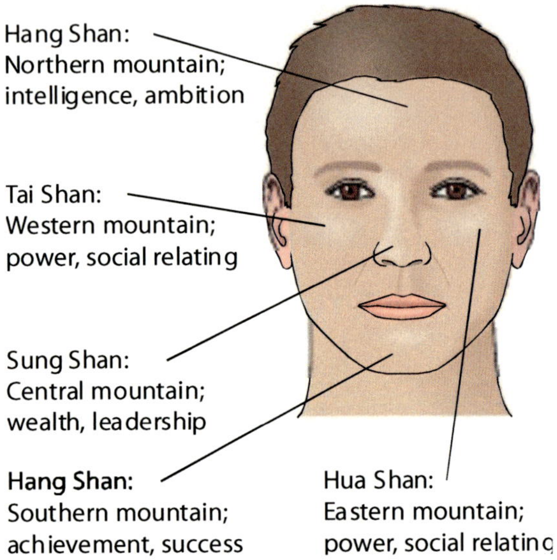

Figure 10.7 : The Five Mountains

1) Forehead

The bulge, height, width, shape, markings, and lines of the forehead are studied. In general, the forehead represents mental activity, the intellect and the tendency to think things over. It also corresponds to ambition and reflects parental influence and education and relates to control as well as ethics and socialization, the capacity to harmonize one's emotions in relation to society (▶ Fig. 10.8).

Width of the forehead	Corresponds to Liver-Blood	
	Wide forehead	Good memory
	Narrow forehead	Poor memory, learning disabilities, learns better from experience rather than schooling
Height of the forehead	Corresponds to Liver-*Yang*; also to the degree of parental education and socialisation; a high forehead indicates freedom from rules and beliefs	
Shape of the forehead	Reflects the inherited energies	
	Bulging right side	Predominant inheritance from the mother's side
	Bulging left side	Predominant inheritance from the father's side
	Dip in the middle	Difficulty integrating the two inheritances
	Flat from profile	Linear thinking

	Slanting back	Good negotiators
Shape of the hairline	Corresponds to the ability to socialise	
	Heart shaped	When symmetrical (▶ Fig. 10.8.a) = good ability to socialise
		Asymmetrical (▶ Fig. 10.8.b) = notion of parental abuse, over-control
	Straight line (▶ Fig. 10.8.c)	Social conformity
	Pointed (▶ Fig. 10.8.d)	"Widows peak" leadership qualities; seductiveness; exuberant Liver-*Qi*; in women possible dysmenorrhea
	Oval, smooth (▶ Fig. 10.8.e)	Diplomatic, good leadership
	Receding hairline (▶ Fig. 10.8.f)	Stomach channel weakness; Blood-*Xu* or Blood-stasis; also the capacity to think outside the established norm, creativity
	Squarish (▶ Fig. 10.8.g)	Anti-conformism, rebelling against rules
	Strong incline (▶ Fig. 10.8.h)	Moralistic; tendency to restlessness
	Rounded sides (▶ Fig. 10.8.i)	Sensuality; difficulties with the emotions

Three regions of the forehead (▶ Fig. 10.9).

Upper region	Liver's relation to Spleen: rationality and understanding; lines, wrinkles or skin bumps indicate Liver over-controlling the Spleen

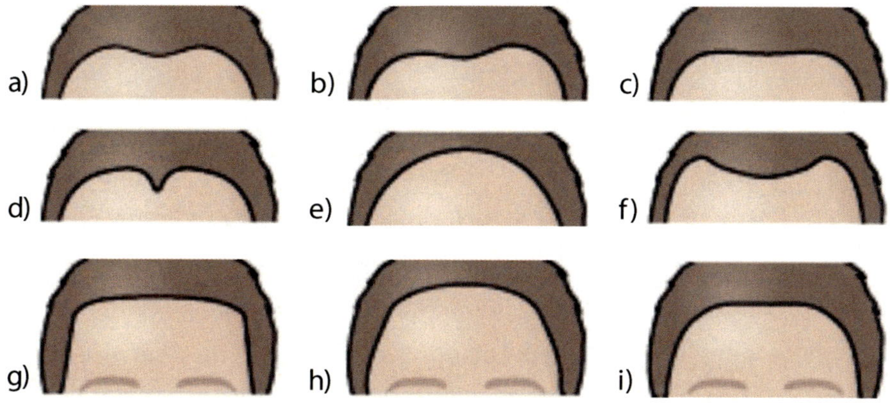

Figure 10.8: Hairline: a) heart-shaped (symmetrical), b)heart-shaped (asymmetrical),c) straight line, d) pointed, e) oval, smooth, f) receding hairline, g) square forehead, h) strong incline, i) rounded sides

Middle region	Liver's relation to Pericardium; emotional expression; lines or wrinkles indicate frustration, anger or suppressed emotions; the deeper the line, the stronger the suppression
Lower region	Liver's relation to Lungs: morality; lines or wrinkles above the eyebrows indicate Lung over-controlling the Liver

Eyebrows reflect the innate impulse and the energy of Liver and Gallbladder. They will be studied with the Eyes.

Brow Bones: reflect the activity of the Liver and of Testosterone, and are usually more prominent in men.

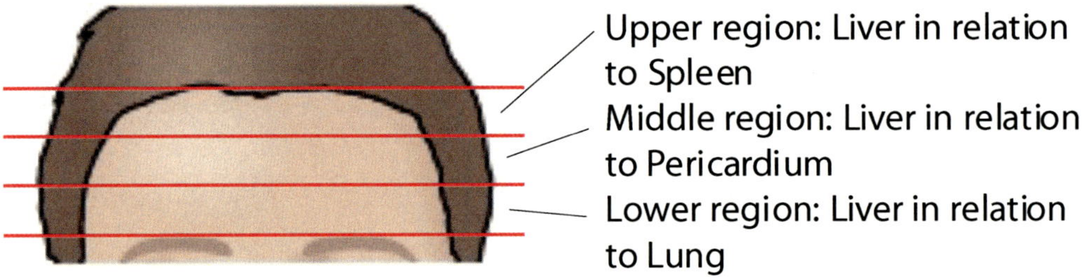

Figure 10.9: Three regions of the forehead

- Prominent brow: Power, leadership, dislike of authority; dogmatism
- Dip in middle: Easier to manage, good overseers

  Between the eyes: "Seat of the Stamp", analyzed further with the eyes

  Temples: Analyzed further with the eyes

2) Ears

Ears reflect the strength of the inherited *Jing* ≈ Essence; they should be flexible, with firm cartilage and should not be translucent in which veins are visible.

Ear shape and size	Reflects the ability to take risks	
	Thin helix	Weak will power; tendency to Liver-*Yang* rising
	Small ears	Fearfulness, shock; conformism
	Large ears	Risk taking; may exhaust the *Jing*
	Fleshy helix	Spleen is supporting the Kidney; good investors
Ear position	Reflects the relation of Wood to Water, and of brain activity	

	Above the eyebrow (► Fig. 10.10)	Early achievers; hyperactivity
	Below the nostril	Brain activity slow to develop and might decline early (Alzheimer)
	Sticking out	Difficulty to hear other people's opinions
	Flat	Good in keeping secrets
Lobes	Are related to the influence of Spleen and family, reflect the relation of Earth to Water	
	Attached lobes	Dependence on family; digestive disorders from Spleen & Kidney-*Yang Xu*
	Detached lobes	Independence; friendships that replace family
	Long lobes	Compassion; taken care of by family members
Ear width (► Fig. 10.10)	Reflects the activity of the Triple Warmer	
	Large upper third	Dominance of Fire: Mental and emotional
	Large middle third	Dominance of Earth and Wood: Physical, athletic
	Large lower third	Dominance of Water: Spiritual
Ear color	The normal ear color is reddish pink, any other color is considered pathological	
	White	Cold; *Yang Xu*
	Bluish or black	Pain
	White or black, dry and thin	Kidney-*Jing Xu*
	Helix brownish, dry	Kidney-*Jing Xu*
	Turbid discharge	Damp-Heat in Liver and Gallbladder

Ears are the portals of the Kidneys and correspond to *Shao Yang* channels (GB and TW).

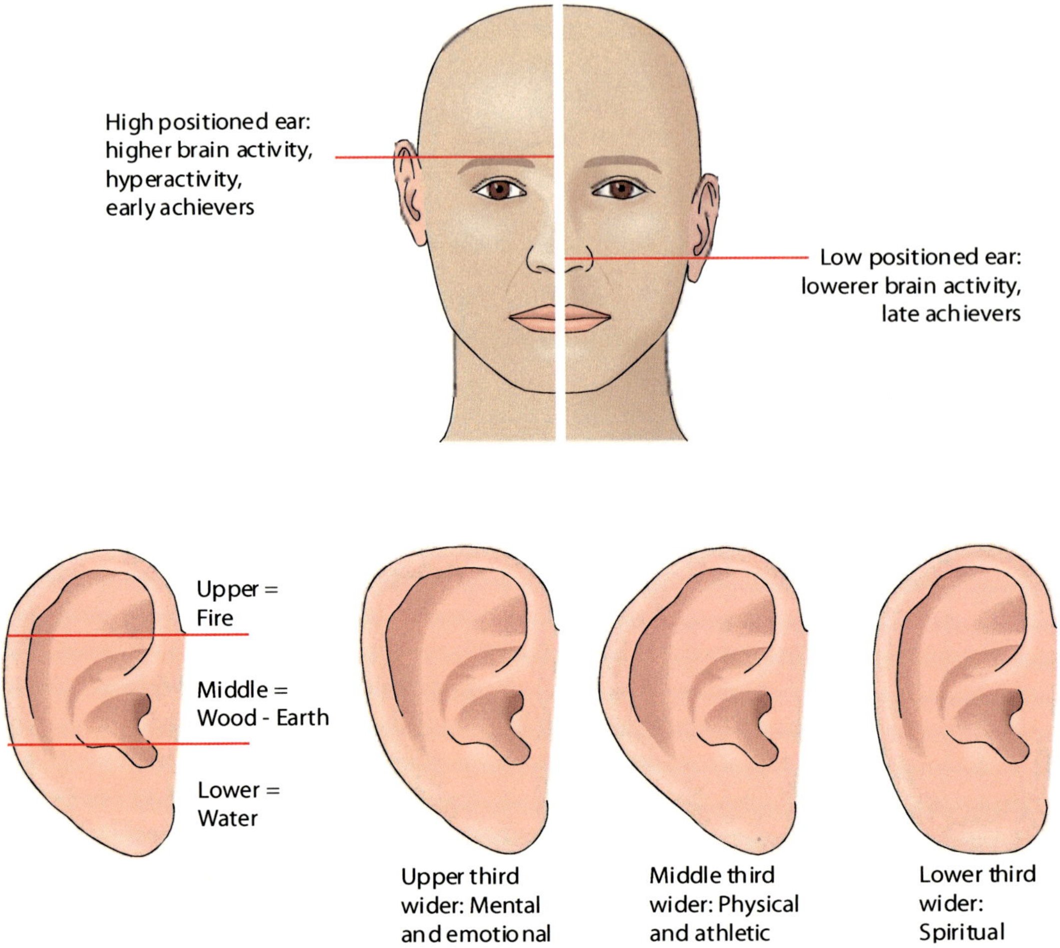

Figure 10.10: Ear size (courage), position (brain, activity), width (Triple Warmer); lobe (related to Spleen); close to the head (Lung), detached (Liver); ear shape: wide upper (mental, emotional), middle wider (physical), lower wider (spiritual).

3) Nose

The nose is the basis of Post-natal *Qi* and of health; it also reflects the social status and wealth, ambition and the necessary drive to succeed.

Length

In relation to the need for discovery.

Long nose	Large mind, interested in knowledge; ambition
Protruding nose	Dislike of routine, need for adventure
Flat nose	Need for stability
Small nose	More playful, need to conform and blend in

Nose-bridge

Reflects the capacity to realize and to create wealth; it also connects to the spine and reflects the spinal alignment. (► Fig. 10.11).

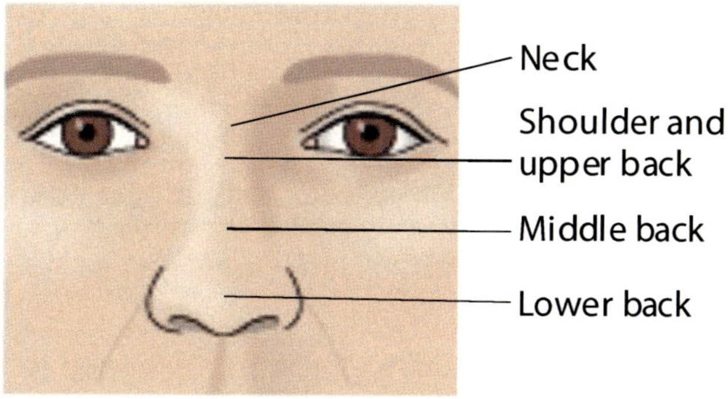

Figure 10.11: Projection of the spine on the bridge of the nose

Large bridge	Facility to make money
Narrow bridge	Less energy for physical work
Bump	Need to control, pride, good leader but bad follower
Striated skin (► Fig. 10.11)	Muscle tension in the related spinal area

Nose Shape

Large, rounded	Physical, tactile, sensual; overindulgence, need to accumulate
Thin nose	Idealistic rather than material; also Stomach-*Yin Xu* or Lung-*Yin Xu*
Thin and bony	Ascetic tendency
Pointed nose	Need for change and travel
Crooked	Failure in relationships
Small, sloped up	Childish and unconventional nature
Long, sloped down	Maturity, Metal quality

Nose Tip

Reflects the activity of Heart or Spleen.

Square tip	Practical character
Rounded tip	Trusting personality
Pointed tip	Curiosity, desire to find out the reasons
Turned up	Sentimental, sensitive
Turned down	Mistrusting, not easily fooled
Large, pimply	Stagnation, Spleen-*Qi Xu*, food stagnation

Large, greasy	Damp-Heat; Spleen-*Qi Xu*, Phlegm
Tip depression	Possibility of hereditary heart weakness
Horizontal line	Weakness of Fire; emotional disappointments
Rhinophyma	Red tumor on the nose: Lung and Stomach-Heat

Nostrils

The larger the nostril, the more tendency to spend or to share knowledge; small nostrils reflect difficulty to bring information out. In general, nostrils correspond to the Lung and the bronchi.

Reddish veins	Lung-Heat
Purplish-white	Lung-*Qi Xu*
Whitish	Normal color
Flaring nostrils	Tendency to purchase esthetical items; also Lung-Heat or Asthmatic condition due to Kidney-*Qi Xu* or Lung-*Qi Xu*

Nose Color

The nose is the opening of the Lung and is on the path of *Yang Ming* channel (ST and LI). In general, the nose reflects the conditions of Spleen and Stomach.

White	Blood-*Xu*
Red	Lung-Heat, Spleen-*Yin-Xu*, Heart-Fire
Grey	Water accumulation
Green or bluish	Abdominal pains
Purplish	Low blood pressure

Nasal Discharge

Clear mucous	External Wind-Cold
Turbid mucous	External Wind-Heat; sinusitis
Turbid and smelly	Accumulated Heat in the Liver and GB channels, chronic sinusitis

Philtrum

Reflects longevity, creativity, and fertility.

Long and large	Long life and good health

Larger on top	Best health in childhood; early creativity
Larger on bottom	Best health later in life; later creativity
Narrow groove	Delicate health
Short philtrum	Decreased fertility
Lines across	Kidney-*Jing Xu*; fertility problems

4) Cheeks

Cheeks represent one's sovereignty, power, authority, and control. Cheekbones are referred to as the "shoulders of the face", in a sense upholding the will and the power.

Cheeks, in general, are related to the Lungs, although the left cheek reflects also the Liver.

Shape	Protruding	Strong authority, bossy
	Large, padded	Authority with softness
	Large, bony	Ruthless authority
	Closer to the ears	Ruthless, destructiveness, self-destruction
	Closer to the nose	Stubbornness; or Hot-Phlegm harassing the heart
	Slanting from the temple to the mouth	Adventurous nature
	Flat or hollow	Issues with self-esteem, lacking of pride in self, dislike of being watched or bossed
	Below cheekbones	Reflects the state of Lung *Qi*, should show a firm skin and a pink color
Moneybags (fleshy area below the cheeks and above the jaw)	Represents reserve energy or wealth	
	Firm but soft and full and pink	Balanced Earth functions
	Cold, hard and white	Accumulation diseases; materialism
	Sagging	Depletion of Spleen-*Qi*
Color	Red right side	Lung-Heat
	Red left side	Liver-Heat
	Blotchy and rosy	Lung congestion, accumulation

	Redness of cheeks, forehead and chin	Floating *Yang* (Heat from *Yin Xu*)
	Pale	Lung-*Qi Xu*
	Pimples	Phlegm accumulation; fat excess

5) Chin

Chin reflects the willpower, supported by the jaw it shows the determination for getting what one wants.

Shape	Strong chin and jaw	Willfulness, stubbornness; if there is no outlet to the will, the person might be prone to ulcers
	Long chin (▶ Fig. 10.12.a + b)	Strong will; also a sign of longevity
	Prominent jaw (▶ Fig. 10.12.e)	Related to the pelvis, possibility of fibroids or hemorrhoids
	Square shaped (▶ Fig. 10.12.c)	Stubbornness, fighting for ones beliefs, practicality; also possible rebellious Stomach-*Qi*
	Weak chin and jaw	Weak will, difficulty holding on to emotions, emotional outbreaks; also weak Kidney *Qi*
	Pointed chin (▶ Fig. 10.12.d)	Weak will, indecisiveness; emotionality
	Rounded chin (▶ Fig. 10.12.b)	Even tempered, diplomacy
	Receding chin (▶ Fig. 10.12.f)	Often dominated; un-fulfillment in family, needing help or service
	Protruding chin (▶ Fig. 10.12.g)	Servitude, needing to give or to help
	Turned up chin (▶ Fig. 10.12.h)	Stubbornness
	Cleft below (▶ Fig. 10.12.i)	Natural performer, need to please, need for recognition, difficulty to mature; also poor protein digestion
	Dimple in chin (▶ Fig. 10.12.e)	Fire in Water; need for attention and recognition, dependence on people; issues with commitment

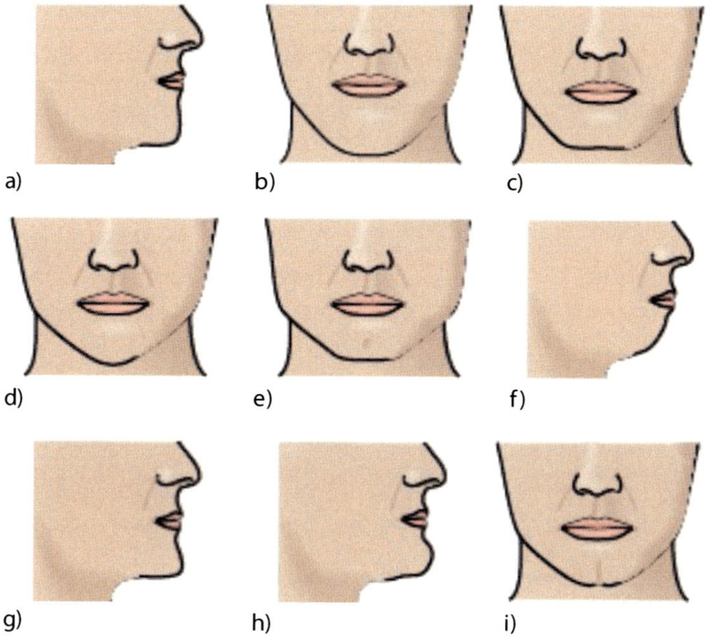

Figure 10.12: Chin shapes:
a) long,
b) long and round,
c) square,
d) pointed,
e) prominent jaw, dimpled chin,
f) receding,
g) protruding,
h) turned-up,
i) cleft in chin.

6) Eyes

The eyes are the portals of the Liver, but also receive energy from the Five *Zang* ≈*Yin* organs (▶ Fig 10.13.a). The brightness reflects the state of *Shen* and *Jing* (*Re Shen*). The left eye is more receptive, the right eye more outgoing.

In general, the openness of the eyes reflects on the openness of the Heart. Openness does not mean having large eyes, rather how open they seem (irrespective of racial diversity).

- Right eye issues: problems with trusting the world (*Yang Qiao Mai*)
- Left eye issues: problems with trusting oneself (*Yin Qiao Mai*)

Eye Size

Reflects the generating quality of Liver Blood in relation to Heart *Qi*.

Large eyes	More Heart-*Qi*, imagination, emotionality, drama
Small eyes	Relates to Pericardium, introspective, cautious, need for control
Squinting	Very cautious, mistrusting, good in keeping secrets

Eye Shape

Round eyes	The upper and lower eye lids are strongly curved with the whole iris showing; saying what they think, easily fascinated,

	reactive, extreme mood swings, bold or even reckless
Broad eyes	Romantic, impulsive, emotional, artistic, charming
Little eyes	Introverted, holding emotions in, sceptical, trustworthy, precise, good with details
Almond eyes	Sensitive but cautious about expressing emotions, common sense
Rectangular	Eyelids are quite horizontal; logical and mental, good in business

Eye Setting

Sunken eyes	Introverted, dreamers, may become delusional
Protruding eyes	Extraverted, might denote hyperthyroidism
Wide-set eyes	More than one eye width between the eyes; open minded, flexible; dislike for detail
Close-set eyes	Observing, analytical, focus on details, narrow perspectives

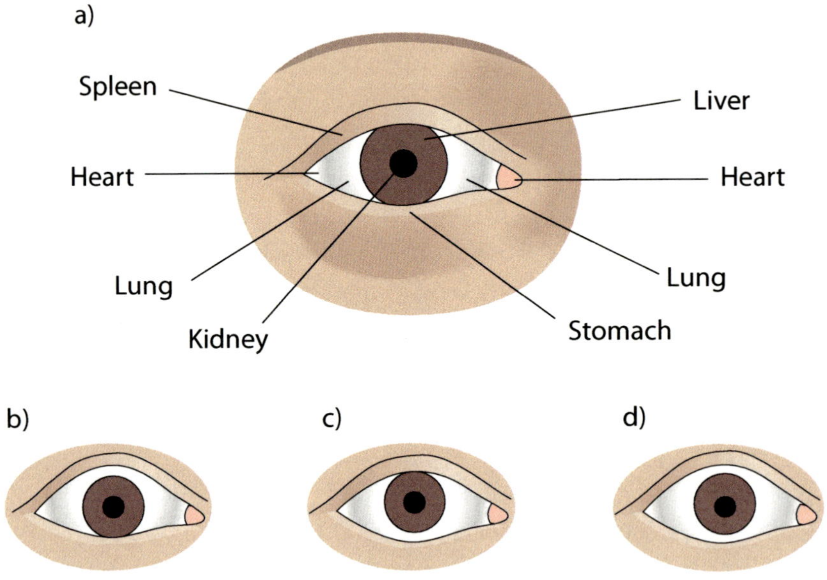

Figure 10.13: a) eye regions in relation to the *Zang-Fu*, b) *Yang San Paku*, c) *Yin San Paku*, d) four whites.

Eye Position

Slanted up	"Cat's eyes" (outer corners are higher), ambitious, over achievers, optimistic, quick and clever minds
Slanted down	"Puppy eyes"; pessimistic, under achievers, trying to please others; also Liver *Qi Xu*, drawing on Spleen and Kidney *Yang*, Adrenal exhaustion

Iris

Is in relation to the Liver.

Dull, veiled	Accumulation of Phlegm or excess acidity
Ring around	Also called cholesterol ring; accumulation of Phlegm, possible arteriosclerosis

Sclera

Is in relation to the Lung, the inner and outer canthus areas relate to the Heart.

Red sclera	Lung-Heat or Liver-Heat, or accumulation of toxins
Red, swollen, painful	(Conjunctivitis)/ external Wind-Heat or Liver-Fire
Pain, itching, lacrimation	External or internal Wind
Itching	Wind and Fire
Ulceration	Keratitis: Dampness
Lacrimation	Sensation of foreign body: Cold
Lacrimation with Wind	External Wind-Cold, or Kidney and Liver-*Qi Xu*
Dry eyes	Sensation of foreign body: Dryness
Yellow or Greenish	Damp-Heat invasion, Liver disease
Cataract	Liver-Fire or Liver-Wind; or Spleen-*Yin Xu*

Pupils

Reflect the state of the Kidneys.

Dilated	Exhaustion of *Jing Qi*

Inner corner/canthus

Sharp canthus	Sharp tongue, accuracy in use of words
Curved down	May use words in order to hurt
Rounded canthus	Tact in the use of words, or even avoidance
Pale canthus	Inner and outer: Blood *Xu*
Red canthus	Inner and outer: Heart-Fire

Upper Lid

Reflects the Spleen, Liver and Gall Bladder as well as the *Tai Yang* channel.

Red and swollen	Wind-Heat (external or internal from the Liver)
Sty, swelling	Damp-Heat in Stomach and Spleen, or Spleen-*Yin Xu*
Puffiness	Spleen-*Qi Xu* with Dampness
Purple lines	Irritable Gallbladder
Pimples	Gallbladder stones
Drooping upper lid Water retention	Dampness
Sunken or lidded	Weak Earth, loss of energy and money
Raised upper lid (► Fig. 10.13.b)	(White showing above), *Yang* excess, excess adrenaline; tendency to panic or hysteria, "3 whites ≈ *San Paku*" eyes

Lower Lid

Is in relation with the Stomach.

Lowered lid (► Fig. 10.13.c)	(white showing below), "3 whites ≈ San Paku" eyes *Yin* excess, exhaustion of Kidney *Yang*; emotional reactivity, temperamental
Four whites (► Fig. 10.13.d)	(white showing above and below the iris), extreme nervous tension, quick reactions; possible manic behaviour, prone to accidents, possibly a short life.
Red rims	Adrenal exhaustion

Below the eye area

Is in relation to Kidney-*Yang* (Adrenals).

Puffiness	Kidney-*Yang Xu*; mineral stagnation (stones) or mineral deficiency (osteoporosis); also denotes nervousness, propensity to accidents
Wrinkles	(Horizontal lines), poor metabolism, dehydration
Darkness	Kidney-*Yang Xu* or external Cold
Chronically dark	Wei-*Qi Xu*, allergies, food intolerance

Vision (► chap. 12.2, page 210 "Sensory Organs")

Movement of the Eyes

Open eyes are considered *Yang*; closed eyes reflect a *Yin* condition.

Deviated	Liver-Wind, or imminent Wind convulsions
Nystagmus	(Uncontrolled movement), Liver-Wind, or imminent convulsions
Strabismus	*Yang* repletion in the neck and shoulders
Open eyes when sleeping in children	Predisposition to internal Wind and convulsion due to Liver-Blood *Xu*; wandering *Hun* (dreaming)
Open eyes when sleeping in adults	Spleen-*Qi Xu* causing Blood-*Xu*

Eye Lashes

Reflect the state of Liver-Blood.

Thick, long	Romantic and emotional tendency
Thin, straight	Realistic and pragmatic character

Eyebrows

Are called the "Leaves of the tree", and reflect the innate drive and impulse and the strength of the Liver.

Thick, bushy	Liver-Blood; assertiveness, reactivity, rigidity in thinking, fanatical; may be aggressive or moody
Bushy and wild	Unusual thinking, inventors, mad scientists
Joined, "unibrow"	Explosive tempers (may be controlled)
Fine, soft hairs	Weak Liver *Qi* but more flexible, easy going, kind
Tapering from thick (medial) to thin (lateral)	Difficulty to finish projects
Tapering from thin (medial) to thick (lateral)	Difficulty starting but enthusiasm to finish; tendency to migraine headaches
Long eyebrows	Strong Liver; creativity, reproductive power; humanitarian and friendly, or judgmental
Short eyebrows	Weakness of Liver and Gallbladder; shyness; difficulty in asking for help, independence, hard working
Regular, orderly	Friendly, assertive, orderly
Irregular, erratic	Unfriendly, aggressive, cruel
Arched	Even-tempered, kind

Straight	Well organized, good manager, even-tempered
Sweeping up	Decisive character, tendency to superiority, arrogance
Slanting down	Low self-esteem, needing help

Between the eyebrows

"Seat of the Stamp", related to issues with anger discipline and reflecting the father's influence.

Broad and clear	Good discipline, good education from the father
Narrow	Impatience, lack of discipline; possible rebel or loner; difficulty in taking criticism
Vertical lines	Irritability, frustration; depth of the line reflects the degree of anger (see under lines and wrinkles)
Horizontal lines	Worry
Bluish color in children	Shock; with possibility of imminent fevers or convulsions

Brow Bones

(► Figure 10.7 "Analysis based on the Mountains and Rivers" / Forehead)

Temples

According to L. Bridges represents the desire for altered states.

Full	Being in the present
Hollow and dark	Tendency to addiction and to self-destruction
Hollow and light	Search for spiritual experiences
Distinct ridge between forehead and temple	Spiritual awakening or realization

7) Mouth and Lips

Represent the earliest stages of human interaction, the lips are the outer appearance of Spleen and they inform on the digestive system function.

Shape

Large mouth (► Fig. 10.14.b)	Strong Earth energy, generosity

Small mouth (▶ Fig. 10.14.c)	Lack of expansion, small boundaries, loner
Thin lips (▶ Fig. 10.14.e)	Difficulty in transitional periods; difficulty in showing feelings, needing intimacy and security
Thick lips (▶ Fig. 10.14.d)	Generosity, sensuality, easy emotional expression, need for external contact and sharing
"Cupid's bow"	Small mouth but thick lips; express emotions only to trusted people; giving to be appreciated
Thick upper lip	Desire for activity, sensuality, more dramatic (▶ Fig. 10.14.f)
Protruding center	Upper lip has extra flesh in the center: tendency to exaggerate all emotions, hypochondriac
Swollen upper lip	Stomach weakness, indigestion
Crooked upper lip	Stomach excess, acidity in stomach
Thick lower lip (▶ Fig. 10.14.g)	Desire for physical pleasure and comfort, holding on to things and collecting, overindulgence; Dampness
Swollen lips	Spleen-*Qi Xu*, Dampness, digestive problems
Swollen sides	Large Intestine-*Qi Xu*, constipation

Lip Tonus and slant

Loose, flaccid	Spleen-*Qi Xu*, searching for more; extra-marital relations, addictions; when mouth stays open (gums are showing), poor boundaries, weak morals, emotional and sexual vulnerability
Flaccid lower lip	Poor self-control, overindulgence in food and sex
Pouting, puffy	Self-indulgence, hedonistic
Firm lips	Good digestion, great discipline
Tight, puckered	Holding on to resentment, judgmental
Angling down	Cynical, pessimistic
Crescent shape	Needing humour, possibly Heart-Blood *Xu*
Raised corners	Optimistic and cheerful personality
Raised and red	Stomach counter-flow *Qi*; if dry: Stomach-Fire
Monkey lips	Vertical wrinkles on both lips), inability of Spleen to hold blood, possible miscarriage; tendency to loose money
Vertical line or dip	(on lower lip), good sense of humour
Lines above the lip	Exhaustion of Spleen-*Qi*; excessive worry; having given too

	much nurturing to others
Lip biting	Lack of confidence, resistance to change

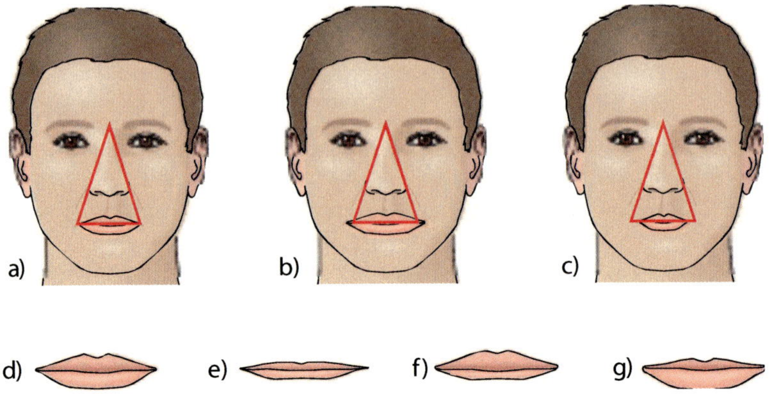

Figure 10.14 : Mouth shapes and sizes: a) average mouth size, b) large mouth, c) small mouth, d) thick lips, e) thin lips, f) thick upper lip, g) thick lower lip.

Color

Pale	Blood *Xu*
Bluish	*Yang Xu* or external Cold
Purple	Blood stasis from Cold
Bright red	Blood-Heat
White corners	Phlegm accumulation in the duodenum
Dark above the lip	Stomach problems
Dark below the lip	Large Intestinal problems

Wrinkles, markings, sores

Ulcers on sides of lips	Toxic accumulation in the Large Intestine
Ulcers in the middle	Small Intestine-*Qi Xu*, mal-absorption
Ulcers in the corners	Duodenal ulcers
Dry, wrinkled and cracked	External Dryness, or Body fluid vacuity from Heat

Mouth ulcers, mouth sores

In general signify Stomach-Heat or Stomach-Fire, or Damp-Heat in Stomach and Spleen, or Heart-Fire.

Pale sores	Stomach-Heat or Heart-*Yin Xu* (Empty-Heat)
Red swollen sores, ulcers, swelling of the jaw	Heart-Fire
Drooling during sleep	Spleen-*Qi Xu* with Dampness, or Stomach-Heat; in children may also signify intestinal worms

8) Teeth and Gums

The Kidneys control the teeth; the Stomach channel feeds the gums.

Teeth	Lack of brightness	Stomach-Heat drying up the body fluids
	Dull color and dry	Kidney-*Jing Xu*
	Dry and sticky upper teeth	Stomach-Fire
	Dry and sticky lower teeth	Large or Small Intestine-Fire
	Decaying teeth	Kidney-*Qi Xu*, Kidney-*Jing Xu*
	Loose teeth	Kidney-*Jing Xu* or Kidney-*Qi Xu*
	Grinding of teeth	Stomach-Heat or intestinal worms
Gums	Pale	Blood *Xu*
	Swollen and red (bleeding easily)	Stomach-Fire
	Bluish	Poisoning

Analysis based on Facial lines and wrinkles

The presence of lines, wrinkles, and discolorations, has specific interpretations and diagnostic values.

1) The 7 Emotions

The emotions leave lines on the face, the more lines the more intense is the emotion. The overall positioning of the lines in relation to the face reflects on severity; the lower the line position the more severe is the emotion.

Anger

Causes a narrowing of the eyes, tightening of the jaws and the mouth, a lowering of the eyebrows and the appearance or deepening of lines between the eyebrows, the *Yin Tang* area.

Deep vertical lines	Frequent anger; Liver-*Yang* rising, Liver-Fire
Suspended sword (single deep line) (▶ Fig. 10.15.a)	Suppressed anger, Liver-*Qi* stagnation, Liver-*Yang* rising
Suspended needle (more shallow line)	Inability to move forward, holding back, Liver-*Qi Xu* or Liver-Qi stagnation
Two lines	Impatience, frustration, irritability; Liver-*Qi* stagnation
More lines	Anger is well managed

Joy

Harmonizes the *Qi* calms the *Shen* and dilates the vessels, it is not to be confused with excessive excitement that disperses the Heart-*Qi* and may cause Heart-*Yin Xu* or Heart-Fire.

Sides of the eyes (▶ Fig. 10.15.b)	Lines ascending around GB-1 area; joyful personality, easy to laughter
Raised sides of lips	Optimistic and cheerful character
Up slanted eyes	Ambitious, optimistic, quick and clever minds

Sadness and grief

Disturbs the Lung-*Qi*, compromises the *Wei Qi* and depresses the *Shen*.

Lateral canthus (▶ Fig. 10.15.c)	Descending lines along GB-1: retained grief
Medial canthus (▶ Fig. 10.15.c)	Descending lines from BL-1: depression and worry
Medial canthus	Descending line from medial canthus towards the nose: pain and severe suffering, risk of suicide
	If red: inflammation
	If Yellow: Damp-Heat
	Pale: stiffness
	Green: toxins
	Dark: Blockage

Fear and anxiety

Depletes the Kidney-*Qi*.

Mouth corners (▶ Fig. 10.15.d)	Descending lines from the corner of the lips: fear
Around ST-4	Descending lines lateral to the mouth corners: fear of death
Medial canthus	Ascending lines from BL-1: Anxiety

Worry and pensiveness

Harm the Spleen-*Qi*, as well as the Lung and the Heart.

Yin Tang area	Horizontal lines between the eyebrows
Side of cheeks (▶ Fig. 10.15.e)	Deep vertical lines: obsession lines

Fright, shock

Can scatter the *Qi*, causing a sudden depletion of Kidney-*Jing* and of Heart-*Qi*.

Ear Lobe	Diagonal line, descending across the earlobe: childhood fright, autism
Across the chin	Several horizontal line along RM-24: PTSD (Post Traumatic Shock)

2) Other lines and wrinkles

Across the chin	Single horizontal line along RM-24: unfulfilled potential, *Yin* is being impeded; considered normal after age 60: retirement line	
Side of nostril (▶ Fig. 10.15.f)	From above the nostril to side of the mouth: Purpose line; if deep: effort to attain purpose; could also reflect general fatigue	
Side of nostril (▶ Fig. 10.15.g)	From above the nostril to the chin: using more effort than is necessary, disappointment lines	
Mouth corner (▶ Fig. 10.15.d)	Towards the chin could also reflect duodenal diseases	
Forehead	Lateral slanting	Looking for shortcuts, tendency to frustrations
	Medial slanting	Spiritual realisation; may also represent chronic intestinal problems, or over-eating, chronic food stagnation
	Horizontal lines	Could signify bladder problems or *Yin* repletion
Side of face (▶ Fig. 10.15.h)	Line from corner of the eye to the cheek: chronic constipation; poor assimilation of food	

Analysis based on Facial Color

The blood and the Qi of the 12 channels concentrate in the face and pass through the portals. — *Ling Shu, chap. 4*

Brightness

Bright colors	Indicate good health or a mild disease (*Biao*)
Dull colors	Indicate a deeper more serious disease (*Li*)

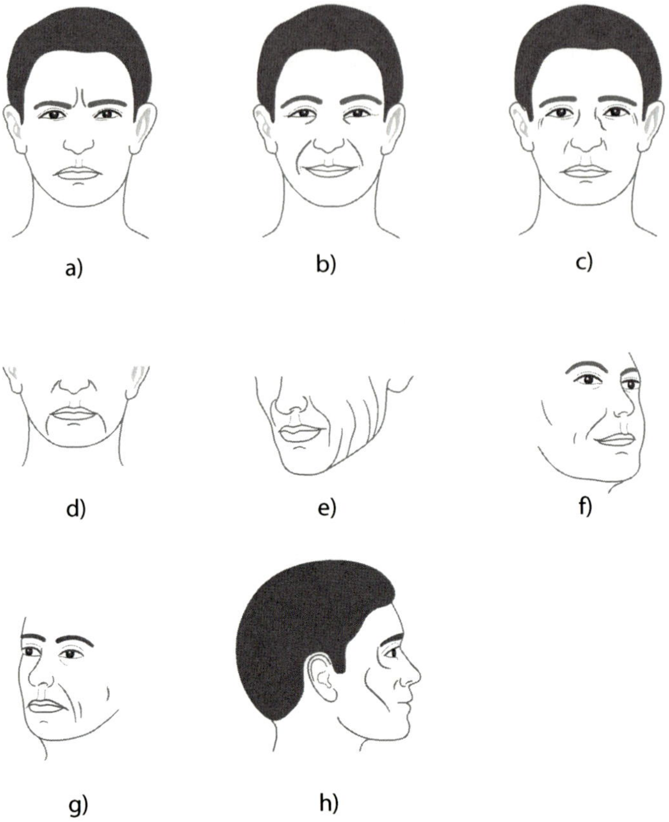

Figure 10.15: Facial lines and wrinkles: a) anger line, b) joy lines, c) grief lines, d) fear lines, e) worry lines, f) purpose line, g) effort line, h) poor assimilation line.

Facial Colors

The overall facial color relates to the Five Phases and reflects the constitution. In this case, the color is bright and the general condition is healthy. The following color tones concern more the Caucasian races and are much harder to distinguish in African populations.

Blue-Green	Wood- Liver
Red	Fire- Heart
Yellow	Earth- Spleen
White	Metal- Lung
Black, dark	Water- Kidney
But the presence of a particular color may also indicate pathology	
Blue-green, black	Could signify pain
Yellow or red	Presence of Heat
White	Could signify Cold

White color or a pale complexion

Indicates a state of the vacuity of *Yang* or of Blood or a Metal constitution.

White, bright	If swollen: *Yang Xu*
White and dull	Blood *Xu*
	In an acute disease: a sudden loss of *Yang*
Pale, greyish, red cheeks and lips	Residual Heat "True Heat false Cold"
Extremely pale	With abdominal pain: internal Cold

Yellow color

Indicates Spleen-*Qi Xu* with an accumulation of Dampness.

Yellow, dull & dry	Spleen-*Qi Xu* with Stomach-Heat or Blood *Xu*
Yellow and swollen	Spleen-*Qi Xu*; internal obstruction by Dampness
Yellow face and Body Jaundice	If the eyes are bright yellow: *Yang* type Jaundice caused by Damp-Heat
	If the eyes are dull smoky-yellow: *Yin* type Jaundice by Damp-Cold

Red color

Indicates either Heat pathology or a Fire-type constitution.

Whole face is red	Fever due to EPF; or a Heat condition from *Yin Xu* in the organs
Cheeks are red	Empty-Heat or "Floating *Yang*" from *Yin Xu*
Malar flush	Red cheeks, forehead and chin: Empty-Heat
Left cheek red	Heat in the Liver
Right cheek red	Heat in the Lung
Chin Red	Heat in the Kidney
Forehead red	Heart-Heat or Heart-Fire
Powdery red	In a chronic and severe disease, a pale face with a reddish powdery appearance signifies: "Inner Cold with apparent Heat" (serious)

Blue-green color

Signifies Cold or Pain or Blood accumulation; in children the possibility of infantile convulsions.

Bluish, pale	With pain in the heart and abdomen: internal Cold
Ash blue	With purple lips: Heart-*Qi Xu* with Blood stasis
Purplish face	In children, with high fever, a, bluish tinge between the eyebrows and around lips signifies imminent convulsions

Black color

Signifies the vacuity of Kidney-*Qi*, or accumulation of Water or of Blood, or the presence of a Cold type disease.

Black and moist	Kidney-*Yang Xu*
Black and dry	Kidney-*Yin Xu* or Kidney-*Jing Xu*
Black under the eyes with swelling	Kidney-*Qi Xu* with water accumulation
Black around the eyes	Liver-*Qi Xu*
Black around the eyes with leucorrhea	Cold and Damp accumulation in the lower TW

Skin texture

Dry	Dehydration, Body fluid vacuity
Oily	Liver-*Qi* stagnation or Liver-Heat

Head

The head is the reunion of all of the *Yang* channels and the most *Yang* part of the body. It contains the brain matter that is governed by the Kidneys.

Uncontrolled swaying of the head	Blood *Xu* and Kidney-*Jing Xu*
Shaking, tremor	Internal Wind
Boils, ulcers	Damp-Heat or Liver-Fire
Itchy scalp	Liver-Blood *Xu* or *Yin Xu* or Fire with Liver-Wind

Hair

The hair is the external manifestation of the Kidney, it also depends on Liver Blood for nourishment and on the Lung's function to nourish the skin.

Hair loss	Kidney-*Qi Xu* or Kidney-*Jing Xu*, Liver- Blood *Xu*, Lung-*Qi Xu*
Sudden alopecia	Blood *Xu* and external Wind
Premature loss	Kidney-*Qi Xu*, or Heat in the Blood
Premature greying	Kidney-*Jing Xu*; anxiety; excess salt and acid
Splitting ends	Blood *Xu*, Lung or Kidney-*Qi Xu*
Brittle hair	Liver-Blood *Xu* or Kidney-*Yin Xu*
Greasy, shapeless	Liver-Blood *Xu* or Liver-*Qi Xu*; Dampness
Dandruff, dry scalp	Lung-Dryness, Liver-Blood *Xu* or Liver-Heat

Throat

The throat area is connected with the Lungs and Stomach, but it also receives ramifications from the Heart, Kidney, Liver, and Spleen channels.

Red, swollen	Painful with pus, or ulcers: Lung-Heat or Stomach-Heat
Bright red	But not painful: *Yin Xu* with repletion of Fire
Sore throat	Without *Biao* symptoms: Kidney-*Yin Xu*, Kidney-Fire
Pale throat	Chronic, no swelling: Kidney-*Yang Xu*
Greyish coating	If easily scraped off: stomach-*Qi Xu*, indigestion
	If very adherent: toxic heat; Diphtheria
Plum pit	Feeling of lump in the throat: Liver-*Qi* stasis, Liver-*Yin Xu* or Liver-Blood and *Qi Xu*

10.2 Body Shape and Movements

The body shape and movements depend on the constitution as well as the state of harmony of the *Zang-Fu*.

The basic constitution depends on Pre-Heaven *Qi* consisting of:

- *Yuan* ≈ Source *Qi*: Life principle
- *Jing Qi* or Essence of the parents, which defines the form and therefore plays an important role in “Constitution”

- *Zong* ≈ Ancestral *Qi*: this is the cosmic *Qi* at the moment of conception and is believed to define the destiny "*Ming*" and influences the basic "Temperament" of the person.

In most cases, the constitution is a combination of several elements that blend together to define the particular characteristics of each person. Each Element will influence the morphology of the person in a particular way.

Elements often combine their influences, the most common combinations being:

- Earth and Metal, these are the most frequent of the combinations and constitute the basic traits of most sedentary populations
- Wood and Fire, to be found more in nomadic populations seeking new lands and adventures, mostly found today in Latin races
- Water and Fire, are more rare, North European or African races

Additionally, a third element may be present and would then modify the shape, in some cases, the person may even manifest all five characteristics, but always with one dominating element.

General Head and Body Shape

The Observation of the general head and body shape gives us several important indications:

- The strength or weakness of the Pre-natal energies, and may give an indications of the complexity of the disease. A transmitted and inherited condition would obviously be more difficult to treat.
- Strength or weakness of Post-natal energy; this may be used to evaluate the prognosis.
- Tolerance to pain and to medication is a further element of prognosis.
- The constitution according to the Five Elements, which will also orient towards certain organic and pathological pre-dispositions.
- The "Temperament", which is assessed by combining the form and the behavior of a person. The temperament reflects also the strength or weakness of the channels and can orient the therapy and help select the most appropriate combinations of acupuncture points.

Strong Pre-natal energy "Jing"

- A broad forehead and Glabella
- The nose is wide and long, with spaced orifices and a long Philtrum
- Full Cheeks
- Long ears with long earlobes
- The facial complexion (five colors) are normal with luster

- Breathing is even and smooth
- Muscles and skin are firm
- Generally, the person may expect a long life
- Diseases are easy to treat, otherwise, the patient is capable of surviving even serious illnesses
- The subject is easily getting away with an unhealthy lifestyle

Weak Pre-natal energy

- Eyes, nose, ears, and mouth are close together
- The forehead is narrow and the Glabella is small
- The nose is narrow with nostrils turned up, with a short Philtrum
- Short and thin ears
- The breathing is coarse
- Skin and muscles are loose
- There is a tendency to suffer from vacuity of *Qi*, Blood, *Yin*, and *Yang*
- Treatment tends to be more difficult

Strong Post-natal energy

- Strong Shen in the eyes
- Ruddy complexion with luster
- Strong body build with solid muscles
- Firm and elastic skin
- Shiny hair
- Vigor and swift movements
- Spleen and Stomach are strong
- *Qi*, Blood, *Yin*, and *Yang* are abundant
- The person is generally easy to treat

Weak Post-natal energy

- Thin and small build
- Little energy with a haggard and sallow complexion
- Dry withered hair
- Loose skin without elasticity
- Spleen and Stomach are weak;
- *Qi*, Blood, *Yin*, and *Yang* are deficient
- Frequently the disease involves vacuity of the substances

10.3 Body Form according to the Five Elements

Fire Types

In general are tall, presenting:

- Long limbs in relation to the body, with the head, carried high
- Broad shoulders and a rigid spine, often a long neck
- Usually, elongated and thin body but could also be heavy set (▶ Fig. 10.16)
- Fast or possibly jerky movements

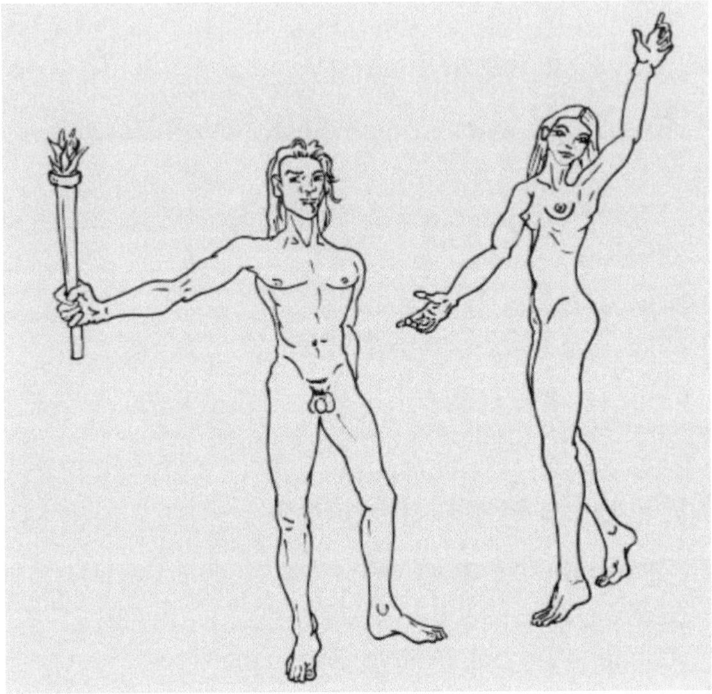

Figure 10.16: Fire-types: often tall with long limbs, broad shoulders, long neck, regal bearing

Fire-type face

- Broad face with high cheekbones (▶ Fig. 10.17)
- A red or dark complexion, or easily blushing
- Wide-set eyes, at times with a hard piercing look
- Voice could be loud or have a high pitch
- Often a dominating presence
- Well dressed, preference for expensive clothing

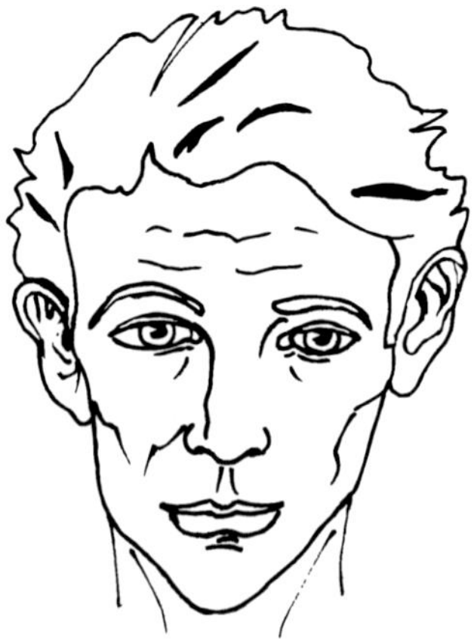

Figure 10.17: Fire-type face: triangular, with a broad forehead and wide-set eyes, piercing look, high cheekbones, strong chin, red or dark complexion

Fire-type hands

Fire-type hands are long and oval, with long fine fingers, very agile, spreading out easily with a hollow palm and even the hooking of the fifth finger when the fingers are spread wide. This is due to the excessive *Qi* in the Heart channel, at times it can even involve the Pericardium channel as well, with hooking of both 4th and 5th fingers. The nails are long, oval, reddish, very convex and naturally quite elegant (▶ Fig. 10.18).

Fire frequently combines with Water or Wood

Even if the Fire-type constitution is not tall, the other Fire element attributes are usually present.

As Fire often combines with Water, quite often the two characteristics may be found in the same person.

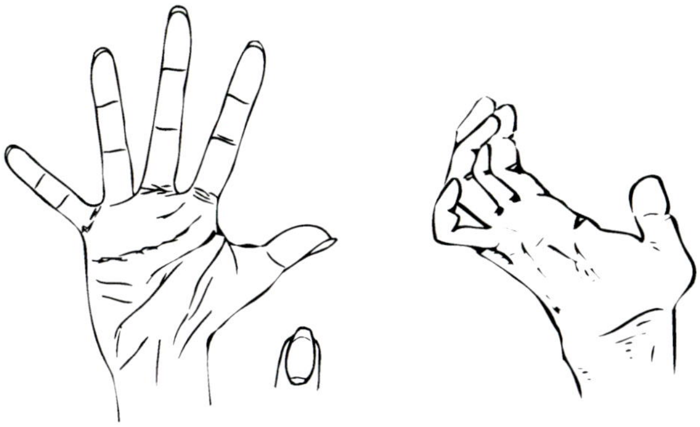

Figure 10.18: Fire-type hand: long, elegant, flexible elongated fingers with pointed tips, hooking of 5th or even 4th fingers when the fingers are in full extension

Fire may also combine with Wood, giving extreme mobility and expansiveness to the already mobile Wood element.

Wood Types

Wood types have an average and a quite proportionate body shape

- Well defined and toned muscles but not bulging (▶ Fig. 10.19)
- Often sportive, agile, or at times quite restless
- Tanned or olive complexion
- With open features, and a warm and expressive look
- Can present either as friendly, easily communicative through speech or body language, with a tendency to be seductive or on the opposite, shy, nervous, nail-biting and prone to tics, or even at times over excited, talkative, loud and quarrelsome.
- Unusual and original clothing or appearance

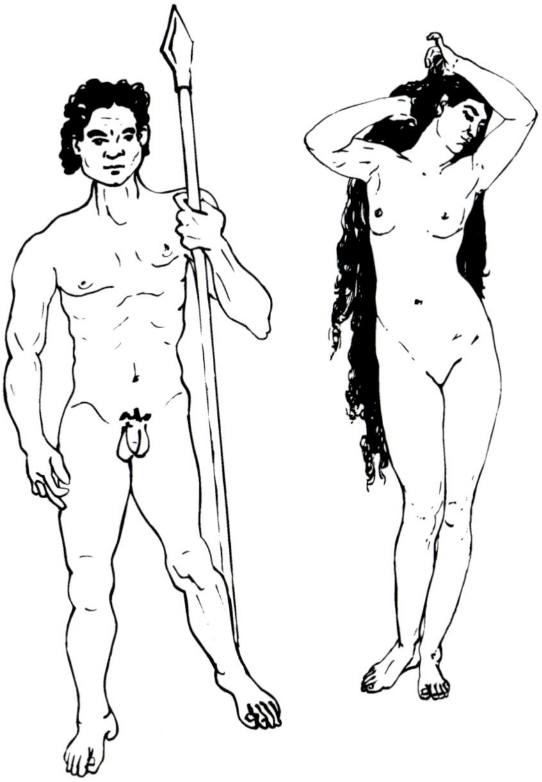

Figure 10.19: Wood types: proportionate body, well-toned muscles, sportive and agile or at times restless

Wood-type face

The facial structure could be larger below or trapezoid with a strong brow and thick eyebrows (▶Fig. 10.20).

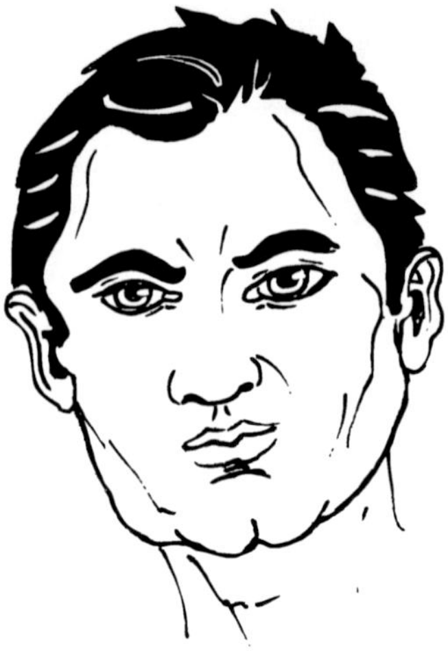

Figure 10.20 : Wood-type face: triangular or trapezoid, prominent jaws, strong brow, thick eyebrows, communicative or seductive

Wood-type hands

Wood type hands are proportionate, knotted, with a very striated palm.

The nails are proportionate, hard and sometimes bitten(▶Fig. 10.21).

The hands are often quite expressive and complement speech.

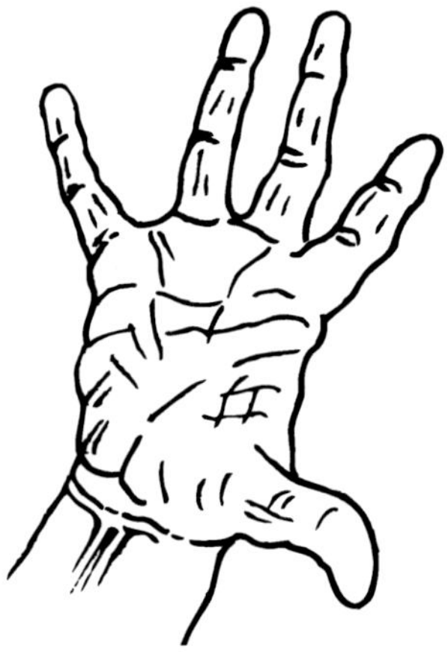

Figure 10.21: Wood type hand: proportionate, abundant palmar lines, well-defined joints, possible nail-biting

Wood may combine with Fire

Wood and Fire elements often combine, lending their *Yang* quality to each other.

Earth Types

Earth types seem balanced and centered, with an earthy look (▶Fig. 10.22).

- Large bone structure, with large shoulders and thighs and a short neck
- Strong but not fast and agile
- The tendency to be overweight
- Friendly and reassuring; great sense of humor
- Possibly an un-kept appearance, clothing is quite secondary

Earth-type face

- A square face with an open and merry expression (▶Fig. 10.23)
- Reddish face color, or of the nose tip and ears; thick lips
- The tendency to hair loss in the front and top of the head

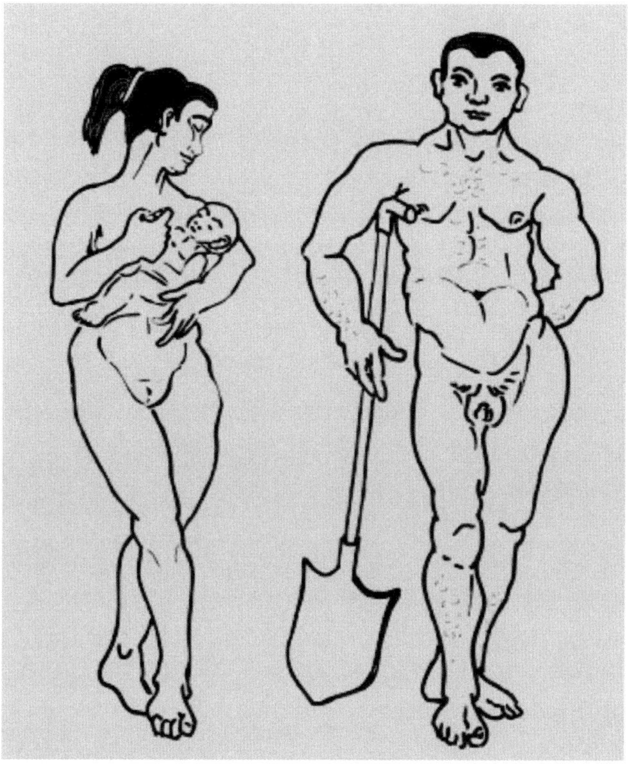

Figure 10.22: Earth types: squarish and strong body, large bones, short neck, and limbs, tendency to be overweight

Earth-type hands

The Earth type hands are short, square and thick, with short and thick fingers. Often lines on the palms are quite simple, and single lines at the interphalangeal joints are quite common.

The nails are triangular, rather flat, with a very thick cuticle that may crack easily, producing hangnails (▶Fig. 10.24).

Earth combines mainly with Metal

Earth and Metal frequently combine; this combination is the most common and by its fixity and stability constitutes the foundation of the society.

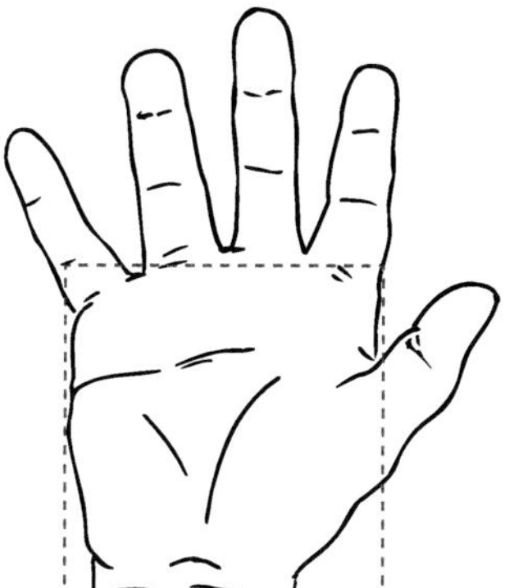

Figure 10.24: Earth type hand: square palm, few lines, thick short fingers, triangular nails, thick cuticle, frequent hang-nail.

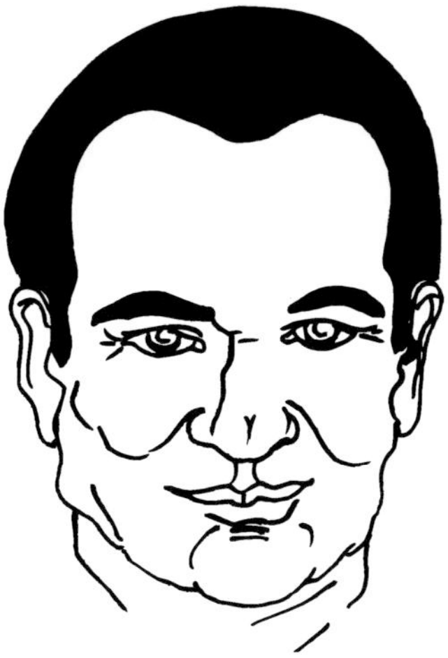

Figure 10.23: Earth-type face: squarish, thick lips and nose tip, merry, friendly and reassuring, tendency to hair loss (front)

Metal Types

Metal types are also tall but with stooping and narrow shoulders, and shorter legs than the Fire types (▶Fig. 10.25).

- In general, the body tends to be rigid, on rare occasions, it could be over-lax
- Generally elegant and neat and precise appearance, with conventional clothing
- Slow and precise movements and speech

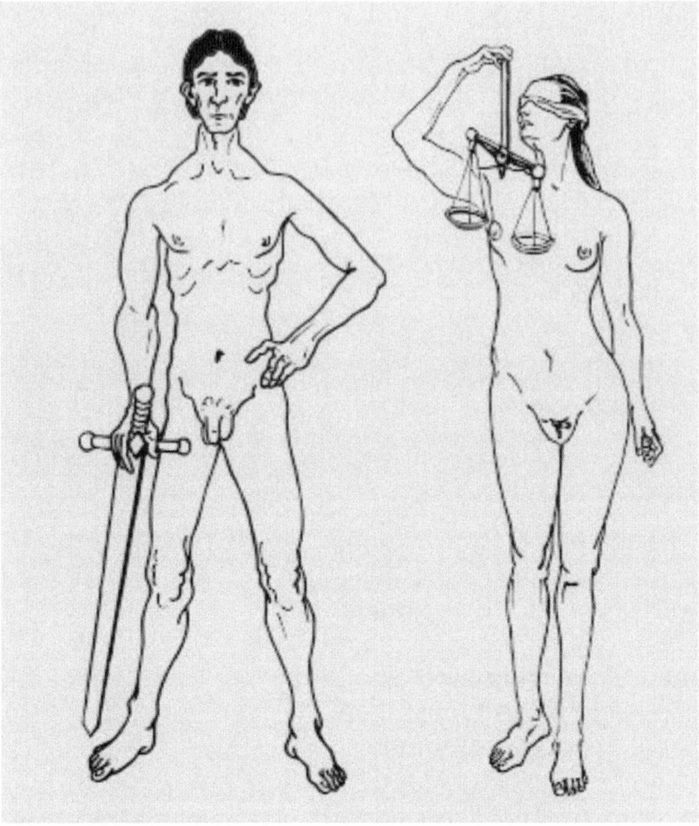

Figure 10.25: Metal types: may be tall or average, narrow shoulders, long trunk, tendency to be rigid

Metal-type face

- A long face with pale, thin lips, long nose
- May have deep wrinkles, square teeth
- May either look friendly and tolerant, or malicious, calculating and wary or at times, distant and bored (▶Fig. 10.26)

Metal-type hands

The Metal type hands are also long, but the palm is longer than the fingers. With the fingers touching, the hand has an oval shape. It could have a pear shape if the Earth element is also present. The fingers are not straight and might even be crooked. There are often 3 inter-phalangeal lines. The nails are rectangular, quite elegant, white and often striated.

Occasionally the nails may be short, quite rounded in both planes resembling drumsticks (▶Fig. 10.27).

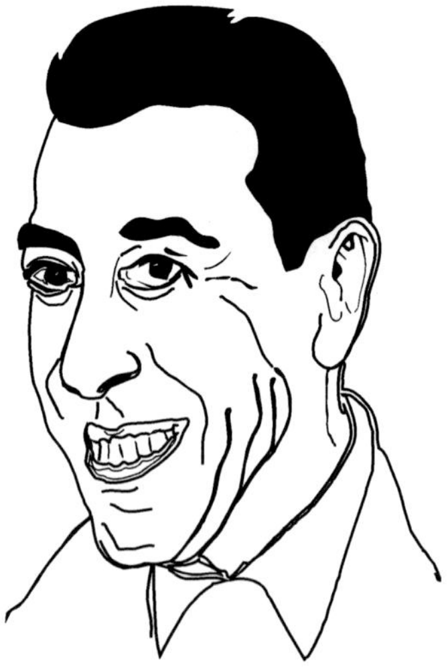

Figure 10.26: Metal-type face: elongated and rectangular shape, vertical lines, prominent nose, large and square teeth, tolerant and patient look

Metal frequently combines with Earth

The precision and orderliness of Metal added to the stability and the centerdness of Earth are the ideal combinations for family and social structures.

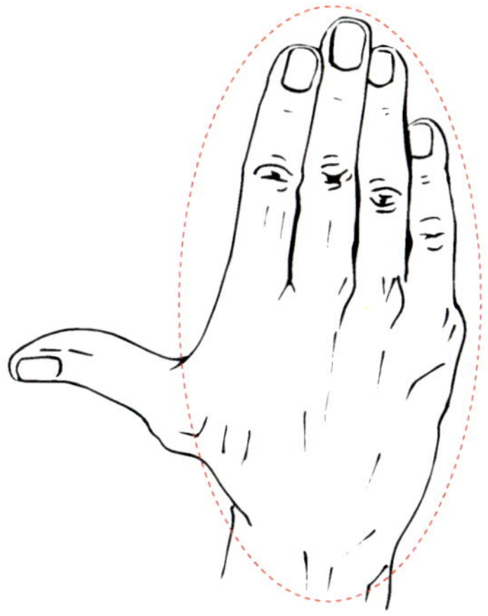

Figure 10.27: Metal type hand: oval shaped hand, long palm, white (ivory colored) rectangular nails

Water Types

Water types often have a rounded body like earth types, but much softer and puffier skin and flesh (►Fig. 10.28).

- Most often short and rounded, the body could also be quite curvaceous; they might also be dry and skinny if the Fire element is stronger
- Often supple but may have choppy movements giving the impression of clumsiness or nervousness
- Often shy, self-effacing with shifty eyes
- Speaking slowly, prone to loss of voice

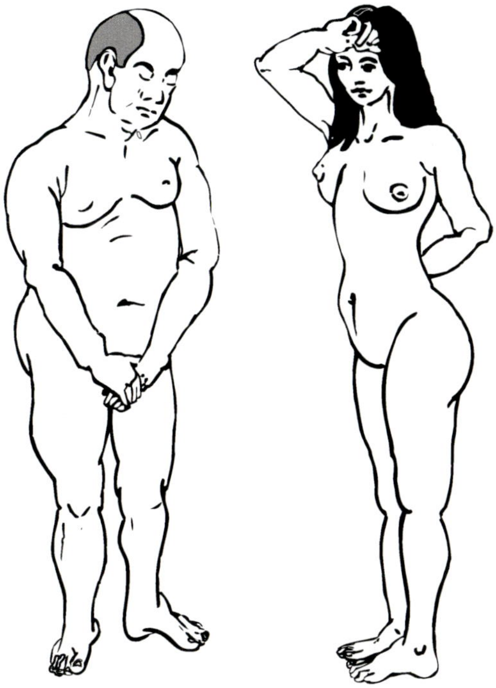

Figure 10.28 Water types: often short and rounded or curvaceous in women, the tendency to shyness, might seem clumsy

Water-type face

- Round face with a darkish complexion, or with red cheeks, blushing easily
- Dark under the eyes, sometimes swollen eyes with red rims

- Frequent baldness (▶ Fig. 10.29).

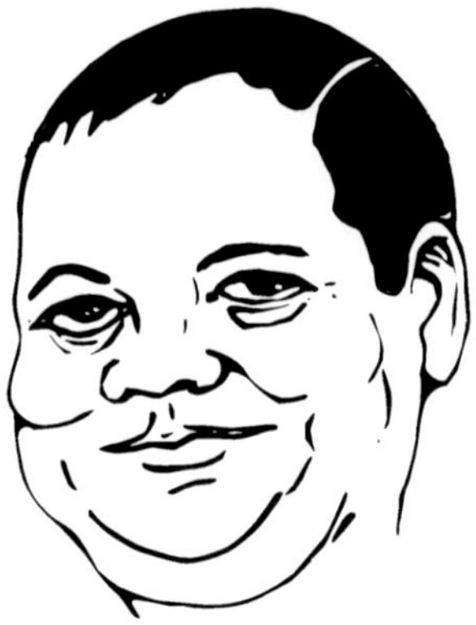

Figure 10.29: Water-type face: round, dark complexion, blushing easily, dark and swollen under the eyes, frequent hair loss

Water type hands

The Water-type hands are short, puffy with loose and soft skin. The fingers are short and present a dimple on the dorsal side of the joints. The nails are trapezoid and very flat or even concave. The limit between nail and skin is not very clear. The nails are soft and tend to grow downwards (▶ Fig. 10.30).

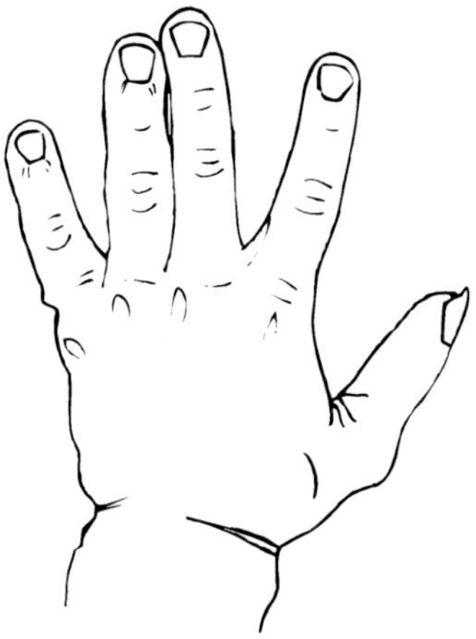

Figure 10.30: Water type hand: puffy skin, flat trapezoid nails, nail and cuticle on one level with skin lines at the corner of the nail, occasional downward growing nails

Water combines with Fire

The combination of Water with Fire brings the expansive quality of Fire into the creative potential of Water, resulting in the blending of intelligence and wisdom.

10.4 Influence of the Six Temperaments on the Morphology and Behavior

As discussed above, the basic anatomical structure of a person depends on their constitutional elements. The concept of the "Five Elements" describes the basic internal rhythm and defines the "Constitution" or the five archetypes that basically depend on the Pre-Heaven parental essence *Jing*. This explains the racial similarities found in a particular country or area of the world. The constitution will further influence the development and activity of the organs *Zang-Fu* and their related "Primary" channels.

The ancestral *Zong Qi* is the cosmic *Qi* at the moment of conception and defines the *Ming* ≈ Destiny of the person and will, therefore, influence the basic "Temperament" of the individual. The "Temperament" will define how a person communicates and responds to the outer world, and is defined by the "Six Great Axis" or channels. The outer manifestations of these "Six Axis" are the twelve "Sinew channels" *Jing-Jin,* controlling amongst other things, the muscles and sinews. The interplay of the muscles, their tension or laxity, will define the outer form/ morphology.

It can be summarized that the "Five Movements" explore the synchronization of the Microcosm with the Macrocosm, the influences of the outer world on a person. The "Six Channel systems or energy levels" constitute the bridge that communicates the constitution "Microcosm" with the constant changes that occur between Heaven and Earth "Macrocosm".

Repletion/ excess in a channel system may indicate the things to which one is drawn to, whereas a Vacuity/ deficiency could underline one's avoidances and inadequacies.

This explains that a person's physiology, as well as their pathology, is not only a reflection of their constitution but also of their "Temperament" and "Behavior".

As long as the temperament is in accordance with the constitution, there is a sense of inner harmony. For example, when a Fire-type constitution has a *Tai Yang* (Fire-Water) or *Shao Yin* (Fire-Water) temperament, they will feel generally "at ease". When the temperament is not adapted, there is a feeling of unease, for example, a Fire-type constitution having any other type of temperament, for instance, a *Tai Yin* (Earth-Metal) temperament, will manifest a discomfort. This situation often arises from external pressures, such as family, society or conditioning. If this dis-adaptation continues for a long time it will cause pathology first on the energetic and later on physical levels. In general, each temperament, when not blocked, has the capacity of moving in and out of their preferential level, in order to respond to the needs of the moment, especially to communicate with their complementary *Yin* or *Yang* levels (▶Fig. 10.31).

When any temperament is blocked in a particular level, pathology arises, manifesting at first psychologically, and over time physically as well. It is important to note that with age, as the individual has less *Qi*, most temperaments tend to either get blocked in their level or in the complementary *Yin* level, which further enhances the development of the corresponding pathologies. In general two temperaments get more easily blocked in their levels: the *Tai Yin* and the *Shao Yin.*

The "Temperament" is evaluated, based on the outer form as well as the habitual "Behaviour" of the person. With some experience, the constitution and the temperament of a patient are evaluated within minutes of having encountered them. This not only helps to better understand the pathology of a person but also orients towards the most appropriate selection of therapy and the best choice of channels and points to treat.

Each constitutional element is related to two channels, and thus to two possible vibrational levels. For example, a Fire-type constitution may present a *Tai Yang* or a *Shao Yin* temperament.

Each individual will blend the two elements in their own and very unique manner. Hence two Fire-types will have similarities but will not be identical. The same applies to temperaments, for example, a Fire-type might present characteristics of Water or vice versa.

Tai Yang Temperament

Usually found in Fire or Water-type constitutions combining the physical characteristics of these two types (▶Fig. 10.32). More frequent in men, especially in the world of business, politics or army. In general, the typical *Tai Yang* types are quite rare.

- Physically, most often presenting the Fire-type bodies, tall, slender and graceful, with elongated limbs. But they could also have Water-type characteristics, shorter and rounder, or even occasionally dried up and ascetic-looking. Even if not tall, the head is being carried high, with a certain rigidity of the spine. Usually presenting impeccably and wearing precise clothing, with a preference for uniforms and outer signs of distinction. The complexion may be red or darkish. Eyes are often hard and dominating or even condescending. Although the *Tai Yang* personalities are quite sensitive, they rarely show their inner feelings, giving an impression of hardness. Their movements are fast or even jerky, they are quite often sportive, liking and needing to win. The *Tai Yang* dislikes winter but

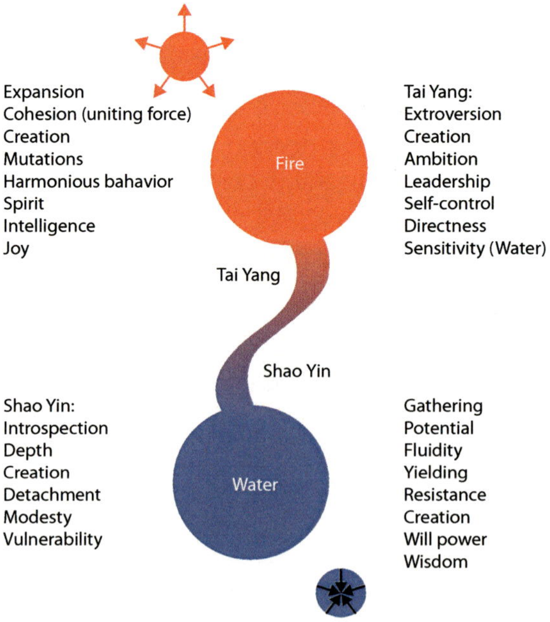

Figure 10.31: *Tai Yang* and *Shao Yin* Temperaments blending the characteristics of Fire and Water

also dislikes excessive heat.

- The strength of *Tai Yang* is their easy communication with the outside; their leadership capacities, good sense of overview; often directing the action. An excellent intellectual and emotional memory, fast minds, with superior intelligence and the facility for learning and high working capacity. Very precise with a good sense of overview and planning.
- Psychologically they are extroverted, have high ambitions and managing to realize them. This ambition and their leadership qualities place them at the head of companies and conglomerates, or as political or army leaders. Often inventors or creators, frequently having a unique passion. When the qualities of Fire and Water combine, the *Tai Yang* are very good leaders, with directness, integrity, sensitivity and vulnerability, good communicators, generous and devoted, with great self-control, capable of self-sacrifice and austerity to reach an ideal or a goal. Issues of family, country, and religion are taken very seriously.
- On the negative side, they tend to become fanatical, with a fixation on a unique passion. When the communication with the *Shao Yin* level is blocked, they tend to have difficulty to integrate with excessive ambition or pretentiousness. Needing to demolish before building. When blocked the *Tai Yang* become quite intolerable and bossy, dominating, insensitive, commanding, controlling even tyrannical, pushing themselves and others, accepting with difficulty any contradiction; intolerant of mistakes and very impatient. They may even become paranoid.
- Pathologically a blocked *Tai Yang* could develop heart and circulation, neurological, osteoarticular or kidney and urinary problems, their sleep is often bad and short.
- *Tai Yang* children have an excitable nervous system, especially if there was a difficult birth. They are easily rebellious, opposing authority, especially if they have a *Tai Yang* parent.
- The *Tai Yang* is quite choosy about their therapists, and have to feel a special connection with them. Once a therapist has been accepted, the *Tai Yang* remains quite faithful and will follow the advised treatments and prescriptions dutifully.
- Examples of *Tai Yang* type temperaments could be found amongst the Scandinavians, certain Slavic races, Germans, and many of the world leaders, presidents or especially dictators.

Shao Yin Temperament

- Physically: Most often short and rounded; in women, the body could also be quite curvaceous. Often supple but may have clumsy or choppy movements. Quite rounded features and face, with smooth skin, redness of cheeks, or easily blushing, may also have a darkish complexion, especially around the eyes. Swollen and moist eyes with red rims, especially in the mornings. Even if the Fire constitution gives them a tall and slender body, the *Shao Yin* personality makes the person, shy and introverted, with a drooping attitude trying not to be noticed. Often introverted, shy, self-effacing, looking down or with shifty eyes, speaking slowly, prone to loss of voice. *Shao Yin* type temperaments in general, avoid action and dislike winters and the cold.

- The *Shao Yin's* capacity for introspection, allows them to recognize their weaknesses and try to change them. Searching for depth and for the essential, which confers great wisdom to the *Shao Yin* types. They are resourceful and creative, self-giving, resigned, modest, vulnerable and detached. In spite of their dislike of action, they are conscientious and serious and will follow through something they have started, they might even come up with ways of doing things with less effort. The *Shao Yin* tend to be quite artistic and romantic.
- Intellectually, they have generally a poor memory, having difficulties in learning by heart; but having an excellent emotional memory and great sensitivity and empathy. They are quite often not good in academic structures but might excel in certain intellectual aptitudes.
- On the negative side, when blocked they tend to become unsatisfied with life, blaming oneself, shy, introverted, easily discouraged, demoralized, not wanting to live, fearful, self-effacing and victimized. Ambitious but not daring to move into action; easily considering oneself a looser and even provoking failure. May also become tricky, sneaky, or even quite clever in business matters. When blocked the *Shao Yin* can become envious, misanthropic, even rejoicing in other's misfortunes; the tendency for guilt or self-destruction, even masochism; or on the opposite side becoming misanthropic, isolating themselves, seeking contact with nature to get recharged and to find serenity.
- As children, they are often fragile, with frequent infections, sore throats, otitis, impetigo, furuncles, rheumatism or even heart problems. In school, other children often pick on them.
- Pathologically, they tend to develop severe infections or chronic diseases, heart and circulation problems, urinary or osteoarticular diseases. Knowing this and being afraid of death, they will often take good care of their health, consulting early and following prescriptions faithfully.
- Examples of *Shao Yin* type temperaments are many of the black races, Russians, Middle Easterners and Semitic races, many philosophers, romantic poets or unconventional scientists.

Shao Yang Temperament

Combines the Wood and Fire characteristics (▶Fig. 10.32).

- Physically: average height, proportionate body shape, martial, fearless even at times reckless, agile, restless, nervous or even prone to tics. With open and frank features, large eyes, open eyebrows, warm and penetrating look, quite expressive, seductive, and extroverted. The *Shao-Yang* is most often quite friendly and open, but may also present as an inhibited and shy type with tics, nail-biting, and nervous wrenching of hands; or on the opposite the agitated type, talkative, wetting of lips, overexcitement, loud or even quarrelsome. The features are tanned or of an olive complexion, but may be pale or blushing. The clothing is often unconventional or quite coquettish. In general, they seek the cold and dislike wind and heat.

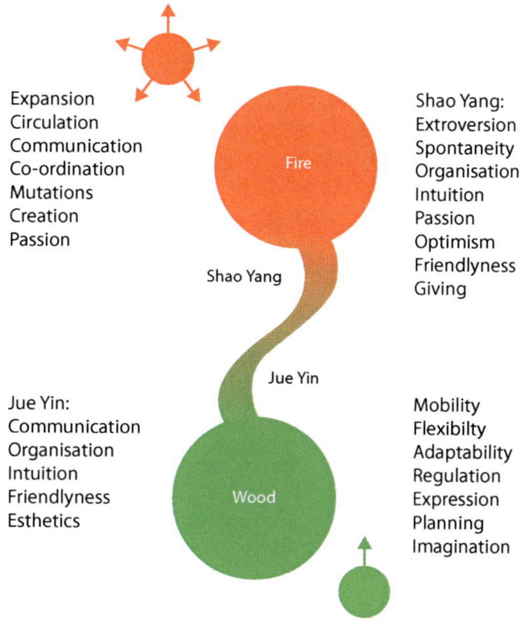

Figure 10.32: *Shao Yang* and *Jue Yin* Temperaments blending the characteristics of Fire and Wood

- The *Shao Yang* temperament is quite spontaneous, intuitive, optimistic, and passionate, living life to the full. They are generous, making friends easily, very charming and cordial, they do not like to hurt others and do not keep grudges and in general, dislike conflicts. They are very sportive, and their sense of coordination gives them the ability to be good at sports or artistic performances. The *Shao Yang* is an excellent coordinator and organizer, their flexibility and friendliness and facility in communication puts them often in positions of negotiation or public relations. Their curiosity and interest in the new explains that most explorers and adventures belong to this type. They like work and starting new projects but have difficulty in finishing them.
- Intellectually they have a good memory that can suddenly decrease with age. Boiling with ideas, imagination, with intense creativity but quite often disorganized intellectually. They are quite active and creative at night but like to sleep late, having difficulty to get going in the morning.
- When blocked the *Shao Yang* has difficulty integrating and becomes insatiable, looking constantly for new adventures or love affairs. Becoming competitive, choleric, reactive, aggressive and vengeful with a tendency to be arrogant, critical, restless and impatient. In some cases, the anger might be interiorized manifesting as anxiety or stress (Liver *Qi* stagnation). There is a tendency to develop liver and gallbladder problems, hypertension, migraine headaches, stress and tension, and various tics or tinnitus.
- In childhood, the *Shao Yang* is often very thin, generally healthy, but sometimes might present with slight liver problems and vomiting (motion sickness) or migraine headaches. In school, they are often the centers of attention, sportive, chief of the band, easily involved in fights.
- Pathologically when blocked the *Shao Yang* might present liver or gallbladder problems, hypertension, migraine headaches, stress and tension, tics, tinnitus and vertigo (Wind). They dislike being sick and usually recover quite fast. In relation to therapy, they might sound very interested and enthusiastic but will follow treatments for a short time only.
- Examples of *Shao Yang* type temperaments are the Mediterranean's, especially Spanish, Greeks, and Corsicans, as well as the North Americans. The *Shao*

Yang temperament is often present amongst explorers, adventurers, in individual sports, extreme sports especially involving danger, martial arts, as well as visual arts, entertainment, and acting.

Jue Yin Temperament

Combines the Wood and Fire characteristics. The *Shao Yang* and *Jue Yin* temperaments can easily be confused, both being very extroverted, spontaneous and emotional. The main difference lies in *Shao Yang*'s love for action.

- Physically: average height, proportionate body shape, very similar to *Shao-Yang* types, but more nervous or even prone to tics, at times difficult to distinguish between the two types. They might either present as a shy type, very nervous, fainting easily, or quite agitated and talkative. Often with open and frank features, large eyes, quite expressive, seductive or mysterious, may be myopic. Often tanned or olive complexion or may be pale. The appearance and clothing attract attention in a provocative or seductive manner, reflecting a passive extraversion. They might be supple and sportive, but get easily exhausted. They dislike wind, heights, airplanes, cars, boats, and crowds. They like spring, but sometimes feel tired at the start of spring.
- The *Jue Yin* temperament is quite spontaneous, intuitive, sensitive, charming, communicative, and may be very seductive. They have a great imagination and creativity with a high aesthetical sense, which combined with their non-conformism, gives them many artistic talents. Their natural charm and communicativeness make them good organizers, mediators and excellent in public relations. Their mental and emotional flexibility gives them, on the one hand, a facility for acting and on the other hand the capacity to be quite at ease in the inner and outer worlds, which combined with their strong intuition, confers to them the necessary tools to be excellent psycho-therapists.
- Intellectually they may have a good memory but may become forgetful because of emotions. They have a very lively imagination, high sense of aesthetics, artistic inspirations as well as intuition. They often have very vivid dreams, which could disturb their sleeping patterns.
- When blocked, which means that they are not able to communicate with their complementary *Yang* level *Shao Yang*, they may become dramatic, hysterical, passionately intense, jealous, pessimistic, with a great tendency to vanity. Emotionally falling in and out of love very quickly. The moods are often inconsistent with swings between anxiety and depression, or dreamy and absent. Their lack of confidence makes them feel conflicts intensely in two possible ways:
  - Inhibition and anxiety "Liver *Qi Xu*": always on the alert, worrying about small things, having difficulty in giving priority to things, with difficulty moving into action; various kinds of phobia, may even be paralyzed by fear. This inhibition can produce great inner tension for even simple daily matters.
  - Evasion: often into imagination, closing their eyes on to reality, dreaming, creating a false identity, a mask; living often in a world of fantasy and pretence, frequently evading into superficiality, excitements, films, whims, exciting love affairs, with a tendency to addictions, drugs, coffee, alcohol (for which they often have a poor tolerance).

- In childhood, the *Jue Yin*, are quite sensitive, may easily feel unloved, needing a lot of assurance and compliments. They tend to be easily jealous of their siblings. Physically they may suffer from liver problems, eye pathologies, and possibly seasonal allergies.
- Pathologically when blocked they can easily develop liver and Gallbladder problems; Liver-*Qi*-stasis; migraines; myopia; tiredness, low blood pressure: various types of spasms (Spasmophilia) and tics. They are difficult patients, as they do not follow through the therapy and the prescriptions, changing often doctors and methods.
- Examples of *Jue Yin* type temperaments are to be found amongst many poets, writers, painters, designers, and actors. The Latin races in particular Italians (more Fire) or French (more Wood).

Yang Ming Temperament

Combines the Earth and Metal characteristics (▶Fig. 10.33). The *Yang Ming* and especially the *Tai Yin* represent the majority of humanity and constitute the backbone and foundation of most societies.

- Physically: Many combinations of Earth and Metal are possible here. If the Earth element predominates the person has a balanced and centered, earthy look. Large bones, large shoulders and thick thighs with a short neck and a roundish or large face open and often jovial features, with thick lips, red face or red tip of nose and ears, with soft, reassuring, slightly protruding merry eyes. Not very agile and fast but quite strong, may be overweight. With age has a tendency to lose hair on the front and top. The general appearance and clothing are often unimportant and might even seem un-kept. They dislike humidity and heat.
- When the Metal is dominant the person tends to be taller, with narrow shoulders, a rounded stooping back with a thin, long and pale face, thin lips and eyebrows, high cheekbones. With age, the face tends to get deep wrinkles. More dry looking, but friendly, calm and patient with slow and precise movements. Naturally elegant, clean and very conventional clothing. Disliking both heat and cold, preferring the Autumn

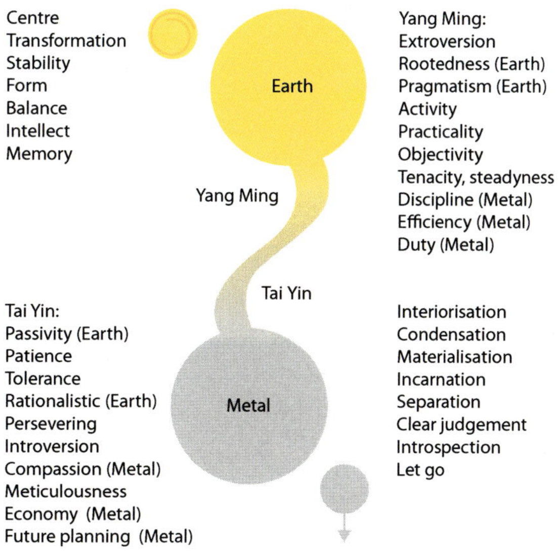

Figure 10.33: *Yang Ming* and *Tai Yin* Temperaments blending the properties of Earth and Metal

season.

- The *Yang Ming* temperament is quite calm, non-reactive and unemotional, with very good objectivity, de-dramatizing situations, seeking harmony, giving support and helping to solve problems in a fair manner. Generally quite diplomatic, loving human relations and company. Practical and non-dogmatic, hard-working, tenacious, completing any project. Optimistic, tolerant, liberal, playful with a good sense of humor.
- Intellectually they tend to have a good memory, inventive and clever, having a very good capacity to break down a problem in order to understand and to integrate it. The Metal type *Yang Ming* has a keen sense of observation, quite comfortable with abstract systems. In general very precise, reliable and punctual, steady and cool, doing a lot with apparent minimum effort.
- When blocked the *Yang Ming* has difficulty communicating with their counterpart level *Tai Yin.* Becoming quite stubborn and obsessive even rigid and intolerant. Lacking comprehension or penetration they deal with their minds rather than with their feelings, they may become quite superficial, ironical, cynical and skeptical. Indulging in all the good things in life, sensual, fun loving, over-optimistic, tending to overspend or overbet. When angry, they complain rather than explode.
- In childhood, the *Yang Ming* Earth types are often in quite good health though they tend to overindulge in food, especially sweets. The Metal type is more delicate, often quite skinny with frequent colds and lung problems.
- Pathologically when blocked the *Yang Ming* Earth types tend to develop digestive problems, with a tendency to obesity, diabetes, gout, excess cholesterol and circulation problems. They are not easy to treat and do not like to follow diets or medical advice. Metal type *Yang Ming's* present more intestinal problems, sinus infections, and teeth decay. They are easy to treat and trust the therapist and follow instructions dutifully.
- Examples of *Yang Ming* Earth types are found amongst, engineers, builders, doctors, and teachers, also the middle-Eastern population, or else the Pre-Victorian British. *Yang Ming* Metal types are to be found amongst a number of scholars, mathematicians, doctors, especially surgeons, as well as the British and the Swiss people.

Tai Yin Temperament

Combines the Earth and Metal characteristics, and as mentioned above is the most frequent in numbers in various societies.

- Physically: Tendency to being large, with a large and fleshy face, quite passive, often "too soft", with thick flesh, very similar to *Yang Ming* but much calmer, with slow deliberate movements. May also be tall and elastic, or on the contrary quite stiff and dry if the Metal predominates, in this case, the face is long and narrow with a long nose and thin lips. Facial color is white or pink with redness of the tip of nose and ears. They dislike the damp and the cold.
- The *Tai Yin* temperament: is very passive, patient, calm, conciliatory and usually a fair referee; often a good listener, unemotional, capable of consoling with great compassion and insight. Rationalistic, persevering, detached, deliberate, moving into action only after considering all the options. When the Metal influence

predominates, they are very organized, strict and meticulous, paying a lot of importance to detail. Planning for the future, economical. They rather prefer an intimate company to groups.

- Intellectually they tend to be quite rationalistic, dogmatic, analytical, and at times judgmental. They need more sleep, getting easily tired.
- When blocked, this level has difficulty exteriorizing towards *Yang Ming*. May become negligent and lazy, passive, introverted, holding their feelings; indifferent and distracted with bouts of asthenia, depression even melancholia. The Earth type tends to eat to compensate, whereas the Metal type becomes even more rigid and fixed in habits and ideas, obsessed with details, perfectionism, introverted and un-expressive, worrying about the future, holding onto things and even becoming stingy.
- In childhood: the Earth types are usually easy children to handle, quite passive, loving to eat. On the opposite the Metal types are often sickly and fragile, lacking appetite and vitality.
- Pathologically when blocked the *Tai Yin* will easily present digestive problems, obesity, diabetes, gout, excess cholesterol as well as lung pathologies, asthma, and constipation. The Earth type *Tai Yin* often will have difficulty in following diets and treatments, whereas the Metal type *Tai Yin* is overly concerned about their health, they will show up at their appointment long before time, will follow the doctors orders to the letter, will never travel without considering all health risks and having the appropriate medication for it.
- Examples of *Tai Yin* type temperaments are found amongst farmers, workers laborers and builders, as well as the Chinese and Mexicans (more Earth), the Indians, the Swiss and Scottish (More Metal), and in most sedentary and farming societies.

Body Shapes according to Yin and Yang

The *Ling Shu* chapters 72 and 67 describe five types of body shape. I have included these descriptions to respect the tradition but personally find them somehow incomplete and even confusing, and much prefer the Five-element approach.

Yang Abundant body shapes: related to Tai Yang

- Strong body build, lively character
- The tendency to a red face
- Preference for cold, intolerance of heat
- The tendency to be a high achiever with assertiveness and self-contentment
- Walking with chest and abdomen projecting forward

The description fits the Fire types and the *Tai Yang* temperament. *Ling Shu* advises to sedate the *Yang* and nourish the *Yin*; results may be expected quickly.

Yin Abundant body shapes: related to Tai Yin

- Tendency to obesity
- Preference for heat and being wrapped warmly
- Having a somber appearance and pretending to be humble, looking down and not showing their feelings easily
- Followers
- Exposed to diseases of Cold, Damp and Phlegm, stagnation of *Yin* and of Blood

This description fits the *Yin* type of Earth or Metal constitutions and especially the *Tai Yin* temperaments. It is advised, in the *Ling Shu*, to reduce *Yin* and supplement *Yang* and move *Qi*; the expected response would be slow.

Yang Deficient: related to Shao Yang[3]

- Overweight with a swollen body,
- Pale or pale-bluish complexion
- Listlessness with a low spirit and easily tired
- Slow movements, weak loose muscles
- Preference to warm and aversion to cold
- A tendency for contracting Cold or Damp type diseases
- The treatment strategy aims at supplementing *Yang*.

Yin Deficient body shape: related to Shao Yin[4]

- A thin, emaciated body
- Sometimes red cheeks and lips
- Maybe tall, long neck with narrow shoulders, bend forward when walking or standing
- Excited look, restless expression
- A feeling of heat and quick movements
- Tend to get diseases of *Yin* or *Jing* vacuity and hyperactivity of *Yang*: Empty-Heat or Dryness

The proposed treatment aims at supplementing *Yin* and reducing *Yang*.

Harmonious Yin-Yang body shape

- Medium built, medium height
- Balanced movements
- Content with themselves, living a quiet life

---

[3] The description here fits better the Water-type and the *Shao Yin* personality and does not seem at all appropriate to *Shao Yang* temperaments.

[4] The description would more easily fit the *Yin*-deficient Metal or Fire types, and the temperament is more suggestive of *Shao Yang* or *Tai Yang* and not at all of *Shao Yin*.

- A stable personality with kind looking eyes
- Adjusting well to change, not often sick
  This constitutional type responds rapidly to treatment.

  The description fits the Earth type constitution and the *Yang Ming* temperament.

Tolerance to Pain and to Medication

The evaluation of tolerance to pain, is very helpful when practicing acupuncture, hence the choice of points and the intensity of the stimulation may be better adapted to the constitution of the person.

- People with a high tolerance for pain have a relatively dark complexion, body build is big and full with a strong skeleton, tendons are soft, muscles relaxed and the skin is firm.
- People with a low tolerance for pain have a thin body, hard muscles, and thin, loose and tender skin.

Particular body shapes in relation to pathology

Thin, emaciated	*Yin Xu*, Blood-*Xu* or *Jing Xu*
Overweight, heavy	Spleen-*Yang Xu*; accumulation of Dampness
Barrel chest	Stomach-*Qi Shi* (repletion)
Heavy thighs	Spleen-*Qi Xu*
Agitated, fast movements	*Yang* condition; Heat repletion
Calm and slow, apathetic	*Yin* condition; Empty-Cold (from *Yang Xu*)
Deformities	Congenital organ weakness, *Jing Xu*
Depressed chest, hunched back	Congenital Lung-*Qi Xu*
Kyphosis, scoliosis	Depends on the area may relate to Lung, Spleen, or Kidney
Inverted nipples	Inherited or childhood Lung diseases
Flat feet, tipped inwards	Spleen-*Qi Xu*
Arched feet; hallux	Liver-*Qi* stasis or repletion
Shoulders not level	Gallbladder problems

Body posture during sickness

Lying on the belly	*Xu* ≈ Vacuity condition; Cold from *Yang Xu*
Cannot stay lying	Heat repletion
Restlessness, impatience	Kidney-*Yin Xu* (Heat from deficiency)
Trembling, tics, convulsions; opistotonos	Internal Wind/ Liver-Wind

Hands

Pale hands	*Yang Xu* or Blood *Xu*
Red dorsum of hands	Heart-Heat (repletion) or Lung and Stomach Heat
Red palms	Heart-Heat or Lung & Stomach-Heat from *Yin Xu*
Thenar eminence	Shows the state of the Stomach Red capillaries: Stomach-Heat Bluish veins: Stomach-Cold Purple veins: Blood stasis
Tremor of hands	Liver-Wind (from Heat or *Yin Xu*); in alcoholics Phlegm-Heat
Contractions of the fingers	"Chicken Claw Wind": Liver- Blood or *Yin Xu* as in Dupuytren's disease Cold in the joints *Qi* stagnation
Spoon-shaped fingers	Shaped as drum sticks: may be constitutional also seen in chronic Lung diseases by Cold-Phlegm or Phlegm-Heat
Thin, pointed fingers	Generally relates to a Stomach pathology from Cold-Damp or Damp-Heat
Swollen fingers	*Bi* ≈ Impediment syndrome, Blood stasis, oedema
Cracked fingers	Blood *Xu* or Blood stasis, Cold from *Yang Xu*

Nails

Nails are related to the Liver but they reflect the general condition, the circulation, and the diet. The growth rate of nails reflects Liver-*Qi and* Liver-Blood; thickening of nails may be in relation to Liver-*Yin Xu,* Liver-Fire or Phlegm; their brittleness would reflect a Vacuity of Liver-Blood or Liver-*Yin.*

Concave nail	*Yin* exuberance
Convex nail	*Yang* exuberance
Lunules (moons)	Relate to circulation, diet and general constitution
	If larger than ¼ of the nail: abundance of *Qi* and Blood; excessive intake of protein
	If small or absent: weak constitution; fatigue; aggravation
White spots	Stress; intake of excess *Yin* or of acidic foods
White cloudiness	Zinc or Silicium or Magnesium deficiency
Brown or black spots	Stomach-Heat or chronic constipation
Thick cuticle	Excess protein intake
Thick cuticle, red and peeling	Lack of animal protein
Pronounced vertical lines	Stress; Blood *Xu*; *Bi* ≈ Impediment syndrome; Lung-*Qi Xu*
Thin and brittle	Blood and *Qi Xu*, Liver-Blood *Xu* or Liver-*Yin Xu*
Cracked	Liver-Blood *Xu*, Liver-*Qi Xu*
Thickening of nails	Liver-Fire, Liver-Blood-stasis or Phlegm
Withered and thickened	Stomach and Spleen vacuity, Liver-Blood *Xu*, Damp-Heat, Toxic Heat
Bulging uneven nail	A sudden change of diet or Vitamin B deficiency
Indented	Onset of a disease from Liver-Blood *Xu*, *Qi Xu* or Heat injuring fluids
Curled	Blood and *Qi Xu* with Blood stasis
Pale nail, that becomes white under pressure and remains white for a while	Blood *Xu*
Red nails	Heat
Purple nails	Stagnant Blood from Cold or Heat or *Qi* stasis
Yellow	Damp-Heat

Diagnosis of Blood-Xu

The hand is put in hyperextension, after a few seconds the nails become white if they remain white after relaxing the hand there is weak Blood. Please note that Blood *Xu* is not identical to the Western notion of anemia, which is equivalent to a combined Blood and *Qi Xu*.

Skin

Skin is the outer appearance of the Lung.

Color

The color modification is studied in relation to the Five Phases.

Red

Signifies Heat.

Red cheeks in the after-noon "malar flush"	Empty-Heat from *Yin Xu* ≈ Vacuity
Blotchy red	Exhaustion of *Qi*
Powdery red	Empty-Heat from *Yin Xu* ≈ Vacuity

Yellow

Signifies Spleen-*Qi Xu* with Dampness.

Bright yellow and moist	Damp-Heat
Dull yellow, old looking	Damp-Cold
Dry and withered	Stomach-Fire

White

Signifies Lung-*Qi Xu* and Cold.

Bright white and puffy	*Yang Xu* and *Qi Xu* after Blood loss
Dull white and thin	Blood *Xu*
Pale, greyish, with red cheeks and lips	Residual Heat "True Heat false Cold"
White patches in front of the ears	Parasites
Pale with dark patches on the forehead	Pregnancy or contraceptive pill

Black

Signifies weak Kidneys or Pathogenic Cold, stagnant Blood, or pain.

Black, dry and thin	*Yin Xu* with Fire (Empty-Fire)
Dull black but with a bright nose	The condition is not severe
Dull black face and nose	Severe condition

Green

Signifies Liver-Wind or Cold.

If there is pain	Stagnation of *Qi* or Blood
Green with white	Internal Wind from Liver *Yin* or Blood *Xu*
Green with red	Liver-Fire

Texture

Skin Rashes

The majority of skin rashes reflect a condition of Heat or Fire. In general, the Pathogenic factor involved is identified by the aspect and other accompanying symptoms:

- Red with a sensation of heat: Heat or Fire
- Itching: Wind
- Oozing with exudate or blistering: Dampness
- Dryness: External Dryness or Cold; Body fluid *Xu;* Liver-Blood *Xu;* Kidney-*Yin Xu*
- Scaling: Dryness; Blood *Xu*, or Heat
- Purplish: Blood stasis
- Dark, bluish: Cold

<table>
<tr><td>Swelling that keeps the pressure marks</td><td colspan="2">"Water edema"; Humidity; Kidney-Yang Xu</td></tr>
<tr><td>Non depressible swelling</td><td colspan="2">"Qi edema" Qi stagnation</td></tr>
<tr><td>Scaly</td><td colspan="2">Poor circulation of Qi</td></tr>
<tr><td>Dry, dull and wrinkled</td><td colspan="2">Body fluid Xu; Lung-Yin Xu, Liver-Blood Xu</td></tr>
<tr><td>Greasy</td><td colspan="2">Dampness, Damp-Heat, Phlegm</td></tr>
<tr><td>Loose, easily damaged</td><td colspan="2">Lung-Qi Xu</td></tr>
<tr><td>Leathery, rough, tough</td><td colspan="2">Lung-Qi Xu</td></tr>
<tr><td>Leathery and painful skin</td><td colspan="2">Blood stasis</td></tr>
<tr><td>Fissures</td><td colspan="2">Blood Xu; Lung or Kidney-Yin Xu</td></tr>
<tr><td rowspan="5">Spider veins; angioma</td><td colspan="2">Fullness in the Luo ≈ Connecting channels</td></tr>
<tr><td>Red</td><td>Heat</td></tr>
<tr><td>Bluish</td><td>Cold</td></tr>
<tr><td>Greenish</td><td>Pain</td></tr>
<tr><td>Purplish</td><td>Blood stasis</td></tr>
</table>

10.5 Examination of Children

The Four Pillars of diagnosis are only partially applicable in small children and infants. Signs tend to change very rapidly. Diagnosis relies on the observation of the facial colors, general head and body movements, the state of the upper orifices and the examination of the index finger in children under the age of three. These signs are combined with the symptoms provided by the parents.

In general children have immature Kidneys, a deficient Spleen, a weak *Yin* and tendency to an exuberance of *Yang*, therefore they are prone to Heat, high fevers and to Liver Wind, convulsions.

The most common etiological factors in infants are the constitution and the diet. In fact in young infants as the Spleen-*Qi* is still not strong enough, the early introduction of animal milk and complex foods is often the main cause for the production of Dampness, frequently manifesting in the lungs and the upper portals, the nose, and the ears. Furthermore, the Spleen and Stomach being overloaded, the production of *Ying* ≈ Nourishing and *Wei* ≈ Defensive-*Qi* is compromised resulting in a propensity to catching frequent colds and upper respiratory infections. In such cases, the unfortunate frequent use of antibiotics, which are Cold in nature, will further damage the Spleen-*Yang* and contribute to maintaining this vicious circle.

Facial Color

Same correspondence as in adults:

Acne	Damp-Heat from SP-*Qi Xu* or Stomach-Heat
"Exanthema": bright red in a patch or isolated	Blood-Heat or *Qi Xu* not retaining the Blood
Rosacea	Lung and Stomach-Heat, Blood-Heat, Blood stasis
Erythema	Blood-Heat
Urticaria	Wind-Heat or Cold; Liver-Blood *Xu* with Wind; Blood-Heat, Stomach-Heat
Psoriasis	Blood-Heat; Liver and Kidney-*Yin Xu*; Blood *Xu*
White patches "Vitiligo"	*Qi* stagnation
Papules	Wind-Heat
Very dark red	Intense Heat
Purple	Blood stasis (from Heat)
Pale red	Blood *Xu* or *Yang Xu*
Dermographism	Wind; Wind-Heat
Tight rash not disappearing under pressure	Intense Pathogenic Heat
Vesicles: small, trans-lucid	Damp-Heat; *Qi* & Blood stasis

and shiny rash (herpes)	
Vesicles: dry, white, empty	Body Fluids have dried up
Abscess, anthrax, ulcers	Heat toxins; Damp-Heat (Stomach and Spleen)
	If large red, hot, painful and superficial: *Yang* condition
	If swollen, deep, no skin color change: *Yin* condition
Warts	Blood-stasis, Blood *Xu*
Moles	Blood stasis, Damp-Heat
Fungal infections	Damp-Heat, Spleen-*Qi Xu*

Head and body

Fontanel

The fontanel should be closed by the age of 18–24 months.

Delayed closing	Kidney-*Qi Xu*
Depressed fontanel	Deficiency; Kidney-*Jing Xu*
Swollen fontanel	Heat
Head too big or small	Kidney-*Jing Xu*
Swaying of the head	Liver-Wind
Weak spinal muscles	Kidney-*Jing Xu*; Spleen-*Qi Xu*
Listless movements	Vacuity≈*Xu* condition
Hyperactivity	Liver-Fire, Heart-Fire, Stomach-Heat
Sweaty head during sleep	Spleen-*Qi Xu*; *Wei-Qi* vacuity

Palpation of the Five Centers

The palpation of the "Five Centers": palms, soles, and chest inform on the balance of Fire and Water.

Colder than rest of body	Kidney-*Qi* or *Yang Xu*
Warmer than the rest	Pathogenic Heat or Kidney-*Yin Xu*

Skin Rash

In general skin rashes have the same significance as for adults.

Macular rash (flat and pale)	Cold; *Yang Xu*
Papular rash (raised)	Heat; small papules could indicate measles, rubella

	or scarlet fever
Pustules	Dampness; a vesicular rash could indicate chicken pox or impetigo

Orifices (Portals) and Eliminations

Valuable information may be gathered by observing the condition of the portals and especially the discharge from the eyes and the nose in children.

Eyes

Watery eyes	External Wind-Cold or Wind-Damp
Red	External Wind-Heat, Internal-Heat
Red corners, cracked	Damp-Heat in Intestines, food retention
Yellow, with discharge	Dampness
Greenish or bluish	Liver-Wind
White haze on the pupil	Malnutrition
Sunken eyes	Dehydration
Dry eyes	Liver-*Yin Xu*
Dark rings, red cheeks	Kidney-*Yin Xu*
Dark rings, pale face	Kidney-*Yang Xu*
Brown rings	Possible steroid poisoning
Eyelids pale	Blood *Xu*
Eyelids puffy	Spleen and Kidney-*Qi Xu*

Nose

Clear, watery discharge	Wind-Cold
Yellow discharge	Wind-Heat
White and chronic	Lung-*Qi Xu*, atopic (allergic) rhinitis
Blocked nose	Dampness
Flaring nostrils	Lung-Heat; Phlegm; Asthma
Dry and irritated	Lung-Heat; Wind-Heat
Sweaty nose	Lung-*Qi Xu*

Ears

Reflect the constitutional *Jing* (please see above under Ears).

Red	Heat
Bluish helix	Abdominal Cold; pain
Discharge	Damp-Heat in Liver or Gallbladder

Mouth

Pale lips	Cold or Spleen-*Qi Xu*
Red lips	Heat in Stomach and Intestines; Heart-Heat
Red lips with white face	Residual Pathogenic factor
Dry, cracked, dark lips	Loss of Body fluids, dehydration
Swollen and red gums	Stomach-Heat, intestinal parasites
Tongue tip, red and raised (strawberry surface)	Blood-Heat
Red throat	Wind-Heat
Chronic red throat	Stomach-Heat, Large Intestine-Heat
Swollen tonsils	Phlegm; Residual Pathogenic factors
Red and swollen tonsils	Wind- Heat, Damp-Heat
Red with exudate	Toxic Heat in Stomach or Intestines
Chronic sore throat	Kidney-*Yin Xu*, Lung-*Yin Xu*
Drooling when sleeping	Spleen-*Qi Xu*
Mouth hanging open	Extreme *Qi Xu*
Protruding lower lip	Spleen-*Qi Xu*; malnutrition
Strong mouth smell	"Halitosis": Stomach-Heat, food stagnation

Examination of the index finger

The capillaries on the palm side of the index finger in children under 3 years of age are studied to determine the type of Pathogenic Factor (PF).

The index finger is held with 2 fingers, right index finger for girls left index finger for boys. With the other hand, the palmar side of the index finger is massaged a few times, moving from the extremity towards the base with average pressure. Some capillaries will appear, if the capillaries are on the surface, this is a superficial disease, deep capillaries signify a deep disease (▶Fig. 10.35).

- The proximal segment is called "*Feng* ≈ Wind Gate" reflects Pathogenic factors or food stagnation: veins in this section signify a superficial disease
- The middle segment is the "*Qi* ≈ Energy Gate", in relation to the channels; congested veins signify a more serious condition of Heat that can lead to *Qi Xu*.

- The distal phalange is called "*Ming* ≈ Life Gate" and reflects the *Zang-Fu* activity; congested veins in this segment signify that Heat may enter the Pericardium resulting in high fever and convulsions. Capillaries that extend all the way to the nail denote extreme severity.
- The color of the veins also indicates the type of pathogen
  - Light red, barely visible: normal
  - Bright red: external Wind (Hot or Cold)
  - Pale: cold disease
  - Purple: Wind-Heat
  - Dark purple: Obstruction by accumulation; Blood stasis
  - Blue: Liver-Wind; pain

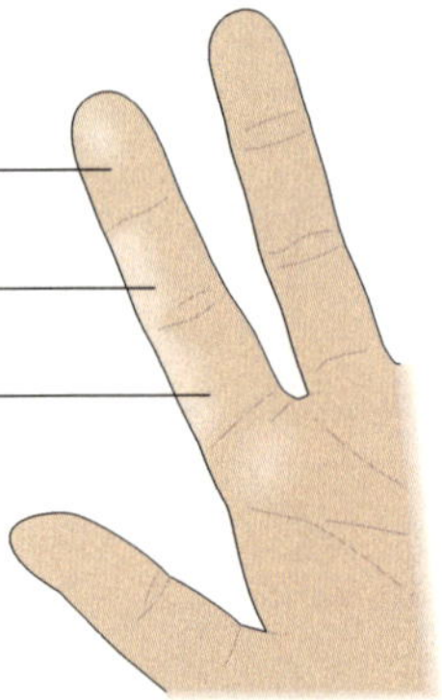

Figure 10.35: Examination of capillaries of the index finger

The Pulses in children

Pulse reading can only be used in children over 4 years of age. A faster pulse rate is normal until puberty: infant: 120–140/min; 1-year-old: 110–120 /min; 4-year-old: 110/min; 8-year-old: 90/ min.

Fullness on surface	Heat
Floating, Wiry or Tight	Biao diseases, allergies, skin problems
Weak moderate pulses	In relation to inappropriate diet or emotions
Wiry or Tight moderate	Accumulation of Dampness or Phlegm
Wiry left moderate level *Guan* (middle position)	Liver-Wind; tics, convulsions, fidgetiness
Wiry deep level on *Guan* (middle position)	May reflect personality issues, learning disabilities, authoritative parents

Comparison of left and right carotid pulses (ST-9) and left and right radial pulses (LU-9): (Please note that in infants only the carotid pulses are compared).

- If the left pulses are stronger than the right: inflammation and heat, possibly excess protein in the diet.
- If the right pulses are stronger: possibly too much sugar or the presence of parasites.

Between the ages of 4 to 8, the radial pulse may be studied on the superficial (*Wei Qi*) and moderate levels (*Ying Qi*).

After the age of 9, the deeper pulse (*Yuan Qi*) is also taken.

Interrogation of the parents

The parental heredity, the age of the parents, the evolution of the pregnancy and the occurrence of diseases during the pregnancy, physical or psychological shocks, intake of alcohol, tobacco or drugs, will inform on the quality of the inherited *Jing*.

The conditions of birth, in particular, cesarean or prolonged labor tend to weaken the Lungs of the child. Furthermore, children's diet plays a very important role in their pathologies and has to be carefully analyzed.

Diet and feeding rhythms

Early weaning	Food stasis; skin problems; rhinorrhoea
Rich foods	Dampness; frequent colds
Thirst, dry lips	Stomach-*Yin Xu*
Thirst but cannot drink	Damp-Heat; Stomach-*Yin Xu*

General symptoms

Sweating easily	*Wei-Qi Xu*
Sweating at night	*Wei-Qi Xu*; *Yin-Xu*
Constipation	Internal Heat or Body fluid *Xu*≈ Vacuity
Poor sleep, nightmares	Heat, or *Yin Xu*, or Blood *Xu*
Sleeping with open eyes	Spleen-*Qi Xu* or wandering *Hun* (difficulty in waking up); Phlegm obstructing the upper parts
Sleeping on the belly	Stomach and Spleen-*Qi Xu*
Disliking to sleep on belly	Food stasis
Sleeping on sides	Lung-*Qi Xu*
Excessive dreaming	Liver and Kidney-*Yin Xu*
Night frights (terror)	Phlegm
Night crying	Food stasis; Spleen-*Qi Xu*

10.6 Tongue Diagnosis

[...] the tongue is the orifice of the Heart.
[...] the tongue is the root of the Spirit.

The tongue itself is in relation with the Heart. The Heart *Qi* manifests in the tongue and if it is in harmony the speech is clear and one can taste the "5 tastes". The surface of the tongue is in relation to the Spleen and Stomach representing the Earth phase and the function of absorption, assimilation, and elimination.

Several channels are connected with the tongue:

- Heart *Jing Bie* ≈ Divergent channel: the root of the tongue
- Spleen: under the tongue
- Kidney: surrounds the base of the tongue
- Liver: follows the base of the tongue
- Bladder and Heart *Jing Jin* ≈ Sinew channels, connect with the root of the tongue.

Thus the changes in the functions of the *Zang* ≈ Organs and *Fu* ≈ Bowels can be observed on the tongue.

Three topographical representations are possible: according to the Triple Warmer theory, the 5 Phase theory, or the Biao-Li (▶ Fig. 10.36).

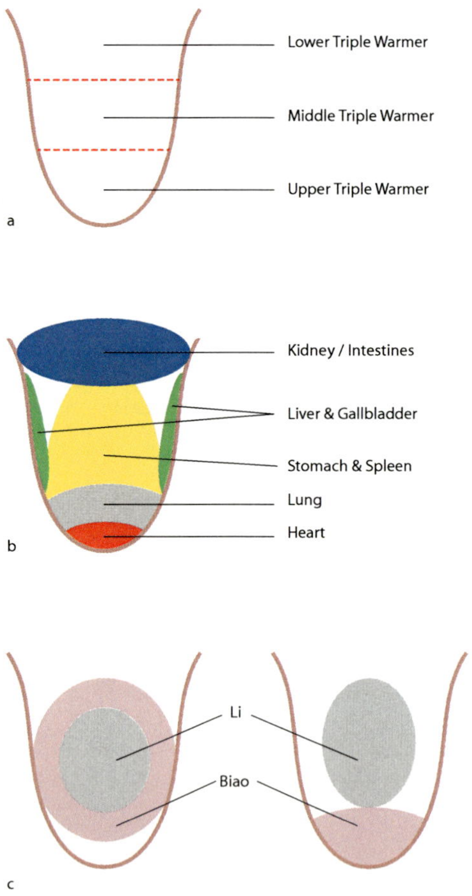

Figure 10.36: Topography of the tongue:
a) according to the Triple Warmer,
b) according to the Organs,
c) according to *Biao-Li*.

Examination Technique

- Light: daylight is preferable, as artificial light does not allow distinguishing between white and yellow coatings, neon light gives a bluish hue.
- Position: the tongue should be pulled out sufficiently and yet not too much. Excessive or prolonged protrusion tends to

give a purple color to the tongue

- False color and texture of the coating can be observed after consumption of:
  - Olives, or licorice: black
  - Orange juice: yellow
  - Vinegar, tobacco, and coffee: grey or brown
  - Antibiotics: brown, grey or black
  - Food coloring in candies, ice cream etc.: various colors
  - Hot drinks make the tongue red.
  - Breathing through the mouth dries up the coating.
- Constitution: the *Qi* of Spleen and Stomach influences the thickness of the coating. A sturdy and strong person may have naturally a thicker coating.
- Tongue scraping: Helps to distinguish the real coating from deposits.
- In general three points should be observed:
  - Tongue texture, body shape, and mobility
  - Tongue body color
  - Texture, color, and distribution of the coating
- The specific sign's that are observed on the tongue should always be integrated with information gathered by the pulse and the synthesis of the symptoms. According to G. Maciocia, the tongue never lies, but Professor Zhou maintains that the tongue is the only organ that may lie!

Texture and the Body of the Tongue

They reflect the activity of the organs.

Normal tongue: a flourishing vitality corresponds to a tongue that has Spirit, is mobile, bright, light red and fresh. (▶ Tab. 10.2, plates-1-2)

Tongue Shapes

Thin and Narrow

If light red (▶ plates 3,12,13, 20)	Heart-*Qi Xu*; Spleen-*Qi Xu*; Blood *Xu*
If red	*Yin Xu* or, Fire repletion (▶plate-3)
Dark or blackish	Severe prognosis (unless due to antibiotics)

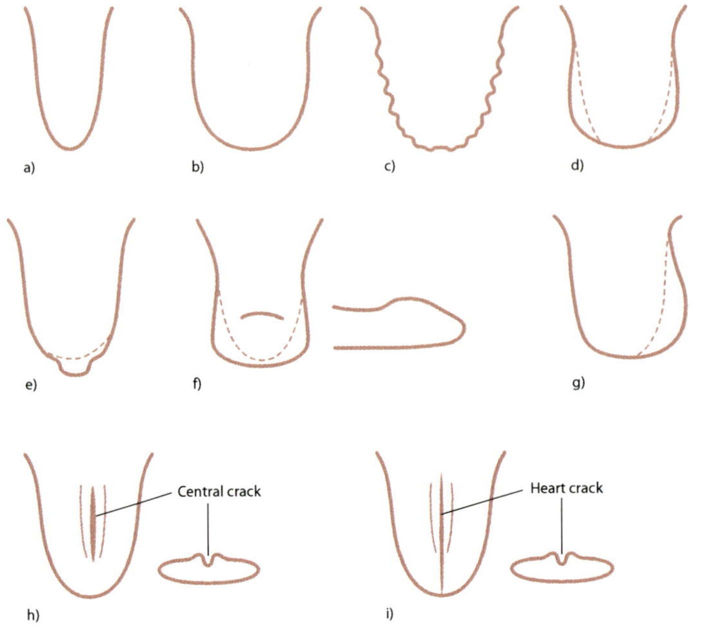

Figure 10.37
Tongue shapes:
a) thin tongue,
b) large tongue,
c) teeth marks,
d) swollen sides,
e) swollen tip,
f) swollen front third,
g) one half swollen,
h) swelling along a central crack,
i) swelling along a long central crack

Large and Big

(▶ plates 5 through 15)

If supple and pale, with teeth marks (▶ plates 7, 9)	Spleen-*Qi Xu*; Kidney-*Yang Xu*; accumulation of Dampness
If swollen and red (▶ plates 17, 18)	Heat repletion in Spleen and/or Heart
If swollen and purple	Intoxication

Teeth marks with a swollen or normal tongue

Teeth marks signify retention of Dampness and reflect a Spleen-*Qi Xu* (▶ plates 6, 7, 12).

Partially Swollen

Edges swollen more in in the mid-section (▶ plates 5, 8)	Spleen-*Qi Xu* or Spleen-*Yang Xu*
Swollen sides and red ▶ plate 18	Liver-Fire or Liver-*Yang* rising
Tip, with normal color (▶ plates 8, 11, 13)	Heart-*Qi Xu*
Tip, with red color (▶ plates 10, 11, 14, 17, 18)	Heart-Fire, severe emotional problems
Behind the tip (▶ plates 5, 10)	Lung-*Qi Xu* with Phlegm accumulation

One half swollen (▶ plate 12)	Blood and *Qi Xu* on that side of the body
Half swollen with Lung symptoms	Lung-*Qi Xu*
Localized swelling (▶ plates 12, 22)	Blood and *Qi* stasis in the related area
Along a central crack (▶ plates 22, 24)	Heart-*Qi Xu*
Swollen along a central crack & red	Heart-Fire
Very swollen with a sticky coating (▶ plates 28, 34)	Shen obstruction by Phlegm
Swollen in front third hammer shaped (▶ plates 11, 13, 28)	Phlegm retention in Lung, or Spleen and Stomach *Qi* exhausted (serious)

Cracks, Fissures

Fissures signify a state of dryness due to *Yin Xu.*

<table>
<tr><td>Superficial cracks (▶ plates 4, 5, 6)</td><td colspan="2">Mild disease</td></tr>
<tr><td>Deep cracks (▶ plates 22, 24, 25, 30)</td><td colspan="2">More severe disease</td></tr>
<tr><td>In a healthy person (▶ plate 6)</td><td colspan="2">No significance</td></tr>
<tr><td>Tongue dark red Fluids (▶ plates 16, 30)</td><td colspan="2">Heat damaging the Body</td></tr>
<tr><td>Pale white tongue</td><td colspan="2">Blood Xu</td></tr>
<tr><td>Horizontal cracks (long or short) (▶ plates 4, 6, 29, 30, 37)</td><td colspan="2">Yin Xu</td></tr>
<tr><td>Horizontal cracks on the sides (▶ plate 23)</td><td colspan="2">Spleen-Qi Xu</td></tr>
<tr><td>Irregular cracks (▶ plates 4,6, 29, 30, 37)</td><td colspan="2">Stomach-Yin Xu</td></tr>
<tr><td>Vertical crack in the center with a coating (▶ plates 16, 22, 26, 27)</td><td colspan="2">Stomach-Qi Xu</td></tr>
<tr><td>Vertical crack in the center with no coating (▶ plates 13, 24, 25)</td><td colspan="2">Stomach-Yin Xu</td></tr>
<tr><td>Vertical crack in the center with a sticky, rough, yellow coating (plate 26)</td><td colspan="2">Stomach-Phlegm-Fire</td></tr>
<tr><td>Deep with horizontal cracks (▶ plates 30, 37)</td><td colspan="2">Kidney-Yin Xu, internal Dryness with possibility of kidney stones</td></tr>
<tr><td rowspan="3">Long vertical crack to the tip (▶ plates 24, 38)</td><td colspan="2">Heart crack</td></tr>
<tr><td>Normal tongue color</td><td>Constitutional Heart weakness</td></tr>
<tr><td>Red tongue (▶plates 24, 30,</td><td>Heart-Fire</td></tr>
</table>

	34)	
	Red no coating (▶ plates 36, 38)	Heart-Fire, Heart and Kidney-*Yin Xu*
Transversal behind the tip (▶ plate 5)	Lung-*Yin Xu*; or childhood lung problems	

Rough and Spiky surface

A rough tongue surface signifies Pathogenic Heat or Fire (▶ plate 31).

According to the zone	Fire in the corresponding system

Ulcers

Red and painful	Heart-Fire
White rim	Heart-Heat from Kidney-*Yin Xu*
Under the tongue	Heat in Spleen or Kidney damaging the Body Fluids

Tongue Mobility

The tongue should normally be flexible and remain steady when protruded.

Stiff	Deep red in external disease	Heat penetration and Phlegm obstruction
	In internal disease	Liver-Wind (apoplexy)
Trembling (fast, small movements)	Pale	*Qi* and Blood *Xu*; Spleen-*Yang Xu*
	Red, dry	Internal Wind from Heat and Fire
Moving (slow movements)	Red in acute diseases	Liver-Wind from Pathogenic Heat
	Deep red, dry	Liver-Wind with Heart-Fire
	Red, swollen, dry	Liver-Wind with Heart-Fire & Spleen-Heat
Flaccid	Limp, atrophic or paralyzed	Exhaustion of *Qi* and of Body Fluids
	Pale	Heart & Spleen-*Qi Xu* with Blood *Xu*
	Red and dry	Body Fluids injured by Heat
Long	Fire type constitution or Heat condition (▶ plates 35, 36)	
Darting in and out	Heart or Spleen-Heat	
	In children	Underdevelopment of intellectual capacity

Deviated to one side	Internal Wind (stroke) or external (palsy); (▶ plates 27, 38)	
Curled (up or down)	Heart-Heat (▶ plates 21, 23, 36, 39)	
Short	Always a severe condition	
	Pale or purple and humid (▶ plates 3, 12, 25)	Internal Cold from *Yang* or *Qi Xu*
	And large (▶ plates 11, 12, 13, 25)	Obstruction by Phlegm
	Red (▶ plates 4, 14, 17)	Internal Heat with Liver-Wind
	Dark red and dry	Body Fluids damaged by internal Heat
Numb	Blood and *Ying Xu* (vacuity)	

Color of the Tongue Body

Mainly informs about the condition of the *Zang ≈ Organs*

Pale or White

Paleness signifies Empty-Cold from *Yang Xu*; Blood *Xu* (▶ plates 3, 7, 11, 12, 13, 15, 20 25); or *Qi Xu*.

Red

A red color is always a sign of Heat:

With yellow coating in an acute disease (▶ plates 18, 31)	External pathogenic Heat
Thin or no coating in a chronic disease (▶ plate 4)	Heat from *Yin* deficiency
Bright red and spiky (▶ plates 16, 18, 23)	Fire penetrating the Triple Warmer
Dull red and dry	Heat damaging the fluids of the Stomach

Purple

A purple color denotes Blood stasis:

If purple in one area (▶ plate 22)	Blood stasis in the related organ

Reddish purple and dry (▶ plates 22, 35)	Heat in Ying and Blood levels; Blood stasis and Body Fluid exhaustion
Pale bluish purple and damp (▶ plates 21, 39)	Blood stasis from internal Cold

Tongue Coating

The tongue coating is produced by the evaporation of Stomach *Qi* and directly informs about the function of the Stomach.

Normally the coating is thin, white and moist and is rooted and cannot be scraped off. A coating without root is called a "False" or "Rootless" coating.

As the Spleen and Stomach produce the three substances, *Qi*, Blood and Fluids, any pathological process, will automatically involve and affect the Stomach's digestive process, which will manifest in a change of coating. Therefore the coating would inform on:

- The type of Pathogenic factor "*Xie Qi*"
- The depth of the disease, "*Biao/ Li*"
- The evolution of the disease "prognosis"
- The integrity of the body's energies
- Internal stagnations accumulations

Texture and Distribution

False coating "rootless" (▶ plates 32, 35)	Stomach-*Qi* or *Yin Xu*; Kidney-*Yin Xu* Spleen-*Yin Xu*
Thick coating (▶ plates 18, 22, 31, 34)	Attack by External Pathogenic "*Xie Qi*"; Food stasis or Damp and phlegm accumulation
Thin coating (▶ plates 1, 2, 3, 5, 12, 15, 20)	Normal or Surface "*Biao*" disease
Going from thin to thick	Aggravation of the disease
Going from thick to thin	Improvement (except when going to too thin)
Dry (▶plates 13, 14, 15, 25)	Heat or Dryness causing Body Fluid *Xu*
Too moist (▶plates 7, 20, 38, 39)	*Yang Xu*; or Cold-Wind Damp pathogen
Slippery, wet, sticky and oily (▶ plate 39)	Dampness and Cold
Greasy (▶ plates 10, 19, 22, 32, 34, 35)	Phlegm accumulation
Mouldy, rotten, rootless (▶ plates 32, 35)	Heat with Stomach-*Yin Xu*

Peeling, patchy coating (▶ plates 16, 19, 30, 32, 35, 37, 38)	Stomach-*Yin Xu*
No coating (▶ plates 4, 6, 13, 17, 37)	Stomach and Kidney-*Yin Xu*

Color of the Coating

White and fine	And moist (▶ plates 1, 2, 7, 9, 12)	Normal; or recent *Biao* disease
	Slippery, bright & shiny	Wind-Damp pathogen
	Dry, normal tongue body	Wind-Dry
	Dry with a pale tongue (▶plates 12,13)	Blood *Xu*
White and thick	And wet	Wind-Cold PF; internal Damp-Cold
	Slippery, greasy (▶ plates 22, 35, 38)	Dampness, Food or Cold stasis in the Stomach
	Moldy (▶ plates 32, 35)	Exhaustion of Stomach and Kidney-*Yin*; internal Phlegm
	Dry (▶ plate 31)	Pathogenic Cold transforms into Heat
	Powdery with a red tongue	Stomach-*Yin Xu* and external or internal Heat
	Spiky and cracked (▶ Plate 31)	Heat pathogen in the *Qi* level
Yellow	Thin	Wind-Heat pathogen
	Slippery, sticky (▶ plates 18, 33)	Damp-Heat
	Greasy (▶ plates 10, 19, 22, 32, 33, 34)	Hot-Phlegm; food stagnation with heat
	Thick, dirty (▶ plate 31)	Damp-Heat in Stomach-intestines
	Dry (▶ plate 31)	Heat drying up the Body Fluids
Grey	Moist and slippery	Cold-Damp in Stomach and Intestines
	Dry	Heat repletion
Black	Slippery and greasy	Cold-Damp in Stomach and Intestines
	White slippery, black in center	Spleen-*Yang Xu* with internal Cold-Damp
	Dry, cracked	Extreme Heat; Body Fluids dried
	Black prickles on a white fur	Cold pathogen transforming in to Heat

Sublingual veins

In normal conditions, the two sublingual veins should be just identifiable (▶ plate 36.a).

Distended	Blood stasis
Distended and light color (▶ plate 41)	Less severe
Distended and dark color (▶ plates 42, 43)	More severe stagnation of Blood
Distended on one side (▶ plate 42)	Stagnation on the corresponding side, as in injury, trauma or surgery
Covered by a white membrane (▶ plate 42)	Phlegm; Phlegm-stasis

10.7 Tongue Examples

Table 10.2: Color Plates of Tongues

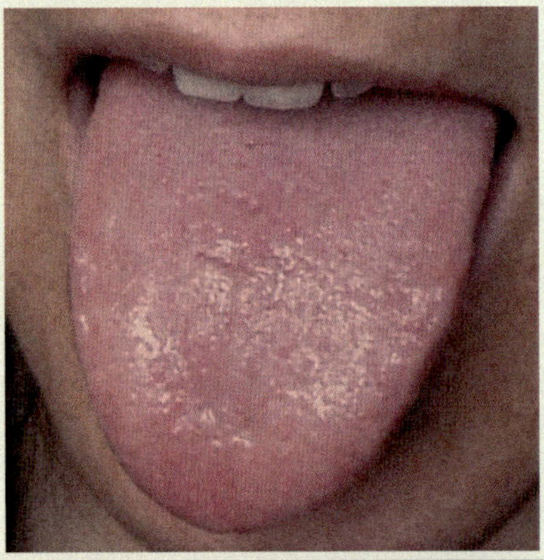	**Plate-1:** Normal pink tongue body, thin and white coating. ▶ A healthy subject.
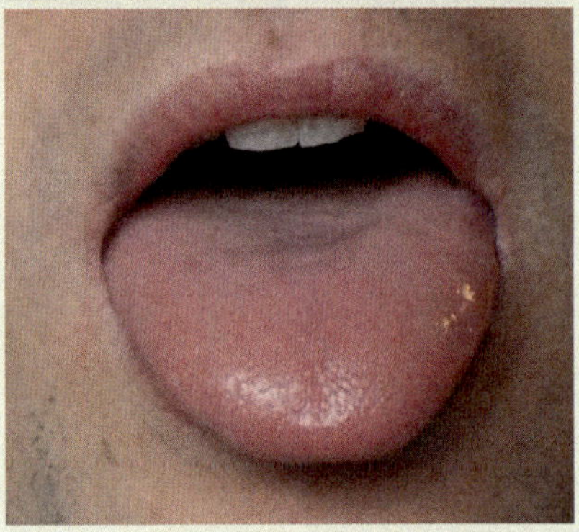	**Plate-2:** Normal tongue, pink, slightly swollen in the front and left sides, thin and white coating. ▶ A healthy subject.

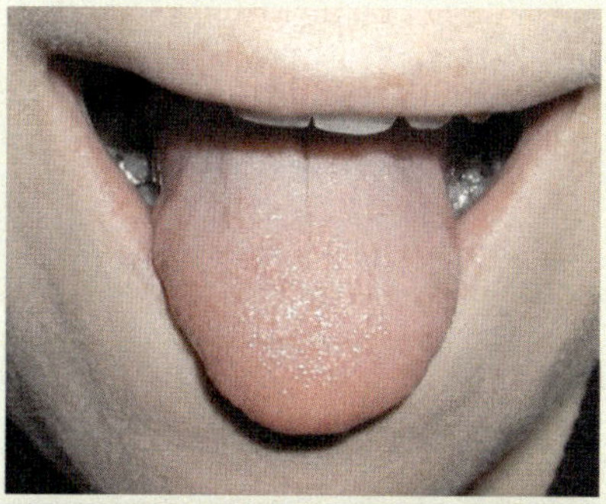

Plate-3:

- Short, narrow and pale, slightly dry ► *Yang*, *Qi* and Blood *Xu*.
- Symptoms: Patient suffering from fatigue, frequent colds and poor sleep.

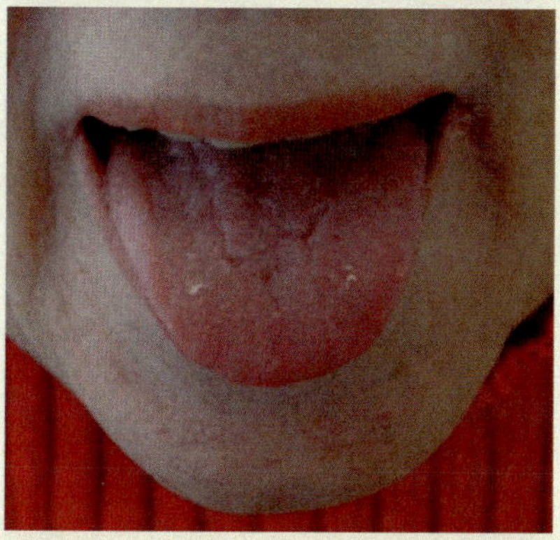

Plate-4:

- Short, thin, light red, dry, no coating with shallow cracks ► Internal Heat, with damage to body fluids.
- Symptoms: Menopausal patient with Empty-Heat (*Yin Xu*).

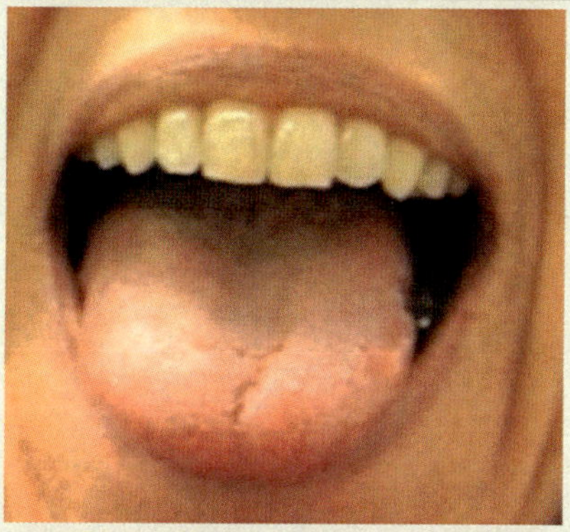

Plate-5:

- Tongue body swollen on the sides and the front; few teeth marks on the left side; cracks on the front third ► Lung and Spleen-*Qi Xu*.
- Symptoms: Propensity to catching colds: constitutional weakness of Lung.

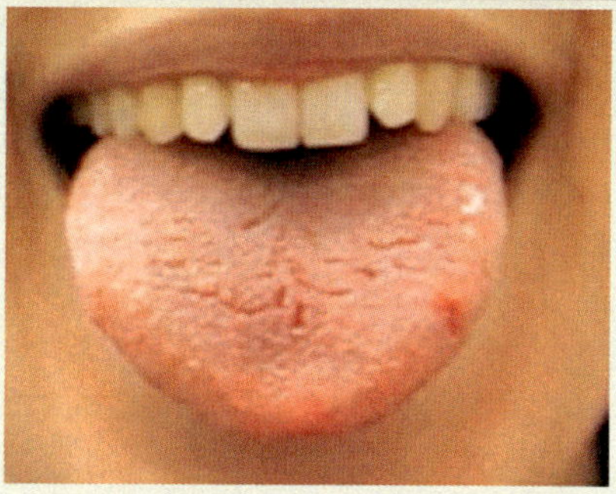

Plate-6:

- Pink tongue, no coating, scalloped surface; multiple horizontal cracks, in a healthy young subject (presenting no symptoms of *Yin Xu*) ► reflecting an episode of a childhood feverish disease.

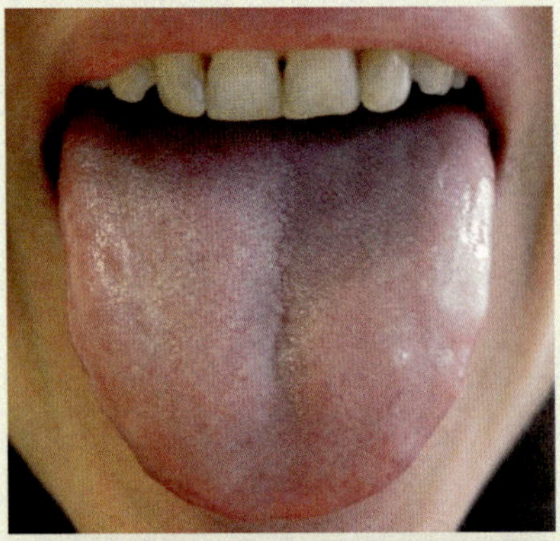

Plate-7:

- Large tongue, pale, slightly bluish and moist ► Spleen and Kidney *Qi* or *Yang Xu*; retention of Dampness);

- Symptoms: fatigue, coldness, lumbar pains, diarrhoea.

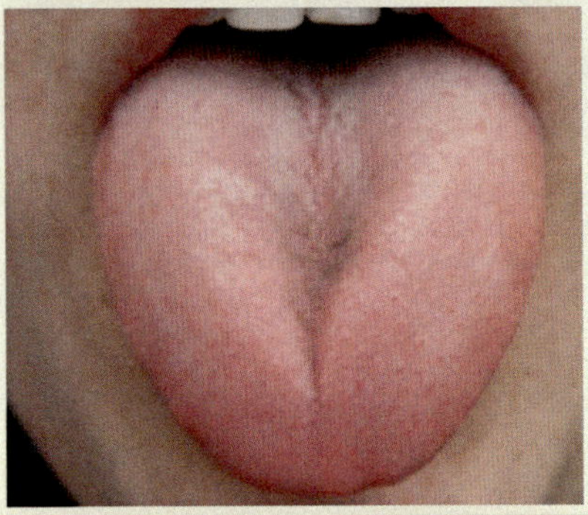

Plate-8:

- Large tongue, with very swollen edges extending to the front ►Spleen and Lung-*Qi Xu*).

- Symptoms: fatigue, shortness of breath, digestive and respiratory allergies, frequent colds.

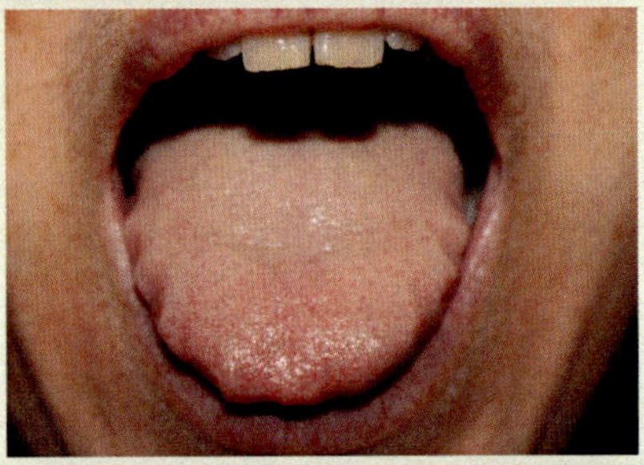

Plate-9:

- Large tongue, with swollen sides and front, teeth marks ► Spleen and Lung Qi-*Xu*; some pale red spots at the front-

- Symptoms: recovery from an external Pathogenic Factor in the Lung; propensity to catching colds.

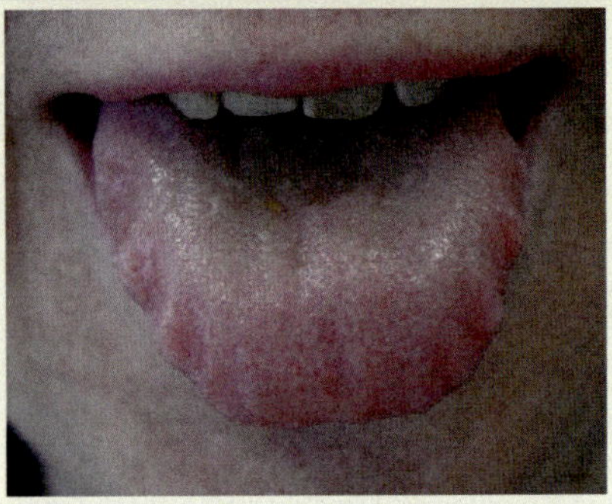

Plate-10:

- Large tongue, with swollen sides and tip, teeth marks; shallow heart-crack, some red spots at the tip; greasy-yellow coating in the centre ►Spleen, Lung and Heart-*Qi Xu*, mild Heart-*Yin Xu*, Damp-Heat in the centre.

- Symptoms: chronic fatigue, palpitations, shortness of breath.

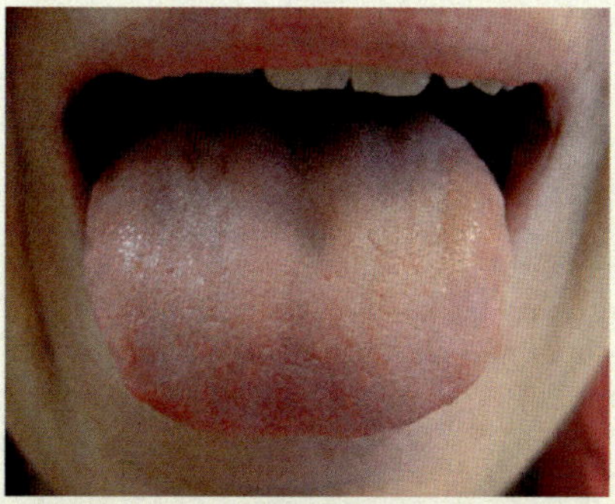

Plate-11:

- Large tongue, pale sides, with swollen front third, red tip ► Heart-*Qi Xu*, Heart Heat, possibly Phlegm misting the Heart; Liver-Blood *Xu*.
- Symptoms: Long standing depression, loss of memory.

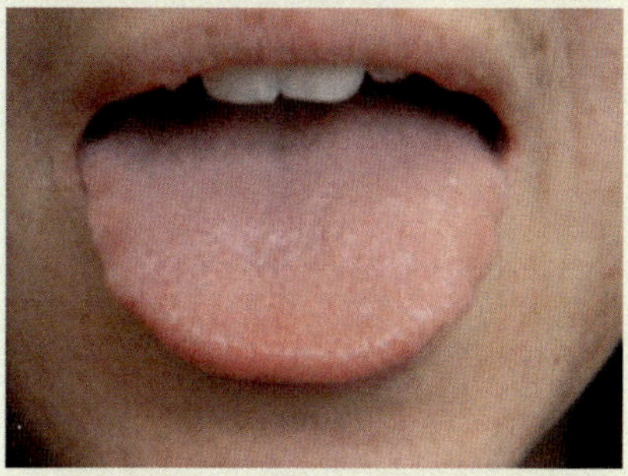

Plate-12:

- Large tongue, pale sides, swollen on the left side; very thin-white coating ► Blood and *Qi Xu* on the left side.
- Symptoms: Weakness and paraesthesia on the left side.

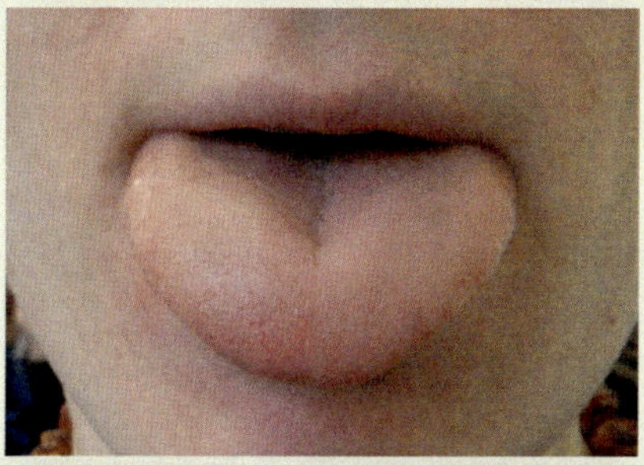

Plate-13:

- Large tongue, pale and dry, with swollen sides and front; no coating, crack in the centre ► Spleen, Lung and Heart *Qi* and Blood *Xu*, Stomach-*Yin Xu*.
- Symptoms: Exhaustion, depression, indigestion; poor sleep.

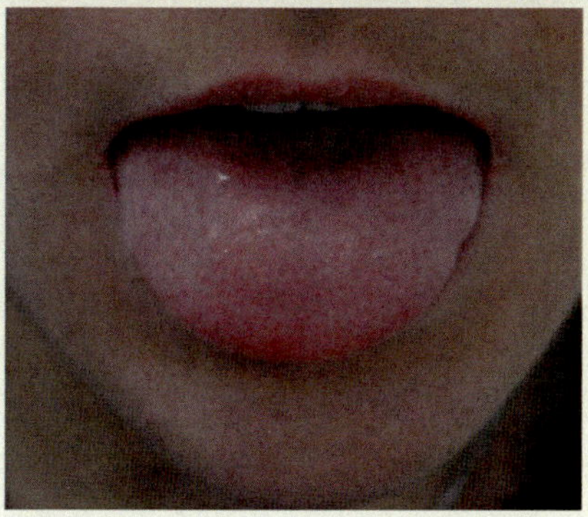

Plate-14:

- Large and short tongue, pale sides, a red tip and red spots on the tongue surface; shallow stomach crack ► Liver Blood *Xu*, Heart-Heat, residual Heat, Stomach-Yin *Xu*.
- Symptoms: Anxiety, gastritis, dream-disturbed sleep, feverishness.

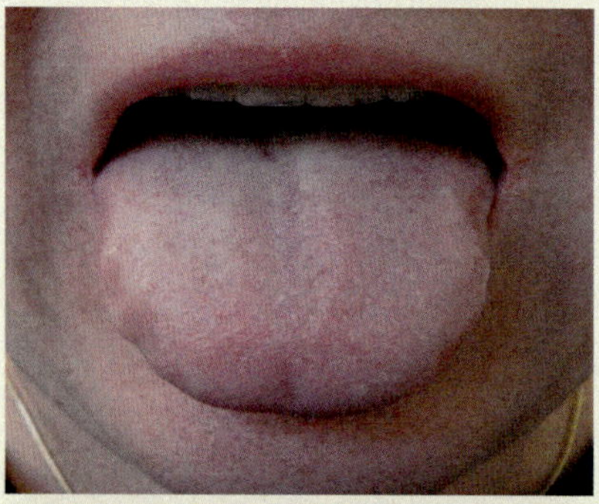

Plate-15:

- Large tongue, with swelling and teeth marks in front; pale-bluish colour; thin coating ► Spleen and Lung-*Qi* and *Yang Xu*.
- Symptoms: Coldness and fatigue, indigestion and respiratory symptoms.

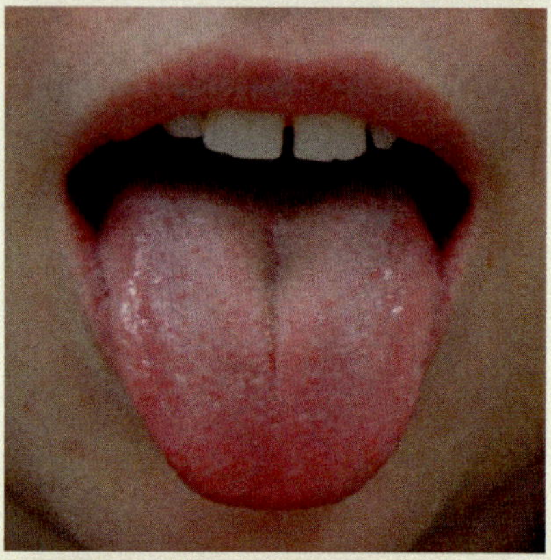

Plate-16:

- Red tongue with redder tip; no coating in front; stomach crack ► Heart-*Yin Xu* with Heat; Liver Heat, Stomach-*Yin Xu*.
- Symptoms: Nervousness, insomnia, gastritis.

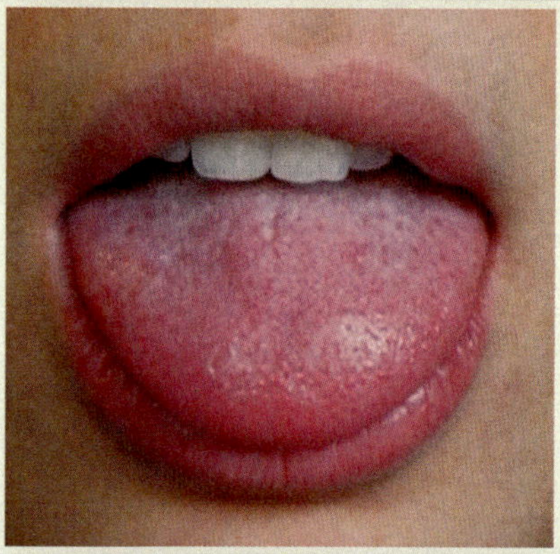

Plate-17:

- Red tongue swollen with no coating in the front; red spots over the surface and tip ► Heart and Lung-*Yin Xu*, Empty Heat.
- Symptoms: Insomnia, restless sleep, palpitations, night sweating; perennial allergies.

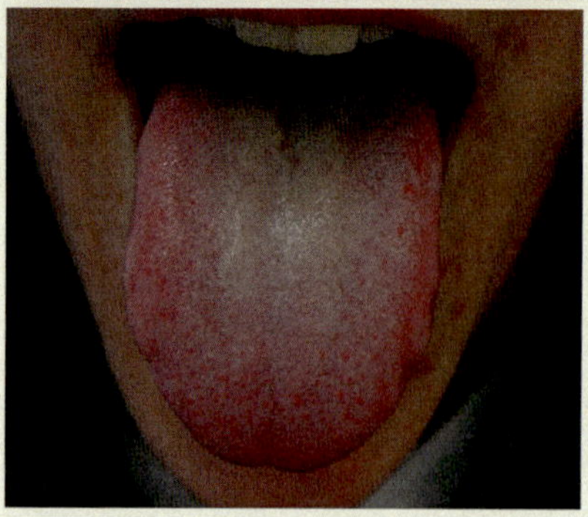

Plate-18:

- Swollen and red tongue with redder tip; red spots, red raised spots at base with sticky yellow coating ► Liver-*Qi* stasis; Heart Fire; Damp-Heat in the lower TW.
- Symptoms: PMS, chronic vaginal discharge, nightmares.

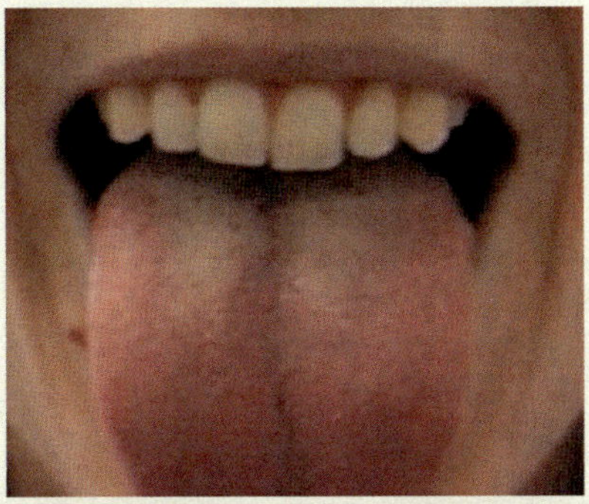

Plate-19:

- Large tongue with peeled coating in the front and a greasy yellow coating at the base with purplish red spots ► *Yin Xu* with Damp-Heat and possibly Blood stasis in the lower TW.
- Symptoms: PMS and recurrent vaginal discharge.

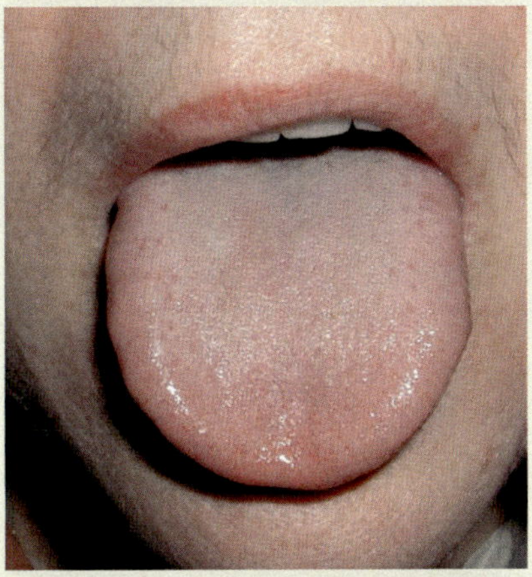

Plate-20:

- Large and pale tongue with paler sides; normal coating, depression in the front ► *Yang Xu*; Blood *Xu*; *Zong Qi Xu*.
- Symptoms: dizziness, fatigue, palpitations, frequent colds.

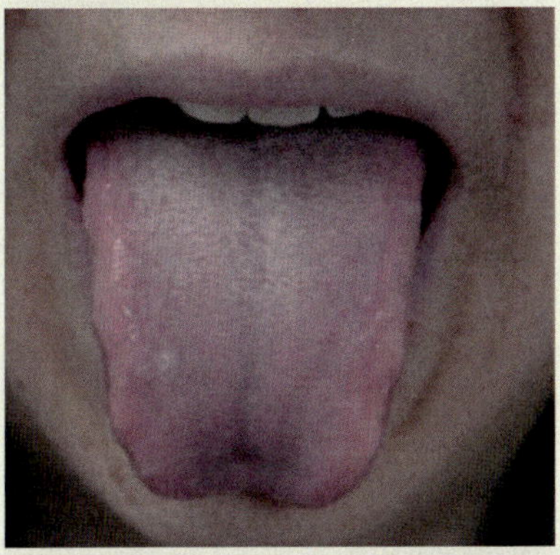

Plate-21:

- Large bluish-purplish tongue; normal coating, depression in the front and curled down ► *Yang Xu; Zong Qi Xu*; Heart-Blood *Xu*, slight blood stasis.
- Symptoms of palpitation, depression, fatigue and coldness.

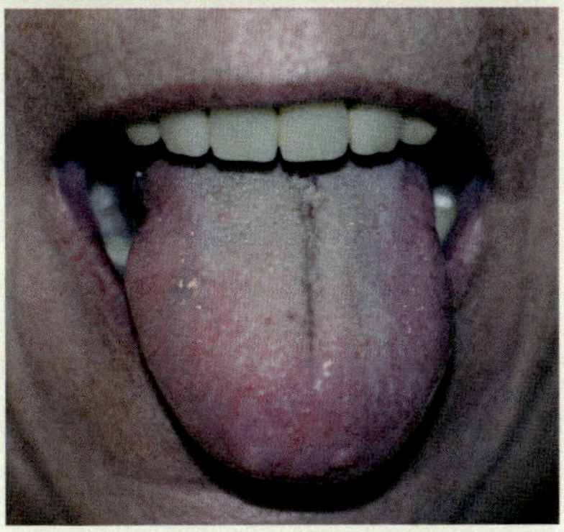

Plate-22:

- Purple colour with swollen sides and front; peeled coating at the tip; greasy yellowish coating along a central crack; purple spot on the right, two outgrowths at tip ►Blood stasis; Phlegm in the chest, Spleen-*Qi Xu*);
- Symptoms: History of extra-uterin pregnancy, lung embolism and varicous veins.

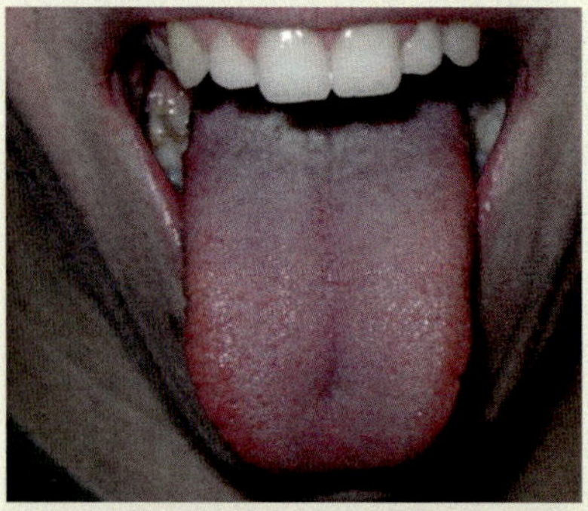

Plate-23:

- Deep-red tongue with a redder and slightly curled tip, cracked sides ► Liver and Heart-Heat, Spleen-*Qi Xu*.

- Symptoms: Irritability, stress, headaches, superficial and restless sleep.

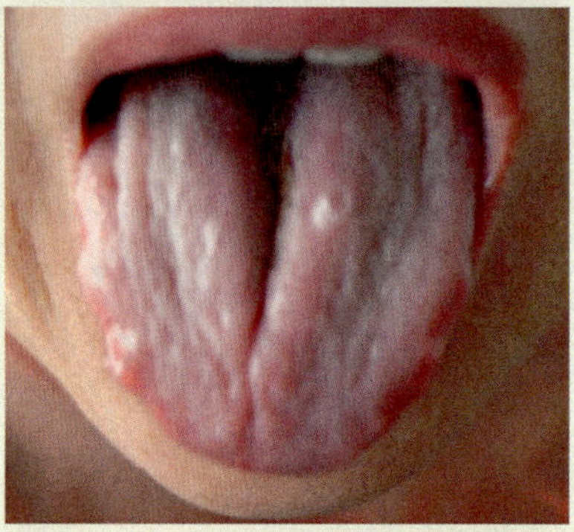

Plate-24:

- Heart crack with swelling along the crack; red sides, teeth marks ► Kidney, Stomach and Heart-*Yin Xu*; Liver-Heat.

- Symptoms: anxiety, restlessness, irregular sleep and eating, digestive problems, in a psychiatric patient.

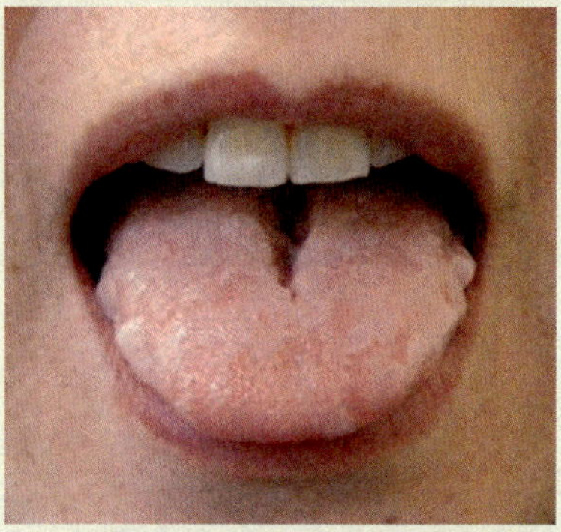

Plate-25:

- Large short and pale tongue with paler sides with teeth marks; deep stomach crack; very thin coating ► Stomach-*Yin Xu*; Blood *Xu*; Spleen-*Qi Xu* with Dampness.

- Symptoms of poor digestion, poor sleep, exhaustion from overwork and irregular eating.

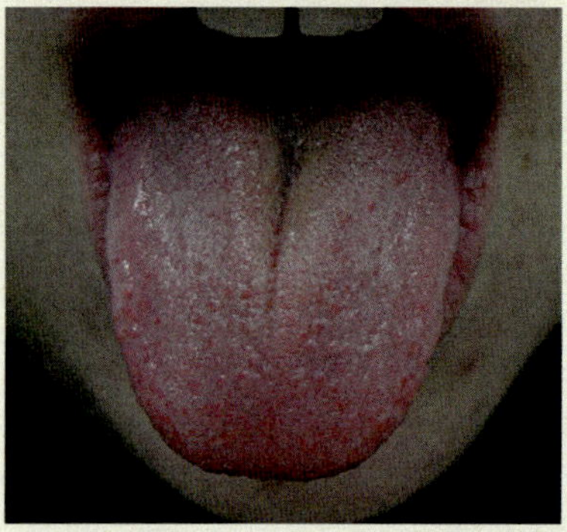

Plate-26:

- Red tip, stomach crack with slight swelling along the crack with sticky yellow coating, the rest of the coating is normal ► Stomach-*Yin Xu*; Damp-Heat in the middle, Heart-Heat.

- Symptoms: Worry, stress, gastritis, bloating, smelly soft stools.

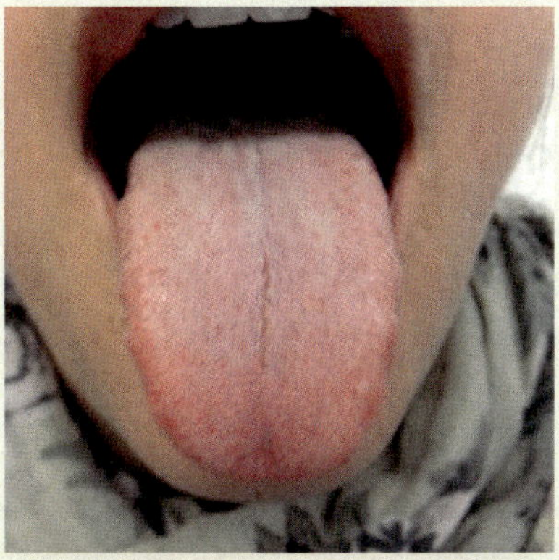

Plate-27:

- Long tongue with a shallow stomach crack; normal coating ▶ Stomach-*Yin Xu*.
- Symptoms: Sudden hunger, tendency to hypoglycemia.

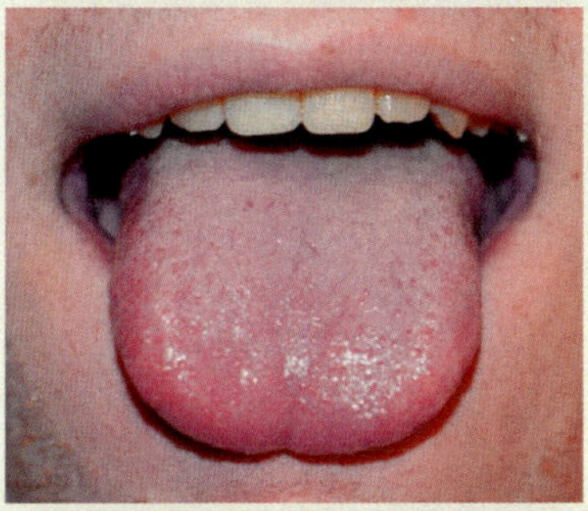

Plate-28:

- Swollen, red peeled and dented tip (hammer shaped), red spots along the sides ▶ constitutional weakness of the Heart; Heart-Fire from *Yin Xu*; Liver-Heat.
- Symptoms: A psychiatric patient (mild autism), with outbursts of anger.

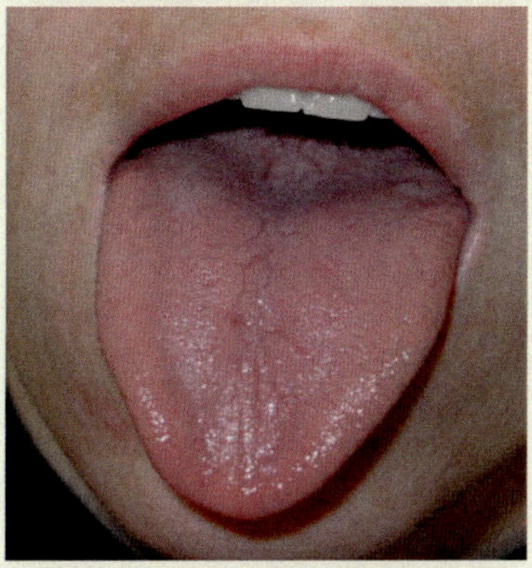

Plate-29:

- Peeled pink tongue with shallow cracks ▶ Stomach-*Yin Xu*.
- Symptoms: Healthy person with a past history of a feverish disease.

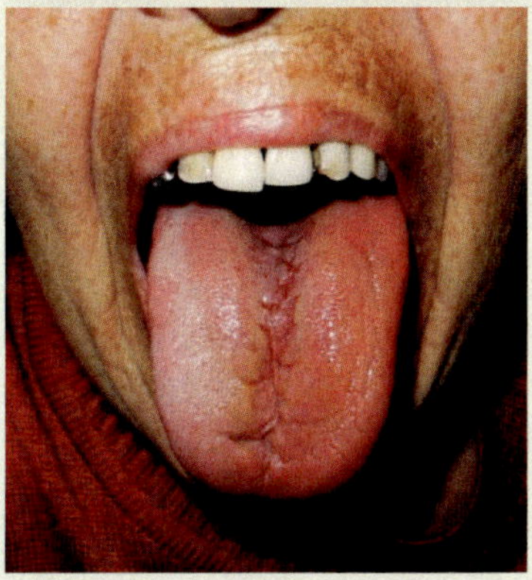

Plate-30:

- Large, red-orange tongue with deep cracks from base to tip; peeled coating from left to right ▶ Kidney, Stomach, Heart and Lung-Yin *Xu*; empty Heat.
- Symptoms: After chemotherapy for intestinal carcinoma.

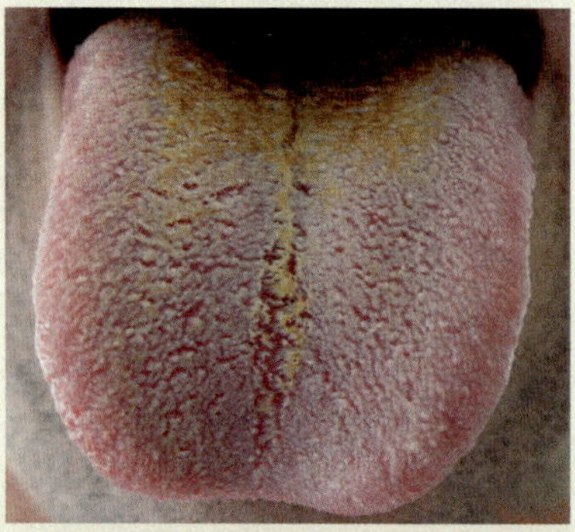

Plate-31:

- Thick, sticky and spiky yellow to brown coating at base, white and dry in front, tongue body is normal ► Damp-Heat in the Stomach and Intestines.

- Symptoms: Recovery from an episode of gastro-enteritis (*Yang Ming* channel level).

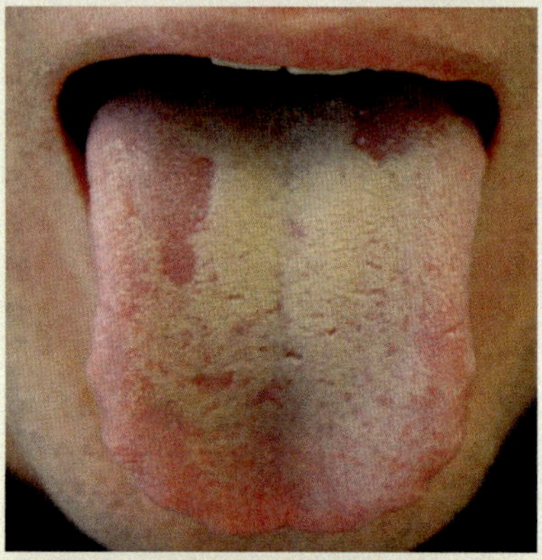

Plate-32:

- Rootless yellow greasy coating, with peeled areas ► Stomach-*Yin Xu*; retention of Damp-Heat.

- Symptoms: Chronic intestinal Candida infection.

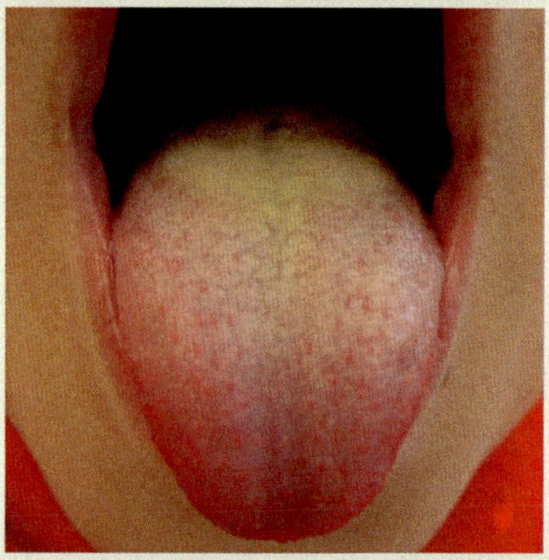

Plate-33:

- Red tongue in front, with red spots along the surface, thick sticky yellow coating at the base ► Heart-Heat; Damp-Heat in the lower TW.

- Symptoms: Restlessness, insomnia, hay fever and irritable bowels.

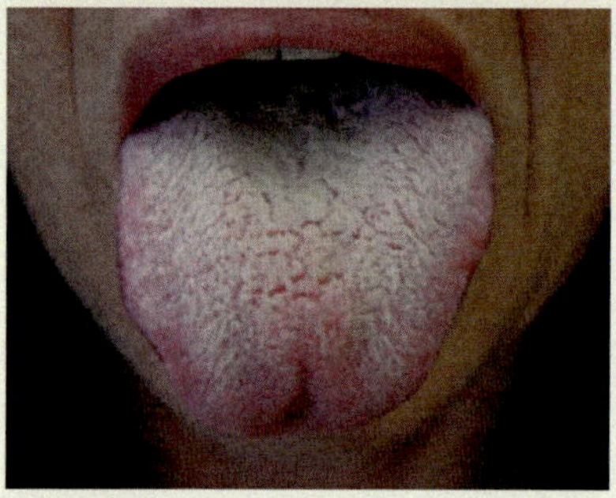

Plate-34:

- Red tongue, swollen with a deep crack at the tip, greasy slightly yellow coating in the middle ► Heart-Fire from *Yin Xu*; Phlegm-Heat in the Stomach.

- Symptoms: Chronic digestive and emotional problems since childhood.

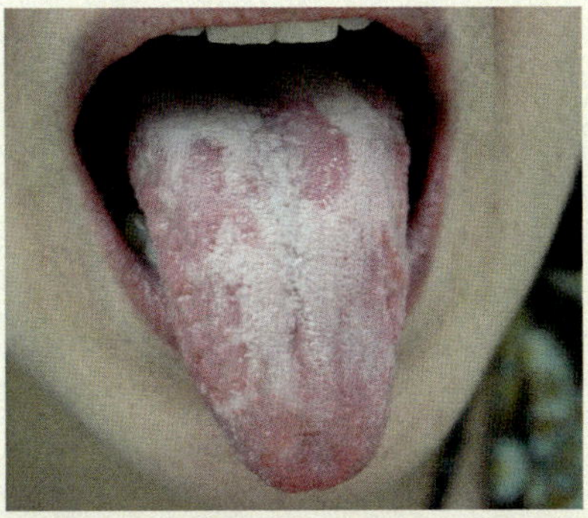

Plate-35:

- Geographic tongue, rootless white greasy coating ► Stomach-*Yin Xu*.

- Symptoms: Irregular eating habits, food allergies with gluten intolerance.

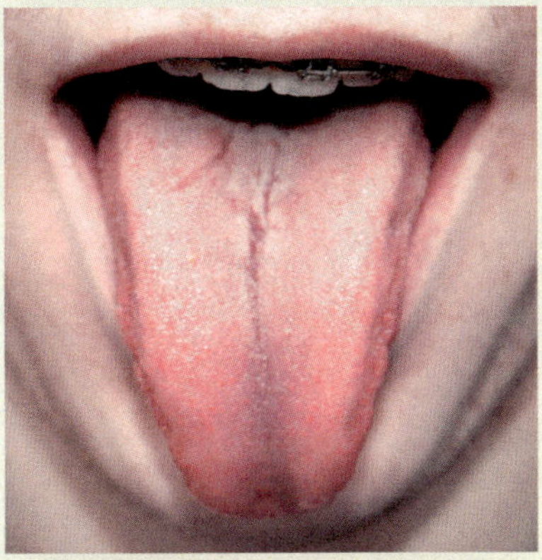

Plate-36:

- Long red tongue, red tip, peeled coating in front, cracks in centre and base ► Heart and Stomach-*Yin Xu,* Kidney-*Yin Xu,* empty-Heat.

-Symptoms: Gastritis, palpitations, frequent waking; short cycles with red watery menses.

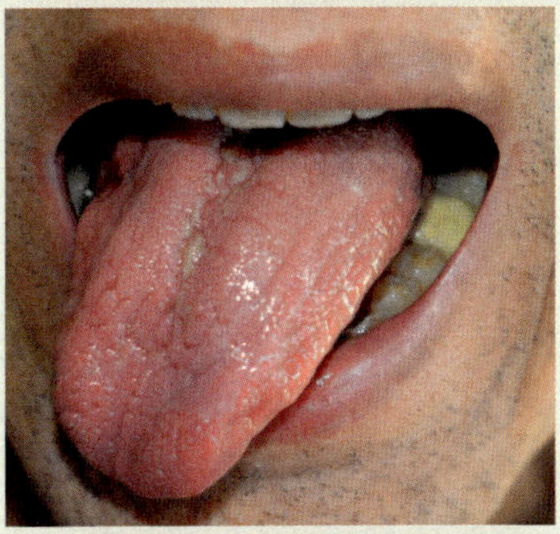

Plate-37:

- Redish, deviated tongue with swollen sides and centre, peeled coating, cracks ► Spleen and Stomach-Qi *Xu,* Stomach-*Yin Xu;* Kidney-*Yin Xu*, Empty-Heat.

- Symptoms: High blood pressure, tinnitus and insomnia.

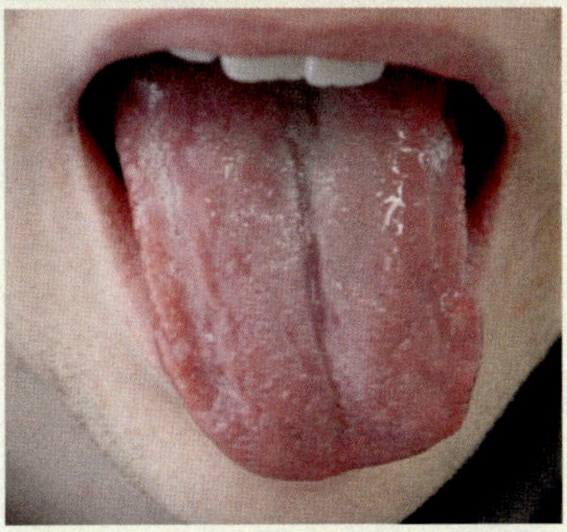

Plate-38:

- Deviated moist tongue with a heart crack, coating is peeled at base ► Kidney, Heart and Stomach-*Yin Xu*, with some *Yang Xu*.

- Symptoms: Severe vertigo, palpitations, fearfulness and coldness.

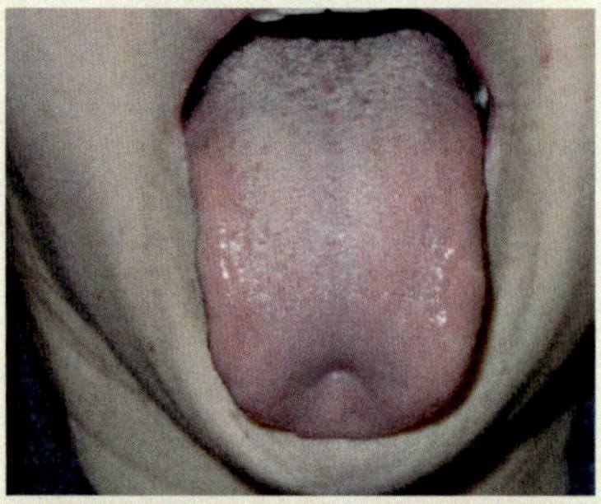

Plate-39:

- Tongue curled under, shiny pale-bluish color, sticky coating with raised reddish spots at base, indentation in Lung area ▶ *Yang Xu*, Heart-*Yang Xu,* Heat in the lower TW.

- Symptoms: Palpitations, shortness of breath, coldness, recurrent cystitis.

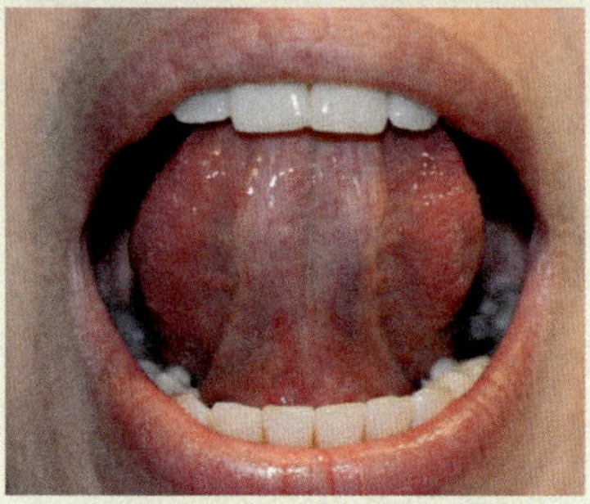

Plate 40:

Normal sub-lingual veins in a healthy subject.

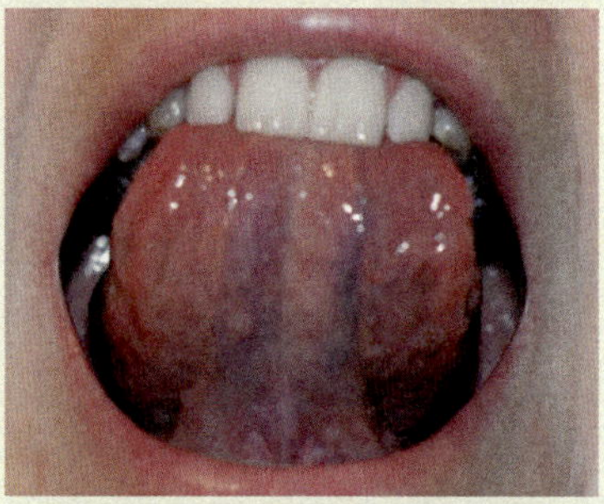

Plate 41:

- Congested bluish sublingual veins, especially on the left side, shiny tongue ▶ Blood stasis from *Yang Xu*.

- Symptoms: PMS and ovulation pains on the left.

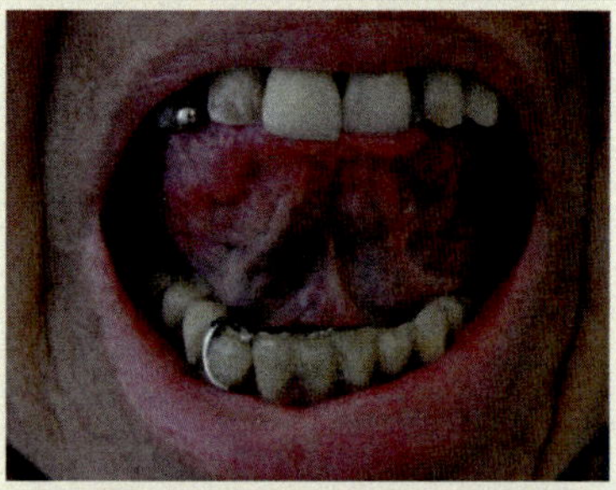

Plate 42:

- Dilated purplish sublingual veins with a white membrane, mainly on the right side ▶ Blood stasis.

- Symptoms: Patient operated for uterine fibromyoma.

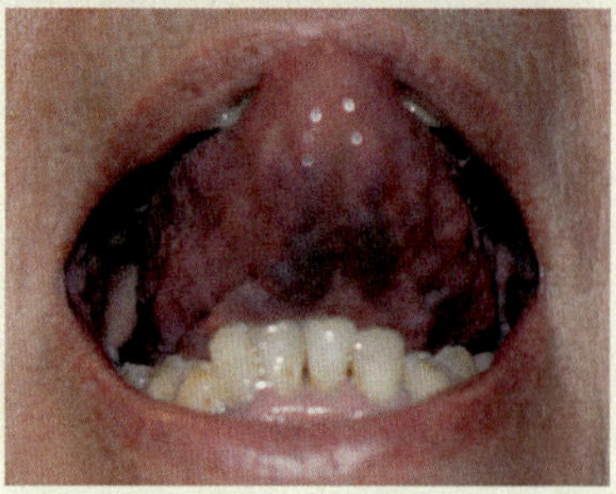

Plate-43:

- Slightly purplish tongue; dilated sublingual veins ▶ Blood stasis.

- Symptoms: Severe varicous veins and a history of Cesarien and gynecological operations and thrombo-phlebitis.

11. To Smell

11.1 Body Smells

Humans have greatly lost the ability to distinguish and interpret smells, although the sense of smell represents the strongest sense in a new-born child. The sense of smell may be reduced by excessive use of perfumes, or tobacco smoking, as well as chronic sinusitis. However, it is possible with some training to recover the smell acuity and to even smell the presence of various pathologies or emotions.

In general, body smells depend on the constitution and the *Zang-Fu* disharmony patterns. Strong smells denote the presence of Heat, lack of smell indicates Cold. Two smells are easier to detect: rotten (related to the Kidney) and rancid (Liver).

- Rancid, oily, greasy smell: Liver-*Qi* stasis or Liver-Damp-Heat; also often present in emotional repression or frustrations
- Burnt, smoky smell: Fire constitution
- Sweet, fragrant: Earth constitution; harmony of the *Zang-Fu*
- Sickly sweet: Spleen Damp-Heat
- Acrid, metallic: Metal constitution
- Decaying leaves or fish: Lung-Damp-Heat; Lung-*Yin Xu*
- Rotten, putrid, decaying flesh smell, especially of the feet or the genital area: Kidney-*Qi Xu* or Kidney-*Jing Xu*; the presence of fear
- Stale smell: Spleen-*Qi Xu*

11.2 Breath

- Foul breath: Heat in the Stomach and Intestines (indigestion or constipation); or decaying teeth from Kidney-*Jing* or Kidney-*Qi Xu*
- Sour smell: Food stagnation in the Stomach
- Acrid, metallic smell: Lung-*Qi Xu* (asthma)
- Strong fishy smell: Lung-Heat

11.3 Eliminations

- Foul smelling stool or gas: Heat; Damp-Heat in the Intestines
- Animal smell (goat or fish): Vacuity and Cold
- Intestinal gas with no smell: Spleen-*Qi Xu*
- Strong smelling urine: Damp-Heat in the Bladder
- Strong smelling vaginal discharge: Heat or Damp-Heat
- Mild fish smelling discharge: Damp-Cold

12. To Listen

In the West, the interrogation of the patient constitutes the most important aspect of diagnosis. Not only do we get important information about the medical history of the person and precisions about their complaints, but also the voice and the way a person expresses themselves to reflect on their constitution and temperament and gives us valuable insights as to the condition of the disease and the best therapeutic approach.

Additionally, learning to listen and perceive a person, establishes a connection between therapist and patient, which is fundamental in the healing process.

Although classically it was stressed that the interrogation should cover the basic "Ten Questions", in practice I believe that all the parts and functions of the body should be covered, including the psyche. It is important to hear the complaint as articulated by the patient, and then evaluate it in terms of Chinese medicine, avoiding the systematic labeling done by a Western diagnosis. The most common error made by Western practitioners is to treat based on diagnosis rather than based on TCM patterns as expressed by the patient. The most common tendency would be to apply a set of acupuncture points for a given Western label, for example, "insomnia". Whereas the type of sleep disturbance should be analyzed, and most importantly evaluated in the context of the patient, and only then to propose a personalized treatment.

In a true Holistic medicine, we treat the patient and not the disease.

12.1 Voice and Sounds

Voice

The pitch of the voice is in relation to the constitution.

High pitched	Fire type constitution
Singing, melodious	Earth type constitution
Monotonous, sad or whining	Metal type constitution
Deep, groaning, moaning	Water type constitution
Loud, shouting, aggressive	Wood type constitution

In pathology

Loud, talkative, agitated, with a hoarse voice	Heat condition; Heat *Shi* ≈ Repletion
Small voice, depressed and quiet	Cold condition; Yang *Xu* ≈ Vacuity

Extinction of voice	Dampness in the Lung
Weak voice with cold extremities	*Zong* ≈ Ancestral Qi-*Xu* ≈ Vacuity
Sudden loss of voice	*Biao* ≈ External Hot-Wind or Cold-Wind
Progressive loss of voice	Lung- and Kidney *Yin-Xu* or Lung-*Qi Xu*
Nasal voice	Presence of Dampness or Phlegm
Hoarse voice	Dryness from Biao≈ External Wind-Heat
Chronic hoarse voice	Lung-*Yin Xu* or Kidney-*Yin Xu*
Sudden hoarse voice; "Plum pit"	Liver-*Qi* stagnation

Speech

Speech, in general, depends on the Heart.

Confused speech, delirium	*Shen* disturbed by Heat, or Phlegm-Fire
Excessive talking and laughter	Heart-Heat or Heart-Fire
Talking to oneself, muttering or difficulty finding words	Heart-*Qi Xu*; Phlegm obstructing the Heart orifices
Repeated, uncontrolled speech and movements	Liver-Wind, as in Tourette's syndrome
Stammering	Heart-Blood *Xu*, Heart-Fire or Heart disturbed by Wind-Damp
Slurred speech	Internal Wind, Wind-stroke, Phlegm

Breathing

Weak breathing, shortness of breath		Lung and/or Kidney-*Qi Xu*
Loud and rough		Heat *Shi* ≈ Repletion
Wheezing		Phlegm obstructing the Lung
Panting	Out-breath is fast	External pathogenic factor in the Lung
	In-breath is fast	Lung and Kidney-*Qi Xu*
Long sighs with chest oppression		Liver-*Qi* stasis
Small and weak sighing		Heart-*Qi Xu*, Spleen-*Qi Xu*
Yawning		Lung-*Qi Xu*; general *Qi Xu*; empty Lung *Luo*
Snoring		Obstruction by Phlegm or Dampness

Cough and Sneezing

Are manifestations of the rebellious/ counter-flow *Qi* of the Lung, in which Lung cannot descend or propagate the *Qi*, which ascends in the opposite direction.

Deep and low cough	*Shi* ≈ Repletion
Weak and hesitant cough	*Xu* ≈ Vacuity
Dry cough	External Dryness or Lung-*Yin Xu*
With sputum	Dampness with Heat or Cold (► chap. 12.2/ sputum)
Loud and acute sneezing	External Wind
Weak sneezing	Lung-*Qi Xu*

Hiccups, Burps, and Vomiting

They result from an upward and rebellious/ counter-flow *Qi* of the Stomach.

Hiccups	Strong and loud	*Shi* ≈ Repletion; Stomach-Heat; Food stasis
	Muffled	Stomach-*Qi Xu* and Cold
	Isolated after food	Exposure to Cold-Wind after eating
	Weak in chronic disease	Exhaustion of *Qi*, a critical sign
Burps	Smelly and acid after eating	Food stagnation
	No smell	Liver and Stomach disharmony, Stomach-*Qi Xu*
Vomiting	Loud	*Shi* ≈ Repletion; Stomach-Heat; Food stasis; Liver-*Qi* stasis

12.2 Interrogation

The Eight Diagnostic Principles "Ba Gang"

The most pertinent diagnostic tool at the disposal of TCM practitioners is the "*Ba Gang*". Every symptom is classified according to eight principles, into four categories:

Yin and Yang	Classifies the type of the disease
Biao ≈ Surface and Li ≈ Lining	Defines the localization and evolution as well as the prognosis of the disease
Hot and Cold	Evaluates the nature of the disease and further confirms the Yin or Yang quality
Shi ≈ Repletion/ excess) and Xu ≈ Vacuity/ deficiency	Analyses the state of the Xie ≈ Pathogenic Qi versus the Zheng ≈ Upright Qi

Biao-Li 表里

The notion of *Biao-Li* is somehow complex to describe. The image of a coat is appropriate, in which we have the outer material whose purpose is to stop the wind and expel the rain, and the lining that is meant to keep the warmth in.

- *Biao*: outside, exterior, surface, is a disease localized in the skin and subcutaneous tissues, the secondary channels or the *Tai Yang* channel territory (the *Tai Yang* primary channel is included here to signify that the most important function of *Tai Yang* is to protect, that it is controlling the largest surface of the body and that it is very rich in *Wei Qi*).
- *Li*: lining, interior, depth: the disease is deeper, in the primary channels or in the *Zang-Fu* organs

	Biao	**Li**
Signs and symptoms	Acute onset; short duration; fever and chills, aversion to wind; little change in urine and stool	Gradual onset, chronic; low grade fever, if fever is higher there is no aversion to wind; presence of urine and stool changes
Etiology	Caused by the six pathogenic factors or mild trauma	Deeper penetration of *Xie Qi* or internal causes: emotions, wrong diet and life-style; heredity; parasites; intoxication, radiation, etc.
Tongue	Only the coating changes or might even be normal	Changes in tongue body, shape, colour and coating
Pulse	Superficial / Floating	Deep

Please note that a manifestation on the skin, like a skin rash, is not automatically a *Biao* ≈ Surface disease, for example, contact urticaria is a *Biao* condition, whereas eczema is a manifestation of Blood-Heat and therefore classified as *Li* ≈ Internal.

Hot – Cold, Fever and Chills

- Fever is a sensation of Heat, either objective with a raised temperature or subjective as felt in the whole or in a part of the body. The intensity of the fever depends on the *Zheng* ≈ Upright *Qi*. Fever is a *Yang* condition.
- Chills are a sensation of Cold often accompanied by an aversion to cold that may or may not be improved by heat. The intensity of chills depends on the strength of the *Xie* ≈ Pathogenic factor. This is a *Yin* symptom.

Fever, aversion to cold not improved by heat, with no sweating	*Biao* ≈ External- Cold-Wind (the cold sensation is stronger than the fever)
Fever, aversion to cold, maybe sweating	*Biao* ≈ External- Hot-Wind
Fever, aversion to heat with Sweating	External Hot or Cold-Wind with underlying *Wei* ≈ Defensive *Qi* vacuity
Cold improved by heat, no fever	*Li* ≈ Internal Cold from *Yang Xu*
Alternating fever and chills	Disease is ½ *Biao*- ½ *Li* in the *Shao Yang* level
Cyclic fevers	Evening fever, with night sweats: *Yin Xu*
	Afternoon fever with oppression: Damp-Heat in the Stomach and Spleen
	Between 3–5 p.m. with stomach pains: Dry-Heat in the *Yang Ming*
Chronic low grade fevers	With fatigue, anorexia: *Qi Xu*

The concept of Hot-Cold is further refined when applied to herbal or dietary principles. In this manner, a condition may be classified as "Hot" or "Warm" as opposed to "Cool" or "Cold". In the absence of particular signs (face, tongue, pulse) and symptoms of heat or coldness, the condition is considered "Neutral". The herbal or dietary treatments will be adapted accordingly:

Nature of the disease	Nature of the herbal or dietary remedy
Hot type disease	Cold inducing
Warm type disease	Cooling
Neutral disease	Neutral treatment
Cool type disease	Warming
Cold type disease	Heating

Shi ≈ Repletion – Xu ≈ Vacuity

The analysis and combination of the signs and symptoms help to evaluate if a given symptom is arising from an invasion of an external pathogenic factor, classified as an external *Shi* ≈ Repletion, or from internal blockage or stagnation, and would be termed as an internal *Shi* condition. Otherwise, symptoms caused by a weakness of one of the five substances, are classified as *Xu* ≈ Vacuity/ empty. In general, a *Shi* ≈ Replete condition gets worse when more *Qi* is added and gets better when *Qi* is removed. For example, an abdominal pain getting worse after eating, or better after vomiting or bowel movement is a *Shi*-type pain. Conditions that get better during pregnancy are *Xu*-type conditions because during pregnancy there is an abundance of Blood and Fluids. Pain is further analyzed below.

Technically speaking, the term *Shi* should only refer to external Pathogenic factors (PF), as the body does not produce excess energy. In fact, all internal *Shi*-conditions are either due to an accumulation of *Qi* or Fluids or Blood or to an exuberance of *Yang* due to a vacuity of *Yin* and vice versa.

Perspiration

Sweat is the liquid of the Heart, but abnormal sweating may be caused by any of the *Zang-Fu* and would signify a weakness of their respective *Qi*. In general, the *Wei* ≈ Defensive-*Qi* is in charge of the opening and closing of the pores. Schematically, the presence of sweat could either signify a *Shi* condition, where the body is attempting to cool down the surface by the evaporation of fluids; or sweating could be the result of a weakness of the *Wei Qi*, unable to close the pores sufficiently, with the sweat leaking out.

In a *Biao* disease	With no sweating	Cold repletion with a strong *Wei Qi*
	With sweating	Wind or Wind-Heat repletion with *Wei Qi Xu*
	Spontaneous sweating	Spleen or Lung-*Qi Xu*; *Ying* ≈ Nourishing and *Wei* ≈ Defensive *Qi* disharmony
With fever	Wind-Damp repletion; *Qi* stage disease	
Abundant sweat, high fever, big thirst, Flooding pulse	*Yang Ming* stage disease	
Abundant, oily with cold limbs	Exhaustion of *Yang-Qi* (critical)	
Night sweats	Kidney-*Yin Xu*; Heart-Blood *Xu*; Spleen-*Qi Xu* with Dampness	
Only on the head	Pathogenic Heat in the upper Triple Warmer	
With fatigue, heaviness, anuria	Damp-Heat in the middle Triple Warmer	
After a serious disease	Critical loss of *Yang* with *Yin-Xu*	

Only on one side ("Hemihidrosis")	Wind-stroke from Blood and *Qi-Xu*; or channel Obstruction by Wind-Cold; *Ying* ≈ Nourishing and *Wei* ≈ Defensive *Qi* disharmony	
Greasy, forehead	Exhaustion of *Yang* (critical)	
Sweaty palms and soles	Damp-Heat in Spleen and Stomach; Spleen and Stomach-*Qi Xu* or *Yin Xu*	
Sweaty feet	Kidney-*Qi Xu*	
Sweaty chest	Heart & Spleen-*Qi Xu*; or Heart & Kidney-*Yin Xu*	
Sweaty underarms	With no smell	Liver-*Yin Xu* with Heat; or Liver-*Qi* stasis
	With smell	Liver and Gallbladder Damp-Heat
Cold sweats	*Yang Xu*, or weakness of *Wei Qi*	
Hot sweats	External Hot-Wind or internal Heat	
Yellow sweat	Internal Damp-Heat	
Lack of sweat	External or Internal Cold	

Pain, paresthesia, hypoesthesia

Pain is always evaluated by the "Eight Diagnostic principles" (► Table 12.2):

- *Yang* type pain: Acute, intense, wrenching, burning, getting worse with heat
- *Yin*-type pain: Chronic, dull, heavy, imprecise, cold; getting worse with cold
- Pain better with Heat: *Yang Xu* or *Yin Shi* or Stagnation
- Pain better with Cold: *Yin Xu* or *Yang Shi*
- Pain worse with pressure: Excess of *Yin* or of *Yang* or Stagnation
- Pain better with pressure: Vacuity of *Yin* or *Yang*
- Better after movement: Stagnation of *Yin* or *Yang*
- Better with soft massage: Stagnation of *Yin* or *Yang*
- Pain worse with rest: Stagnation of *Yin* or *Yang*
- Pain worse at night: *Yin* stagnation

Table 12.2 Characteristics of *Yang* Pain and *Yin* Pain.

Yang Pain	*Yang* repletion (Excess)	Better with cold Worse with heat Worse with pressure
	Yin vacuity (Deficiency)	Better with cold Worse with heat Better with pressure

	Yang stagnation	Better with heat and movement Worse with cold and rest Worse with pressure Worse during the day
Yin Pain	*Yin* repletion (Excess)	Better with heat Worse with cold Worse with pressure
	Yang vacuity (Deficiency)	Better with heat Worse with cold Better with pressure
	Yin stagnation	Better with heat and movement Worse with cold and rest Worse with pressure Worse during the night

Analysis of Pain and Numbness:

Better with rest	*Qi Xu*	
Worse with movement	*Qi Xu* or mechanical pain	
Pain with swelling	Fixed and stabbing	Blood stasis
	Mobile, cramping	*Qi* stasis
Irradiating	Channel obstruction; Wind	
Paresthesia "pins and needles"	Blood *Xu* or Dampness blocking the channels	
Unilateral paresthesia	Internal Wind and/or internal Dampness	
Paresthesia and hypoesthesia (numbness)	Blood *Xu*	
Hypoesthesia	With paralysis	*Wei* ≈ Atrophy syndrome
	No paralysis	Vacuity in the *Jing Jin* ≈ Sinew channels
Head aches and pains	Neck area	*Tai Yang* from external pathogenic factors or Kidney-*Qi Xu*
	Forehead	*Yang Ming* from Stomach-Heat or Liver-Blood *Xu*
	Temples and sides	*Shao Yang* from external pathogenic factors; or Liver-*Yang* rising or Liver-

		Heat
	Vertex	*Jue Yin* from Liver-Blood *Xu* (dull ache) or *Tai Yang* (intense pain)
	Whole head	*Biao* ≈ External Cold-Wind penetration
	Heavy feeling (dull)	Dampness, Phlegm
	Internal	Kidney-*Qi Xu*
Joint pains with limitation of movement: *Bi* ≈ Impediment syndrome	Erratic, mobile pains	Wind-*Bi* ≈ Impediment
	Intense and fixed	Cold-*Bi*
	Inflamed red and hot	Heat-*Bi*
	Fixed, swollen with joint deformity	Damp-*Bi*
Lumbar pains	Chronic	Kidney-*Qi* or *Yin* or *Yang* or *Jing Xu*
	Acute	Pathogenic Cold-Damp
	Lumbago	Blood stasis or *Qi* stasis
Chest pains	Heart-Blood stasis; Lung Damp-Heat	
Side pains	Liver *Qi* stasis	
Abdomen, epigastric area	Burning	Stomach Heat or food stasis
	Dull	Stomach Cold from *Yang Xu*
	With bloating	Spleen-*Qi Xu*; Dampness
Abdomen, hypogastrium	Above the naval	Relates to Spleen or Stomach
	Bellow the naval	Kidney, Bladder, Large or Small Intestine, Uterus

Eliminations

Sputum

The expectoration of sputum (visible Phlegm) always signifies a condition of *Shi* ≈ Repletion, even if it is due to an underlying *Xu*≈ Vacuity pattern. The color and consistency will inform on the type of *Xie Qi* ≈ Pathogenic Factor.

White and thin and loose	Cold condition
Yellow or white and thick	Heat condition
Scarce, hard to bring up	Fire and Dryness
Abundant, easy to bring up	If white: Damp-Cold
	If yellow or green: Damp-Heat
Coughing up blood or blood with pus	Lung-Heat or Lung-Fire

Nasal Discharge

Rhinorrhea may be due to a condition of *Shi* ≈ Repletion or *Xu* ≈ Vacuity.

Clear rhinorrhea	Cold-Wind	
Yellow, green	Hot-Wind; Damp-Heat	
Acute rhinitis	External Wind (*Wei Qi Xu*)	
Chronic rhinitis	Liver-*Qi* Repletion (Liver-*Yang* rising) or Lung-*Qi Xu*; involves the *Yang Ming* channel	
Hay fever (allergic rhinitis)	Liver-*Yang* rising	
Sinusitis	Maxillary sinuses	Heat or Cold in *Yang Ming* channel
	Ethmoidal sinuses	Heat or Cold in *Shao Yang* channel
	Frontal sinuses	Heat or Cold in *Tai Yang* channel
Nose bleeds (epistaxis)	Mild bleeding	External Wind-Heat or Wind-Cold
	Frequent but mild	Spleen-*Qi Xu* or Blood *Xu* with Heat; Kidney-*Yin Xu*
	Abundant	Blood-Heat from Liver-Fire; or Heat in *Yang Ming* from Stomach-Fire

Vomiting

Is the Stomach counter-flow *Qi*.

Fluid, clear mucous	Stomach-Cold
Turbid, acid, foul smelling	Stomach-Heat or indigestion (Food stagnation)
Yellow and bitter	Heat in the Liver and Gallbladder
Blood and digested food	Liver-Fire attacking the Stomach

Stool, Bowel movement, Abdominal bloating

Bowel movements inform about the digestive system and the function of the Triple Warmer:

Symptoms better after bowel movement	*Shi* ≈ Repletion	
Symptoms worse after bowel movement	*Xu* ≈ Vacuity	
Stool Color	Pale or yellow	Dampness or Damp-Heat
	Dark	Heat
	Green in children	Cold
Constipation	Hard, difficult, with dry stools	Body Fluid *Xu*; Kidney-*Yin Xu*, Stomach-*Yin Xu*
	Acute with thirst	Heat in Stomach and Large Intestine
	After delivery or in the elderly patients	Blood *Xu*
	Small hard pellets	Liver-*Qi* stasis
	Difficult, soft and thin	*Qi Xu*; Spleen-*Qi Xu*
	Wet stools, abdominal pains	Internal Cold from *Yang-Xu*
Soft stools	Diarrhea	Spleen-*Qi Xu* or Spleen-*Yang Xu*; Small Intestine-*Qi Xu*
	Sunrise diarrhea "cock-crow diarrhea"	Kidney and Spleen-*Yang Xu*
	With undigested food	Spleen-*Yang Xu*; Small Intestine-*Qi-Yang Xu*
	Yellow and smelly	Damp-Heat in Large Intestine
	Smelly with pain that is better after bowels	Food stagnation
	Watery, painful, no smell	Cold in Large Intestine
	With mucous	Dampness or Phlegm in Large Intestine
	With blood and mucous	Damp-Heat in Large Intestine
	Fresh Blood	Heat in Blood or hemorrhoids
	Black (occult bleeding)	Blood stasis
Frequent stools, anal	Sinking of Central *Qi*; *Chong Mai*; Spleen-*Qi Xu*	

prolapse, incontinence		
Alternating diarrhea and constipation	Liver *Qi* stasis	
Bloating, flatulence with Borborygmus (noises)	After eating	Spleen-*Qi Xu*
	Without soft stools	Liver-*Qi* stasis
	Foul smell	Damp-Heat in Spleen and Stomach
	No smell	Cold from Spleen-*Yang Xu*
Anal burning pain, fissures	Heat	
Hemorrhoids	With hard small stools	Blood stasis from Liver-*Qi* stasis
	With anal prolapse	Sinking of Central *Qi*; *Chong Mai*; Spleen-*Qi Xu*

Urine

Urination mainly indicates the functions of the Kidney and Bladder.

Abundant urine ("polyuria"), Incontinence	Kidney-*Yang Xu*	
Frequency ("pollakiuria")	Kidney-*Yang Xu*; Lung and Spleen-*Qi Xu*; Damp-Heat in the Bladder	
Frequency, night urination	Kidney-*Qi Xu*	
Frequency, urgency, dark urine	Damp-Heat in the lower Triple Warmer (Bladder)	
Scanty urine ("oliguria")	Kidney-*Yin Xu*, Lung-*Yin* or Lung-*Qi Xu*, Spleen-*Yang Xu* with Dampness; Damp-Heat in Bladder	
Urinary retention ("anuria")	Kidney-*Yang Xu*; Kidney-*Yin Xu*; Damp-Heat in the lower Triple Warmer	
Incontinence	Kidney-*Yang Xu* or Kidney-*Qi Xu*; sinking of Central *Qi* (Spleen-*Qi*)	
Colour of urine	Dark yellow	Heat
	Yellow and turbid	Damp-Heat in the Bladder
	Pale urine	External Cold or Kidney-*Yang Xu*
	Bloody "hematuria"	Blood-Heat or Spleen-*Qi Xu*
Painful urination	Before urination	*Qi* stasis
	During urination	Heat or Damp-Heat

	After urination	*Qi Xu*
	Burning	Heat
	Stabbing pain	Blood stasis
	Distending	*Qi* stasis
	Sacrum and back	Kidney-*Qi Xu*
Difficulty with pain and dribbling is called a *Lin* ≈ Strangury syndrome	Burning, scanty but frequent urine	Hot-*Lin* from Liver-Fire or Heart-Fire or *Biao* Cold
	With sand and blood	Stone-*Lin* from Hot-Phlegm or Dryness
	Distending pain with irritability	*Qi-Lin* from Liver-*Qi* stasis
	Weak stream, fatigue	*Qi-Lin* from sinking *Qi* or Spleen-*Qi Xu*
	Bloody urine, burning	Blood-*Lin* from Liver-Fire; Kidney-*Yin Xu* or Kidney-*Qi Xu*
	Cloudy urine, difficulty prostatitis	Turbid *Lin* from Dampness or Kidney-*Qi Xu*
	Difficulty, frequency, prostatic adenoma	Fatigue *Lin* from Kidney-*Qi Xu*
Incomplete urination	Kidney-*Qi Xu* or Spleen-*Qi Xu*	

Menstruation

The menstrual cycle is a reflection of the state of *Xue* ≈ Blood, the free flow of Liver-*Qi*, as well as the coordination by the Extraordinary Vessels.

Short cycles, early periods	Blood-Heat or *Qi Xu*; Liver and Kidney-*Yin Xu*; or Blood stasis in the uterus
Long cycles	Blood *Xu* or Blood stasis in the uterus from Cold; Damp-Phlegm in the uterus; Kidney-*Qi* or *Yang Xu*
Irregular cycles	Liver-*Qi* or Blood stasis; Kidney and Spleen-*Qi Xu*; Heart-Blood *Xu*
Bleeding in between periods	Injury of *Chong* and *Ren Mai*; *Qi-Xu*; Blood stasis; Damp-Heat
Heavy periods	Blood-Heat, Liver-Fire or Spleen and Kidney-*Qi Xu*; Liver and Kidney-*Yin Xu* with empty Heat; Blood stasis in the uterus
Scanty periods	Blood *Xu*; uterine Blood stasis from Cold; Phlegm obstructing the uterus; Kidney-*Yin* or *Yang Xu*

Periods that stop & start	Blood stasis from Cold; Liver-*Qi* stasis	
Absence of periods ("amenorrhea")	Blood *Xu*; Liver and Kidney-*Yin Xu*; Heart and Kidney-*Yin Xu*; Heart-Blood and Spleen-*Qi Xu*; Blood-stagnation	
Menses after menopause	Liver and Kidney-*Yin Xu* with empty Heat; Liver-Fire; Toxic-Heat; Spleen-*Qi Xu*	
Color of menses	Dark or bright red	Blood Heat
	Light red or pale	Blood *Xu*
	Very dark, blackish	Blood stasis
	Purplish	Blood stasis from pathogenic Cold
	Brownish	Blood stasis from *Yang Xu*
Clots	Dark dull and large	Blood stasis in the uterus
	Dark, shiny	Blood-Heat
	Small, dark	Cold in the uterus
Watery menses	Blood *Xu* or Cold-Dampness in the uterus from Spleen & Kidney-*Yang Xu*; Liver & Kidney-*Yin Xu*	
Sticky menses	Damp-Heat in the uterus	
Pain ("Dysmenorrhea")	Pre-menstrual	Liver-*Qi* stasis or Blood stasis
	During the period	Blood stasis from Cold or Blood-Heat; Damp-Heat in the uterus
	Post-menstrual	Blood *Xu*
	Mild	Blood *Xu* or Blood-Heat
	Intense, stabbing	Blood stasis
	Intense, cramping, better with heat	Cold accumulation
	Bearing down feeling	Sinking of Central *Qi*
	Heaviness	Damp-Heat
	With backache	Kidney-*Qi Xu*; *Dai Mai* vessel
	Unilateral pain	Blood or *Qi* stasis; *Yin Qiao Mai*
	With sensation of *Qi* rising	*Chong Mai*
Pain during ovulation	Damp-Heat	
Pre-menstrual ("PMS")	Liver-*Qi* stasis	
	Headaches	Liver-*Yang* rising; Heat in Blood
	Edema	Kidney- or Spleen-*Yang Xu*; Liver-*Qi*

		stagnation
	Cramps in limbs	Liver-Blood *Xu*
	Body aches	Liver-Blood *Xu*; Blood stasis
	Insomnia	Blood-Heat; Liver-Fire; Heart-Fire; Heart-*Yin Xu*
	Breast tension and pain	Liver-*Qi* stasis; Liver-Fire; Liver-Blood-stasis; Phlegm accumulation from Liver or Lung-*Qi* stasis
	Diarrhea	Spleen-*Qi Xu*; Kidney-*Yang Xu*; Liver-*Qi* stagnation invading the Spleen
	Constipation	Liver-*Qi* stagnation invading the Large Intestine; Liver-Blood *Xu*; Kidney-*Yang Xu*
Mastitis	Liver-*Qi* stasis; Damp-Heat in the Stomach channel	
Infertility	Kidney-*Jing Xu*; Blood *Xu*; Damp-Heat in the lower Triple Warmer; Blood stasis in the uterus	
Miscarriage	First 3 months	Blood *Xu* or Kidney-*Jing Xu*
	After the 3rd month	Liver-*Qi* stasis; Blood-Heat; Spleen-*Qi Xu*
Morning sickness	Slight, diluted fluids, with fatigue	Stomach-*Qi Xu* with Cold (from *Yang* deficiency)
	Thirst but no desire to drink	Stomach-*Yin Xu*
	Severe, sour taste, with irritability	Liver-*Qi* stagnation invading the Stomach; ST-Heat; Stomach-Fire
	After food, thirst, and stomatitis	Stomach-Fire; Heart-Fire
	Abundant, with chest oppression	Phlegm stagnation in the Stomach
Pregnancy with palpitation or depression	Heart-*Qi Xu*	
Pregnancy with thirst, restlessness & insomnia	Heart-Fire	
Post-partum	Bleeding, nausea	*Chong Mai* weakness; Spleen-*Qi Xu*; Blood-Heat
	Fever, sweats	Invasion of external pathogenic factors from exhaustion of *Qi* and Blood

	Sweating	Kidney-*Qi Xu*; Kidney-*Yin Xu*
	Depression	Heart-Blood *Xu*; Heart-*Yin Xu*; Heart-Blood stasis; Liver-Blood or *Yin-Xu*
	Discharge of lochia	*Qi Xu*; Blood stasis; Blood-Heat
	Insufficient lactation	*Qi* and Blood *Xu*; Liver-*Qi* stasis

Genital Organs

The genital organs mainly reflect on the conditions of the Kidney, the Liver, and the Spleen.

Vaginal discharge	White, watery	Pathogenic Damp-Cold, Spleen & Kidney-*Yang Xu*
	White, thick or yellow	Damp-Heat in the lower Triple Warmer
	Greenish or red and smelly	Damp-Heat in the Liver channel
	Fishy smell	Cold-Damp
	Cheesy (animal) or leathery smell	Damp-Heat
Orchitis; cervicitis, vaginitis, venereal disease; genital eczema; herpes	Damp-Heat in the Liver channel	
Inguinal hernia; varicocele; torsion of the testicle	Cold in the Liver or Small Intestine channels	
Prostatitis	Damp-Heat in the Bladder	
Sexuality	Reduced sex drive, lack of desire	Kidney, Spleen & Heart-*Qi Xu*; Kidney & Spleen-*Yang Xu*; Liver-*Qi* stagnation; Kidney-*Jing* or *Yin Xu* (physical); Heart-*Yin Xu* (emotional)
	Impotence	Kidney-*Yang*, *Qi* or *Yin Xu*; Heart & Spleen-*Qi Xu*; Liver-*Qi* stagnation; Damp-Heat or in the lower Triple Warmer; Blood stasis
	Slow arousal	Kidney-*Yang Xu*; Liver-Blood *Xu*; Damp-Heat or Phlegm in the lower Triple Warmer
	Exaggerated desire, over-	Kidney-*Yin Xu*; Liver-Heat

	stimulation	
	Premature ejaculation	Kidney-*Qi Xu*; Heart & Kidney-*Qi* or *Yin Xu*; Kidney-*Yin Xu*/ Empty-Fire; Heart & Spleen-*Qi Xu*; Liver-Fire; Damp-Heat in the Lower Triple Warmer and the Liver channel; Liver-*Qi* Stasis
	Needing special types of stimulation	Liver-*Qi* stasis
	Difficulty in erection or lubrification	Liver-Blood *Xu*
	Spermatorrhea	Kidney-*Qi* or *Jing* or *Yin Xu*; Kidney & Heart-*Qi* or *Yin Xu*; Heart-Fire; Heart & Spleen-*Qi Xu*; Liver-Fire; Damp-Heat in the Lower TW

Sensory Organs

The sensory functions depend primarily on the *Zang* ≈ Organs they are related to, but also to the local channels involved.

Ears, Hearing, Tinnitus

Hearing depends on the Kidney-*Qi* or *Jing;* Tinnitus is a manifestation of Internal Wind.

Sudden deafness: *Shi* ≈ Repletion	Pathogenic Cold in the *Shao Yang* channel; physical trauma or emotional shock
Progressive deafness: *Xu* ≈ Vacuity	Kidney-*Jing* or Kidney-*Qi Xu*; Heart-Blood *Xu*
Whistling, worse with pressure on the ear	Liver-*Yang* rising, Liver-Fire or Liver-Wind
Rushing water, better with pressure on the ear	Kidney-*Qi Xu* or Kidney-*Jing Xu*
Sudden ringing or deafness, headache, agitation, chest oppression	Liver-*Qi* stagnation and Blood stasis
Sound of cicada or ringing, reduced hearing, blocked ears, vertigo, heavy	Damp-Heat in the head; Liver-Blood *Xu*

<table>
<tr><td colspan="2">head</td><td></td></tr>
<tr><td colspan="2">Intermittent mild murmur, worse with insomnia; deafness; palpitations, vertigo, anxiety; loss of memory</td><td>Heart-Blood Xu with Kidney-Qi or Jing Xu</td></tr>
<tr><td colspan="2">Tinnitus & deafness worse with over work, ears feeling cold; weakness</td><td>Stomach and Spleen-Qi Xu</td></tr>
<tr><td colspan="2">Cicada sound, worse at night with fatigue and coldness</td><td>Kidney-Qi Xu</td></tr>
<tr><td colspan="2">Intermittent mild murmur, shortness of breath, spontaneous sweating</td><td>Lung Qi Xu</td></tr>
<tr><td rowspan="3">Acute otitis</td><td colspan="2">External Wind-Cold; Wind-Heat</td></tr>
<tr><td>With discharge (pus)</td><td>Damp-Heat</td></tr>
<tr><td>No discharge</td><td>Liver-Yang rising</td></tr>
<tr><td>Chronic otitis</td><td colspan="2">Liver-Yang rising; Gallbladder Damp-Heat</td></tr>
<tr><td rowspan="3">Ear pruritus</td><td colspan="2">External Wind-Damp-Heat</td></tr>
<tr><td>With dryness & peeling</td><td>Blood Xu</td></tr>
<tr><td>With redness</td><td>Kidney-Yin Xu with empty-Fire</td></tr>
</table>

Eye, Vision

The external pathogenic factor may be assessed by the condition of the eye:

- Itching, lacrimation, pain: Wind
- Redness, heat, pain: Heat
- Discharge, ulceration, keratitis: Dampness
- Lacrimation, pain, feeling of a foreign body: Cold
- Dry eye, feeling of a foreign body: Dryness

Red and painful eyes ("conjunctivitis")	External Wind-Heat; Liver and Gallbladder-Fire or Damp-Heat
Itchy eyes	External Wind, Wind-Heat or Wind-Cold; Liver-Fire or Damp-Heat
Tearing with the wind	External Wind-Cold; Kidney or Liver-*Yin Xu*; Liver-*Yang* rising
Light sensitivity with no swelling ("Photophobia")	Liver-*Yin Xu* from Kidney-*Yin Xu*
Photophobia with swelling	Liver-Heat or Fire
Blurred Vision	Exhaustion of *Yin* and Blood
Double vision	Liver-*Qi Xu* and Kidney-*Qi Xu*

Short-sightedness ("myopia") (*Yin-Shi* with *Yang-Xu*)	Liver and Kidney-*Yin Xu*; Spleen and Stomach-*Qi Xu*; Heart-*Yang Xu*; *Shen* obstructed by Phlegm	
Farsightedness ("hyperopia") or "hypermetropia"	Liver-*Yin* or Blood *Xu*; Kidney-*Yin* or *Yang Xu*; Spleen-*Qi* or Blood *Xu*	
Night blindness (hemeralopia")	Liver-Blood *Xu* and Kidney-*Jing Xu*; Spleen and Stomach-*Qi Xu*	
Color blindness ("dyschromatopsia")	Prenatal-*Jing* or *Zong-Qi* weakness	
Strabismus	convergent (*Yang* type), divergent (*Yin* type)	
	In infants	*Yang* excess in the neck; Liver and Kidney-*Yin Xu*
	Essential	Liver-*Qi* stagnation invading the Spleen
	Traumatic	Blood and *Qi* stasis
Glaucoma	Liver-Blood and Kidney-*Jing Xu* with *Yang* rising; Liver-Blood or *Yin Xu* with Liver-Wind	
Stye, chalazion, pterygium "surfer's eye"	Stomach and Spleen Damp-Heat or Hot-Phlegm; Spleen-*Yin Xu*	

Nose, Smell

The nose and acuity of smell are related to the Lung, but the *Yang Ming* channels (ST-LI), as well as the inner pathway of the Liver channel, also play an important role in the pathologies of the nose and the sinuses.

Loss of smell ("anosmia")	*Yang Ming* channel vacuity; Lung-*Qi Xu*; Phlegm obstructing the Heart orifices	
Acute anosmia	External Wind-Heat or Gallbladder Damp-Heat	
Anosmia with Chronic Sinusitis	*Qi* & Blood stasis; Stomach & Spleen Damp-Heat	
Rhinitis/ sinusitis	► "Nasal discharge"	
Allergic rhinitis ("hay fever")	Liver-*Qi* invading the Lung	
	Worse with heat	Excess of *Wei Qi* on the surface
	Better with heat	The vacuity of *Wei Qi* on the surface
Stuffy nose	External Wind-Cold or Wind-Heat; residual Damp-Heat (sinusitis); Lung and Spleen-*Qi Xu*	
Polyps	Dampness or Phlegm from Lung, Spleen or	

	Stomach-*Qi Xu;* Stomach or Spleen Damp-Heat

Mouth, Speech, and Throat

The mouth reflects primarily the Stomach and Spleen physiology, although the Heart channel's inner branch ends at the tongue, hence the Heart is responsible for speech. The strength of the voice reflects, on the one hand, the strength of Lung and *Zong Qi* ≈ Ancestral energy and on the other hand the *Yang Ming* channels (LI-ST).

Stomatitis	Pale sores "aphtha"	Heart and Kidney-*Yin Xu* with empty Heat; Spleen and Kidney-*Yang Xu*
	Red sores, raised	Heart-Fire; Stomach-Damp-Heat
A sore throat, angina	External Wind-Heat or Wind-Cold; Lung-*Yin* or Kidney-*Yin Xu*	
Tonsillitis	Stomach-Heat or Fire	
Loss of voice ("aphonia")	External Wind-Heat or Wind-Cold	
Hoarse voice	Stomach-Heat and Dryness	
	Worse after talking	Lung and Kidney-*Yin Xu*
	Worse in the evening	Lung and Spleen-*Qi Xu*
Throat "Plum pit" feeling	Liver-*Qi* stagnation; Phlegm obstruction	
Stuttering	Heart-Fire	

Skin (▶ chap. 10.2, page 170)

Sleep and Dreams

Sleeping is the *Yin* counterpart to activity *(Yang)*. After air, water, and food, sleep is the most important factor in the preservation of health. Dreams are also indispensable to health and are the domain of *Hun* ≈ Ethereal soul.

Insomnia

Insomnia is a *Yang* condition and may be due to *Yang Shi* ≈ Repletion, *Yin Xu*-Vacuity or Blood-*Xu.*

Difficulty falling asleep	Heart-Blood *Xu*; Heart and Kidney-*Yin Xu*; Heart-Fire

Frequent waking	Kidney-*Yin Xu*; Heart-Blood or Heart-*Yin Xu*
Superficial sleep, frequent dreams	Heart-Blood *Xu*, or Liver-Blood *Xu*
Superficial sleep, anxiety	Heart-*Qi Xu*; Heart-*Yang Xu*; Kidney-*Yang Xu*
Restless sleep, nightmares	Liver-Fire; Heart-Fire; Phlegm harassing the mind; Stomach-Fire; Blood stasis; Liver & Heart-Blood *Xu*; Liver-*Yin Xu* with *Yang* rising
Restlessness, nightmares, early waking	Liver-*Yin Xu* with *Yang* rising; Liver-Blood *Xu*
Light sleep from insecurity, shyness	Gallbladder-*Qi Xu*; Damp-Heat in the Gallbladder
Needing to eat to fall asleep	Stomach-Heat or Damp-Heat; Stomach-*Yin Xu*
Feeling of not having slept, nightmares	Stomach-Fire
Waking at 3 am	Spleen- or Lung-*Qi Xu*; Lung-Heat
Jerks during sleep	Liver-*Qi* stasis
Teeth grinding	Large Intestine Heat or stagnation of food
Sleep-walking	Heart-Blood *Xu*; Heart-Blood stasis; Spleen-*Qi Xu*; Phlegm-Fire harassing the mind; Liver-Blood *Xu* with Liver-*Qi* stasis or -*Yin Xu* or -Wind or -Fire
Sleep-talking	Heart-Fire, Heart-Blood-stasis; Liver-*Yin Xu*; Food stasis
Sleep apnea with snoring	Spleen-*Qi Xu*; Phlegm misting the mind; Kidney and Spleen-*Yang Xu*
Night terrors	Phlegm-Fire harassing or Phlegm misting the mind
Crusting around the eyes, drooling	Damp-Heat in the Triple Warmer

Hypersomnia

Hypersomnia or excessive sleeping is a *Yin* condition.

A constant need for sleep ("narcolepsy")	Kidney-*Yang Xu*; Phlegm obstructing the mind; Blood-stasis; Heart and Spleen-*Qi Xu*
Sleepiness after eating	Spleen-*Qi Xu*
Stupor	Pericardium-Heat

Dreams

Dreams are part of the normal functions of *Hun* ≈ Ethereal soul and primarily reflect on the functions of the Liver. The nature and the content of the dreams further inform on the state of all of the *Zang-Fu.*

Excessive dreaming	Heart-Blood *Xu*; Liver-Blood *Xu*; Liver-*Yin Xu*; Heart & Gallbladder-*Qi Xu*; Heart & Kidney-*Yin Xu*; Liver-Fire; Phlegm-Fire harassing the mind
Nightmares	Liver-Fire; Heart-Fire; Phlegm-Fire harassing the mind; Liver and Heart-Blood *Xu*; Liver-*Yin Xu* with Liver-*Yang* rising; Heart & Gallbladder-*Qi Xu*; Stomach-Heat or Fire; Heart-Blood-stasis
Dream of vast waters	*Yin* repletion
Drowning; sinking ships; fear; death	Kidney-*Qi Xu*
Spine detaching; worms; wounds	Repletion of pathogenic factor in the Kidney
Erotic dreams with spermatorrhea	Kidney-*Yin Xu*
Fire, burns, volcanoes, explosions, calamities	Heart-*Yin Xu*; Heart and Kidney not harmonized
Joy and laughter	Repletion of pathogenic factor in the Heart
Saved from fire; sun; success	Heart-*Qi Xu*
Frequent nightmares, anger, aggression	Liver-Fire
Green pastures, plants, mushrooms	Liver-*Qi Xu*, Liver-Blood *Xu*
Inability to reach a destination; obstacles; break down	Liver-*Qi* stasis; Liver-Blood *Xu* or stasis
Flying; white objects; bloody wars; beheading; precipice; nakedness, vulnerability	Lung-*Qi Xu*; Lung-*Yin Xu*
Grief; crying; flying over metallic structures	Repletion of pathogenic factor in the Lung
Flying	Excess above; pathogenic factor in the Lung
Falling	Excess below; sinking Spleen-*Qi*
Oppression; heavy body singing, music; ruins	Repletion of pathogenic factor in the Spleen
Being buried	Spleen-*Qi Xu* with Dampness

Starvation; building walls and houses; swamps and fog; loss of property	Spleen-*Qi Xu*
Conflict, lawsuits; self-destruction	Gallbladder-*Qi Xu*
Crowds or fights	Intestinal Worms
Crowds, busy roads	Small Intestine-*Qi Xu*
Large meals	Stomach-*Qi Xu*
Foreign lands, fields	Large Intestine-*Qi Xu*
Wandering, travel	Bladder-*Qi Xu*

Diet, Appetite, Thirst

Appetite and thirst primarily reflect the *Qi* and *Yang* of the Stomach and Spleen, although the choice of foods and tastes is in relation with the other *Zang-Fu* in the Five Phase system.

Eating habits and tastes	Relate to the Five Phases	
Taste in the mouth	Sour	Food stasis or Liver attacking the Spleen
	Bitter in the morning	Heart-Heat or Gallbladder-*Qi Xu*
	Constant bitter taste	Liver-Heat, Liver-Fire
	Sweetish or greasy	Spleen-*Qi Xu* or Damp-Heat
	Acrid	Lung-Heat
	Salty	Kidney-*Yin Xu*
	Bland, no taste	Spleen-*Qi Xu*
Lack of appetite	Spleen-Qi Xu; Dampness	
Excessive appetite	Stomach-Heat	
Hunger but no desire to eat	Stomach-Yin Xu	
Thirst for cold drinks	Body Fluid deficiency; Pathogenic Heat	
Thirst, drinking lukewarm water in small sips	Stomach-Yin Xu, or Kidney-Yin Xu	
Thirst but no desire to drink	Stomach-Damp-Heat; Heat in the Ying ≈ Nourishing level	
No thirst	Cold from Stomach and Spleen-Yang Xu	

13. Pattern Identification

Pattern identification constitutes the core of Chinese diagnosis and leads to the appropriate therapeutic principle. Symptoms and signs are collected and grouped to form a picture and to lead to a particular style of treatment.

- Identification according to *Yin-Yang* disharmony patterns and the Eight Principles
- Identification according to the Five substance disharmony patterns
- Identification according to the *Zang-Fu* disharmony patterns
- Identification according to the Six Stages, Four levels or Three Burners disharmony patterns
- Identification according to the *Jing-Luo* channel system disharmony patterns, including the *Qi Jing Ba Mai* ≈ Eight Extraordinary vessels, the *Jing-Jin*≈ Sinew channels, the *Luo Mai* ≈ Connecting vessels and the *Jing-Bie* ≈ Divergent channels
- Constitutional assessment according to the Five Phases (Elements) and related patterns
- Assessment of the Temperaments according to the Six Levels and their related patterns

It is important to underline that in identifying a pattern, only the manifestation or site and the causative factors are revealed. To discover the roots of a disease, the constitution, and the temperament has to be also considered and investigated.

13.1 Identification of patterns according to Yin-Yang disharmony criterion

Every symptom should first be analyzed according to the *Ba Gang* ≈ Eight Diagnostic principles, the first two being *Yin-Yang* (► chap. 12.2, page 198).

Table 13.1 *Yin-Yang* disharmony patterns.

Symptoms	Yin	Yang
General	Pale face; the feeling of cold and aversion to cold; discomfort relieved by warmth; no thirst or preferring warm drinks	Red face and feeling hot, aversion to Heat; thirst and preference for cool drinks
Energy	Tired, weak	Forceful, restless
Behavior	Underactive, quiet, withdrawn	Overactive, noisy, outgoing
Breathing and voice	Weak shallow breathing, weak voice	Deep heavy breathing; a loud and rough voice

Digestion	Reduced appetite, abdominal distension	increased appetite, burning pain in epigastrium
Eliminations	Copious clear urine; diarrhea	Scanty dark urine; constipation
Sexuality and Gynecology	Reduced sexual desire, frigidity; scanty pale menses; white or clear leucorrhoea	Sexually overactive; profuse red menses, yellow leucorrhoea
Pulses	Deep, slow, empty	Superficial, rapid, full
Tongue	Pale tongue body; moist, with a thin white coating	Red tongue body; dry, with a thick yellow coating

13.2 Identification of patterns according to Repletion & Vacuity, Cold & Heat

After establishing the *Yin-Yang* nature of a symptom, Cold and Hot is evaluated either by the clear manifestation of heat and cold or by the question if hot or cold improve or aggravate the condition (▶ chap. 12.2); (▶ Table 13.2).

Table 13.2 Patterns based on *Shi* ≈ Repletion/ Excess, *Xu* ≈ Vacuity/ Deficiency, and Cold & Heat.

	Yin Conditions		Yang Conditions	
	+++	+	+	+++
Pattern	"Full Cold" (*Yin* Repletion)	"Empty Cold" (*Yang* Vacuity)	"Empty Heat" (*Yin* Vacuity)	"Full Heat" (*Yang* Repletion)
General body temperature	Cold limbs, aversion to cold	Cold limbs, aversion to cold	Afternoon fever, malar flush, feverish sensation in palms and soles	High fever, body red and hot
Pain	Pain relieved by heat worse with cold and pressure	Pain relieved by heat worse with cold, better with pressure	Pain worse with heat, relieved by cold, better with pressure	Pain relieved by cold, aggravated by heat and pressure
Movements and Energy	Forceful but slow movements	Weak and slow movements, lassitude	Weak but rapid movements, restlessness	Forceful and rapid gestures, restlessness agitation

Sleep	Sleepiness	Hypersomnia, lethargy	Insomnia	Insomnia with agitation
Sweat	No sweating	Daytime sweating	Night sweating	Excessive sweating
Urine	Clear and copious	Clear and copious	Dark and scanty	Dark and scanty
Stool	Soft stools	Soft stools	Constipation	Constipation
Pulses	Deep, slow, full	Slow, empty	Rapid, thin, floating	Rapid, full
Tongue	Pale tongue, thick white coating	Pale tongue, thick white coating	Red tongue, little or no coating	Dark red tongue, thick yellow coating

13.3 Identification according to the "Five Substance" disharmony patterns

The "Five Substances" are *Qi* ≈ Energy, *Xue* ≈ Blood, *Jin Ye* ≈ Body fluids, *Shen* ≈ Spirit/ mind, and *Jing* ≈ Essence. In daily practice, the most common patterns that we encounter involve *Qi* and Blood.

Pathologies of Qi

Qi Xu ≈ Vacuity is by far the most common complaint. (► Table 13.3).

Qi Xu ≈ Vacuity (Deficiency)

Table 13.3 *Qi Xu* ≈ Vacuity

Pattern	Symptoms	Specific symptoms	Tongue	Pulse
General Qi Xu (Cardinal symptoms)	• General fatigue • Depressed spirit • Shortness of Breath • Aversion to movement • Low weak voice • Aversion to speech • Spontaneous sweating		Pale, Enlarged	Empty, Soft, Weak

Lung-Qi Xu	• General *Qi Xu* • + Respiratory Symptoms	• A weak Cough • Asthma • Phlegm • Whitish face	Pale and swollen in the front one third	Empty, Weak, Soft
Heart-Qi Xu	• General *Qi Xu* • + Palpitations • + Sweating from chest and armpits	• Palpitations • Anxiety • Pale face	Pale and swollen	Empty, Weak, Soft, Knotted, Intermit-tent
Spleen & Stomach-Qi Xu	• General Qi Xu • + Digestive symptoms • + Loss of appetite	• Heavy limbs • Lethargy • Tired and bloated after meals • Indigestion • Soft stools • Organ prolapse • Easy bleeding • Dull yellow face	Pale and swollen with teeth marks	Empty, weak, soft
Kidney-Qi Xu	• General *Qi-Xu* • + Lumbar symptoms • + Urinary dysfunctions • + Sexual dysfunctions	• Lumbar & knee pains • Sweaty feet • Fearfulness • Night urination; incontinence • Impotence; premature ejaculation • Tinnitus; deafness	Pale and swollen	Empty, Weak and Deep

Qi Stagnation

The Liver is in charge of the smooth flow of *Qi* and would be most involved in patterns of *Qi* stagnation. But also most Spleen disharmony patterns result in the production of Dampness, which by its sticky and cloying nature will hamper the flow of *Qi.* (▶ Table 13.4).

Table 13.4: *Qi* Stagnation.

Pattern	Symptoms	Specific symptoms	Tongue	Pulse
General Qi Stasis (Cardinal symptoms)	• Swelling, distention • Moving pains • Depression, moodiness • Irritability		Possible redness	Wiry, Tight
Liver-Qi Stagnation	• Depression; moodiness • Distension or pain of solar plexus, chest, breasts, sides • Sighing, hiccups • Menstrual irregularities; • Digestive disturbances: nausea, vomiting belching, acidity • Bloating, borborygmus; indigestion (fats, alcohol...)	• Irritability, inner stress • Plum pit feeling in the throat • Pre-menstrual breast distention	Normal or purplish with red sides	Wiry or Tight
Spleen-Qi Stasis	• Bloating & gas, • Mild pain (better with heat and movement) • Indigestion • Loose stools • Low appetite • Mental and emotional stagnation • Dampness and Phlegm	• Bloating and gas • Indigestion • Worry, obsession, fixation	Swollen, Sticky coating	Slippery, or empty or soft

Counter-flow, Rebellious Qi

Counter-flow *Qi* is energy going the wrong way; this mainly involves Stomach-*Qi or Lung-Qi* going upwards instead of down, or the Spleen-*Qi* dropping instead of rising. (► Table 13.5).

Table 13.5 : Counter-flow, Rebellious *Qi.*

Pattern	Symptoms	Specific symptoms	Tongue	Pulse
Stomach Counterflow Qi	• Nausea • Vomiting • Burping • Reflux	• Vomiting	Depends on the pattern	Depends on the pattern
Lung Counterflow Qi	• Shortness of breath • Cough • Sneezing • Asthma	• Cough	Depends on the pattern	Depends on the pattern
Chong Mai Counter-flow Qi (Kidney Counter-flow Qi)	• Shortness of breath, oppression • Energy rushing up to the head	• Cold feet, hot head • Panic attack	Depends on the pattern	Firm on all positions Hard on both middle positions

Other types of Abnormal Qi

The following patterns are sometimes also classified as Counter-flow *Qi*, although technically they differ from the above patterns (▶ Table 13.6):

Table 13.6: Other types of Abnormal *Qi*

Pattern	Symptoms	Specific symptoms	Tongue	Pulse
Spleen-Qi Sinking	• Bearing down feeling, urinary or bowel frequency and urgency • Hemorrhoids • Varicose veins • Organ prolapse	• Hernia and prolapse • Bearing down feeling	Depends on the pattern	Depends on the pattern
Liver-Qi not smooth	• Liver-*Qi* stasis symptoms	• (see above)	Red Sides	Wiry, Tight
Liver-Yang rising	• + Head symptoms	• Headaches • High blood pressure	Red, dry, redder sides	Rapid, Full
Liver invading the Stomach	• + Stomach symptoms	• Vomiting • Ulcers	Central swelling and crack	–

Liver invading the Spleen	• + Digestive symptoms	• Fatigue • Diarrhea	Swollen, teeth marks	Empty Earth
Liver invading the Intestines	• + Intestinal symptoms	• Constipation • Colitis	A sticky, or greasy coating	–
Liver-Heat in the lower TW	• + Bladder and genital symptoms	• Discharge • Cystitis • Urethritis	Yellow and greasy coating at the base	–
Kidney not grasping the Qi	• Shortness of breath • Edema	• Asthma • Facial edema	Pale and swollen	Deep and weak
Heart-Qi unsettled	• Restlessness • Mental agitation	• Insomnia	Red tip, yellow coating	Thin, Fast, Knotted, Choppy

Pathologies of Blood

After *Qi* pathologies, Blood pathologies are the most common patterns observed in daily practice.

Blood Xu ≈ Vacuity

Blood *Xu* is much more common in women and should not be confused with the Western notion of anemia, the latter combines patterns of both *Blood Xu and Qi Xu:*

Table 13.7 : Blood *Xu* ≈ Vacuity

Pattern	Symptoms	Specific symptoms	Tongue	Pulse
General Blood Xu (Cardinal symptoms)	• Paleness • Dizziness • Numbness • Palpitations • Insomnia (dreams) • Poor memory • Blurred vision • Dryness • Depression, tiredness	• Paleness of face, lips, nails and the inner side of the eyelid	Pale and dry	Thready, Weak (Choppy if recent blood loss)

Heart-Blood Xu	• General Blood *Xu* • + Palpitations (more pronounced) • + Insomnia (more pronounced)	• Palpitations • Restless-ness and insomnia with dreams	Pale and dry	Thready, Weak
Liver-Blood Xu	• General Blood *Xu* • + Numbness of limbs • + Dryness of skin and nails (brittle)	• Numbness • Night blindness • Color blindness • Blurred vision • Muscle cramps • Irregular menses	Pale or orange on the sides, dry	Choppy; Fine

Blood Stagnation

Blood stagnation in Chinese medicine includes a broad spectrum of Western pathologies such as hematoma, traumatic injuries, blood clots, and angina pectoris, a number of gynecological conditions such as premenstrual pains, fibromyoma, and endometriosis as well as certain ulcers, tumors and even cancer (▶ Table 13.8).

Table 13.8 : Blood Stagnation

Pattern	Symptoms	Specific symptoms	Tongue	Pulse
General Blood Stasis (Cardinal symptoms)	• Fixed and stabbing pain • Swelling • Bleeding (dark blood and clots) • Purple • Spots on the body (purple, red or bleeding)	• Stabbing pain • Bleeding • Purple lips, nails, tongue, spots	Purple or purple spots, with swollen sub-lingual veins	Choppy, Firm or Wiry
Heart-Blood Stasis	• General Blood Stasis • + Chest pains • + Oppression • + Cold hands • + Purple Lips	• Stabbing chest pains radiating to the left arm • Purple Lips	Purple tip	Knotted
Liver-Blood Stasis	• General Blood Stasis • + Dysmenorrhea • + Abdominal masses • + Purple nails	• Painful periods with dark clots • Purple nails	Purple on the sides	Wiry or Firm
Lung-Blood Stasis	• General Blood Stasis	• Tight chest • Cough with a	Purple on tip	Choppy

	• + Chest pain and tightness • + Hemoptysis	bloody sputum	and sides	
Stomach-Blood Stasis	• General Blood Stasis • + Epigastric pains • + Vomiting of blood • + Dark stools (blood)	• Sharp, stabbing epigastric pains • Stomach ulcer or cancer	Purple center	Choppy or Wiry
Uterine-Blood Stasis	• General Blood Stasis • + Dysmenorrhea • + Amenorrhea • + Abdominal masses	• Pre-menstrual cramps • Irregular periods, stopping in the middle	Purple sides	Wiry or Choppy

Blood Heat

When Heat reaches the *Xue* ≈ Blood level, it agitates the Blood manifesting with either an intense red skin rash, bleeding or mental agitation. In the presence of bleeding and *Shen* disturbances, it is customary to define the condition as Fire rather than just Heat (▶ Table 13.9).

Table 13.9: Blood Heat

Pattern	Symptoms	Specific symptoms	Tongue	Pulse
General Blood Heat (Cardinal symptoms)	• Skin Rashes • Bleeding • Agitation, madness • Dry mouth, thirst	• Bleeding • Shen disturbance, agitation	Red and dry	Fast, Full
Heart-Blood Heat	• General Blood Heat • + Agitation, anxiety • + Mouth ulcers	• Insomnia, nightmares • Impulsiveness Manic-depression	Red tip	Fast, Full
Liver-Blood Heat	• General Blood Heat • + Intense skin rashes • + Irritability	• Nosebleeds • Explosive anger • Nightmares • Eczema	Red sides and tip	Fast, Wiry, Full
Uterine-Blood Heat	• General Blood Heat • + Meno-Metrorrhagia • + Short cycles	• Uterine with abundant and scarlet blood • Long periods	Red	Fast, Full

Bleeding

Two patterns dominate the etiology of bleeding, Blood-Heat (Fire), a *Shi* ≈ Repletion/ excess condition, or Spleen-*Qi Xu* ≈ Vacuity, the Spleen being unable to contain the Blood with easy bruising or bleeding. It is customary to say that *Shi* conditions manifest more easily from above (i.e. epistaxis, hematemesis), whereas *Xu* conditions manifest below (hematuria, menometrorrhagia). Please note that this distinction is far from accurate and requires further investigation (▶ Table 13.10).

Table 13.10: Bleeding

Pattern	Symptoms	Specific symptoms	Tongue	Pulse
Spleen-Qi Xu	• Sudden, prolonged bleeding • Pale blood	• Menstrual spotting • Easy bruising	Pale, swollen, Teeth marks	Empty
Blood-Heat	• Abundant bleeding • Dark red blood	• Hemorrhage • Dark red clots	Red	Fast, Full
Blood-Stasis	• Scanty bleeding • Very dark blood	• Dark blood with brown or black clots	Purple	Wiry or Choppy
Yin Xu	• Scanty bleeding • Bright red blood	• Night sweating • Five heart heat	Peeled, maybe red	Fast, Thin, Floating

Pathology of Body Fluids

The *Jin Ye* ≈ Body fluid pathologies involve deficiency patterns with symptoms of dryness or accumulation patterns.

Body-Fluid Xu ≈ Vacuity

The dominant symptoms are dryness and thirst (▶ Table 13.11).

Table 13.11: Body-Fluid *Xu*≈ Vacuity

Pattern	Symptoms	Specific symptoms	Tongue	Pulse
General Body-Fluid Xu (Cardinal symptoms)	• Dryness • Thirst • Constipation with dry stools • No sweating	• Dryness of skin, mouth, nose, eyes, lungs, intestines, vagina	Dry	Empty or Thin
Lung Body-Fluid Xu	• General Dryness • + Thirst • + Dry skin	• A dry cough • Hoarse voice	Dry	Empty or Thin

Stomach Body-Fluid Xu	• General Dryness • + Thirst • + Constipation • + Epigastric pains	• Dry mouth • Thirst but difficulty to drink • Constipation with very dry stools	Dry, red, peeled or rootless in the center	Floating, Empty
Kidney Body-Fluid Xu	• General Dryness • + Thirst • + Scanty urine • + Kidney stones	• Dry mouth at night • Concentrated urine, sand	Dry	Thin or Empty
Intestinal Body-Fluid Xu	• General dryness • + Thirst • + Constipation	• Constipation with very dry stools • Dry, dull skin	Dry, red	Floating, Empty

Body-Fluid Accumulation (Edema)

The Chinese concept of Body fluid accumulation is quite similar to the Western definition of edema (► Table 13.12).

Table 13.12: Body-Fluid Accumulation (Oedema)

Pattern	**Symptoms**	**Specific symptoms**	**Tongue**	**Pulse**
Yang Edema	• Sudden onset • Starting above • Scanty urine	• Pitting edema • *Yang* symptoms • Strong patient	Swollen	–
Yin Edema	• Gradual onset • Starting below • Scanty urine	• Pitting edema • *Yin* symptoms • Weak patient	Swollen	–
Lung Edema	• *Yang* Edema • Cough, frothy sputum • Short breath	• Edema of face (eyelids) and hands • A frothy cough	Dry	–
	• + if Wind-Cold	• Achy body, • scanty urine		Tight
	• + if Wind-Heat	• Sore throat, • Dark urine		Fast
	• + if Damp-Heat	• Fullness of chest and abdomen; • Thirst, scanty urine, constipation		Slippery
Spleen Edema (Damp-Cold)	• *Yin* Edema • Lethargy	• Edema of ankles and trunk	A white, greasy	Deep, Slow,

	• Loss of taste • Clear scanty urine	• Ascitis • Heavy body	coating	Slippery
Spleen Edema (Yang Xu)	• *Yin* Edema • Lethargy, sleepiness • Loss of taste • Clear scanty urine	• Edema below the waist • Cold limbs • Heavy body	A white, greasy coating	Deep, Slow, Slippery
Kidney Edema (Yang Xu)	• *Yin* Edema • Cold body • Reduced libido • Clear scanty urine • Paleness	• Edema of ankle • Lumbar and knee pains • Dark circles below the eyes	Pale, flabby swollen; with a thin white coating	Deep, Slow, Weak or Thready
Qi and Blood Xu Edema	• *Yin* Edema • Tiredness • Paleness • Dizziness • Shortness of breath	• Edema of face and limbs • Paleness • Palpitations	Pale	Weak or Thready

Condensing of Body-Fluids (Dampness and Phlegm)

The condensation or accumulation of Fluids is termed "Dampness", and always involves the Spleen's loss of capacity to transform the Fluids. Dampness may also result from Heat that condenses the fluids or more rarely from Cold disrupting their normal flow. Dampness by its sticky nature further slows down the movements of *Qi.* Phlegm is a further condensation of Fluids.

The concept of *Tan* ≈ Phlegm is quite particular to Chinese medicine including a very large spectrum of chronic conditions ranging from sputum, nasal or vaginal discharge, to cysts and tumors as well as stones, osteo-articular calcifications, and vascular atheroma. Phlegm manifestations may even include certain psychotic conditions.

According to the *Ming Men* School, the etiology of Phlegm involves, not only the Spleen but also the Kidneys. It is customary to state that "all paradoxical symptoms involve Phlegm" (▶ Table 13.13).

Table 13.13: Condensing of Body-Fluids (Phlegm)

Pattern	Symptoms	Specific symptoms	Tongue	Pulse
Visible Phlegm	• Sputum • Nasal Phlegm • Vaginal discharge	• Thick, white, yellow, green or brown discharge	Swollen; Sticky coating	Slippery, Wiry
Invisible Phlegm	• Skin: nodules, lumps	• Lymph nodes • Numbness	Swollen	Slippery, Wiry,

	• Channels: numbness • Heart orifices: disorientation • Gallbladder: gallstones • Kidney: kidney stones • Articulations: arthrosis, swelling	• Disorienta-tion • Gallstones • Kidney stones • Deformity, arthrosis		Tight
Phlegm (Cardinal symptoms)	• Nausea, vomiting • Difficulty swallowing, • Stickiness in mouth • Heavy head, dizziness, fainting • Chest oppression • Anxiety, easily startled, insomnia, or lethargy & sleepiness • Nodules or tumors • Local heat or cold • Chronic sores, ulcers	• Plum pit feeling • Dry mouth with Difficulty to drink • A cottony feeling in the head • Heavy body • Chest tightness (worst with damp) • Discharge or oozing sores • Obesity, greasy skin, smelly sweat	Flabby with a white greasy coating	Slippery and Deep or Wiry, or Soft
Wind-Phlegm	• Dizziness • Nausea, vomiting • Numbness • Coughing up phlegm • Aphasia • Disorientation • Coma	• Rattling sound when breathing • Disorientation amnesia •	Swollen with a greasy coating	Slippery
Hot-Phlegm Affecting Lung, Stomach, Heart	• Red face • Coughing up phlegm • Shortness of breath • Nausea, vomiting • Dementia • Coma	• Sticky yellow sputum • Dry sticky mouth • Restlessness, disorientation, dementia	Red with a sticky greasy-yellow coating	Fast, Slippery
Cold-Phlegm Affecting Lung and Stomach	• Nausea, vomiting • Shortness of breath • Coldness	• White watery sputum • The coldness of back and limbs	Pale, with a white and wet coating	Deep, Slow, Slippery

Damp-Phlegm Affecting the Lung	• A productive cough • Chest oppression and tightness • Epigastric tightness • Lack of appetite	• White abundant sticky phlegm • Shortness of breath	Swollen, with a white, wet coating	Slippery, Soft
Qi-Phlegm Affecting the Liver	• Liver-Qi stagnation symptoms • Tight flanks	• Plum pit sensation in the throat	Red sides, greasy, yellow coating	Wiry
Phlegm misting the Heart	• Disorientation • Manic depression • Psychosis	• Amnesia • Reduced sensory functions	Swollen; white, wet coating	Slippery, Soft

Pathology of Jing: Jing-Qi Xu

Jing ≈ Essence has two origins, the parental *Jing* inherited at conception, and one's personal *Jing* produced after puberty by the Kidneys. The weakness of the inherited *Jing* manifests most often in childhood, ranging from growth retardation and minor conditions in relation with a weak constitution to more serious and permanent conditions of mental retardation or various handicaps. The personal *Jing* deficiency will manifest after puberty mainly concerning the Extraordinary *Fu,* in particular, the bones (and teeth), the uterus (and the gonads), and the Brain, the "Sea of Marrow". Thus the pathologies typically involve infertility and problems in relation to early aging and senility:

Pattern	Symptoms	Specific symptoms	Tongue	Pulse
In Children	• Growth retardation	• Delayed ossification	–	–
In Adults	• Lumbar pain • Weak knees, legs • Impotence • Loose teeth • Early greying or loss of hair • Poor memory • Dizziness • Tinnitus	• Infertility • Early menopause • Osteoporosis • Receding gums, poor teeth	–	Leathery and weak or Floating and Empty

Pathology of Shen

The concept of *Shen* ≈ Spirit/ mind was explored in chapter 4.4, the mental-emotional effects were discussed under the "Internal causes of disease" in chapter 7. The pathologies of *Shen* cover a vast area ranging from mild psycho-emotional disturbances to more severe neurotic and psychiatric conditions. Schematically they can be summarised into three categories (▶ Table 13.15).

Table 13.15: Pathology of *Shen* ≈ Spirit/ mind

Pattern	Symptoms	Specific symptoms	Tongue	Pulse
Weakened Shen	• Depression • Physical and mental exhaustion • Dislike to speak • Anxiety • Poor memory • Insomnia • Pessimism	• Depression • Lack of initiative and will • Dull Shen in the eyes	Swollen tip (hammer-shaped)	Weak, Short, with no wave
Unsettled Shen	• Anxiety • Insomnia • Irritability • Absent-mindedness • Depression • Worry, shortness of breath • Itching and skin rashes	• Insomnia with agitation and nightmares • Mental restlessness	Pale, dry; or Heart-crack	Thin, weak
Obstructed Shen "Misting of the Mind"	• Mental confusion • Dizziness, nausea • Lack of concentration, slow thinking • Emotional numbness • Irritability • Absent-mindedness • Coma	• Amnesia • Reduced sensory functions • Disorientation • Psychosis, mania, dementia • Rattling breathing	Swollen; with a white slippery of greasy coating	Slippery, Soft

13.4 Identification according to the Zang-Fu disharmony patterns

Heart and Small Intestine disharmony patterns

From a Western medical perspective, Heart patterns cover quite different specialties. Patterns of Heart-*Qi* and *Yang Xu* are quite equivalent to the notions of heart failure and congestive heart failure. Heart-Blood *Xu* is more often seen in certain types of insomnia. Heart-*Yin Xu* is a common occurrence in the menopausal syndromes. Heart-Blood stasis is equivalent to angina pectoris, whereas the patterns of Heart-Fire, Phlegm-Fire, Phlegm misting the Heart orifices are in the domain of psychiatric conditions (▶ Table 13.16).

Table 13.16: Heart and Small Intestine disharmony patterns

Pattern	Symptoms	Specific symptoms	Tongue	Pulse
Heart-Qi Xu	• Pale face • Fatigue • Short breath • Spontaneous sweating	• Palpitations	Pale	Empty or Knotted
Heart-Yang Xu	• Same as Heart-*Qi Xu* • Severe fatigue and shortness of breath • Palpitations	• Cold limbs • Aversion to cold	Pale, wet	Deep, Slow, Weak, or Knotted
Collapse of Heart-*Yang*	• Same as Heart-*Yang Xu* • Profuse sweating • Cyanosis • Coma	• Very cold limbs • Bluish lips	Bluish-purple, short	Minute, Hidden, Knotted
Heart-Blood Stagnation	• Stabbing pain in the heart region • Cyanosis • Palpitations	• Heart pain like a knife • Purple face, lips, and nails	Purple or purple spots, swollen veins	Choppy, Knotted or Wiry
Heart-Blood Xu	• Pale face • Unease • Insomnia • Poor memory • Dizziness • Easily startled	• Dream disturbed sleep • Palpitations	Pale, dry	Thin, Choppy

Heart-Yin Xu	• Malar flush • Night Sweats • Palpitations	• Insomnia • Agitation • Five heart heat	Peeled, red, dry	Thin, Fast, Floating
Heart-Fire	• Red face • Extreme agitation • Thirst • Blood in urine	• Tongue ulcers • Agitation • Palpitations • Nightmares	Red; yellow coating	Full, Fast, Over-flowing
Heart Agitated by Phlegm-Fire	• Mental confusion • Insanity, hysteria, mania • Palpitation	• Incoherent speech • Laughing and crying	Red, with a sticky yellow coating	Slippery Fast, Full
Phlegm Misting the Heart (Mind)	• Mental confusion • Dizziness • Lack of concentration, slow thinking • Emotional numbness • Absent-minded • Coma • Chest pain, palpitation • Hoarse breathing • Nausea	• Amnesia • Reduced sensory functions • Disorientation • Psychosis, mania, dementia • Rattling breathing	Swollen; with a white, slippery or greasy coating	Slippery, Soft
Small Intestine-Qi Obstructed	• Abdominal pains with no gas or feces • Vomiting • Bloating	• Violent intestinal pains • Occlusion	Greasy white coating	Wiry, Full
Heat Repletion in the Small Intestine	• Lower abdominal pain • Scanty urine • Painful urination • Blood in urine • Irritability • A sore throat • + Heart-Fire symptoms	• Pain and fullness in the lower abdomen • Hot Lin or Blood Lin symptoms • Agitation	Red tongue with a slippery yellow coating	Rapid, Over-flowing, Slippery

Spleen and Stomach disharmony patterns

The Spleen and Stomach disharmony patterns mainly involve digestive symptoms and disturbances in the production or transformation of the "Vital Substances", in particular, *Qi* and Blood. Spleen-*Qi Xu* is the most common pattern seen in the industrialized societies, caused by over-work, cogitation and worry, but mainly due to wrong eating habits (cold and damp producing foods) (▶ Table 13.17).

Table 13.17: Spleen and Stomach disharmony patterns

Pattern	Symptoms	Specific symptoms	Tongue	Pulse
Spleen-Qi Xu	• General lassitude • Weak muscles • Pale complexion • Loss of appetite • Bloating • Edema • Loose stools • Spontaneous sweating	• Fatigue, with heavy limbs • Bloating and sleepiness after meals • Sticky stools	Pale, teeth marks; white coating	Empty
Spleen-Yang Xu	• Same as Spleen-*Qi Xu* • Abdominal pain better with heat • Watery stools	• Very cold limbs • Diarrhea with undigested food	Pale, swollen and wet	Empty, Slow, Deep
Spleen unable to Control Blood	• Same as Spleen-*Qi Xu* • Rectal or uterine bleeding • Purpura	• Easy bruising • Spotting during the period	Pale and swollen	Thin, Empty
The sinking of Spleen Qi/ Central Qi	• Same as Spleen-*Qi Xu* • Prolapse of anus, stomach, uterus • Hemorrhoids • Varicose veins • Chronic diarrhea	• Hernia and organ prolapse • Bearing down feeling • Urgent urination	Swollen	Empty, Weak
Damp-Cold in invading the Spleen	• Same as Spleen-*Qi Xu* • Heaviness • Chest oppression	• Heavy limbs, head, and chest • Leucorrhoea	Pale; thick white greasy coating	Slippery, Slow

Damp-Heat in invading the Spleen	• Fullness in chest and abdomen • Nausea • Scanty yellow urine • Dysentery • Fever, headache • Bitter taste	• Thirst but difficulty to drink • Jaundice • Smelly, burning stools	Red, Sticky-yellow coating	Slippery, Fast
Exhaustion of Spleen Yin	• Similar to Spleen-*Qi Xu* and Stomach-*Yin Xu* • Fatigue, weak limbs • Anorexia • Soft stools, • Dry mouth and lips • Emaciation	• Dry mouth and lips • Long-standing disease • Chronic weight - loss	Reddish, peeled coating; cracks on the sides	Thin, Empty
Stomach-Qi Xu	• Same as Spleen-*Qi Xu* • Lack of appetite	• Tired in the mornings	Pale; maybe rootless coating	Empty
Stomach Cold and Deficient	• Same as Spleen-*Yang Xu* • Epigastric pains, better with pressure and heat, worse after a bowel movement	• Vomiting of clear fluids • Absence of thirst • Lack of appetite	Pale and wet	Deep, Weak, Slow
Food Retention in the Stomach	• Epigastric pain and distention • Sour reflux • Poor appetite • Insomnia	• Foul smelling burping • Foul breath	Swollen; with a white, slippery or greasy coating	Slippery, Soft
Stomach invaded by Cold	• Epigastric pain worse with cold • Nausea • Preference for warm drinks	• Sudden severe pain • Vomiting of clear fluids	Thick white coating	Deep, Tight, Slow
Stomach-Yin Xu	• Anorexia or bulimia	• Sudden hunger • Little thirst	Red and peeled in the	This, Fast; or Floating

	• Dry mouth and lips in the afternoon • Vomiting • Malar flush • Restlessness, anxiety	• Insomnia	centre	and Empty
Stomach-Fire or Phlegm-Fire	• Burning epigastric pain • Thirst • Constant hunger • Bleeding gums • Constipation	• Desire for cold drinks • Foul breath • Insomnia with nightmares	Red with a thick and dry yellow coating	Full and Fast, or Slippery and Fast
Stomach-Blood Stasis	• General Blood Stasis • + Epigastric pains • + Vomiting of blood • + Dark stools (blood)	• Sharp, stabbing epigastric pains • Stomach ulcer or cancer	Purple center	Choppy or Wiry

Lung and Large Intestine disharmony patterns

Lung, as the first *Zang* ≈ Organ is in direct contact with the outer world, therefore it is the most likely to be invaded by *Xie Qi* ≈ External Pathogenic factors (EPF). Furthermore, modern lifestyle, smoking, exposure to pollution, exhaust fumes and in particular micro-particles (pollen, sand, polymers), is taking its toll on the lungs. It has been established that the incidence of respiratory diseases is much higher in cities than in rural areas (▶ Table 13.18).

Table 13.18: Lung and Large Intestine disharmony patterns

Pattern	Symptoms	Specific symptoms	Tongue	Pulse
Lung-Qi Xu	• Lassitude • Shortness of breath • White, dull face • Asthma • Spontaneous sweating	• Cough, worse with effort • Weak voice	Pale, swollen in the front one third	Empty on the front right position

Lung-Yang Xu	• Same as Lung-*Qi Xu* • + Catching colds easily	• Feeling cold, cold hands • Aversion to cold	Pale, swollen and wet	Weak, Slow, Deep
Lung-Yin Xu	• An unproductive cough • Hoarse voice • Malar flush • Night sweating • Insomnia	• Dry, cough • Afternoon Fever • Dryness	Red, with a peeled and dry coating	Thin, Fast, Floating
Lung Invaded by Wind-Cold	• A cough, clear sputum • Stuffy or a runny nose • Body aches • Chills, aversion to cold • No sweating	• Itchy throat • Sneezing • Chills	Thin and white coating	Floating, Tight
Lung Invaded by Wind-Water	• A cough • Swollen, bright face • Shortness of breath • Scanty urine • Chest oppression	• Sudden swelling of face, eyes, and body	Slippery, white coating	Floating, Slippery
Lung Invaded by Wind-Heat	• A sore throat • Stuffy or a runny nose • Fever, headache • Slight sweating • Slight thirst	• Red swollen throat • Yellow nasal discharge	Red in the front part, thin yellow coating	Floating, Fast
Lung Damp-Phlegm	• A cough, profuse sticky white sputum • Nausea • Chest oppression • Dislike of lying down	• A chronic cough • Watery sputum • Wheezing • Coldness	Swollen, sticky white coating	Slippery

Lung Cold-Phlegm	• Cough, profuse clear sputum • White, pasty face • Chest oppression • Dislike of lying down	• A chronic cough • Sputum easy to expectorate • Wheezing	Swollen, sticky white coating	Slippery, Slow
Lung Hot-Phlegm	• A cough, thick yellow sputum • Shortness of breath • Chest oppression • Heat and thirst • Insomnia, agitation	• Barking cough • Sputum difficult to expectorate • Wheezing	Swollen, thick yellow, greasy coating	Slippery, Full, Fast
Large Intestine-Yin Xu	• Constipation • Dry mouth and throat	• Dry and hard stools	Red, dry with no coating	Thin
Large Intestine Heat	• Constipation • Dry mouth and throat • Scanty dark urine	• Dry and hard stools • Burning anus	Red, thick brown coating	Full, Fast
Large Intestine Cold	• Abdominal pains • Diarrhea • Borborygmus • Pale urine	• Loose stools, duck droppings • Coldness	Pale tongue	Deep, Weak, Slow
Large Intestine Invaded by Cold	• Sudden abdominal pains • Diarrhea with pain	• Cold abdomen better with heat • Chills	Thick white coating	Deep, Wiry or Tight
Large Intestine Invaded by Heat	• High fever or tidal fever • Abundant sweat • Constipation • Vomiting • Thirst • Delirium	• Abdominal pain worse with pressure • A desire for climbing to sing, or running naked	Red, thick dry, yellow coating	Full, Fast, Big, Flooding

Kidney and Bladder disharmony patterns

The Kidneys, being the root of *Yin* and *Yang* of the body, can manifest patterns of *Qi, Yin, Yang* and *Jing Xu* ≈ Vacuity. In general, as the Kidneys are the reservoir of the inherited energies, it is believed that they cannot present *Shi* ≈ Repletion type patterns (► Table 13.19).

Table 13.19: Kidney and Bladder disharmony patterns

Pattern	Symptoms	Specific symptoms	Tongue	Pulse
Kidney-Qi Xu	• General *Qi-Xu* (► Table 13.3) • + Mental fatigue • + Lumbar symptoms • + Urinary dysfunctions • + Sexual dysfunctions	• Lumbar and knee pains • Sweaty feet • Fearfulness • Night urination, incontinence • Impotence; premature ejaculation • Tinnitus; deafness	Pale and swollen	Empty, Weak and Deep
Kidney-Yang Xu	• Same as Kidney-*Qi Xu* • + Impotence • + Infertility • + Clear, abundant urine • + Soft stools • + Edema	• Reduced libido • Coldness	Pale, swollen and wet	Weak, Slow, Deep
Kidney Unable to Receive Qi	• Same as Kidney-*Yang Xu* • + Asthma • + Cough • + Shortness of breath	• Asthma worst with cold in older patients • Aversion to cold	Pale and swollen	Empty, Weak and Deep
Kidney-Yang Xu Water Over-flowing	• Same as Kidney-*Yang Xu* • + Reduced urination • + Edema • + Palpitations (Heart) • + Copious sputum, asthma (Lung)	• Pitting edema starting below • May affect the Heart or Lung	Pale, swollen and wet	Weak, Slow, Deep

Kidney-Yin Xu	• Lumbar pains • Weak knees • Scanty dark urine • Constipation • Thirst • Premature ejaculation • Spermatorrhea	• Night sweating • 5 Heart heat	Red; peeled with cracks	Thin, Fast, Floating
Kidney-Jing Xu	• Lumbar soreness • Weak knee & legs • Impotence • Fatigue • Loose teeth • Early greying or loss of hair • Poor memory • Dizziness • Tinnitus	• Infertility • Early menopause • Osteoporosis • Receding gums, poor teeth	Red and peeled	Floating and Empty, or Leathery and Weak
Bladder Damp-Cold	• Urinary frequency • Clear urine • Heaviness in the lower abdomen	• Coldness • Urinary urgency	White sticky coating	Slippery, Slow
Bladder Damp-Heat	• Urinary urgency, frequency, and difficulty • Fever • Thirst • Lumbar pains	• Painful urination, retention • Turbid urine	Red; Sticky-yellow coating	Slippery, Fast or Wiry
Bladder Cold and Deficient	• Same as Kidney *Yang Xu* • + Abundant, pale urine • + Dizziness	• Incontinence • Nocturia	Pale; wet	Deep, Weak

Liver and Gallbladder disharmony patterns

Liver patterns, in particular, Liver-*Qi* stagnation, have become increasingly more common in modern-day life. The Liver is responsible for adaptation, today's accelerated life challenges are hugely taxing this capacity. Furthermore, the Liver has to detoxify the Blood, affected by external toxins in the form of chemicals, pollution, and radiation as well as internally generated heat caused by frustrations and repressed emotions (▶ Table 13.20).

Table 13.20: Liver and Gallbladder disharmony patterns

Pattern	Symptoms	Specific symptoms	Tongue	Pulse
Liver-Qi Stagnation	• Hypochondriac or epigastric distention • Chest oppression • Premenstrual tension • Irregular periods • Moodiness • Irritability	• Thoracic block • Throat plum pit • Premenstrual breast distention • Depression • Sighing	Reddish sides	Wiry (left middle position)
Liver-Yang Rising	• Headaches: eyes, temples, or vertex • Irritability and anger • Blurred vision • Stiff neck • Insomnia • Dry throat & mouth	• Visual spots • High blood pressure • Minor symptoms of Wind (tinnitus, dizziness)	Red (if *Yin-Xu*), or pale (if Blood-*Xu*); reddish sides	Wiry
Liver-Fire	• Same as Liver-*Yang* Rising • + Bitter taste • + Red eyes and face • + Insomnia	• Explosive anger • Intense headaches • Nightmares	Red, redder sides; dry, yellow coating	Fast, Wiry
Liver-Wind*	• Tremors, tics • Numbness, paralysis • Convulsions • Stroke; hemiplegia • Coma	• Dizziness • Spasms, tremors, convulsions • Tinnitus	Deviated or trembling*	Wiry*
Liver-Yin Xu	• Same as Liver-*Yang* Rising • + Eye floaters • + Weak muscles • + Dry skin and hair	• Dry eyes • Malar flush	Red; peeled with cracks	Thin, Fast, Floating

Liver-Blood Xu	• Pale face • Blurred vision • Numbness and cramps • Poor memory • Dizziness • Tinnitus • Amenorrhea, reduced menses • Dry hair, hair loss	• Reduced night vision • Dream disturbed sleep • Restlessness • Depression, feeling spaced out • Brittle nails	Pale, dry or orange on the sides	Thin or Choppy
Cold Stagnation in the Liver channel	• Pain and distension of the lower abdomen, better with heat • Genital distension and pain	• Coldness • Genital swelling or retraction	Pale and wet	Deep, Wiry, Slow
Damp- Heat in the Liver and Gall-bladder	• Hypochondrial pain and distension • Bitter taste • Fever • Nausea and vomiting • Genital or urinary infections and rashes • Dark-yellow urine	• Jaundice • Thirst but unable to drink • Burning urination • Genital rash • Yellow vaginal discharge	Red; Sticky-yellow coating	Slippery, Fast, Wiry
Damp-Cold in the Gall-bladder	• Jaundice • Nausea, vomiting • No thirst • Dull headaches	• Dull-yellow coloring • Inability to digest fats	Sticky, white coating	Slippery, Slow, Wiry
Gall-bladder Deficient and Cold	• Timidity, indecision • Fearfulness • Dizziness, vertigo • Blurred vision • Sighing	• Lack of courage • Insomnia from insecurity	Pale	Weak

* Liver-Wind may arise from Liver-*Yang* rising (red tongue, no coating; Wiry and fast pulse) or from Liver-Fire (Stiff and very red tongue with yellow coating, fast and Full pulse; or from Liver Blood-*Xu* (Pale, trembling tongue, Choppy pulses).

13.5 Identification of Patterns according to the Six Stages

This theory was formulated by "*Zhang Zhong Jing*" famous physician (160 A.D) in the *"Shang Han Lun*" (Febrile Diseases caused by Cold).

The different patterns are classified into 3 *Yang* and 3 *Yin* stages:

- The *Yang* channels reflect the disease in the *Yang* zones and the *Fu* ≈ Bowels. Here the body's *Zheng* ≈ Upright *Qi* is strong enough to contain the *Xie Qi*≈ Pathogenic factor. Hence, in general, the symptoms are of *Shi* ≈ Repletion/excess and of "Hot" type. The treatment aims at dispersing the pathogenic *Qi*.
  - *Tai Yang* (SI-BL): controls the surface "*Biao*", including the skin and the muscles.
  - *Shao Yang* (TW-GB): is considered half inside/ half outside, manifesting in the chest and the hypochondrium. The symptoms reflect at times the Cold *Xie* ≈ Pathogenic factor (chills) and at times the *Wei Qi* ≈ Defensive energy (heat).
  - *Yang Ming* (LI-ST): the symptoms concern the stomach and the intestines. Here the progressive penetration of the Cold Pathogenic factor is transformed into Full-Heat.
- The *Yin* channels group the pathologies of the *Zang* ≈ Organs. The *Zheng* ≈ Upright *Qi* is weak, the symptoms are of *Xu* ≈ Vacuity/deficiency and "Cold" type. The treatment aims at "Supplementing" the *Qi*.
  - *Tai Yin* (LU-SP): mainly manifest in the digestive system; the Pathogenic Cold invades the Middle Triple Warmer in the presence of Spleen-*Qi* vacuity.
  - *Shao Yin* (HE-KI): concerns the circulation system. There are two syndromes: Hot and Cold.
  - *Jue Yin* (PE-LR): involves the neurological system.

It is important to understand that most of the clinical manifestations are due to the struggle between the Xie Qi ≈ External pathogenic factor and the body's Zheng Qi≈ Upright energy.

- *Shi* ≈ Repletion/ excess syndrome signifies a strong *Xie Qi* ≈ Pathogenic factor as well as a strong *Wei* ≈ Defensive *Qi*
- *Xu* ≈ Vacuity/ deficiency syndrome signifies weakness of the *Zheng Qi*

Table 13.21: Patterns according to the Six Stages *(Shang Han Lun)*

Pattern	Symptoms	Specific symptoms	Tongue	Pulse
Tai Yang Channel stage **Cold-Wind (Pre-dominant**	• A headache and severe • Stiff neck and spine • Body aches • Nasal congestion	• Chills with fever • Aversion to cold • No sweating • Clear nasal discharge	Normal; thin and white coating	Floating, Tight

Cold)	or a runny nose (clear) • Sneezing, cough, sore throat • Nausea • Absence of thirst			
Wind-Cold Predominant Wind = Weakness of the Biao	• Same symptoms as above but less severe • + Itchy throat • + Aversion to Wind	• Sneezing • Slight fever • Sweating	Normal; thin and white coating	Floating, Empty
Wind-Heat (Pre-dominant Heat)	• Similar symptoms • + Fever • + Angina, cough • + Thirst • + Yellow mucous • + Aversion to Wind	• A sore throat, swollen tonsils • Sweating	Reddish tip or sides; thin and white coating	Floating, Fast
Tai Yang Organ stage with Water accumula-tion: Wind-Edema	• Slight fever and sweat • Slight thirst • Vomiting fluids soon after drinking • Aversion to Wind	• Urine retention • Edema in the upper parts	Normal or slightly swollen	Floating, Fast
Tai Yang Organ stage with Blood accumula-tion	• Urinary urgency, incontinence • Pelvic pains and masses • Fever • Mental restlessness	• Blood in urine	Purplish red; yellow coating	Deep, Fine, Rapid or Choppy
Shao Yang stage	• Alternating heat and cold • Irritability, • Hypochondriac fullness • Nausea • Dislike to eat or drink • Bitter taste in mouth, Dry throat • Blurred vision • Vertigo	• Alternating fever and chills	Coating white and slippery on one side only	Wiry, Tight or Fine
Yang Ming stage	• High fever • Profuse sweating	• Full heat: fever, sweat, thirst	Red with a yellow, dry	Fast, Big,

	• Intense thirst • Red face • Agitation, anxiety		coating	Over-flowing
Yang Ming Organ stage	• Fever worse in the afternoons • Profuse sweating • Intense thirst • Abdominal pains worse with pressure • Constipation* • Restlessness and in severe cases: delirium	• Four "Bigs": fever, sweat, thirst, and pulse • The desire to run naked or to climb up and sing	Red with a thick, dry yellow or brown coating	Deep, Fast, Full
Tai Yin stage	• Painful bloating • Vomiting • Lack of appetite and thirst • Diarrhea • Fatigue • Feeling of cold	• Pain better with pressure and heat • Symptoms of Spleen-*Qi Xu*	Pale, with a white sticky coating	Deep, Weak, Slow
Shao Yin stage **Cold pattern (Yang Xu)**	• Chills, aversion to cold, cold limbs • Mental fatigue • Sleepiness • Absence of thirst • Diarrhea with undigested food • Clear abundant urine	• Huddled up • A desire for heat, small amounts of warm drink	Pale, wet; white coating	Deep, Weak, Fine, Slow
Shao Yin stage **Heat pattern (Yin Xu)**	• Fever • Night sweating • Dry mouth and throat worse at night • Mouth ulcers • Agitation, anxiety • Insomnia • Scanty, dark urine	• Night fever and sweat • Five "heart" heat	Red; peeled coating	Rapid and Fine
Jue Yin stage	• Heat rushing towards the chest • Constant hunger but cannot eat • Vomiting	• Cold below, hot above • Thirst but inability to drink	Red spots; white and slippery coating	Deep, Hidden maybe Tight or Wiry

	(roundworms) • Cold abdomen and limbs • Diarrhea • Headache (vertex)			
* There is a possible variation with diarrhea and dysentery as seen in acute gastroenteritis (not described in the *Shang Han Lun*).				

13.6 Identification of Patterns according to the Four Levels or Layers

A gradual evolution between the years 160 and 1500, on the theories of "Feverish Diseases" led to the formation of the *Wen Bing* school of thought as separate from the *Shang Han* School. The important texts are *Xin Kan Wen Bing* by *Wang Chi*; *Wen Yi Xue* by *Wu You Ko*; *Wen Bing Tiao Pen* by *Wu Ju Tong*; *Wen Je Ping Pien* by *Xue Sheng Pi*; *Shi Ping Lun* by *Lei Feng* and *Wen Je Ching Wei* by *Wang Shi Xiung*. The main reference book is the *Wen Je Lun*: Treatise on Feverish Diseases by *Ye Tian Shi* circa 1700, exploring the invasion by pathogenic Heat in 4 stages.

- The *Wei* ≈ Defensive Level: corresponds to the *Biao* ≈ Surface, the Lung, and the skin.
- The *Qi* Level corresponds to the *Li* ≈ Inside, the chest, Lung, Stomach, Intestines, and the Gallbladder. The invasion of the *Qi* level indicates a rather good body resistance but a slight impairment of the organic functions by the outside factors.
- The *Ying* ≈ Nourishing Level: describes an advanced stage of disease with Heat disturbing the *Yin* of the Heart and Pericardium, producing a deficiency of *JinYe* ≈ Body fluids and the consequent mental symptoms.
- The *Xue* ≈ Blood level: concerns a deeper invasion and the involvement of Heart, Liver, and Kidneys.

Table 13.22: Patterns according to the Four Levels or Layers *(Wen Bing)*

Pattern	Symptoms	Specific symptoms	Tongue	Pulse
Wei Qi ≈ Defensive Level **Wind-Heat**	• Fever (with or without sweating) • Aversion to wind or cold • Body aches • Headache • Stuffy or runny nose, Sore throat, • Cough • Thirst	• Fever with chills • Slight sweating	Red tip and borders; thin white or yellow coating	Floating, Fast

Wei Qi ≈ Defensive Level **Summer-Heat**	• Fever • Absence of sweat • Aversion to cold • Headache • Irritability • Thirst	• Fever with no sweating	Red with white, sticky coating	Floating, Fast, Weak
Wei Qi ≈ Defensive Level **Dry-Heat**	• Same as above • + Dry skin, nose and mouth • + Sore throat • + Cough	• Fever with slight sweating • Dryness	Red and dry	Floating, Fast
Wei-Qi ≈ Defensive Level **Damp-Heat**	• Fever • Absence of sweating • Aversion to cold and damp • Headache • Chest oppression • Abdominal fullness • Body aches • Lack of thirst	• Fever worse in the afternoon • General heaviness • Cottony feeling in the head	White and sticky coating	Weak, Floating and Soft
Qi Level	• Fever • Aversion to Heat • Thirst • Anxiety and agitation • Dark urine	• Full heat	Red with a yellow coating	Fast, Big, Over-flowing
Qi Level **Lung-Heat (Chest and Diaphragm)**	• Same as above • + Burning sensation in the epigastrium • + Cough, with yellow phlegm • + Shortness of breath	• High fever • Sweating • Cough	Red with a yellow or brown, thick, dry coating	Fast, Slippery
Qi Level **Stomach-Heat (Yang-Ming)**	• Same as above • + High fever • + Intense thirst • + Irritability	• Afternoon fever • Profuse sweating • Desire for cold drinks	Red with a thick yellow, dry coating	Fast, Slippery Over-flowing

Qi Level **Intestinal-Heat (Yang-Ming)**	• Same as above • + High fever • + Constipation • + Irritability • + Delirium	• Afternoon fever • Dry stools, burning in the anus	Red with a yellow or brown, thick, dry coating	Fast, Full, Slippery, Deep
Qi Level **Gallbladder-Heat (Shao-Yang)**	• Same as above • + Alternating fever and chills • + Bitter taste and dry throat • + Nausea • + Hypochondriac pain & epigastric fullness	• Alternating chills and fever (more heat than cold)	Red with a sticky yellow coating on one side only	Fast, Wiry
Ying ≈ Nutritive Level	• Fever worse at night, hot body, cold extremities • Dry mouth but no desire to drink • Irritability, anxiety • Insomnia • Aphasia or delirium in severe cases • Faint skin eruptions: petechia or maculae	• Night fever • Inability to drink • Macular skin rashes	Deep red, with no coating	Fast, Fine
Ying ≈ Nutritive Level **Pericardium-Heat**	• Same as above • + Mental confusion • + Aphasia or delirium	• Night fever • Delirium	Deep red, with no coating	Fast, Fine
Xue ≈ Blood Level	• High Fever • Delirium; mania • Skin eruptions: purple or black • Bleeding	• Dark skin rash • Bleeding: nose, lungs, uterine, urine, intestines	Deep red, with no coating	Fast, Fine
Xue ≈ Blood Level **Liver-Wind from Heat**	• Same as above • + Convulsions • + Coma	• Convulsions, opistotonus, nystagmus, lockjaw	Deep red, with no coating	Wiry, Fast

Xue ≈ Blood Level **Liver-Wind from Yin Xu**	• Same as above • + Emaciation • + Tremors, twitching • + Malar flush	• Lower fever • Tremors, itching	Deep red, with no coating	Fine, Fast
Xue ≈ Blood Level **Collapse of Yin**	• Same as above • + Night sweating • + Dry mouth • + Irritability • + Insomnia	• Five "heart" heat • Malar flush • Emaciatioin	Deep red, with no coating	Fine, Fast
Xue ≈ Blood Level **Collapse of Yang**	• Cold • Aversion to Cold • Profuse sweat • Absence of thirst • White face	• Oily sweat on forehead • Cold limbs, not improved by heat	Swollen, pale and wet	Hidden, Slow, Minute, Scat-tered

13.7 Identification of Patterns according to the Triple Warmer

Developed by *Wu Ju Tong* in *Wen Bing Tiao Pien*: Detailed analysis of Feverish Diseases, circa 1800. Hot diseases are analyzed in relation to different seasons. These pathologies may be grouped into 2 categories: *Wen Re*- Warm-Heat, *Shi Re* - Damp-Heat.

- The Upper Triple Warmer: represents the *Biao* ≈ Surface, concerning the Lung, the skin, but also the Spleen and flesh as well as the Stomach. Damp-Heat may also affect the Pericardium causing a much more severe condition with psychotic or neurological conditions.
- The Middle Triple Warmer: concerns the digestive system, but there is often the persistence of Upper Triple Warmer symptoms.
- The Lower triple Warmer involves pathologies of Kidney, Bladder, Large Intestine as well as Liver-Wind.

Table 13.23 Patterns according to the Triple Warmer *(Wen Bing Tiao Pien)*

Pattern	Symptoms	Specific symptoms	Tongue	Pulse
Upper Triple Warmer Wind-Heat or Damp-Heat	• Mild evening fever • Aversion to cold • Slight or no sweating • Headache	• Fever with chills • Slight sweating • Yellow nasal discharge	Red tip and borders; thin white or yellow coating	Floating, Fast

(In the Biao-Surface)	• Body aches • Slight thirst • Runny nose			
Upper Triple Warmer Lung-Heat or Damp-Heat	• Fever • Sweating • Thirst • Cough • Shortness of breath • Chest oppression	• Cough, yellow Phlegm • Wheezing	Red; yellow coating	Fast, Over-flowing
Upper Triple Warmer Pericardium-Heat or Damp-Heat	• High fever • Epigastric pain • Mental fatigue • Cold limbs • Delirium or coma	• Fever at night • Aphasia • Delirium	Purple, stiff; no coating	Fast, Fine
Middle Triple Warmer Yang Ming-Heat	• Evening fever • Sallow face • Heavy head • Thirst • Anorexia, stuffiness of the chest, • Scanty urine • Mental confusion	• Cyclic fever • Inability to drink in spite of intense thirst	Red with white, sticky coating	Fast, Over-flowing
Middle Triple Warmer Spleen Damp-Heat	• Fever • Sallow face • Epigastric fullness • Anorexia • Stuffiness of the chest • Diarrhoea • Nausea, vomiting	• Lack of appetite	Red with yellow, sticky or greasy coating	Fast, Slippery, Soft
Lower Triple Warmer Kidney-Heat	• Lingering fever • Thirst • Lassitude • Deafness • Urine retention	• Five "heart" Heat • Night sweating • Thirst but unable to drink	Red and peeled tongue	Fine and Fast; or Floating and Empty
Lower Triple Warmer	• Same as above	• High fever	Deep red with no	Fast, Thin,

Liver-Wind from Heat	• + High fever • + Convulsions • + Coma	• Sweating • Cough	coating	Wiry
Lower Triple Warmer Liver-Wind from Yin Xu	• Low grade fever • Cold limbs • Cracked lips • Black teeth • Convulsion, tremor	• Low fever • Tremors • Dryness	Deep red with no coating	Deep, Fine, Fast
Lower Triple Warmer Large Intestine-Heat	• Fever • Abdominal pain • Constipation	• Constipation • Abdominal pain worse with pressure	Red with greasy-yellow coating	Deep, Slippery Fast

13.8 Comparison between the Six Stages, the Four Levels and the Three Heaters

These three systems, all deal with the different stages of an externally contracted disease. The reasons for the coexistence of three systems is most probably geographical. The Six Stages described in the *Shang Han Lun* deals mainly with a Cold Pathogenic factor predominant in the Northern regions. As the "Heat" patterns were not completely covered, the *Wen Bing* school developed a complementary approach. Whereas in Southern China, the predominant external Pathogenic Factor was "Damp-Heat" for which both systems were lacking in a comprehensive approach, hence, the appearance of *Wen Bing Tiao Pien* to cover the "Heat" and "Damp-Heat" patterns. As many of the patterns described by the three schools are identical, this has often been an issue for the beginner, as to which concept to follow (▶ Fig. 13.1).

Although, a Western idisease, such as bronchitis, or gastro-enteritis, could be approached by all three systems, the *Wen Bing* seems to offer a more comprehensive description of the various infections in general. The historical *Shang Han Lun* retains its originality in describing the stage-by-stage aggravation of an external pathogen in relation to the body's defensive system, and especially the diagnostic and therapeutic refinements, as well as possible medical errors.

Important Diagnostic note on "Retained Pathogenic Factors":

The various patterns as discribed above, concern an acute episode of a feverish condition, are quite often easy to identify with a rigourous anamnesis. It is a very different situation when the patient has been having a chronic sub-febrile disease. This is often the case in conditions such as Post-viral Fatigue Syndrome, Lime's Diasease, Chronic or recurrent Mononucleosis, chronic Hepatitis, Bronchitis, Tonsillitis, Nephritis and even Herpes, Shingles, or Multiple Sclerosis, etc...

In Chinese medicine, these conditions are called "Retained Pathogenic Factors", signifying a lingering PF. These pathologies often involve a weakness of the defensive mechanisms combined with a strong pathogen. Fever, which would be the primary symptom, might be replaced by a feeling of feverishness, not manifested by the doctor's thermometer. At times the temperature might even be sub-normal, signifying a weakness of the *Wei Qi.* Unfortunately in daiy medical practice, after exhausting the routine lab-tests, many patients are prescribed one or more courses of antibiotics. As antibiotics are "Cold" in nature, they further damage the Spleen's capacity to produce *Qi*. For most patients, the chief complaint reflects Qi Vacuity (fatigue, loss of motivation,depression). Here the biggest therapeutic mistake, for the Chinese therapist, would be to start by supplementing Qi before expelling the pathogenic factor. Hence the treatment of "Retained Pathogenic Factors" remains a challenge for the Chinese practitioner. It involves an excellent diagnostic approach to correctly identify the affected level, as well as calling upon other Chinese therapeutic tools, for example: The use of the *Jing Bie* - Divergent channels, indicated for chronic and recurrent condition, or the Chinese Pharmacopea and Diet

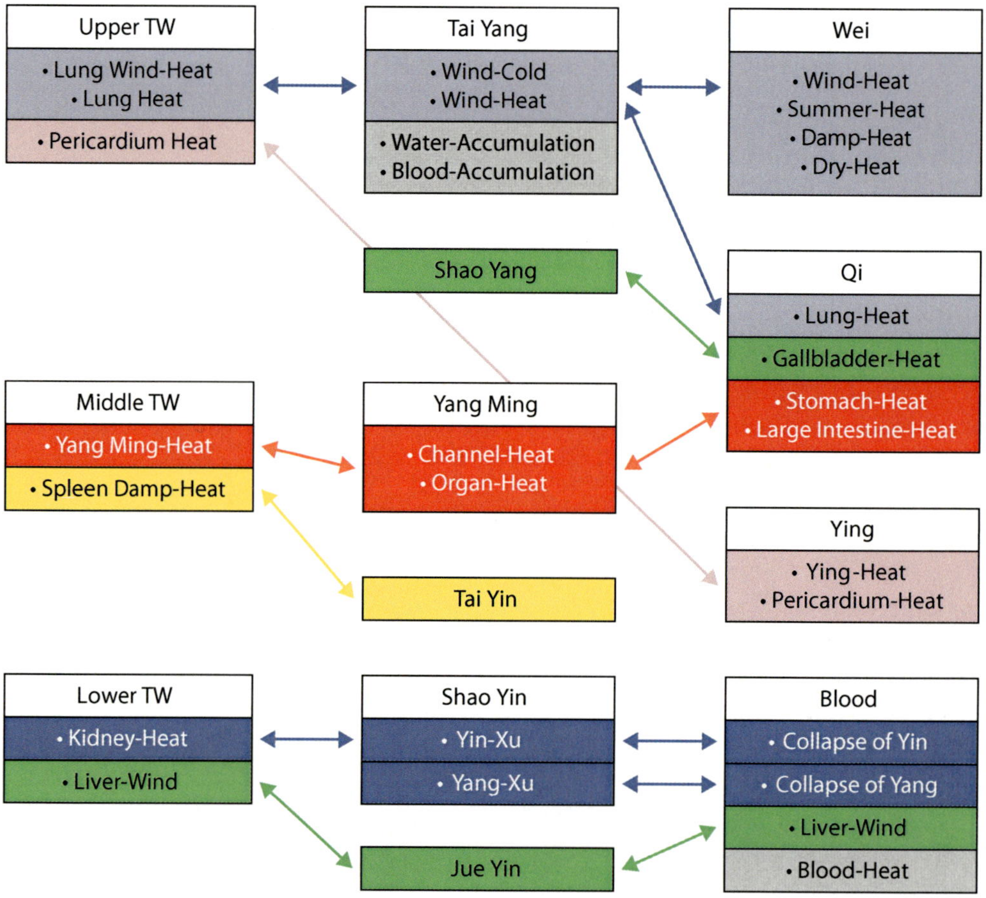

Figure 13.1: Comparatif table; many of the patterns described by the 3 schools are identical although coming from a different perspective.

13.9 Identification according to the Jing-Luo channel system disharmony patterns

The channel disharmony is based on the identification of the symptoms and the reactivity of certain channel points such as *Xi* ≈ Cleft or *Yuan* ≈ Source.

The 12 Primary Channel symptoms

The Primary channel affections combine symptoms of the trajectory as well as the related *Zang-Fu.*

Shou (Hand) Tai Yin: Lung (LU)

Fullness in the chest, cough, dyspnoea, asthma, hemoptysis, sore throat, common cold, chills and pain of the shoulder and back, pain along the pathway of the channel.

Shou (Hand) Yang Ming

Large Intestine (LI): Abdominal pain (which usually signifies the presence of Cold), abdominal bloating (considered as Wind), borborygmus (the presence of Dampness), diarrhoea or dysentery (due to Damp-Heat), constipation (usually from Heat), also fever, dry mouth, sore throat, toothache, serous nasal discharge or epistaxis, pain along the course of the channel.

Zu (Foot) Yang Ming: Stomach (ST)

Abdominal distension, borborygmus, gastralgia, edema, vomiting, febrile diseases, mania, facial paralysis, sore throat, epistaxis, pain along the trajectory of the channel.

Zu (Foot) Tai Yin

Spleen/ Pancreas (SP): Stiffness and pain of the tongue, gastric pain, abdominal distension, vomiting, jaundice, general weakness and heaviness of the body, pain and swelling along the course of the channel.

Shou (Hand) Shao Yin: Heart (HE)

Dryness of the throat, thirst, fever, pain in the chest and upper back regions, jaundice, red eyes, heat in the palms (fidgety hands), stiff tongue, pain along the course of the channel.

These are symptoms of Heat having reached the Blood level. This Heat in the chest may move to the scapulae at *Gaohuangshu* BL-43 via *Geshu* BL-17, then down to the lower Triple Warmer and to the Bladder. Or else the Heart Heat may be redirected to the Small intestine, to be eliminated by the Bladder.

Shou (Hand) Tai Yang

Small Intestine (SI): Nausea, pain in the lower abdomen, diarrhoea with smelly stools (duck droppings), deafness, jaundice, eye degeneration, tearing, eye pressure (glaucoma), swelling of the cheek, sore throat, stiff neck worst in the morning, pain along the course of the channel.

Zu (Foot) Tai Yang: Bladder (BL)

Susceptibility to external Cold with chills and fever, stiff neck, spine and joints, headache (usually a rushing sensation), eye pain, nasal congestion, lumbago, blockage of the knees, pain, and weakness along the trajectory; retention of urine, enuresis, mania.

Zu (Foot) Shao Yin: Kidney (KI)

Hemoptysis, dyspnea, dizziness, nausea, vomiting, diarrhea, constipation with difficult dry stools, incontinence, grayish tinge around the eyes; impotence; facial swelling, abdominal swelling, oedema; dryness of tongue and lips, sore throat, dry skin with wrinkles, malar flush, heat in the sole of the feet. weakness and numbness of lower limbs, lower back, motor impairment and muscular atrophy of the lower extremities, pain along the course of the channel.

Shou (Hand) Jue Yin: Pericardium (PE)

Originally the symptoms were associated with Heat in the Blood level (*Nue* ≈ Malaria), resulting in irritability, restlessness, mania, speech impairment, angina pectoris, a fullness of the chest, palpitation and *Jue* ≈ Inversion/ collapse syndrome. The heat spreading to the face causing a red face, bloodshot eyes, spasm and tremors of the elbow and the arm, heat in the palm, and pain along the course of the channel, as well as stiffness of limbs and neck (meningitis in children).

Shou (Hand) Shao Yang

Triple Warmer (TW): The accumulation of dampness to suppress internal heat manifests as distention, fullness, and hardness in the middle or lower abdomen with frequent urination, incontinence or enuresis and facial and/or limbic edema. Deterioration of the sensory portals, the eyes with redness, pain, poor vision, macular degeneration, the ears with pain behind the ear, deafness, tinnitus; pain along the trajectory, especially the posterior aspect of the shoulder, upper arm, cheek, and throat.

Zu Shao Yang: Gallbladder (GB)

Loss of sensory acuity, deafness or blindness, due to damp-heat or phlegm blocking the blood and Ye-thick fluids to the portals and head; dark complexion (dark rings around the eyes or nostrils), headache, eye or ear pain; lymph swellings in the throat (hypothyroidism) or armpit and breasts, pain along the course of the channel (channel pathology). Intermittent fevers or alternating chills and fevers or tidal fevers due to *Li* ≈ Pestilent factors resulting in *Nue* ≈ Malaria, epidemics (Severe Acute Respiratory Syndrome-SARS). The disruption of *Qi* in the Middle *Jiao*

≈ Warmer causes: vomiting, chest and lateral costal pains, and a bitter taste in the mouth (Fu ≈ Organ pathology).

Zu (Foot) Jue Yin: Liver (LR)

Involves Heat symptoms, from *Yin* and Blood consumption, and ascending of Liver *Yang* with fever, headaches, tinnitus, blurred vision and muscular spasms; in case of Liver-Fire, there is also flushing, nosebleed, emotional outbursts and running piglet syndrome "*Ben Tun*" (today understood as a panic attack). When more extreme, the stirring of wind will cause epilepsy, Bell's palsy, stroke and loss of consciousness. The lack of consolidation causes counterflow *Qi* affecting the Triple Warmer system:

- Lower TW: with enuresis, retention of urine, urinary tract infections, hernia; constipation, diarrhea, or lumbago;
- Middle TW: with jaundice, vomiting;
- Upper TW: with a fullness of the chest and oppression.

13.10 Identification according to the Eight Extraordinary Vessel patterns

Diagnostic particularities

The signs and symptoms are mostly based on the trajectory. This, as well as the psychological profiles inherent to each "Extraordinary Vessel", is presented below. There are some general diagnostic particularities to be considered:

- The symptoms involve chronic conditions.
- There is a relation to some aspects of *Jing* ≈ Essence and the Kidneys.
- Pulses for the 8 Extraordinary vessels according to *Li Shi Zhen* (▶ Fig. 13.2):
  - *Chong Mai*: Deep, Wiry and Firm
  - *Du Mai*: Floating, Wiry and Long
  - *Ren Mai*: Deep, Long, Tight and Thin, especially *Guan* and *Cun* positions
  - *Yin Wei Mai*: Deep, Big, Full that rolls to the thumb or to the *Cun* position
  - *Yang Wei*: Floating, Big, Full, the pulse that rolls to the *Qi* position
  - *Dai Mai*: There are a left-right vibration and Tightness on the *Guan* position
  - *Yang Qiao*: Left-right vibration and Tight on the *Cun* position

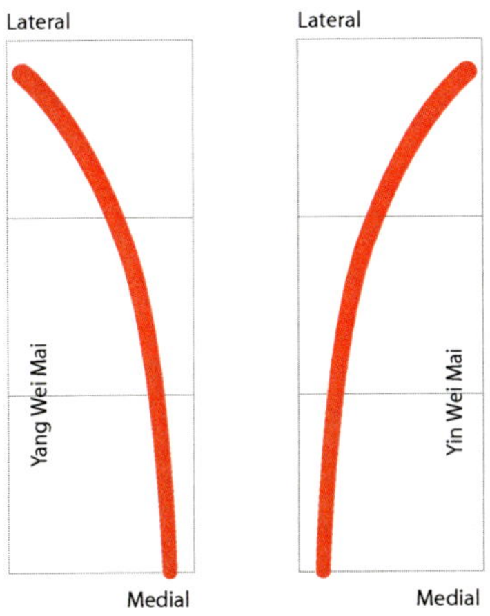

Figure 13.2: Pulses of *Yin* and *Yang Wei Mai*

- *Yin Qiao Mai*: Left-right vibration and Tight on the *Qi* position

- Palpational diagnosis: Four of the Extraordinary vessels have been described to have Xi≈ Cleft points, similar to the primary channels. As a *Xi* -Cleft point's function is to de-obstruct or to unblock, on the one hand, this indicates that these channels have a possibility of getting obstructed, on the other hand, the sensitivity of these *Xi*≈ Cleft points, when palpated, would be an excellent indicator of the disturbance of these vessels.
  - *Jiaoxin* KI-8 on the *Yin Qiao* (*Yin* Motility) vessel.
  - *Fuyang* BL-59 on the *Yang Qiao* (*Yang* Motility) vessel.
  - *Zhubin* KI-9 on the *Yin Wei* (*Yin* Linking) vessel.
  - *Yangjiao* GB-35 on the *Yang Wei* (*Yang* Linking) vessel.

Pain or sensitivity of the confluent or constituent points could also be used diagnostically when combined with other cardinal symptoms of the corresponding vessel.

Some authors have proposed the sensitivity of the opening points as a diagnostic

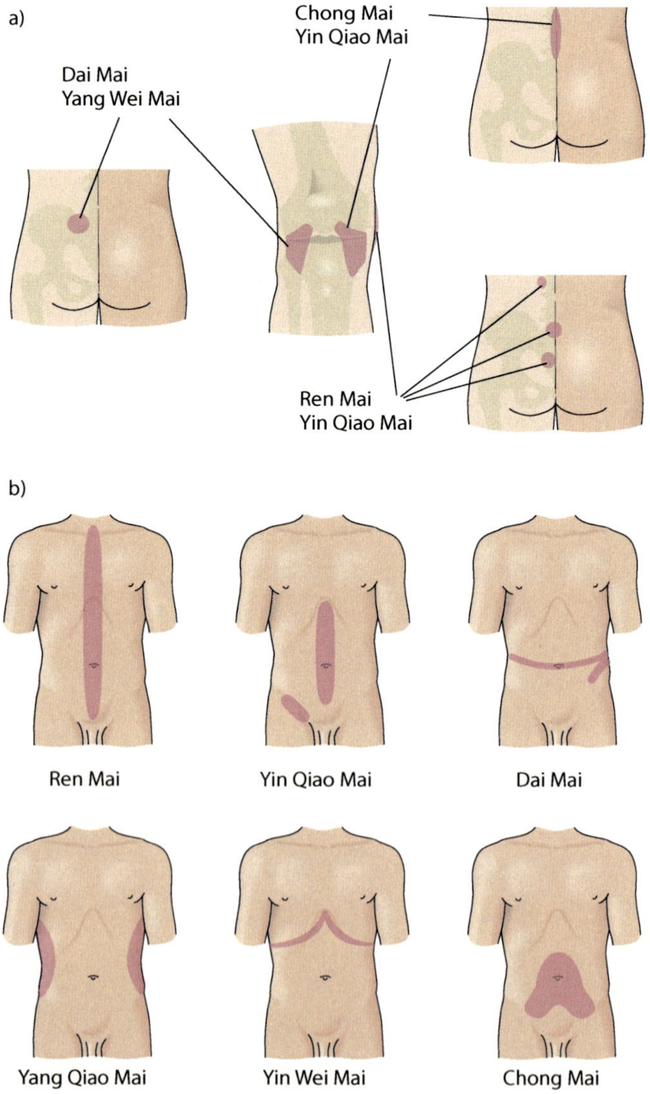

Figure 13.3 : Japanese palpation diagnostic system:

a) Tension zones and the Extraordinary vessels according to Manaka,

b) Diagnosis of the Extraordinary vessels according to Ito.

modality. Personally, I do not agree with this approach, as four of the opening points are *Luo* ≈ Connecting points (SP-4, PE-6, LU-7, TW-5), and the sensitivity of these points denotes a *Luo* ≈ Connecting/ network channel pathology and not an Extraordinary vessel pathology.

The Japanese school has developed an elaborate palpation diagnostic system for the Extraordinary Vessels (▶ Fig 13.3).

Symptoms of the Eight Extraordinary Vessels

Ren Mai ≈ Conception Vessel

Ren ≈ Conception by its name refers to pregnancy and conception: dealing with menstruation, reproduction and the urogenital system. According to the *Nan Jing*: "the Symptoms of *Ren Mai* are the seven *Shan*", referring particularly to accumulations.

- For men, this could represent a hernia, swollen testicles, prostatitis, child bed-wetting (overly dependent on the mother).
- For women, *Zheng-Jia* refers to a fibroid, ovarian cysts, endometriosis, leucorrhea and *Yin* stasis in the lower *San Jiao*≈ Triple Warmer (TW).

The main symptoms of *Ren Mai* concern *Yin* Stasis with *Yin* Vacuity (this may include some types of cancers). The classical symptoms involve conditions especially after delivery, lumbago, depression, retention of lochia, but also digestive disorders, food stasis with vomiting, eating disorders, constipation, diarrhea, hemorrhoids, Spleen *Lao* ≈ Consumption (wasting and thirsting, as in diabetes). Also, 5 types of neck nodules (Goiters) are associated with *Ren Mai*. Other symptoms include a cough and dyspnea. The personality traits in relation to *Ren Mai* are: bonding issues, co-dependency, addictions; compensations, eating disorders; also issues with control (inner milieu, sphincters; or outer world) and faith; issues with identity, gender or race.

Du Mai ≈ Governing Vessel

Febrile diseases, mental disorders, stiffness and pain of the spinal column, opisthotonos. In general *Du Mai* mostly deals with symptoms of *Yang* repletion (excess) generally in the form of Wind and Heat: epilepsy, malaria, disturbed *Shen* with irritability and restlessness, high fever; or sometimes also for vacuity (deficiency) of *Yang* with paralysis, stiffness, numbness, and frigidity. Other classical symptoms include loss of voice, throat *Bi* ≈ Impediment (inability to articulate), red and swollen eyes, head-wind, headaches, Bell's Palsy, Trigeminal neuralgia, neuralgia, Parkinson's disease, numbness of the limbs, stroke, epilepsy; hemorrhoids or prolapse of the uterus, tightness, weakness, spasms of the lower limbs. *Du Mai* is also involved with sexual libido (*Yang* aspects): impotence and infertility (sperm motility, reduced sexual drive).

Du Mai affects the Sea of Marrow: amnesia, loss of memory (frontal brain), lack of coordination (midbrain), as well as affecting respiration and digestion (lower brain).

In repletion (excess) certain personality traits could manifest: being overly independent early in life, difficulty with commitment, overachieving. In vacuity (deficiency) there could be a tendency to timidity and shyness (vacuity in the GB) and an overly dependent personality.

Chong Mai ≈ Penetrating Vessel

Counter-flow *Qi*, wheezing, palpitations, "Running piglet" syndrome (*Ben Tun*) with energy rushing up, panic attacks, internal heat; hot head, cold feet; nine kinds of Heart pains; Spleen-*Qi* or Spleen-*Yang Xu* with digestive symptoms, four types of abdominal fullness; fatigue; sinking of Spleen-*Qi* with prolapse, ptosis or hernia; edema and water retention in the legs, varicose veins. Leakage of Kidney-*Qi*: spermatorrhea, leucorrhoea, incontinence; asthma. Bi-obstruction symptoms, especially from early years (polio); horizontal lumbar pains, after lifting a heavy object, discus hernia; helping consolidation after fractures, osteoporosis, Raynaud's syndrome. The *Bi*-Impediment/ obstruction is often secondary to Blood stasis in the uterus, affecting the *Dai Mai*, further blocking the *Yang* in the *Du Mai*. Gynecological conditions: blood stasis, premenstrual syndrome, myoma, endometriosis; also sterility, miscarriage. Genital pains, prostatic adenoma. Shen disturbances: anxiety, restlessness, paranoia, or deep fear and even severe depression.

Psychologically *Chong Mai* manifests with a lack of a "Central Axis"; lack of connection to the body or emotions; lack of a sense of purpose in life; pessimism; the idealization of relations. It is often a depressive personality, extremely tired, both physically and psychologically, with no desire for anything, sleeping a lot and frequently presenting gynecological, digestive or lumbar problems, with the tendency to sterility or miscarriage. These subjects have often difficulties in finding meaning in their lives, difficulties to express their dislikes, and are prone to stress-related wheezing or cardiovascular conditions.

Dai Mai ≈ Belt Vessel

Abdominal fullness, flaccidity of the waist, Lumbar coldness with the sensation of sitting in water from the waist down; general tendency to coldness; heavy legs; dysmenorrhea with white and red discharge; uterine bleeding, miscarriage or prolapse. Belt-like lumbar pains irradiating to the perineum. Patterns of Excess above/ Deficiency below, manifesting as temporal headaches, Head-wind, head pruritus, dandruff, conjunctivitis, cataract, glaucoma, otitis, throat pain and breast pains, which might be combined with patterns of deficiency below: paralysis, weakness, numbness of legs, frequent ankle sprains; purplish legs or edema. Patterns of Dampness: Edema; ascitis, leucorrhea, cystitis, vaginitis, ovarian cyst; feeling heavy with rain. *Bi* ≈ Impediment/ obstruction syndrome of hips, legs or shoulder involving Damp-Heat and belt-like lumbar pains. Wei atrophy: Paralysis, weakness, hemiplegia as well as paraplegia.

Psychologically *Dai Mai* is involved in holding back and the suppression of past violations; disconnection or rejection of the lower parts; loss of creativity.

Yin Wei Mai ≈ Yang Binding Vessel

Chest oppression, palpitations; nine kinds of Heart pains, intense headaches, hypertension; energy shooting up; panic attacks; intestinal bloating and gas; lumbar pains after a shock; insomnia from fear; depression; irritability; and regrets.

The psychological profile includes an inability to let go of a past event, heartbreaks inability to remain in the present moment; day-dreaming; psychosomatic diseases; oppression and panic attack.

Yang Wei Mai ≈ Yin Binding Vessel

Alternating Fever and chills; sensitivity to weather change; chronic and frequent colds; headaches with wind or storm or snow; superficial body pains; unstable emotions.

Psychologically the person has an inability to let go of a past status; self-identification with the social position, with over-reactiveness to external stimuli or criticism.

Yin Qiao Mai≈ Yin Motility/ Stepping Vessel

In general *Yin* and *Yang Qiao Mai* present the opposite conditions, that is a repletion of the *Yin Qiao,* accompanies a vacuity of *Yang Qiao* and vice versa. The *Yin Qiao* pathologies get aggravated at night and improve during the day, it is the opposite for *Yang Qiao*. Somnolence, fatigue, pelvic heaviness, fibroids, PMS; leucorrhoea, genital swellings pain or hernia, urinary frequency, incontinence; loss of libido; lumbar pains radiating to the genitals; pain or flaccidity along the medial side of the leg; chest tightness, palpitations; throat dryness or tightness; eye dryness, redness.

Psychological profile: lack of self-acceptance and self-love, lack of self-confidence.

Yang Qiao Mai ≈ Yang Motility/ Stepping Vessel

Insomnia; Pain or tightness along the lateral side of the leg; unilateral headaches; unilateral lumbo-sciatica pains; unilateral *Bi* ≈ Impediment or *Wei* ≈ Atrophy; stroke, epilepsy, and hyperthyroidism.

Psychologically: non-acceptance or rejection of the outer conditions, reactivity, political activism, dissatisfaction, and indignation.

13.11 Identification according to the 12 Jing Jin ≈ Sinew channels

Involves mainly the disturbance of mobility, with either muscle or tendon pains, spasms, tightness, and stiffness, or flaccidity and weakness.

The main symptom is the pain. The channel involved is diagnosed by the:

- *Jing Jin* ≈ Sinew channel symptoms
- Palpation along the Sinew channel revealing the *Ah Shi* ≈ Painful points
- Evaluation of the range of motion of the muscle groups
- Palpation of the four convergence points

Jing Jin-Sinew channel symptoms

Channel	Symptoms
Zu Tai Yang **(BL)**	Pain along the trajectory. Inability to support the little toe; pain and spasms of the heel, popliteal region, neck; tension headaches, occipital area: BL-10, GB-20; Inability to raise the arms (extension), GB 21; Supra-clavicular or axillary muscles strain; facial neuralgia
Zu Shao Yang **(GB)**	Inability to support the 4th toe; strain and sprain of the outer aspect of the knee. Inability to bend or extend the knee; spasm of the popliteal fossa; pain and tension of the lateral and posterior aspect of the thigh; strain in the pelvic region in front of the sacro-coccygeal region. Sciatalgia and nodules along the piriformis m. Pain or tension in the lateral costal, the supra-clavicular region, the chest or the neck (inability to open the opposite eye when turning the head). Cluster headaches.
Zu Yang Ming **(ST)**	Spasms of the middle toes and the leg; Weakness of the Tibialis m. causing a collapse of the arch and flat feet, halux valgus. Weakness of the Quadriceps m. accompanied by uro-genital symptoms, with frequency; including Shan in men: uro-genital dysfunctions & hernias. Counter flow *Qi* with nausea, vomiting or bloating; throat obstruction, sudden loss of voice. Difficulty in closing or opening the eyes, acute facial paralysis (Bell's Palsey).
Shou Tai Yang **(SI)**	Pain or strain along the trajectory; inability to support the little finger, medial pain of the elbow, upper arm and the axilla; inability to raise or pull the arm forward, difficult abduction of the arm. Axillary pain radiating to the scapula and neck. Ear pain extending to the jaw; tinnitus, deafness. Needing to close the eyes to get them to focus. Neck spasm or tension causing swelling or atony.
Shou Shao Yang **(TW)**	Pain or strain along the trajectory, ring finger, rotation of the elbow or arm; inability to raise the arm, neck tension, difficulty opening the jaw and chewing, curled tongue. Weight changes (loss or gain), associated with thyroid problems; xophtalmia. Crying easily.

	Surface temperature and skin integrity problems.
Shou Yang Ming **(LI)**	Spasm, stiffness, pain or strain along the trajectory; inability to raise the arm; inability to turn the neck to left or right. Difficulty supporting the weight of an object. Chronic respiratory problems
Zu Tai Yin **(SP)**	Pain or strain along the trajectory (big toe): hammer or trigger toe; pain at the medial malleolus, Gastrocnemius cramp; medial side knee pain, bow legged knee "Genu varum": contraction of the Spleen sinew; pain of the inner thigh and the inguinal region; sharp genital pains radiating to the navel, abdomen, chest or back.
Zu Shao Yin **(KI)**	Cramping of the foot, spasms, twitching or pain along the channel (calve muscles). Foot in medial rotation, and pulling the pelvis down causing lumbar pains, scanty urination, *Lin* ≈ Strangury syndrome (5 *Lin*). Hammer or mallet toes. Knee in rotation. Tendency to lean forward when the Soleus is weak. Convulsions and spasms associated with epileptic diseases. With Yang excess: difficulty bending forward, lower back pains (*Biao*≈ Surface disease). With *Yin* excess: difficulty leaning backward with a sensation of heaviness in the abdomen and chest (*Li* ≈ *Internal* disease)
Zu Jue Yin **(LR)**	Inability to support the big toe; ain at the medial malleolus; cramping and pain in the Gastrognemius; medial knee pain. Inner thigh and inguinal pain. Sharp genital pains irradiating to the navel, ribs or back. In case of Cold in the channel: retraction of the genitals: difficulty in arousal, impotence. In case of Heat in the channel: persistent erection (priapism).
Shou Tai Yin **(LU)**	Cramping and pain along the trajectory. When the condition is severe there is an accumulation of lumps below the ribs, with tension along the ribs with coughing and spitting of blood.
Shou Jue Yin **(PC)**	Spasm or stiffness and pain along the course of the channel. Axillary pains. Chest pains with oppression and a feeling of an "inverted cup" below the lower ribs.
Shou Shao Yin **(HE)**	Internal tension, oppression below the heart; acid reflux. Angina pectoris. Pain or cramping along the pathway of the channel.

Evaluating the movement of the muscle groups

Shoulder	Abduction	TW - LI - BL + KI
	Flexion	LU
	Extension	SI - TW - LI
Shoulder and arm	Adduction and external rotation	LU - PE - HE
	Abduction	TW – LI – BI – KI
	Horizontal abduction	TW - SI

	External rotation	SI
Elbow and forearm	Flexion	HE - PE
	Extension	SI - TW - LI
	Supination	LU - PE
	Pronation	HE
Wrist and hand	Flexion	HE - PE
	Extension	SI - TW - LI
	Adduction	SI - TW
	Abduction	LI
Fingers	Extension or abduction	SI - TW - LI
	Flexion or adduction	LU - PE - HE
	Extension, opposition of 1st finger	LU
	Opposition of the 5th finger	HE

Evaluating the muscle groups motion range

The range of movement further confirms the affected *Jing Jin* ≈ Sinew channel. This is done by establishing which movement causes or aggravates the pain: standing, walking, rotating, holding, etc. *Yang* sinews are evaluated in extension:

- *Tai Yang*: Pain when the joint is in full extension
- *Shao Yang*: Pain when rotating the joint in extension
- *Yang Ming*: Pain when grasping, lifting with resistance or holding
- The *Yin* sinews are evaluated with the joint in flexion:
- *Tai Yin*: Pain upon flexion (retraction)
- *Shao Yin*: Pain when rotating in flexion
- *Jue Yin*: Paralysis

Palpation of the Confluent points

The reactivity/ sensitivity of the confluent point further helps the diagnosis:

Arm *Yang*	Corner of the forehead	ST-1 or GB-13
Leg *Yang*	Below the cheek bone	SI-18 or ST-3
Arm *Yin*	Below the axilla	GB-22
Leg *Yin*	Above the pubic bone	RM-3

Jing Jin Territories and muscle groups

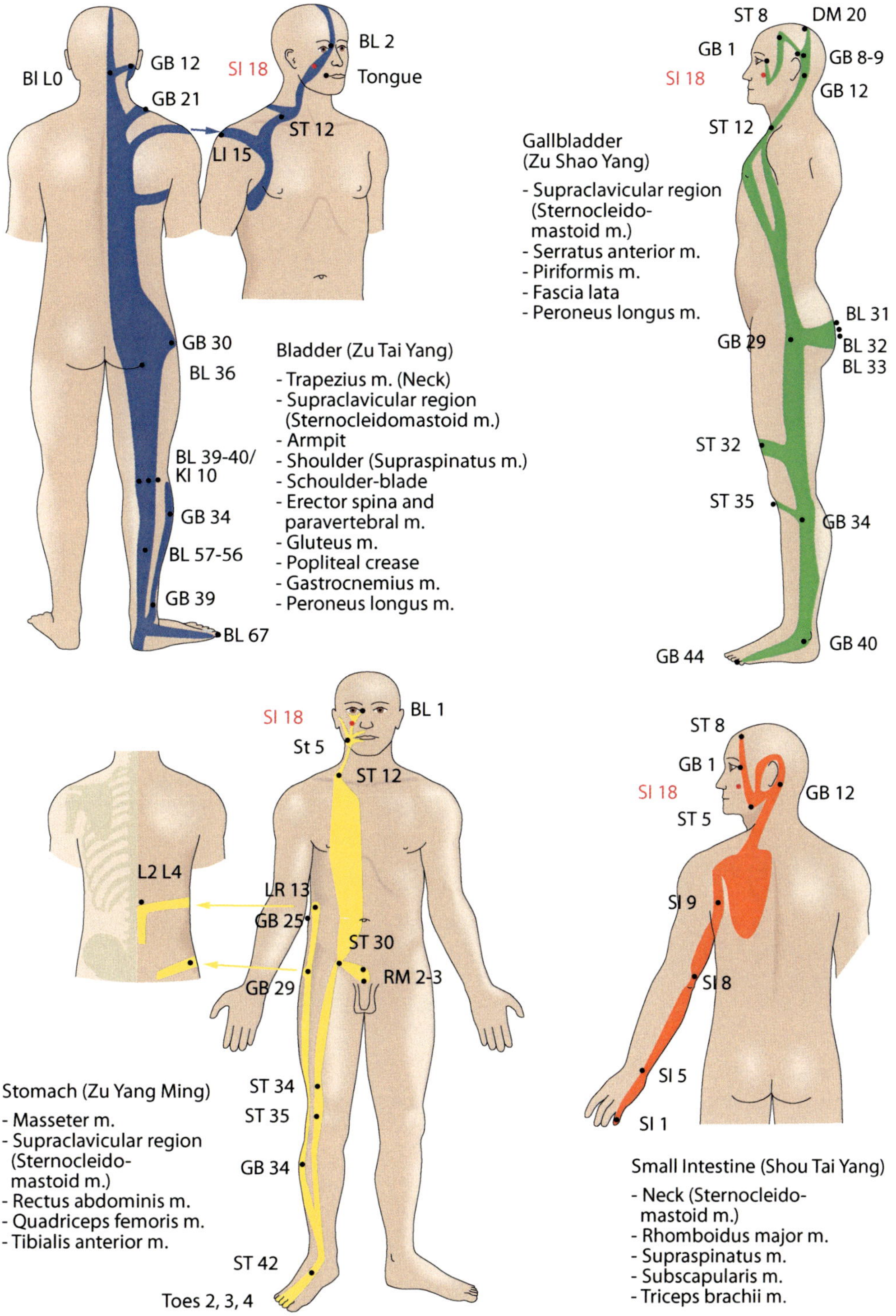

Figure 13.4: ***Jing Jin*** **≈ Sinew channel territories and muscle groups I.**

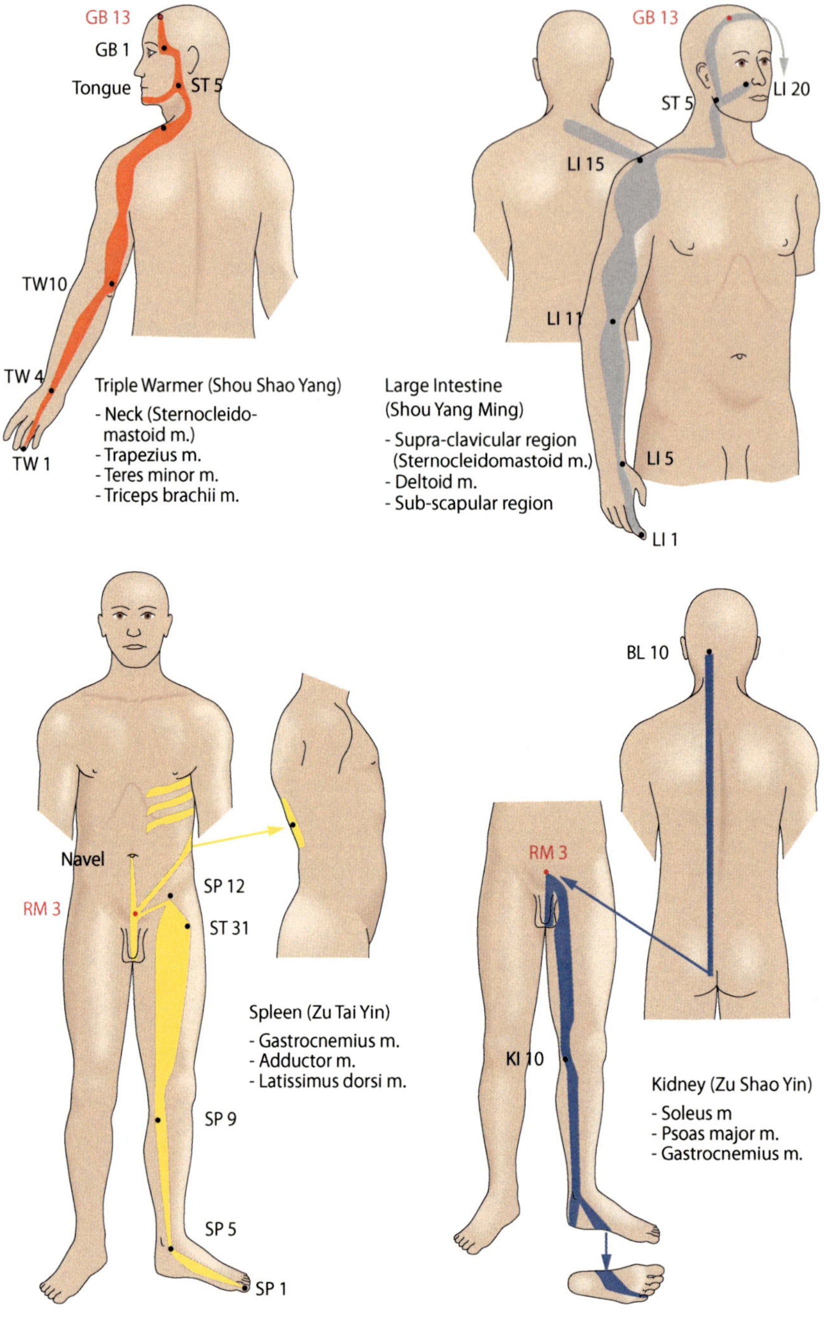

Figure 13.5: *Jing Jin* ≈ Sinew channel territories and muscle groups II.

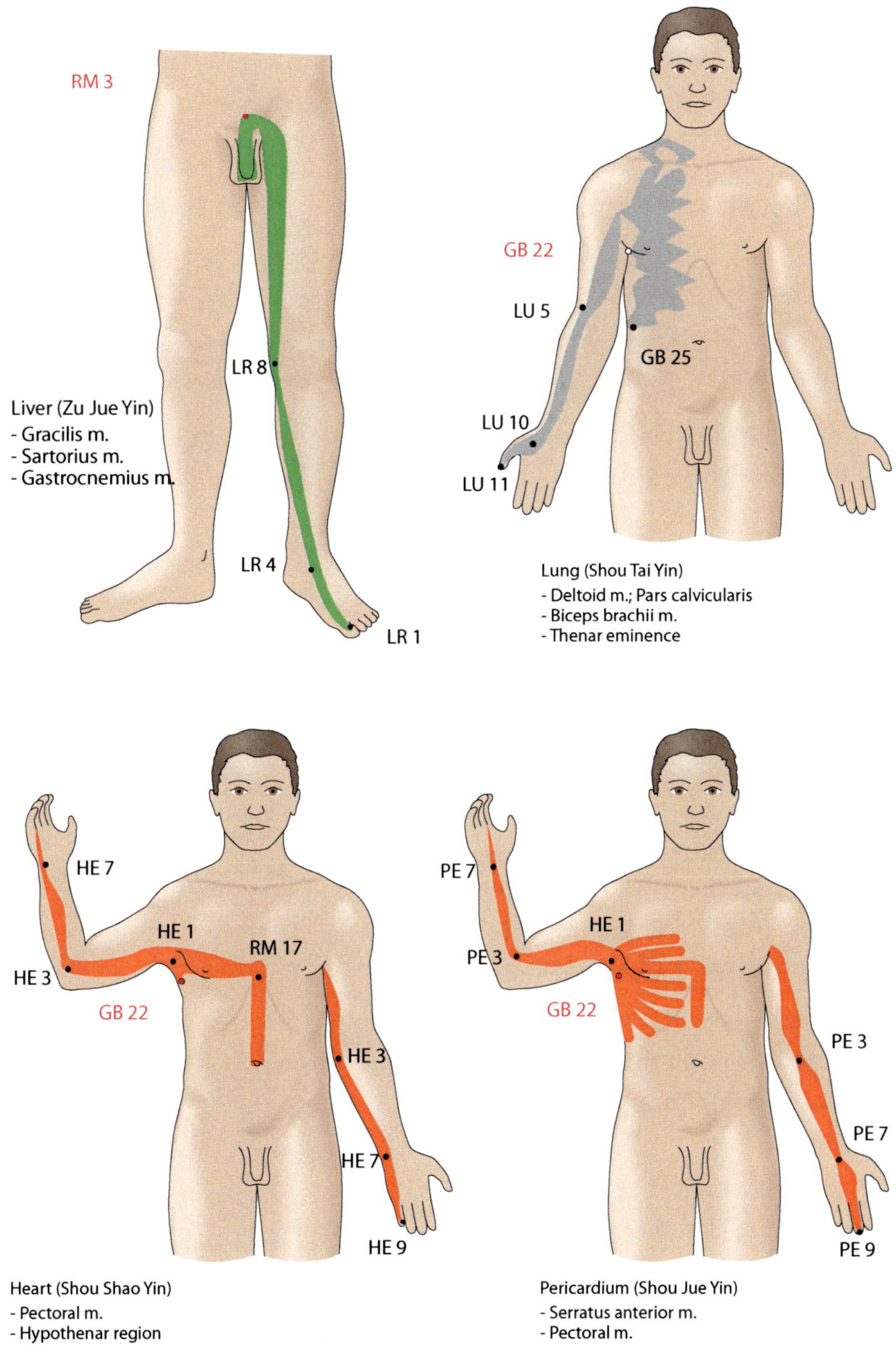

Figure 13.6: *Jing Jin* ≈ Sinew channel territories and muscle groups III.

13.12 Identification of patterns according to the 15 Longitudinal and 12 Transversal Luo ≈ Connecting Vessels

The *Luo* ≈ Connecting/ Network vessels present two distinct pathways, hence the French school has categorized them as "Longitudinal *Luo"* and "Transversal *Luo"*.

The symptom descriptions, as they appear in the ancient Chinese classical texts, refer to the Longitudinal portion (► Table 13.27):

Longitudinal Luo

Aside from the pathological symptoms, there are two main diagnostic elements concerning the state of repletion of the Longitudinal Luo:

- The Luo become visible: this visibility depends on the anatomical layer involved and could manifest as:
  - On the skin: maculopapular eruptions
  - In the sinews: masses, tumors (invisible phlegm)
  - Vessels: varicosity; the color of varicosity further indicates the type of the pathogenic factor involved:
    - Reddish signifies: Heat
    - Bluish signifies Cold and pain
    - Purplish signifies Blood stasis, which implies an underlying *Qi-Xu*-vacuity and the possibility of chronicity and Bi-obstruction syndrome.
- The *Luo* point becomes painful to palpation and swollen
- There are also often acute counter-flow *Qi* patterns:
  - Sighing, yawning, frequent urine: LU-*Luo*
  - Frequent bowels, flatulence: LI-*Luo*
  - Sinking SP-*Qi*, bloating: SP-*Luo*
  - Nausea, vomiting: ST-*Luo*
  - Palpitations, angina: HE-*Luo*
  - Mouth, throat ulcers; reflux: SI-*Luo*
  - Anuria: BL-*Luo*
  - Wheezing: KI-*Luo*
  - Fibrillation, palpitation: PE-*Luo*
  - Alternating chills and fevers: TW-*Luo*
  - Alternating above/below/sides: GB-*Luo*
  - LR-*Yang* rising: LR-*Luo*

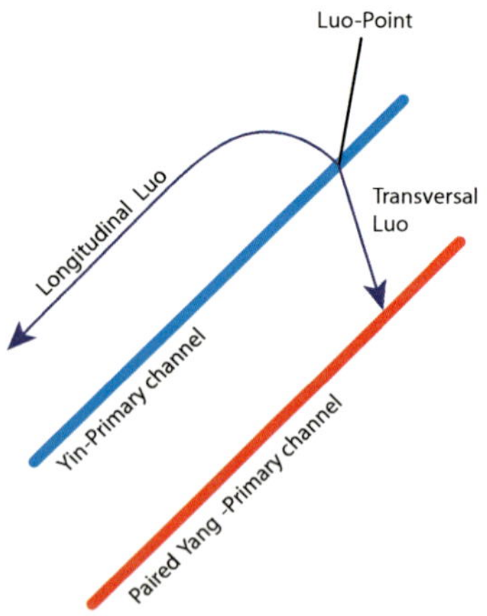

Figure 13.7: Two branches of *Luo* ≈ Connecting vessel: Longitudinal and

Master Yuen recommends taking the moderate pulse (between the surface and the depth) to evaluate the state of repletion or vacuity.

Table 13.27 Symptoms of the Longitudinal *Luo*

Luo Vessel	Repletion (Excess)	Vacuity (Deficiency)
Shou Tai Yin (LU)	Heat in the palm of the hands (same as for HE and PE); inability to let go	Counter-flow *Qi*, yawning, sighing, cough, frequent urination or incontinence
Shou Shao Yin (HE)	Discomfort and pain in the chest, includes palpitations and angina pectoris	Impossibility to speak, aphasia; incapacity to to connect emotionally with the other or to express feelings
Shou Jue Yin (PC)	Repletion: pain in heart area, oppression, inability to let go	Discomfort and stiffness in the neck
Shou Tai Yang (SI)	Discomfort in the elbow and shoulder joints; loose joints	Furunculosis, warts, acne, small and itchy swellings
Shou Yang Ming (LI)	Pain in the teeth and gums, tooth decay, bruxism, deafness	Cold sensation in the teeth, pain and oppression in the chest; hyperventilation, dyspnea
Shou Shao Yang (TW)	Spasm of the elbow joint; dominating personality	Discomfort and laxity in the elbow, weak personality
Zu Tai Yang (BL)	Stuffy nose; head and back pain; cannot "take anymore"	Nose bleed, clear rhinorrhoea
Zu Shao Yang (GB)	Very cold feet and legs; loss of consciousness in more severe cases	Weak legs, difficulty in walking or getting up; rigidity; lack of motivation, emotional blindness.
Zu Yang Ming (ST)	Sudden mutism; sudden loss of voice, plum pit, goitre; *Kuang*≈Madness; excessive excitement	Laxity of the leg articulations, muscle atrophy or spasms; loss of excitement.
Zu Tai Yin (SP)	Intense intestinal pains, intestinal parasites, dysentery and vomiting; obsessiveness, intellectual fixity	Abdominal bloating, ascites; inability to recognise feelings
Zu Shao Yin (KI)	Constipation and anuria; shyness; holding on to fear	Lumbar and dorsal pains; self destructiveness
Zu Jue Yin (LR)	Swelling of scrotum and penis, priapism; multiple personalities but unaware (J. Yuen)	Sudden itching in the scrotum and penis; cruelty, schizoid behaviour but aware of it (J. Yuen)
Ren Mai	Superficial abdominal pains;	Abdominal pruritus; difficulty

	obsessions	assimilating new ideas
Du Mai	Spinal stiffness, headache; inability to let go	Heavy head, vertigo, trembling
Da Bao (Great Luo of Spleen)	Diffuse pain in the whole body; great emotional suffering	Weakness and laxity of all the joints
Great Luo of Stomach (Su Wen)	Epigastric and thoracic pain and congestion, respiratory difficulties, rapid and irregular breathing	Pain around *Rugen* ST-18 on the left side, palpitations

The Horizontal or Transversal Luo and the Five Movements (5 Elements)

The Transversal *Luo* maintain the equilibrium between two coupled *Zang-Fu* by establishing a connection between their respective channels (an inner connections is established by the deep pathways of the channels) (▶ Table 13.28):

Table 13.28 Symptoms of the Transversal *Luo* dysfunction

LU	Chest fullness, cough, asthma, hot palms
LI	Dry lips, mouth, and throat
ST	Fever with sweat, epigastric distention, phlegm; pain along the pathway with heat rising above to affect the other *Yang Luo*
SP	Heart pain, tongue pain, stiff body, frequent bowel movements
HT	Yellow eyes, pain along the pathway, Raynaud's syndrome, heart failure
SI	Tinnitus, deafness, submaxillary swelling
BL	Yellow eyes, watery eyes, head and neck pain, hemorrhoids
KI	Cold and numbness along the legs, cockcrow diarrhea or stools with undigested food, depression-introversion, running piglet syndrome (*Ben Tun*)
PC	Heart pain, depression, hot palms, circulatory problems
TH	Sweating and pain along the pathway
GB	Sweating and achiness of the joints
LR	Nausea, vomiting, loss of appetite, diaphragmatic constriction, loose stools, incontinence or anuria

In any case, the predominant consequence of a disturbance of the Transversal *Luo* is the impact on the related movement in the Five Phase theory. The following symptoms are suggestive of a Phase disturbance, especially if there are other symptoms such as reactivity to specific climates, tastes, colors or seasons, reflecting a microcosm-macrocosm dysfunction (▶ Table 13.29):

Table 13.29: Impact of the Transversal *Luo* on the Five Phases

Wood	**LR - GB**	Bitter taste in the mouth, gallstones, difficulty in the digesting fats (damp heat)
Fire	**HT - SI**	Tongue ulcers with burning; dark yellow urine, palpitations, anemia
Earth	**SP - ST**	Weak digestion with symptoms of fullness, bloating, flatulence, loss of appetite, loose stools; phlegm (sluggish lymphatic system)
Metal	**LU - LI**	Constipation, wheezing, breathlessness
Water	**KI - BL**	Frequent urination or urinary retention, edema, brittle bones and joints deposits (arthrosis)

13.13 Identification of patterns according to the Jing Bie ≈ Divergent Channels

Jing Bie complement the Primary channels, by maintaining the internal rhythms and communication between the body and the organs (Earth) with the head (Heaven), they function in pairs (▶ Fig. 13.8).

The *Jing Bie* pathology often involves "Residual pathogenic factors" (RPF) manifesting as chronic and recurring conditions in the form of *Bi* ≈ Impediment/ obstruction or *Wei* ≈ Atrophy syndromes with underlying Blood and *Yin* vacuity and the presence of Heat.

Diagnosis is based on a combination of elements:

- Chronic intermittent or cyclic symptoms, often combining osteoarticular complaints of proximal joints, combined with chest, throat and head symptoms.
- The *Zu Tai Yang*-BL *Jing Bie* draws the pathogen to the *Shou Tai Yang*-SI *Jing Bie* in the shoulder area: hence the sensitivity of Naoshu SI-10 and *Bingfeng* SI-12
- The *Zu Shao Yang*-GB *Jing Bie* draws the pathogen to the *Shu Shao Yang*-TW and via *Baihui* DM-20 into the brain manifesting with chronic headaches, allergies; or into the spine with scoliosis, ankylosing spondylitis.
- The *Zu Yang Ming*-ST *Jing Bie* draws the pathogen to the *Shou Yang Ming*-LI in the shoulders at *Jianyu* LI-I5 and *Dazhui* DM-14.
- According to the French school, the palpation sensitivity of the

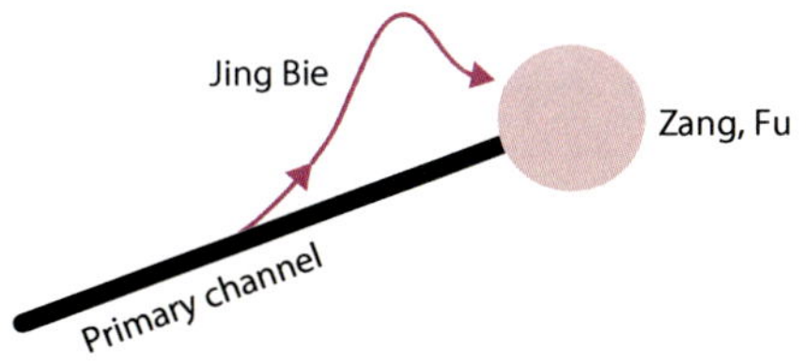

Figure 13.8: *Jing Bie* ≈ Divergent channel

related Window of Heaven points would be a further confirmation of the involvement of the corresponding *Jing Bie.*

Table 13.30 Symptoms of the Six *Jing Bie* ≈ Divergent Channel groups

Zu Tai Yang (BL) and Zu Shao Yin (KI)	• Heart pains, abdominal and diaphragmatic distension; throat pain, anger with no reason; Ben Tun ≈ Running piglet syndrome (panic attacks); anus and urethra problems; dryness of the throat and the mouth; floating Yang conditions • Liver-Yang rising: dizziness, vertigo, high blood pressure • Kidney-Yang from Yin Xu: dizziness, a tendency to faint • Excess Yang from Heat: headaches. • Neck, shoulder and back pains; weakness of the legs, lack of coordination
Zu Shao Yang (GB) and Zu Jue Yin (LR)	• Chest or rib pains; hip pains; dyspnea with sweating; Blood pathologies; eyes, ears, uterus and prostate problems; spine pathologies; swelling of neck and gums; speech difficulties, cough, throat irritation; dizziness (Yin Xu, or Yang Shi), heaviness (Yin Shi, or Yang Xu), hypertension (Yin or Yang Shi), migraines; relationship to Liver Luo: • Repletion: abnormal sexual arousal • Vacuity: genital swelling and itch • 3 types of consumption: physical, mental or sexual. Pathologies of accumulation of Dampness (compensation for Dryness of Yin-Xu)
Zu Yang Ming (ST) and Zu Tai Yin (SP)	• Chronic and recurrent lumbar pains, abdominal distension, dyspnea. Clear Yang not reaching the head: head not clear, dizziness; dryness of the orifices. Sneezing, nasal discharge, nose-bleed, the coldness of upper teeth. • Internal Wind in the head and face with loss of latency: tremors, seizures, optic neuritis. Lack of tongue coating. Symptoms in connection with Renying St-9: dyspnea, hoarse voice, sore throat, goiter. Food toxicity or food stasis (as one of the "Six accumulations": Qi- Blood- Water/Phlegm-Heat-Cold- Food)
Shou Tai Yang (SI) and Shou Shao Yin (HE)	• Heat trapped in the head: • *Wei* ≈ Atrophy: stroke, paralysis • Psychosis (*Dian Kuang*) • Stuttering, aphasia. • Connection with *Tianchuang* SI-16: • lack of coordination • pain and swelling of throat (Cold-Wind) • eye, ear and throat problems

	• Lower abdominal pains radiating to the back and genitalia. Diarrhea or constipation. Chest and rib pains, palpitations, dyspnea when lying down. Disturbed sleep, dizziness; numbness of the 4 limbs
Shou Shao Yang (TW) and Shou Jue Yin (PC)	• Heat and Dampness in the deep sinews or joints: rheumatoid arthritis; osteoporosis. Chronic Dryness; opportunistic infections; emaciation (Heat consuming the Jing). Nodules (Phlegm); skin rashes, moles, herpes, bleeding. • Connection with TW 16: Yin stagnation in the head: • headaches, facial edema • sudden mutism; vision problems • dream of falling • Throat pains, dry mouth; restlessness, irritability, oppression, palpitations, delirium (Phlegm harassing the Heart). Difficulty lifting the head and the arms; wrist pains: carpal tunnel syndrome
Shou Yang Ming (LI) and Shou Tai Yin (LU)	• Chronic and recurrent pathologies of the shoulder, breasts, thyroid, pituitary (hormonal) and tumors. A fullness of chest and sides, dyspnea; cough, wheezing, restlessness, palm heat. Intermittent deafness. Sudden mutism or loss of vision. Sudden dyspnea, noises in the throat; hoarse voice, goiter, tonsilitis; excess salivation; trembling lips

14. To Touch

Although palpation constitutes the fourth pillar of diagnosis, the ancient Chinese considered touching offensive as demonstrated by the saying: "the superior doctor diagnoses by looking, the average doctor by looking and hearing, and only the inferior doctor has to take the pulses" in other words to actually touch a patient!

Besides taking the pulses, the palpation of specific acupuncture points, such as the back *Shu* ≈ Transport points or the front *Mu* ≈ Alarm points, had been recommended in the classics as a means of diagnosis. Somehow the palpatory diagnosis never really developed in the Chinese medical tradition. By opposition the Japanese acupuncture traditions had no taboo in touching and palpating the body points and zones, therefore the majority of palpational diagnostic methods used today in the West come from the Japanese school.

14.1 Palpational Diagnosis

All pathological phenomena produce a change in the local balance of *Qi* and Blood.

In diagnosis, this local modification of *Qi* and Blood will manifest as a change in color, temperature, and sensitivity.

Temperature

- Local heat: Accumulation of *Yang* usually from Damp-Heat
- Local coldness: Accumulation of *Yin*
- Heat or cold of the 3 zones of the Triple Warmer: hyper or hypoactivity of the zone
- Surface Heat:
  - If heat sensation gets less after holding: External pathogenic Heat
  - If heat increases: Internal Heat
- Heat is inside and does not come to the surface: Heat from *Yin Xu*≈ Vacuity

Moisture, Dryness

Indicates the balance between the local *Ying* ≈ Nourishing *Qi* and *Wei* ≈ Defensive-*Qi*; *Wei Qi* is more *Yang*, therefore, more drying in nature.

An excellent method of discovering areas of dysfunction is to lightly slide the fingers along the inner branch of the Bladder channel on the back and to note the areas where the fingers seem to stick a little. Invariably these areas will correspond to the Back *Shu* of the organ and/ or the vertebrae, which is out of balance.

Swelling, Tightness, Lumps

Swellings indicate an accumulation of *Qi* or of Body Fluids.

- Hot swelling: Heat, Damp-Heat; toxic Heat (abscess)
- Cold swelling: Water edema; *Yin* stagnation, Phlegm
- Swelling holding the pressure marks: "Water edema"; Humidity; Kidney-*Yang Xu*
- Non-depressible swelling: "*Qi* edema"; *Qi* stagnation
- Firm lumps, swollen lymph glands; cysts, tumors: Phlegm; Cold-Phlegm
- Boils, abscesses: Hot-Phlegm; toxic Heat
- Purplish swelling, bruises: Blood stagnation

Tightness or looseness of muscles in an area reflects on the state of repletion or vacuity of the *Jing Jin* ≈ Sinew channels. The state of repletion usually causes a painful tightness, cramping or twitching of the muscles controlled by a specific Sinew channel, the vacuity would cause flaccidity or even paralysis.

The 12 Sinew channels control the following muscle groups:

***Zu* (foot) *Tai Yang* - Bladder**	Long Peroneus m., Gastrocnemius m. and Achilles tendon; Popliteal crease; Gluteus; Rectus and Paravertebral m; Trapezius; Supraspinatus; neck, shoulder and shoulder-blade, axillary and supraclavicular areas
***Zu Shao Yang* - Gallbladder**	Long Peroneus m., Fascia lata, Piriformis m. anterior Serratus; axillary and Sternocleidomastoid areas
***Zu Yang Ming* - Stomach**	Tibialis m., Quadriceps; Abdominal rectus supraclavicular areas and Sterno-cleido-mastoid m.; Masseter m.
***Shou* (arm) *Tai Yang* - Small Intestine**	Triceps m.; Sub-scapularis; Supraspinatus; Rhomboids
***Shou Sha Yyang* - Triple Warmer**	Triceps m.; Terris minor and Trapezius m.
***Zu Yang Ming* - Large Intestine**	Adductor & abductor Policis, Extensor carpi longus & brevis; Supinator m.; Subscapularis area; Deltoid m; Supraclavicular area
***Zu* (foot) *Tai Yin* - Spleen**	Gastrognemius; Adductor muscles; Latisimus dorsei
***Shou* (arm) *Tai Yin* - Lung**	Thenar eminence; Bracial radialis; Biceps; anterior Deltoid
***Zu Shao Yin* - Kidney**	Gastrognemius; Psoas and Solas muscles
***Shou Shao Yin* - Heart**	Hypothenar region; Pectoralis m.
***Zu Jue Yin* - Liver**	Gastrocnemius, Sartorius and Gracilis muscles
***Shou Jue Yin* - Pericard**	Pectoralis and Serratus muscles

Pain

Pain signifies a change in the local balance between Blood and *Qi* and primarily denotes an obstruction of *Qi* and Blood.

Any point that becomes painful to pressure is called an *Ah Shi* point

Pain that is felt spontaneously could be caused by the following:

- Articulations and bones, tendons and ligaments
- Trigger points, and myo-facial structures
- Organic or neurological pains
- Pain that may not be felt spontaneously and is only discovered by pressure:
- Scar tissue, or reflex zones: in this case, the pain increases with pressure and massage until there is numbness.
- *Ah Shi* point in which *Qi* is stagnating: the pain improves with manipulation. In the case of a *Shi* ≈ Repletion/ excess, the pain might increase at first but would eventually improve.

Pain is always evaluated according to the "Eight Diagnostic Principles" (*Ba Gang*) (▶ chap. 12.2).

The significance of Painful zones and Lumps

- The 5 areas in "Abdominal diagnosis"
- The tight zones or Kori in "Hara diagnosis"
- Tightness and stiffness in bands in "Body Armors"

The significance of Painful Points

A painful acupuncture point does not always have a diagnostic significance but mainly reflects a local dysfunction of *Qi* and Blood (*Ah Shi*).

Some points though, do indicate a specific disturbance of the corresponding channel system or organic function. Globally the point reactivity may be grouped to indicate a functional problem of a particular system:

"Four Phases", the Internal Structure	Diagnosed by *Mu* ≈ Alarm point sensitivity
The "Five Phases" and the *Zang-Fu* the "12 Officials"	By Specific organ points; Back *Shu* ≈ Transporting, *Xi* ≈ Cleft, and *Yuan* ≈ Source points
The 12 Primary channel	By *Xi* ≈ Cleft and *Yuan* ≈ Source point pain
***Jing Jin* ≈ Sinew channels**	Will manifest with "*Ah Shi*" points in their respective territories and the reactivity of the 4 meeting points (see below)
The 6 channel layers	With *Luo* ≈ Connecting, Knot, *Xi* ≈ Cleft and, *Yuan* ≈ Source point sensitivity

Triple Warmer problems	Will cause the tenderness of some distal points, such as *Neiguan* PE-6 (upper TW), *Lieque* LU-7 (middle TW) and *Dazhong* KI-4 (lower TW), as well as local points: *Xiawan* RM-10, *Jianli* RM-11, *Shangwan* RM-13 and globally *Zhongwan* RM-12
***Jing Bie* ≈ Divergent channels**	Could manifest by the reactivity of the corresponding Window of Heaven
8 Extraordinary Vessels	Four of them have *Xi* ≈ Cleft points, their tenderness would signify a disturbance

Mu (Mo) ≈ Collecting or Alarm points 募

Mu points were outlined in the *Tai Su*, further complemented by the *Nan Jing*.

The concept of *Mu* ≈ Collecting/accumulation or concentration refers to *Shi* ≈ Repletion/ excess pathology in case of an external pathogenic factor as well as physiological overactivity, in which case these points become sensitive, hence their name "Alarm". They are all situated on the front, chest, and abdomen.

They seem to be in direct connection with the *Zang-Fu* ≈ Organs-bowels.

Only 3 *Mu* points are situated on channels corresponding to their respective organs: *Zhongfu* LU-1, *Zhejin* GB-23 or *Riyue* GB-24 and *Qimen* LR-14. For the Gallbladder, there has been a debate about the actual *Mu* point being GB-23 and not GB-24 (both share the same secondary names).

As for the Triple Warmer, it would have two *Mu* points, some even use the whole area between *Shimen* RM-5 and *Yinjiao* RM-7.

The *Mu* points seem to affect more the *Qi* or *Yang* aspect of the organ. They are used for re-enforcing the "*Qi* function" of the organ. As they are situated on the *Yin* part of the body, they are indicated for the treatment of *Yang* diseases *(Nan Jing).*

The French school (J. M. Kespi; Schatz), refutes the organic connection of the *Mu* points, favoring rather the relation to the 5 Elements in their "Cosmogenic" representation. In this manner, the *Mu* are not reflecting an organic function, but rather govern the five movements. According to Kespi, only this correspondence can explain their names and their symptoms:

Mu Point	Zang-Fu	Significance in Relation to the Five Elements
Zhongfu LU-1	Mu of Lung	Interiorization of *Yin*
Tianshu ST-25	Mu of Large Intestine	Interiorization of *Yang*
Zhongwan RM-12	Mu of Stomach	Production and distribution of *Yang*
Zhangmen LR-13	Mu of Spleen	Production and distribution of *Yin*
Juque RM-14	Mu of Heart	Fire "Source" ; "Life Principle"

Guanyuan RM-4	Mu of Small Intestine	Birth and mobilization of *Yin*
Zhongji RM-3	Mu of Bladder	Maximum of *Yin*
Jingmen GB 25	Mu of Kidney	Mobilization of *Yang*
Shanzhong RM-17	Mu of Pericardium	*Yang* Expansion "Superficialization"
Shimen RM-5 and *Yinjiao* RM-7	Mu of Triple Warmer	Exteriorization of *Yang*
Zhejin GB-23 and *Riyue* GB-24	Mu of Gall Bladder	Movement of *Yin* towards the *Yang*
Qimen LR-14	Mu of Liver	Exteriorization of *Yin*

I have extensively verified the above theories. The systematic palpation of the *Mu* points in patients diagnosed with specific organic conditions such as heart diseases (*Juque* RM-14), hepatitis (*Qimen* LR-14), bronchitis or pneumonia (*Zhongfu* LU-1), colitis (*Tianshu* ST-25) etc., revealed on average a sensitivity of only about 60%. On the other hand, using these points in relation to the elemental movements has yielded very interesting results as well as explaining their classical indications.

In this aspect, the *Mo* points reflect the organic function in relation to the "Four Phases-internal structure" rather than the "Five Movements"; their sensitivity would, therefore, signify a disturbance of the corresponding movement rather than an organic disease.

Combining the two systems gives us a clearer view of the situation, for example, the tenderness of *Qimen* LR-14 reflects a surplus of function "stagnation" in the Liver, but also a problem of movement, the non-exteriorisation of *Yin*.

Rather than palpating the *Mu* points, the dysfunctions of the *Zang-Fu* could more easily be demonstrated by the sensitivity of their respective Back *Shu* ≈ Transport, *Yuan* ≈ Source and *Xi* ≈ Cleft points, as well as the "Specific Organ" points.

Specific Organ Points

These points have only been described by the French school, no mention has been made as such in the Chinese classics. Their specific grouping is mainly based on the classical and traditional indications that have been attributed to these points.

These points could be assimilated to the *Mu* ≈ Accumulation/ alarm points, reacting especially to excess energy from external pathogenic factors, and becoming tender.

Henggu KI-11 and *Siman* KI-14	For the Kidneys
Shangqu KI-17	For the Spleen
Youmen KI-21	For the Liver
Bulang KI-22	For the Lung
Shenfeng KI-23	For the Heart

Liangmen ST-21	For the Stomach
Guanmen ST-22	For the Gall Bladder
Huaroumen ST-24	For the Small Intestine
Wailing ST-26	For the Large Intestine
Shuidao ST-28	For the Bladder

There seems to be an intimate correlation between these points and the abdominal and thoracic trajectory of *Chong Mai*, especially if we refer to the ancient description of its pathway as running between the Stomach and Kidney channels. This would possibly corroborate the French school concept.

In any event, in clinical practice, I have found most of these points to be extremely useful, especially *Henggu* KI-11, *Siman* KI-14, *Youmen* KI-21, *Shenfeng* KI-23, and *Liangmen* ST-21, *Wailing* ST-26, *Shuidao* ST-28.

Back Shu ≈ Transporting (Associated) Points 俞/ 背俞

Located on the medial branch of the *Zu Tai Yang*/ Bladder channel on the back, they are directly connected with the *Zang-Fu*, they seem to affect more the *Yin* and Blood of the organs. Their tenderness has diagnostic value, indicating more often a condition of *Shi*≈ Repletion/ excess such as:

- Residual pathogenic factor in the *Zang-Fu*
- Excess from stagnation

The 12 back *Shu* of the *Zang-Fu* are:

Feishu BL-13	**Lung**
Jueyinshu BL-14	**Pericardium**
Xinshu BL-15	**Heart**
Ganshu BL-18	**Liver**
Danshu BL-19	**Gallbladder**
Pishu BL-20	**Spleen**
Weishu BL-21	**Stomach**
Sanjiaoshu BL-22	**Triple Warmer**
Shenshu BL-23	**Kidney**
Dachangshu BL-25	**Large Intestine**
Xiaochangshu BL-27	**Small Intestine**
Pangguangshu BL-28	**Bladder**

There are also some additional Back Shu points that are not related to the *Zang-Fu*:

Dushu BL-16	*Du Mai* ≈ Governing Vessel
Geshu BL-17	Diaphragm; Hui ≈ Meeting point of Blood
Qihaishu BL-24	Upper region of the lower back, second branch of the Dai Mai
Guanyuanshu BL-26	Lower region of the lower back, third branch of the Dai Mai
Zhonggushu BL-29	Spine and Sacro-iliac regions
Baihuanshu BL-30	Sphincter muscles
Gaohuangshu BL-43	All the Huang ≈ Nourishing membranes

Xi ≈ Cleft/ Accumulation Points 郗 (郄)

They become painful in case of disturbance and stasis. More specifically Cold produces pain, Wind causes distension, Dampness causes a sensation of fullness. In general, the sensitivity of the *Xi* -Cleft point suggests a disturbance of the channel and/or of the 5 movements: *Sheng* ≈ Nourishing and *Ke* ≈ Control cycles: LU-6/ Kong Zui; LI-7/ Wen Liu; ST-34/ Liang Qiu; SP-8/ Di Ji; HE-6/ Yin Xi; SI-6/ Yang Lao; BL-63/ Jin Men; KI-5/ Shui Quan; PE-4/ Xi Men; TW-7/ Hui Zong; GB-36/ Wai Qiu.

Besides the 12 *Xi* ≈ Cleft points related to the 12 primary channels, there are four *Xi* ≈ Cleft points in relation to four of the eight Extraordinary vessels, their sensitivity signifies a disturbance of the corresponding vessel:

Zhubin KI-9	**Yin Wei Mai**
Yangjiao GB-35	**Yang Wei Mai**
Jiaoxin KI-8	**Yin Qiao Mai**
Fuyang BL-59	**Yang Qiao Mai**

Luo ≈ Connecting Points 絡

Informs on a disturbance of the longitudinal *Luo* system. When the *Luo* channel is in Repletion/ excess the *Luo* point becomes painful and may even be swollen and change color and temperature. The sensitivity of *Luo* points could signify:

- If red: External pathogenic factor Heat
- If bluish: Cold pathogenic factor
- If purplish: Blood stasis and *Bi* ≈ Impediment/ obstruction of smaller joints ; Trauma: physical or emotional

In general, a painful *Luo* point may also reflect difficulties in terms of connecting to the outer world, the nine portals, zones of contact or articulations and psycho-emotional conditions.

The sensitivity of the Luo should be analyzed according to the overall context:

Lieque LU-7	Lung Luo; hand and wrist pathologies; disturbances of the middle Triple Warmer; boredom; difficulty to let go
Pianli LI-6	Large Intestine Luo; pathologies of ears and mouth; blood circulation problems of arm and face; presence of grief and sadness
Fenglong ST-40	Stomach Luo; Bi ≈ Impediment of the leg joints; circulation problems of the legs or the head; pathologies of the throat and of speech; issues with worry; strong likes and dislikes
Gongsun SP-4	Spleen Luo; abdominal blood circulation problems; fixity and obsessions
Tongli HE-5	Heart Luo; pathologies of the eye portal and speech; superficial blood circulation problems; stuttering, difficulty to express or to connect
Zhizheng SI-7	Small Intestine Luo; skin problems; arm pathologies; blood circulation problems of the arm; issues with anxiety or excitement; difficulty with criticism
Feiyang BL-58	Bladder Luo; pathologies of the nose portal; blood circulation problems of the legs; presence of fear or shock, inability to take on more pressure
Dazhong KI-4	Kidney Luo; problems of the lower Triple Warmer; lumbar or anal pathologies; pelvic blood circulation problems
Neiguan PE-6	Pericardium Luo; problems of the upper Triple Warmer and neck; internal blood circulation problems; withholding emotions
Waiguan TW-5	Triple Warmer Luo; pathologies of the elbow; blood circulation problems of the arm; personality problems
Guangming GB-37	Gallbladder Luo; pathologies of the feet and ankles; blood circulation problems of the leg; irritability and anger
Ligou LR-5	Liver Luo; pathologies of the uro-genital portals; blood circulation problems of the pelvis
Jiuwei RM-15	Luo of Ren Mai; superficial abdominal pain or itching; obsessions
Changqiang DM-1	Luo of Du Mai; spine problems; cannot let go
Dabao SP-21	Great Luo of Spleen; general articular problems; general blood circulation; notion of great suffering
Rugen ST-18	Great Luo of Stomach; issues with breast-feeding

There are 4 points called "Group *Luo*" which are not really "*Luo*" points but more exactly "*Jia*" crossing points:

- *Sanyinjiao* SP-6: Crossing of the 3 lower *Yin*
- *Xuanzhong* GB-39: Crossing of the 3 lower *Yang*
- *Jianshi* PE-5: Crossing of the 3 upper *Yin*
- *Sanyangluo* TW-8: Crossing of the 3 upper *Yang*

Yuan ≈ Source points 原

Their sensitivity may indicate either organ disturbance or a loss of balance between two *Biao-Li* coupled channels.

Taiyuan LU-9	For the Lung or Large intestine channel disbalance
Hegu LI-4	For the large Intestine or Lung channel disbalance
Chongyang ST-42	For the Stomach or Spleen channel disbalance
Taibai SP-3	For the Spleen or the Stomach channel disbalance
Shenmen HE-7	For the Heart or Small Intestine channel disbalance
Wangu SI-4	For the Small Intestine or Heart channel disbalance
Jinggu BL-64	For the Bladder or Kidney channel disbalance
Taixi KI-3	For the Kidney or Bladder channel disbalance
Daling PE-7	For Pericardium or Triple Warmer channel disbalance
Yangchi TW-4	For Triple Warmer, or Pericardium channel disbalance
Qiuxu GB-40	For the Gall Bladder or Liver channel disbalance
Taichong LR-3	For the Liver or Gallbladder channel disbalance

Taichong LR-3 and *Hegu* LI-4 are called the "Four Gates" and control all the *Yuan* -Source points.

The 4 meeting points of the Jing Jin ≈ Sinew channels

- Their sensitivity signifies the presence of *Xie*≈ Pathogenic *Qi* in the corresponding group of Sinew channels:
- *Quanliao* SI-18: meeting of arm *Yang Jing-Jin* ≈ Sinew channels
- *Benshen* GB-13: meeting of leg *Yang Jing Jin*
- *Yuanye* GB-22: meeting of arm *Yin Jing Jin*
- *Zhongji* RM-3: meeting of leg *Yin Jing Jin*

Special He ≈ Sea or Lower He ≈ Sea points Xia He Xue 下合穴

Their sensitivity signifies the presence of *Xie* ≈ Pathogenic *Qi* in the *Fu* organs.

- *Shangjuxu* St-37: Pathogenic factor in the Large Intestine
- *Xiajuxu* St-39: Pathogenic factor in the Small Intestine
- *Weiyang* BL-39: Pathogenic factor in the Triple Warmer

Jie ≈ Knot Points

Each of the 6 Grand Channels has a concentration point, called the “Knot” point. These points may become painful, signifying a disturbance of the corresponding channel:

Zhongwan RM-12	Knot of Tai Yin; dysfunction of the Lung & Spleen channels
Yutang RM-18	Knot of Jue Yin; disturbance in the Pericardium and Liver channels
Lianquan RM-23	Knot of Shao Yin; dysfunction in the Heart & Kidney channels
Jingming BL-1	Knot of Tai Yang; dysfunction in the Small Intestine and Bladder channels
Tinggong SI-19 or possibly *Tinghui* GB2 or *Ermen* TW-21	Knot of Shao Yang; dysfunction in the Triple Warmer and Gallbladder channels
Chengqi ST-1 or possibly *Touwei* ST-8	Knot of Yang Ming; dysfunction in the Large Intestine and Stomach channels

The Ba Hui Xue ≈ Eight Master/ Influential Points 八会穴

These points control some general functions and have a special influence on the *Zang-Fu* organs, their sensitivity may inform on the "Vital substances".

Shanzhong RM-17	Hui of Qi
Geshu BL-17	Hui of Blood
Dazhu BL-11	Hui of Bones
Xuanzhong GB-39	Hui of Marrow
Zhongwan RM-12	Hui of Fu ≈ Bowels
Zhangmen LR-13	Hui of Zang ≈ Organs
Taiyuan LU-9	Hui of arteries
Yanglingquan GB-34	Hui of tendons

The Zhi ≈ Will or the five Sian points

On the outer branch of the *Zu Tai Yang*-Bladder channel on the back, there is a set of points corresponding to an area of accumulation of psycho-emotional energy. Usually, in the presence of emotion, the point becomes painful to pressure.

Pohu BL-42	Relates to *Po* ≈ Corporeal soul; blockage of *Qi* through loss, sadness and grief
Shentang BL-44	Relates to *Shen* ≈ Spirit; blockage of *Qi* through excessive excitement or incoherence
Hunmen BL-47	Relates to *Hun* ≈ Ethereal soul; blockage of *Qi* through frustration, anger or indecision
Yishe BL-49	Relates to *Yi* ≈ Intellect; blockage of *Qi* through excessive cogitation, worry and obsessive thinking
Zhishi BL-52	Relates to *Zhi* ≈ Will power: blockage of *Qi* through anxiety, especially fear of the unknown
Gaohuangshu BL-43	Relates to the self; blockage of *Qi* due to rejection, self doubt or lack of self love

Ling ≈ Soul/ Transformation Points 靈

The reactivity of these points may denote difficulties with life passages or issues with the acceptance of change:

Chengling GB-18	Difficulty assuming ones spirituality
Lingdao HE-4	Difficulty in ones spiritual path
Lingtai DM-10	Difficulty in grasping ones becoming
Lingxu KI-24	Difficulty being in this world
Qingling HE-2	Difficulty in waking ones spirituality

Shen ≈ Spirit Points 神

The sensitivity of the *Shen* points mostly reflects on difficulties with the outer world and *Shen* disturbances. There is no specific indication as to the significance of the reactivity of each point:

Shenmen HE-7	Spirit Door
Shentang BL-44	Spirit Hall
Shenfeng KI-23	Spirit Seal
Shencang KI-25	Spirit Storage
Shendao DM-11	Spirit Path
Shenting DM-24	Spirit Court
Shenque RM-8	Spirit Gate
Benshen GB-13	Spirit Root

Gate Points

When these points become painful they reflect difficulties in transformation or mutation through a particular stage of life. This often indicates issues pertaining to non-acceptance or of blockage of that particular stage:

Pucan BL-61: Heel Gate	"Gate of childhood"; issues with growth, standing on one's own feet
Juliao GB-29: Hip Gate	Gate of adolescence"; issues with sexuality and gender
Naoshu SI-10: Shoulder Gate	"Gate of maturity"; issues with responsibility and position in the outer world
Qixue KI-13	Also "Gate of childhood", in relation to procreation and fertility
Lianquan RM-23	"Gate of the tonsils", dealing with recapitulation, issues of expression and creativity
Yamen DM-15	"Gate of the ears" in relation to the inner silence

The Tian Chuang Xue ≈ Window of the Sky/ Heaven Points 天窗穴

The sensitivity or reactivity of a Window of Heaven point, on the one hand, signifies a disturbance of its specific energetic movement, and on the other hand, may indicate a problem with the associated *Jing Bie* ≈ Divergent channel.

Fengfu DM-16 and *Tiantu* RM-22	Entry and exit of *Qi* from the chest
Tianchi PE-1 and *Tianfu* LU-3	Movements of *Qi* and Blood to the head
Tianzhu BL-10	Descent of *Yang* from the head; also Bladder and Kidney *Jing Bie*
Renying ST-9	Ascent of *Yang* and *Qi* to the head; also Stomach and Spleen *Jing Bie*
Tianchuang SI-16	Descent of *Yang*; also Heart and Small Intestine *Jing Bie*
Tianrong SI-17	Ascent of Blood and *Yin* to the head; also Gallbladder and Liver *Jing Bie*
Tianding LI-17 or *Futu* LI-18	Ascent and diffusion of *Yang Qi* and *Wei Qi*; also Lung and Large Intestine *Jing Bie*
Tianyu TW 17	Mobilization of *Yin* and Blood in the head; also Triple Warmer and Pericardium *Jing Bie*

Men or Guan ≈ Doorways of the Earth 門關

Not as popular as the Windows of Heaven and not described specifically in the classics. Their names do not always carry the notion of door or gate.

As the Windows of Heaven mainly deal with the head and the *Shen* disorders, the Doorways of the Earth reflect more the *Jing* ≈ Essence pathologies. There is no clear indication of their diagnostic significance:

Weizhong BL-40	Henggu KI-11
Huantiao GB-30	Jimai LR-12
Qichong ST-30	Chongmen SP-12
Mingmen DU-4	Guanyuan RM-4
Changqiang DM-1	Huiyin RM-1 (Jinmen)
Huiyang BL-35	Qihai RM-6 (Cimen or Mingmen)

Huang ≈ Vital Membranes 肓

These points relate to the protective and nourishing membrane surrounding the *Zang-Fu*. As such they seem to reflect various types and stages of nourishment. When painful to the pressure they signify an issue with an aspect of nourishment:

Gaohuangshu BL-43	In relation to self-nourishment, self-respect and the notion of rejection (broken heart point)
Huangmen BL-51	In relation to breast nourishments; issues of early age under-nourishment or under-protection
Baohuang BL-53	Relating to sexual issues and frustrations
Huangshu KI-16	Reflecting foetal maternal under-nourishment
Qihai RM-6	General under-nourishment

Feng ≈ Wind Points 風

Six acupuncture points contain the word *Feng* ≈ Wind in their names. When painful, they could indicate accumulation of Wind or stasis of *Qi* and Blood: *Fengfu* DM-16: Wind Palace; *Bingfeng* SI-12: Receiving Wind; *Fengchi* GB-20: Wind Pond; *Fengmen* BL-12: Wind Gate; *Yifeng* TW-17: Wind Screen; *Fengshi* GB-31: Wind Market

General Facilitating Points for the Movements of Yin and Yang

A set of points help the descent of *Yang* from the head towards the body and the feet, or vice versa the ascent of *Yin* from the feet towards the head. Other points facilitate these movements by mobilizing the *Yang* or the *Yin*. In general, the points that facilitate the movements of *Yin* and *Yang* become painful when the corresponding flow is hampered.

Facilitating the descent of Yang

Tianzhu BL-10	For Yang repletion in the head with Yang vacuity below
Xuanzhong GB-39	Brings Yang from the head and shoulders to the feet
Yanglingquan GB-34	For upper body and Biao ≈ External conditions, weakness in the legs
Tianshu ST-25	Brings surface Yang inwards

Mobilising Yang

All the *Yang Xi* ≈ Cleft and *Ying* ≈ Spring points as well as Group *Luo*'s: *Sanyangluo* TW-8; *Xuanzhong* GB-39 mobilize *Yang*. The following points become tender under palpation when there is a stagnation of *Yang*.

Jingmen GB-25	Yang stagnation
Zhongwan RM-12	Qi and Yang stagnation in the centre
Zhejin GB-23 and *Riyue* GB-24	Facilitate the exteriorization of Yang

Facilitating the ascent of Yin

The following points become reactive in the presence of *Yin* accumulation below.

Sanyinjiao SP-6	Yin accumulation in the lower parts, legs and pelvis
Jianshi PE-5	For Yin accumulation below (uterine blood stasis or phlegm nodules in the throat area), with Yin vacuity above: i.e. insomnia
Baihui DM-20	Helps pull Yin up and harmonize Yin and Yang in the head
Qimen LR-14	For exteriorization of Yin

Mobilising Yin

All the *Yin Xi* ≈ Cleft and *Ying* ≈ Spring points as well as Group *Luo*'s: *Sanyinjiao* SP-6, *Jianshi* PE-5, help to mobilize *Yin*. Generally, the following points become painful with pressure in the presence of *Yin* stagnation.

Guanyuan RM-4	Pelvic Yin accumulation
Zhangmen LR-13	Abdominal Yin stagnation
Qimen LR-14	Facilitate the exteriorisation of Yin

The movement of Yang and Yin between the front and the back

Zhiyang DM-9	Exuberant Yang in the back
Guanyuan RM-4 with *Zhongwan* RM-12 and *Tiantu* RM-22	Exuberant Yin in the front

Local Barrier and Mobilisation Points (▶ Fig. 14.1)

The concept of "Barrier Points" was originally proposed by the French school, and has been enriched by several decades of clinical application. Personally, I find it most useful in diagnosing and treating local pains.

Definitions

A “Barrier point” is a point that can selectively unblock a particular flow (*Yin* or *Yang* obstruction). These sets of points facilitate the movements of *Yin* and *Yang* from one area of the body to another. Usually, each body area is sub-divided into three segments, therefore three points are often found that help this movement. Usually, a blockage of *Qi* in a segment will cause an accumulation on one side of the blockage and a vacuity on the other side. Barrier points are most indicated in acute painful conditions, although they may also be used in more chronic pathologies.

A local "Mobilisation point" would be defined as a point specifically mobilizing *Yin* or *Yang* in a particular area of the body. These points become more easily reactive in chronic conditions.

The "Barrier" system is ideal for the treatment of local pain or paralysis.

A local obstruction of *Qi* most often causes pain, which is always first analyzed according to the *Ba Gang* ≈ Eight Diagnostic Principles (see above).

The local palpation of the Barrier points confirms the condition and indicates the best local therapeutic point.

Based on the spatial disposition of the 6 layers (▶ chap. 2.5), the movements of *Yin* or *Yang* are subject to the following order: *Tai Yang – Shao Yang – Yang Ming – – Tai Yin – Jue Yin – Shao Yin*. In other words, when *Yang* moves from one area to another, it will follow the *Tai Yang – Shao Yang – Yang Ming* sequence, and for the *Yin*, it would be *Tai Yin – Jue Yin – Shao Yin.* Hence the facilitating points would be found on the corresponding channels.

Arm Yin Barriers

3 points facilitate the exit of *Yin* from the chest into the arm, and 3 points help its return into the chest (▶ Fig. 14.1):

Yunmen LU-2 (*Tai Yin*)	Excess Yin in the chest and shoulder (frozen shoulder), with Yin Xu ≈ Vacuity in the arm
Ximen PE-4 (*Jue Yin*)	Excess Yin in the arm and shoulder, with Yin Xu in the forearm
Yinxi HE-6 (*Shao Yin*)	Excess Yin in the forearm, and Yin Xu in the hand
Kongzui LU-6 (*Tai Yin*)	Excess Yin in the hand (swelling, coldness, numbness, Arthrosis, Dupuytren's) and Yin Xu in the forearm
Tianquan PE-2 (*Jue Yin*)	Excess Yin in the forearm and hand (lymphoedema), and Yin Xu in the arm
Yinxi HE-6 (*Shao Yin*)	Excess Yin in the arm (lymphoedema), and Yin Xu in the chest (dry cough, palpitations). Note that HE-6 has a dual action on exiting of Yin to the hand and entering of Yin in to the chest.

For example, if the ascent of *Yin* is hampered at the wrist, there would be an accumulation/ repletion of *Yin* in the hand accompanied with symptoms of *Yin Xu* ≈ Vacuity in the arm, confirmed by *Kongzui* LU-6 becoming sensitive to pressure; whereas if the blockage is at the level of the elbow, the *Yin* accumulation would be in the forearm and hand with *Yin* Vacuity above with *Tianquan* PE-2 becoming painful.

Mobilization of Yin in the upper limbs

Jiquan HE-1: General mobiliser of Yin in the arm; Yin stasis, (frozen shoulder, lymphoedema, adenopathy, osteoarthritis, arthrosis).

Arm Yang Barriers

3 points facilitate the exit of *Yang* from the trunk into the arm, and 3 points help its return into the trunk (► Fig. 14.1).

Tianzong SI-11 (*Tai Yang*)	Excess Yang in the upper thorax and shoulder, (pain in the scapula, periarthritis of the shoulder), with Yang Xu in the arm (weakness, numbness)
Tianjing TW-10 & *Naohui* TW-13 (*Shao Yang*)	Excess Yang in the arm and shoulder (periarthritis, tendinitis), with Yang Xu in the forearm
Xialian LI-8 (*Yang Ming*)	Excess Yang in the forearm (tendinitis), and Yang Xu in the hand (coldness, weakness, paresia)
Yanglao SI-6 (*Tai Yang*)	Excess Yang in the hand (pain, inflammation, heat) Yang Xu in the forearm
Huizong TW-7 (*Shao Yang*)	Excess Yang in the forearm (tendinitis), and Yang Xu in the arm
Jianyu LI-15 (*Yang Ming*)	Excess Yang in the arm and shoulder (Yang type periarthritis), and Yang Xu in the chest (Heart & Lung)

Mobilization of Yang in the upper limbs

Jianliao TW-14: General Yang mobiliser of the arm, chronic Yang stasis (periarthritis, shoulder or elbow tendinitis)

Leg Yin Barriers

3 points facilitate the exit of *Yin* from the pelvis into the leg, and 3 points help its return into the pelvic region (▶ Fig. 14.1).

Chongmen SP-12 (Tai Yin)	Excess Yin in the abdomen and pelvis (cold in the uterus or intestines, inguinal adenopathia, hernia), with Yin Xu in the leg (hot, restless legs, Yin pain)
Xiguan LR-7 (Jue Yin)	Excess Yin in the knee (swollen knee, knee arthrosis), and Yin Xu in the lower leg
Shuiquan KI-5 (Shao Yin)	Excess Yin in the leg, with Yin deficiency in the foot (hot painful feet, better with pressure)
Diji SP-8 (Tai Yin)	Controls the return of Yin from the foot in to the leg, excess Yin in the foot (swelling, coldness, heaviness, numbness, Arthrosis) and Yin Xu in the leg
Yinlian LR-11 (Jue Yin)	Excess Yin in the leg (heavy, swollen legs), and Yin Xu in the thigh
Qixue KI-13 (Shao Yin)	Excess Yin in the lower limbs (heavy, swollen or cold legs), and Yin Xu in the pelvis (dryness, heat)

Mobilization of Yin in the leg:

Jiaoxin KI-8: Is the general mobilization point of Yin in the leg; chronic Yin stasis (heavy swollen legs, oedema, varicous veins, osteoarthritis, arthrosis).

Leg Yang Barriers

3 points facilitate the exit of *Yang* from the pelvis into the leg, and 3 points help its return into the pelvis (▶ Fig. 14.1).

Chengfu BL-36 (Tai Yang)	Excess Yang in the pelvis and sacro-iliacregion (lumbago, acute constipation), with Yang Xu in the leg (weakness, numbness, Yin pains)
Xiyangguan GB-33(Shao Yang)	Excess Yang in the upper thigh and Yang Xu in the leg (paresia or paralysis)
Xiajuxu ST-39 (Yang Ming)	Excess Yang in the leg and Yang deficiency in the foot (coldness, numbness, Yin type pains)
Chengfu BL-63 and *Zhonglushu* BL-29 (Tai	Excess Yang in the foot (pain, inflammation, heat, tendinitis) and Yang Xu in the leg

Yang)	Note that Zhonglushu BL-29 controls the exit of Yang from the pelvis in both directions downwards and upwards
Waiqiu GB-36 (Shao Yang)	Excess Yang in the leg (pains, tendinitis of the knee), and Yang vacuity in the thigh
Biguan ST-31 (Yang Ming)	Excess Yang in the lower limbs (hot, restless legs, Yang pains), and Yang Xu in the pelvis (coldness, premenstrual pains better with heat)

Mobilization of Yang in the leg:

Huantiao GB-30: General Yang mobilization in the lower limbs, chronic Yang stasis (pains which get worse with rest and cold and improve with heat and movement).

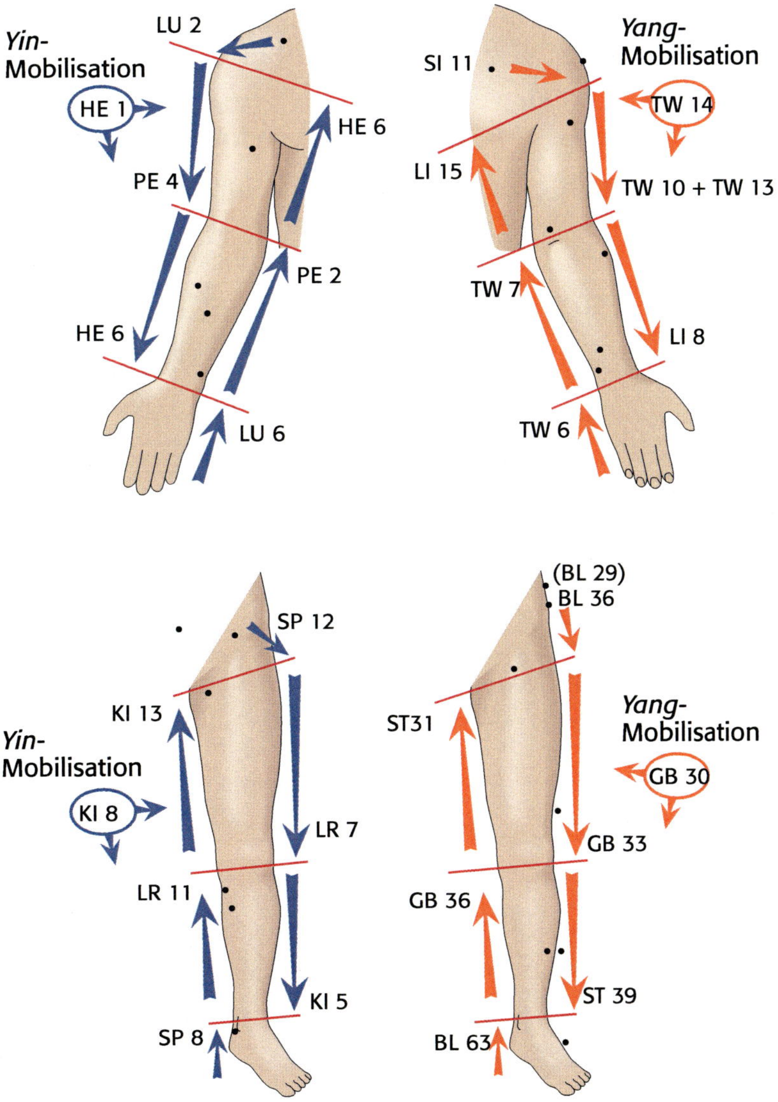

Figure 14.1: Local Barriers and Mobilization points of the limbs

Yin Barrier Points of Chest and Abdomen (▶ Fig. 14.2)

Yunmen LU-2 and *Chongmen* SP-12 (Tai Yin)	Control the general exit of Yin from the trunk towards the limbs with Yin accumulation inside (Dampness, Phlegm, tumours, Yin type Asthma, constipation or diarrhoea, difficulty expressing feelings), with Yin deficiency in the periphery (dryness, peripheral heat, dermatitis)
Zhongzhu KI-15 and *Yuzhong* KI-26 (Shao Yin)	Control the general entrance of Yin from the limbs in to the trunk, Yin accumulation in the limbs (heavy limbs, swelling, coldness), with Yin vacuity inside (empty-Heat, difficulty putting on weight, insomnia, restless mind

Yin movements between the pelvis and the chest (▶ Fig. 14.2)

3 points control the ascent of *Yin* and help bring the pelvic *Yin* to the chest. The points controlling the descent of *Yin* from the chest to the abdomen are not known.

Fujie SP-14 (Tai Yin)	Excess Yin in the pelvis (diarrhoea, coldness in the pelvis with Yin Xu in the abdomen (gastritis)
Qimen LR-14 (Jue Yin)	Yin excess in the abdomen (coldness, abdominal pains and bloating worse with pressure and better with heat), with Yin vacuity in the chest (heat, palpitations)
Futonggu KI-20 (Shao Yin)	Yin accumulation in the chest and abdomen (bloating and pain, dyspnoea, asthma, vomiting), with Yin Xu above

Yang Barrier Points of Chest and Abdomen (▶ Fig. 14.2)

Tianzong SI-11 and *Chengfu* BL-36 (Tai Yang)	Control the general exteriorization of Yangfrom the trunk towards the limbs, with Yang repletion inside (tension and pain in the back or lumbar regions, cramps, heat, restlessness, Qi stagnation, hypertension), with Yang Xu in the limbs (coldness, weakness, paralysis)
Wuyi ST-15 and *Daju* ST-27 (Yang Ming)	Facilitate the entrance of Yang from the limbs towards the trunk, with Yang repletion in the limbs (heat, restless legs, pains worse with heat and pressure), and Yang Xu inside (coldness, stasis, pains better with heat and pressure)

Yang movements between the pelvis and the chest (▶ Fig. 14.2)

3 points control the ascent of *Yang* and help bring the pelvic *Yang* to the chest. Only one point is known for the descent of *Yang* from chest to pelvis (ST-27).

Zhonglushu BL-29 (Tai Yang)	Moves Yang out of the pelvis, Yang repletion in the pelvic and lumbo-sacral regions (acute lumbago, constipation, heat in the lower Triple Warmer)

Figure 14.2: Local Barriers and Mobilization points of the trunk.

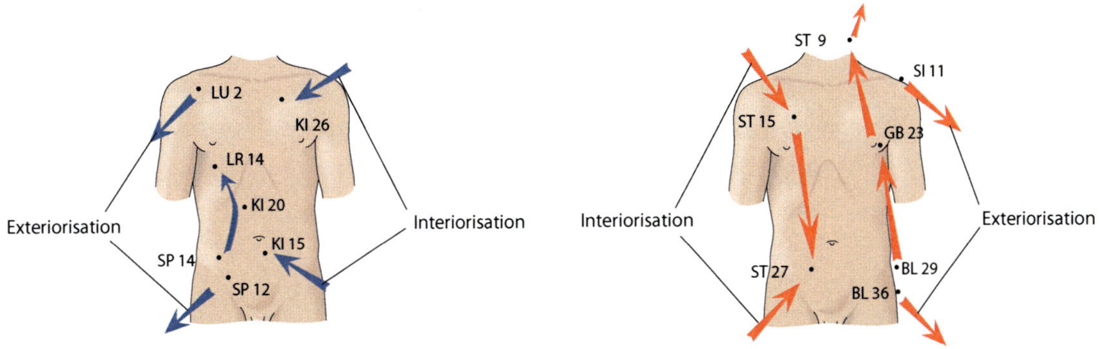

Zhejin GB-23 (Shao Yang)	Yang repletion below the diaphragm (Stomach stagnation) and Intestinal heat, Liver-Qi
Renying ST-9 (Yang Ming)	Helps Yang to move from the chest upwards: dyspnea, hoarse voice; sore throat, goiter, energy shooting up and down
Daju ST-27	*Yang* excess in the chest (palpitations, heat nervousness,) with pelvic *Yang Xu* (pre-menstrual pains improved by heat and pressure, constipation or diarrhoea, *Yin* stasis in the lower TW

Yang Barrier Points of the Neck (▶ Fig. 14.3)

In the neck and head areas, there are only *Yang* points controlling the movements of *Yang*. Few points affect the movements of *Yin* in the head, such as *Jianshi* PE-5, which brings *Yin* to the upper parts and the head, *Tianrong* SI-17, helps bring *Yin* to the head, and *Baihui* DM-20 that helps ascend *Yin* and *Yang*, *Qi* and Blood up to the head.

Yang movements between the head and the chest

3 points control the descent of *Yang* from above into the trunk (▶ Fig. 14.3).

Tianzhu BL-10 (Tai Yang)	Excess Yang above (heat, hypertension, pain worse with pressure), with Yang Xu below (vertigo with weak legs, stiff neck, shoulders and back, lack of co-ordination)
Jianjing GB-21 (Shao Yang)	Excess Yang in the neck (neck tensions and cramps, torticolis, cervico-brachial neuralgia on the Shaoyang channels), with Yang Xu below (phlegm in the throat; melancholia)
Qishe ST-11 (Yang Ming)	Excess Yang above (neck tensions and pains, sore throat, aphtha, cervicobrachial neuralgia on Yang Ming channels), with Yang Xu below

Yang movements between the trunk and the head

3 points control the ascent of *Yang* from the chest upwards (▶ Fig. 14.3).

Jianwaishu SI-14 (Tai Yang)	Yang accumulation in the shoulder area(cervico-brachial neuralgia on SI channel and some types of epitrochleitis, with Yang Xu above (cold feeling in the neck, stiffness)
Tianliao TW-15 (Shao Yang)	Yang accumulation in the chest, shoulder and neck (cervico-brachial neuralgia on the Shao Yang channels, stiff neck), with Yang Xu above
Juliao ST-3 (Yang Ming)	Excess Yang in the neck, lips and cheeks (trijeminal neuralgia) with Yang Xu in the eye, nose, and sinuses

Yang movements on the Head and the face

There are only *Yang* channels on the head; therefore only *Yang* movements are taken into account. The head being the most complex energetic area of the body, the *Yang* movements have to be considered in relation to the cranium and the face, the endocranium, and the outside, the front, and the back and the middle and the sides. The diagnosis of *Shi* ≈ Repletion and *Xu* ≈ Vacuity is not always easy, hence the importance of the information given by the palpation of the relevant "Barrier" and "Mobilisation" points.

Yang movement from the Cranium towards the Face (▶ Fig. 14.3)

Chengguang BL-6 (Tai Yang)	Yang excess in the head with empty symptoms in the Ear, Eye, Nose, face and teeth
Shangguan GB-3 (Shao Yang)	Yang excess in the head (visual and auditory hallucinations), vacuity below (Xu type tinnitus, deafness)
Xiaguan ST-7 (Yang Ming)	Yang repletion above (tinnitus, vertigo; blurred vision), with Yang Xu below (facial palsy, neuralgia, toothache)

Mobilization point: *Hanyan* GB-4: Stagnation of Yang (headaches) with vacuity symptoms in the ear.

Yang movement from the Face towards the Cranium (▶ Fig. 14.3)

Zanzhu BL-2 (Tai Yang)	Yang excess above the eyebrow (headache, sneezing with the sun and the wind), with Yang Xu below: eye pains
Yangbai GB-14 (Shao Yang)	Yang excess in the eye; Yang Xu below
Touwei ST-8 (Yang Ming)	Yang repletion in the eye and the eyebrow

Mobilization point: *Sizhukong* TW-23: Yang stagnation in the eye (congestion headaches, neuralgia worse with wind; hypoesthesia)

Yang movement from the side of the Face towards the nose (▶ Fig. 14.3)

Tinggong SI-19 (Tai Yang)	Yang accumulation in the ear (sound of cicada, deafness, stuffed ear, madness), with Yang Xu in the eye and nose
Sizhukong TW-23 (Shao Yang)	Yang repletion in the eye (congestion, blurred vision, in-growing eye lashes)
Yingxiang LI-20 (Yang Ming)	Yang repletion in the eye, Yang Xu in the nose

Yang movement from the Occiput towards the Face (▶ Fig. 14.3)

Yuzhen BL-9 (Tai Yang)	Yang accumulation in the occipital area (intense neck and headaches, vertigo)
Xuanlu GB-5 or *Wangu* GB-12 (Shao Yang)	Yang repletion in the occiput and ear (headaches, otitis), with Yang Xu in the face
Chengqi ST-1 (Yang Ming)	Yang repletion in the ear, with Yang Xu in the face and the eye

Mobilization point: *Tinghui* GB-2: Yang stagnation (deafness, tinnitus, otalgia, pruritus of the ear, facial palsy, hypoesthesia, gum and cheek problems)

Yang movement from the Face towards the Occiput (▶ Fig. 14.3)

Only one point is known: *Meichong* BL-3: *Yang* accumulation (epilepsy, internal headaches, nose symptoms)

Mobilization point: *Tongziliao* GB-1: Yang stagnation in the face and eye (congestion, pruritus, lacrimation, photophobia, blurred vision), with vacuity in the ear and the occipital region

Yang movement from the Endocranium /inside towards the surface (▶ Fig. 14.3)

Luoque BL-8	Yang repletion in the head (repressed worry, over excitement, fugue, false ideas, vertigo, myopia, tinnitus, deafness
Touwei ST-8	Yang repletion in the head (intense internal headaches, wrenching pain in the eyes)

Mobilization point: *Naokong* GB-19: Yang excess in the head (intense internal headaches, diplopia caused by shock, vertigo, lack of coordination and balance, tinnitus, deafness).

Yang movement from the outside towards the inside (Endocranium) (► Fig. 14.3)

Only one point corresponds to this movement:

Jingming BL-1: Superficial Yang repletion (pain, congestion, visual veil, lacrimation, photophobia, hay fever), with Yang Xu inside (Xu headache, dizziness).

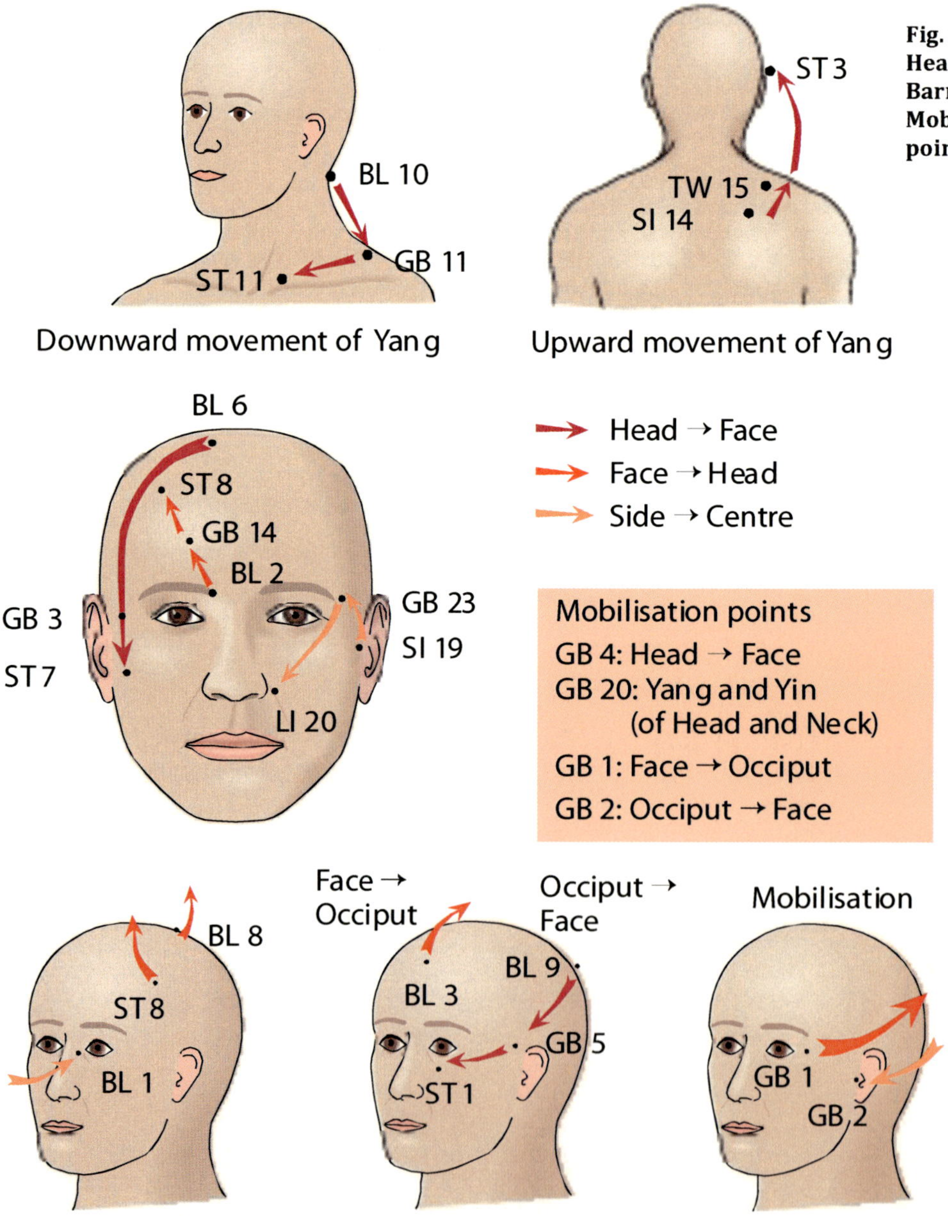

Fig. 14.3: Head Barriers and Mobilization points

14.2 Abdominal Diagnosis

General Palpation

- Comparison of the temperature of the three zones of the Triple Warmer
- Evaluation of heat and coldness of the organ zones
- Appreciation of the elasticity, firmness, and sensitivity of the abdomen.

The normal abdomen: presents a shiny skin, is not sensitive to touch, the muscles have a normal tone, and no aortic pulsation is felt. The upper epigastric area (*Jiuwei* RM-15) should be relaxed. The lower epigastric zone (*Zhongwan* RM-12) should be firm but not tense and the hypogastric area (*Qihai* RM-6) should be firm and tonic.

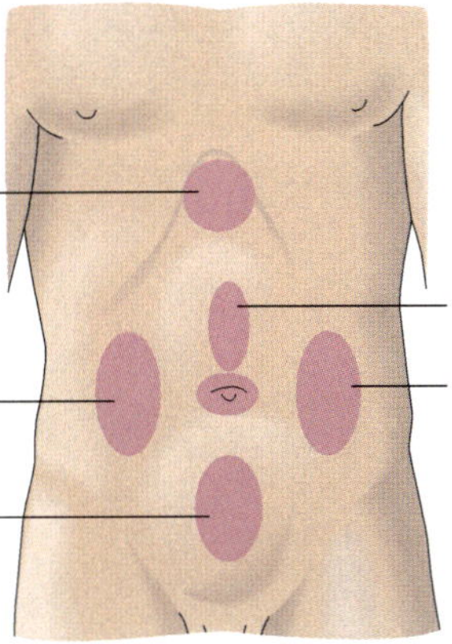

Figure 14.4: Abdominal tension areas and the five *Zang*

Tension and Pain (▶ Fig. 14.4)

Tension and pain	Shi ≈ Repletion (Excess)
Loose skin, thin, pale	Xu ≈ Vacuity (Deficiency)
Upper Epigastrium hard, tight, painful	Repletion of Heart or Lung Qi or Heat; nervous tension
Lower Epigastrium tense, hard and painful	Repletion of Cold or stagnation of Qi or food in the Stomach and Spleen Qi
Hypogastrium loose, non elastic	Yuan Qi Xu; Kidney-Qi Xu
Mobile lumps and pain	Qi stasis
Fixed and hard lumps	Blood stasis

Aortic pulsations (▶ Fig. 14.5)

Felt in the hypogastrium	Normal state of *Yuan Qi* ≈ Inherited energy
Umbilical, superficial	State of *Xu* ≈ Vacuity
Umbilical, deep	State of *Shi* ≈ Repletion
At *Jiuwei* RM-15	Heart-*Qi Xu*
At *Zhongwa* RM-12	Spleen and Stomach-*Qi Xu*

At *Shuifen* RM-9	Kidney and Liver-*Qi Xu* or *Yin Xu*
At *Tianshu* St-25	Stagnation
Lateral to *Zhongji* RM-3 & *Guanyuan* RM -4	Kidney-*Yin Xu*

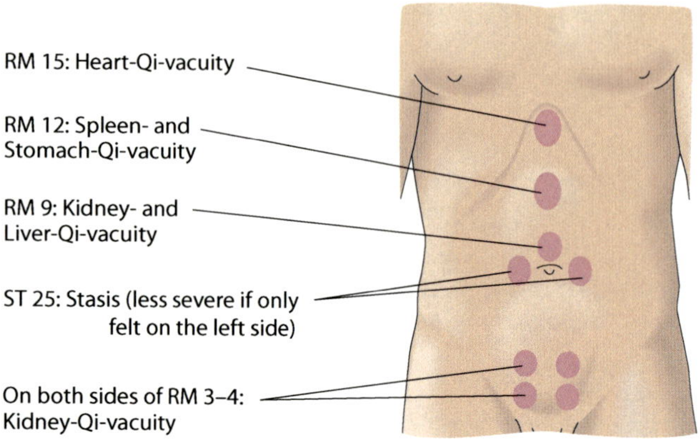

Figure 14.5: Aortic pulsation areas and the five *Zang* ≈ Organ *Xu* ≈ Vacuity

Organ Knots

Organ Knots are pressure sensitive hard knots in the area of the organs and signifying a state of repletion (excess). They usually appear in the season that they dominate according to the *Ke* ≈ Control cycle i.e. Heart in autumn, Lung in spring, Kidney in summer etc.

Solar plexus knot	Heart knot
Left side of the navel; small turtle shaped	Liver knot
Mid-abdominal; small bowl shaped	Spleen knot: Spleen Damp-Cold
Right side of the navel; mobile bowl	Lung knot: Cold-Wind in Lung
Sensation of a moving ball going from the lower abdomen to the upper or even to the throat	Kidney knot: Kidney-*Yin Xu*

Japanese Abdominal palpation

Tension areas on the abdomen are utilized to detect pathology of the Extraordinary Channels. These tension areas are most often combined with other palpational areas (▶ chap. 13.9, Fig. 13.3.b).

14.3 Pulse Diagnosis

[...] the heavens have given us the pulse and the complexion

through these, the old sage is informing us [...].

Pulse Localisation

Pulse of the "Three Regions"

- Heaven: on the carotid artery, *Renying* ST-9
- Earth: the radial pulse, *Taiyuan* LU-9
- Man: Tibial pulse, *Taixi* KI-3, and the foot dorsal artery pulse, *Chongyang* ST-42
- *Taiyuan* LU-9 reflects on the *Qi* of air, *Renying* ST-9 and *Chongyang* ST-42 reflect on the *Qi* of food, and *Taixi* KI-3 represents the hereditary *Qi*. These three regions inform on the quality of *Ying*≈ Nourishing *Qi*, and of *Wei*≈ Defensive *Qi*.

Pulses of the "Nine Regions"

Also referred to as the "Revealing pulses", described in the *Su Wen*; these pulses are taken on different arteries.

- Superior section:
  - Heaven: temple area, *Taiyang* (extra point), for the head *Qi*
  - Earth: cheek area, *Juliao* ST-3, for mouth *Qi*
  - Human: in front of the tragus, *Ermen* TW-21, and *Tiangong* SI-19, for the eye and the ear *Qi*
- Middle section:
  - Heaven: radial area, *Jingqu* LU-8, for Lung *Qi*
  - Earth: hand area, *Hegu* LI-4, for Large Intestine *Qi*
  - Human: cubital pulse, *Shenmen* HE-7, for the Heart *Qi*
- Lower section:
  - Heaven: inguinal pulse, *Zuwuli* LR-10 and *Yinlian* LR-11 for Liver *Qi*, or *Taichong* LR-3 in women
  - Earth: tibial pulse, *Taixi* KI-3, for Kidney *Qi*
  - Human: femoral pulse, *Jimen* SP-11, for the Spleen *Qi,* or the foot dorsal artery, *Chongyang* ST-42 for Stomach *Qi*

The twelve Radial Pulses

This is the most utilized pulse position. *Su Wen* chapter 21 explains the reason for the pulse position: "...the *Qi* of food is extracted by the Stomach, enters the Heart, circulates in the channels; the *Qi* of the 12 channels reaches the Lung; ...the *Qi* portal becomes the *Cun* pulse..."

The radial pulse is situated on the radial artery, below the styloid process. Each pulse is divided into three sections:

- Rear *Chi* ≈ Cubit/ foot: 1 cun from the wrist crease
- Middle *Guan* ≈ Bar or Barrier: right below the styloid corresponding to LU-8
- Front *Cun* ≈ Inch: on the wrist crease corresponding to LU-9

Technique

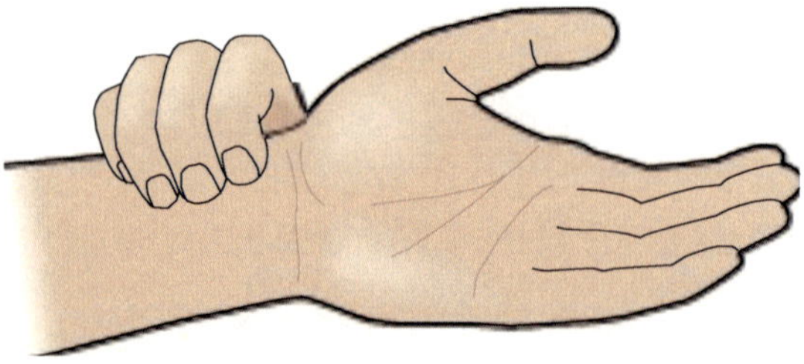

Figure 14.6: Taking the radial pulses

- The patient should either be sitting comfortably, hands on a cushion, or better lying down. Quiet, breathing normally, all constricting objects being removed from the arms, avoid the crossing of the legs
- The practitioner should be relaxed, quiet, preferably with eyes closed. Remembering that we are not taking the pulse but listening to it.
- The right wrist pulse is taken with the left hand and vice-versa.
- The 2nd, 3rd, and 4th fingers are used. The middle finger is placed on the radial artery right below the radial styloid process, the index and ring fingers on either side. (► Fig. 14.6 and 14.7)
- For individual evaluation, starting with the Earth pulses, Stomach and Spleen, on the right middle *Guan* ≈ Bar/ Barrier position.
- Comparing each position with the corresponding position on the opposite side

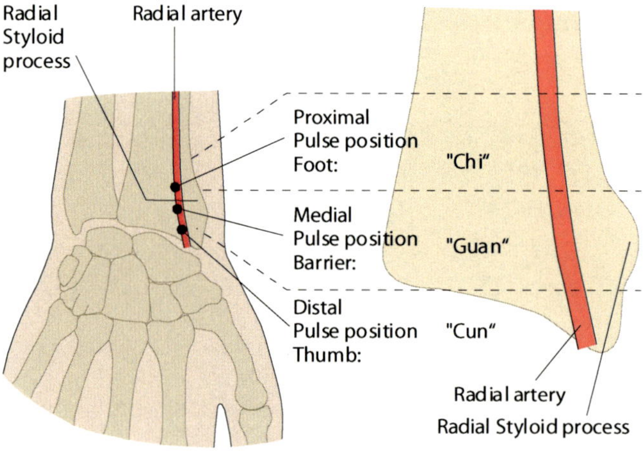

Figure 14.7: The three pulse positions:
***Cun* ≈ Inch/ distal,**
***Guan*≈ Bar/ Barrier/ middle,**
***Chi*≈ Cubit/ proximal**

Depth

The palpation reveals various depths: there are several possible interpretations, according to the method used:

- 2 levels (▶ Fig. 14.8):
  - Surface: *Yang-Fu* ≈ Bowels
  - Depth: *Yin- Zang* ≈ Organs
- 3 levels (▶ Fig. 14.9):
  - Surface: *Qi* in relation with the Lung (= *Wei Qi*)
  - Middle: *Xue* ≈ Blood in relation with the Spleen (= *Ying Qi*)
  - Deep: *Jing* ≈ Essence in relation with the Kidney (= *Zang-Fu)*
- 5 Depths (▶ Fig. 14.10): all five *Zang* ≈ Organs are evaluated on the same point. This method is quite complicated to master and is not commonly used.

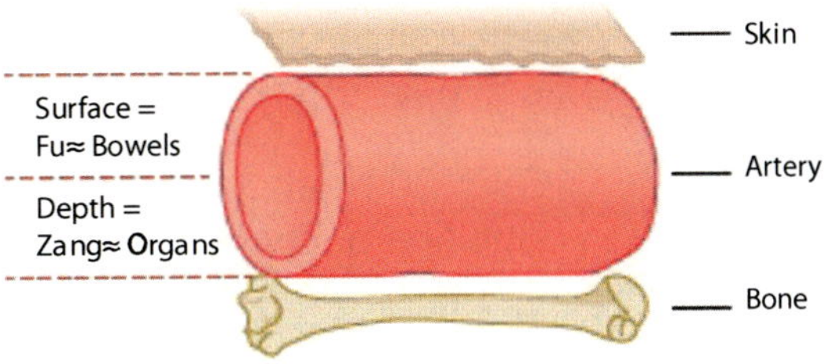

Figure 14.8: Two level pulse reading: *Fu* ≈ Bowels and *Zang* ≈ Organs

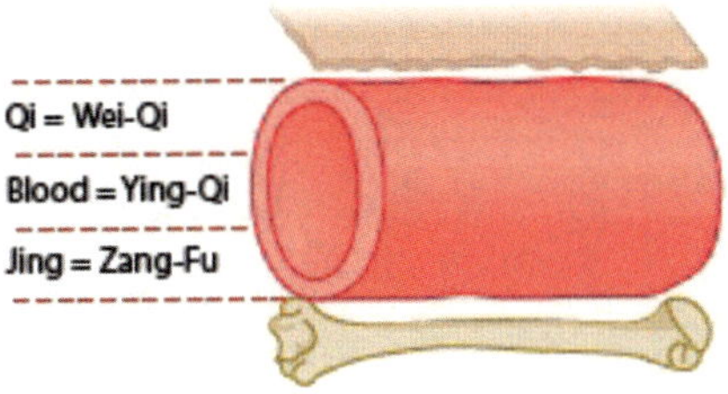

Figure 14.9: Three level pulses reading: *Qi*, Blood, and *Jing*

Qualities

- General pulse qualities are appreciated with all three fingers together.
- Individual qualities are felt by one finger at a time on each pulse position.

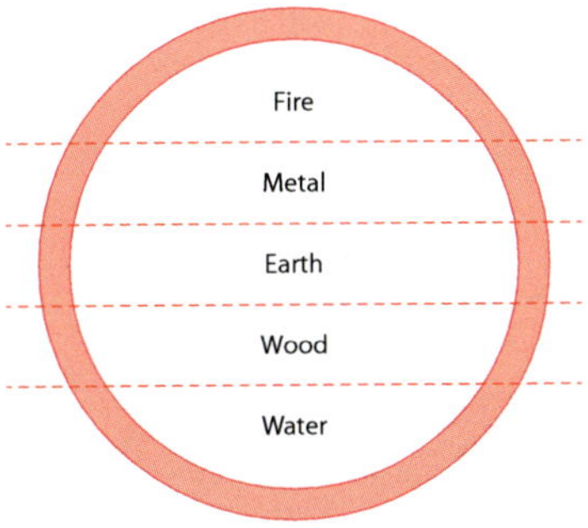

Figure 14.10: Five levels of pulses: Fire-Metal-Earth-Wood-Water.

Interpretation

The results should be compiled through 3 consecutive stages.

Stage I

With all three fingers, appreciate the strength, rhythm, frequency, and root. Compare the Surface/ Depth, Right/ Left; and the three depths.

- Surface and Left: *Yang*
- Depth and Right: *Yin*

In general, the right pulses are more reflective of *Qi*, the left pulses of Blood. In spite of this, in a healthy person, a man's pulse is often stronger on the left side and on the *Cun* ≈ Inch/ distal position, a woman's on the right and *Chi* ≈ Cubit/ proximal position.

There are eight pulse categories that are the most common and could be detected with this simple three-finger pulse taking:

Rapid	Over 80 beats per minute or over 6 beats per breathing cycle: it signifies a *Yang* condition, Heat; nervousness
Slow	Inferior to 65 beats per minute or less than 6 beats per breathing cycle: signifies a *Yin* condition; internal Cold; *Xu*≈ Vacuity/ deficiency. Please note that a slow pulse could also be observed in a healthy person practicing regular sports
Full	Gives an impression of fullness, abundance, and hardness: signifying a *Yang* condition; Heat repletion, Cold or Damp
Empty	The pulse does not offer much resistance to are less distinct and can disappear under pressure; signifies the lack of *Qi* and denotes a *Yin* condition; *Qi*-this pulse pressure, the edges *Xu* ≈ Vacuity or Blood and *Qi Xu*
Floating	This pulse is mainly felt on the surface when the finger is barely touching the skin, often disappearing under pressure: it denotes a *Yang* condition and can be felt mostly in a *Biao*≈ External disease, although it could also signify a "Floating *Yang*" from *Yin* deficiency
Deep	The pulse is submerged in the depth, the fingers have to press almost to the bone in order to feel the pulse: signifying a *Yin* condition, an internal disease, quite often in relation to a Kidney weakness
Slippery	This pulse is said to be rolling like a pearl in water; the pulse presents a roundness and firmness in all of its dimensions: It signifies a fullness of both *Qi* and Blood, it denotes a state of *Shi*≈ Repletion/ excess or stagnation of Dampness, Phlegm, food or of Blood, hence it is considered normal during the menses and pregnancy
Choppy	This pulse is a little more difficult to feel, it is described as fine, short, rough and not flowing. The fingers are placed in a manner as to feel the surface of the pulse, the intensity of the pulse beat is not even and regular, giving the impression that the pulse disappears at times: this pulse denotes a vacuity/deficiency condition of Blood, *Qi* or *Jing*; it may be found after recent blood-loss or after a shock

Stage II

With each finger compare the 3 zones on both sides.

- *Cun* ≈ Inch (distal): Reflects the upper Triple Warmer
- *Guan* ≈ Barrier/ Bar (middle): Represents the middle Triple Warmer
- *Chi* ≈ Cubit (proximal): Represents the lower Triple Warmer

- Also, the comparison of Inch and Bar gives the relation between *Qi* and Blood.

Stage III

With one finger, each pulse position is evaluated on two or three levels, depending on the style of pulse reading.

The pulse quality is noted for each division and depth. It is possible to feel combinations of the pulse qualities, for example, Rapid and Floating, signifying an external Wind-Heat, or Deep and Slow, signifying an internal Cold from *Yang* vacuity. It is recommended to always start with the Earth (Stomach and Spleen) pulses, on the right *Guan* ≈ *Bar* position, using this pulse as a reference (▶ Fig. 14.11).

A comprehensive method of notation should be applied.

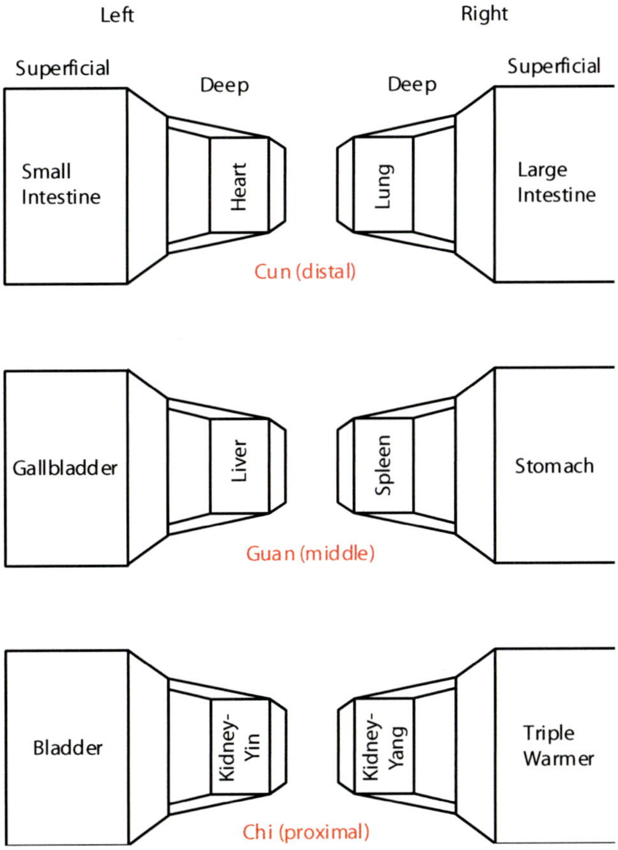

Figure 14.11: *Zang-Fu* Pulse positions according to the Pulse Classic *Wang Shu He* (2nd century)

The Terminology of the 28 Pulses

Table 14.1: Terminology of the 28 Pulses

Pin Yin	Chinese	English	Other names	Yin-Yang	Pulse Quality
Fǔ	浮	Floating	Superficial	*Yang*	Depth
Chén	沉	Deep	Sinking	*Yin*	
Fù	伏	Hidden	Buried	*Yin*	
Shí	實	Full	Replete	*Yang*	Strength
Hóng	洪	Flooding	Overflowing	*Yang*	
Dà	大	Big	Large/ Wide	*Yang*	
Xū	虛	Empty	Vacuous/ Deplete	*Yin*	
Rú	濡	Soft	Soggy	*Yin*	
Wēi	微	Minute	Faint	*Yin*	
Sàn	散	Scattered	Dissipated/ Dispersed	*Yin*	
Ruò	弱	Weak	Frail	*Yin*	
Xì	細	Fine	Thin / Minute	*Yin*	
Xián	弦	Wiry	Bowstring	*Yang* of *Yin*	Tension
Jǐn	緊	Tight	Tense	*Yang*	
Gé	革	Leathery	Drum-skin	*Yang*	
Kōu	芤	Hollow	Onion stalk (stem)	*Yin* of *Yang*	
Láo	牢	Firm	Confined	*Yang* of *Yin*	
Huá	滑	Slippery	–	*Yin* of *Yang*	
Dòng	動	Moving	Stirring (Bean)	*Yang*	
Chí	遲	Slow	–	*Yin*	

Huǎn	緩	Retarded	Slowed-down/ Moderate	*Yin*	Speed, Rhythm
Sè	澀	Choppy	Rough	*Yin*	
Shùo	數	Rapid	Fast/ Accelerated	*Yang*	
Cù	促	Hasty	Agitated/ Skipping	*Yang*	
Jié	結	Knotted		*Yin*	
Dài	代	Intermittent	Interrupted	*Yin*	
Cháng	長	Long	–	*Yang*	Length
Duǎn	短	Short	Brief	*Yin*	

Classification and Description of the 28 Pathological Pulse Qualities

Superficial and Floating pulse categories

Fǔ ≈ Floating Pulse 浮 (Yang)

- Description: Very superficial, it disappears under pressure. (▶ Fig. 14.12.a to ▶ Fig. 14.14.a)
- Significance:
  - External disease
  - In autumn this is a normal seasonal pulse
  - Floating and Tight: *Biao* Wind-Cold or Wind-Heat
  - Floating and empty: Blood and *Jing Xu*
- Differential diagnosis:
  - *Xu* ≈ Empty pulse: is larger and softer
  - *Kou* ≈ Hollow: under pressure disappears but reappears
  - *Ru* ≈ Soft: is without strength

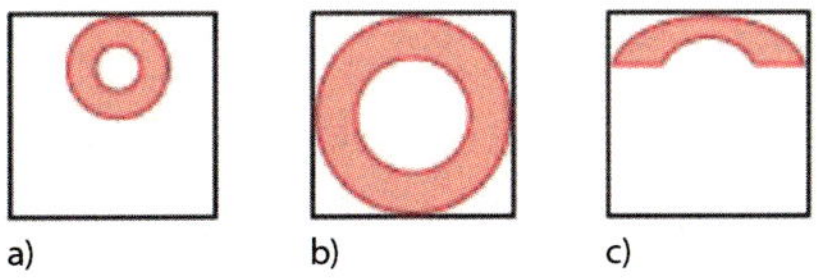

Figure 14.12. Superficial and Floating pulse categories: a) floating pulse, b) hollow pulse, c) drum-skin pulse

Kōu ≈ Hollow Pulse 芤 (Yin of Yang)

- Description: Superficial, big and soft, disappears under pressure and reappears in the depth. The middle is empty the sides full, like an onion stem. (▶ Fig. 14.12.b, and ▶ Fig. 14.14.b)
- Significance

- Loss of Blood or liquids
- *Yin Xu* ≈ Vacuity with apparent Heat

- Differential diagnosis: *Xu*/Empty: is larger and softer and disappears under stronger pressure

Gé ≈ Leathery, Drum-skin Pulse 革 (Yang)

- Description: It is tight and hollow at the same time, and vibrates like the skin of a drum. (▶ Fig. 14.12.c, ▶ Fig. 14.14.c)
- Significance: loss of Blood or *Yin*; in a man could also signify a loss of *Jing*
- Differential diagnosis:
  - *Jin* ≈ Tight pulse: is stronger and firmer
  - *Xian* ≈ Wiry pulse does not disappear under pressure
  - *Lao* ≈ Firm pulse is not felt on the surface and is hard inside

Deep / Sinking pulse categories

Chén ≈ Deep Pulse 沉 (Yin)

- Description: It is sunken and only or mainly felt at the deep level, with stronger pressure. (▶ Fig. 14.13.a and ▶ Fig. 14.14.d)
- Significance:
  - Normal pulse in winter and for the Kidneys
  - Deep and Tight: internal Cold repletion
  - Deep and Empty and Slow: *Yang* and *Qi Xu* ≈ Vacuity
- Differential diagnosis:
  - *Lao* ≈ Firm pulse is also felt on the surface
  - *Fu* ≈ Hidden pulse is difficult to feel

Láo ≈ Firm, Hard, Confined Pulse 牢 (Yang of Yin)

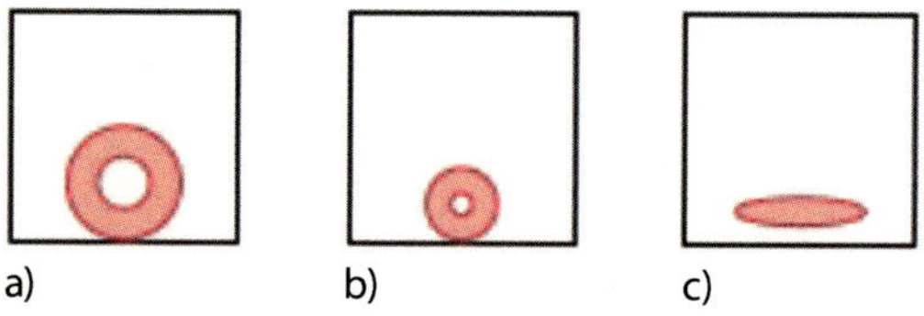

Figure 14.13: Deep, sinking pulse categories:
a) deep pulse,
b) firm (hard, confined) pulse,
c) hidden pulse.

- Description: Fine, long, full, like a string; felt in the Deep position. (▶ Fig. 14.13.b, and ▶ Fig. 14.14.e)
- Significance:
  - Internal repletion of Cold
  - Painful masses, hernia
- Differential Diagnosis:
  - *Shi* ≈ Full pulse is felt on all levels
  - *Fu* ≈ Hidden pulse is hard to feel
  - *Ge* ≈ Leathery pulse has hardness only on the surface

Fù ≈ Hidden Pulse 伏 (Yin)

- Description: It is felt weakly against the bone under strong pressure. (▶ Fig. 14.13.c, ▶ and Fig. 14.14.f)
- Significance:
  - Cold blocking the circulation of *Qi* and Blood
  - Exhaustion of *Yin* and *Yang*
  - Fainting, *Jue* ≈ Reversal
- Differential Diagnosis:
  - *Chen* ≈ Deep pulse is clearly felt under pressure
  - Duan ≈ Short pulse is only short and clearly felt in the *Guan* ≈ Bar zone

Slow pulse categories

Chí ≈ Slow Pulse 遲 (Yin)

- Description: Very slow, less than 4 beats per breath (<65/min), small and weak. (▶ Fig. 14.14.g)
- Significance:
  - Disease of *Yin Zang* ≈ Organs
  - Cold repletion; Internal Cold, *Yang Xu* ≈ Vacuity
- Differential Diagnosis:
  - *Se* ≈ Choppy pulse is slow but rough
  - *Jie* ≈ Knotted pulse has irregular stops
  - *Xu* ≈ Empty pulse is floating and soft.

Huǎn ≈ Relaxed, Moderate Pulse 緩 (Yin)

- Description: Harmonious flow, 4 beats/ breath, soft like a loose rope. (▶ Fig. 14.14.h)
- Significance:
  - Normal pulse for Spleen, and the Fifth Season
  - External Dampness; Spleen and Stomach-*Qi Xu* ≈ Vacuity
- Differential Diagnosis:
  - *Chi* ≈ Slow: is slower and less soft
  - *Jie* ≈ Knotted: has irregular stops

Jié ≈ Knotted Pulse 結 (Yin)

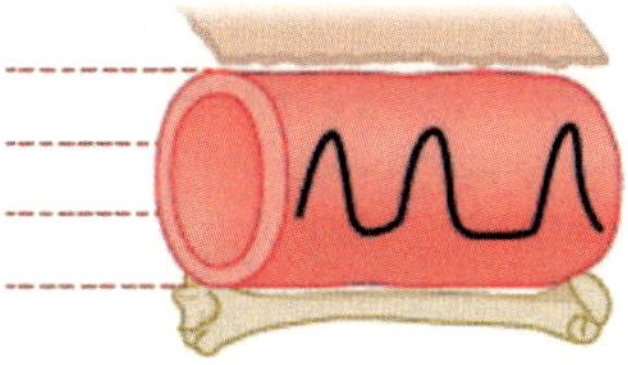

Figure 14.15: Knotted pulse.

- Description: Slow pulse with occasional (irregular) stops. (▶ Fig. 14.15 and ▶ Fig. 14.19.a)
- Significance:
  - Blood stasis from Cold-Damp
  - *Qi* stasis from *Yin Shi* ≈ Repletion
- Differential Diagnosis: *Dai* ≈ Intermittent pulse stops at regular intervals

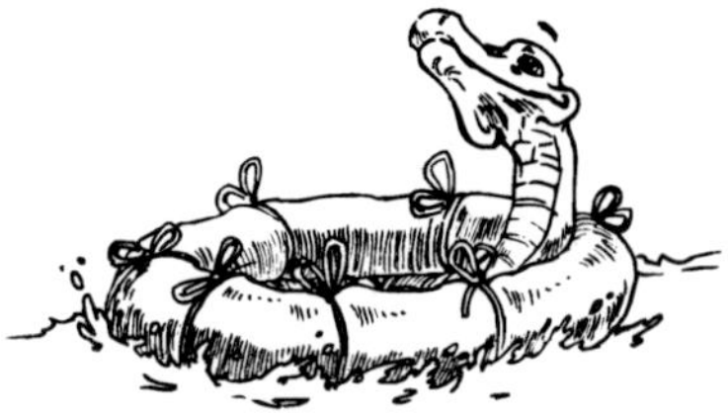

a- Floating Pulse - Fŭ

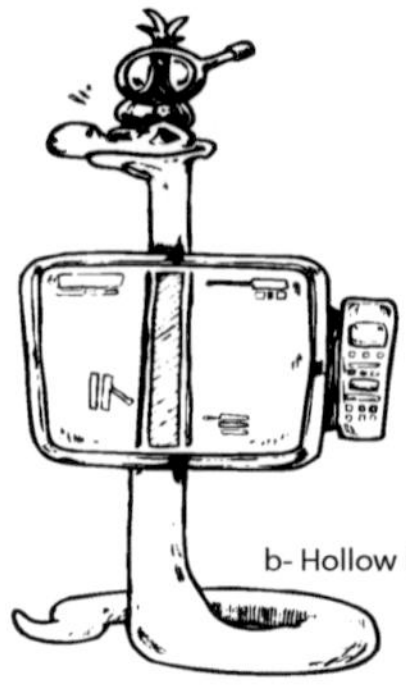

b- Hollow Pulse - Kōu

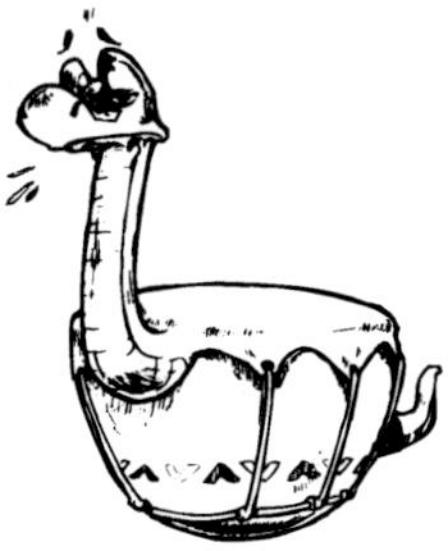

c- Leathery/ Drum-skin Pulse -Gé

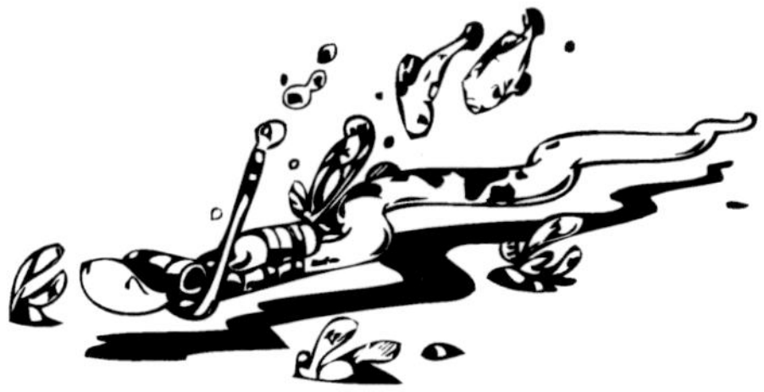

d- Deep Pulse - Chén

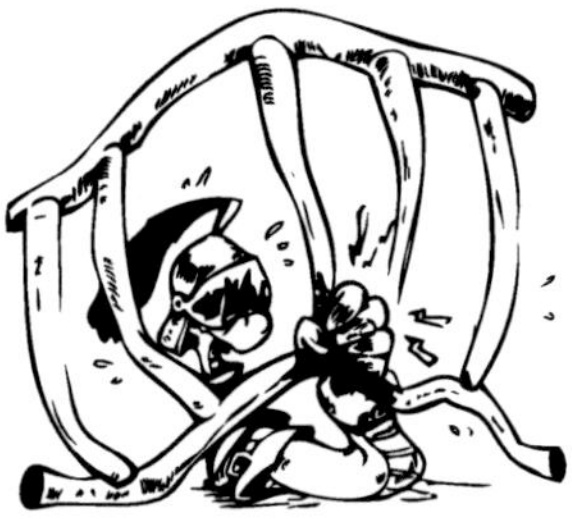

e- Firm/ Hard/ Confined Pulse - Láo

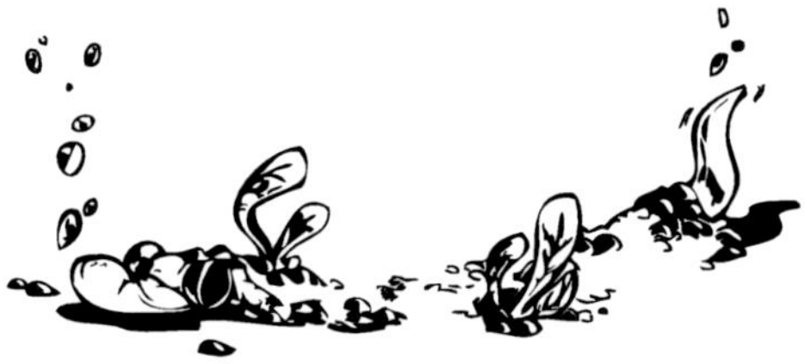

f- Hidden Pulse - Fù

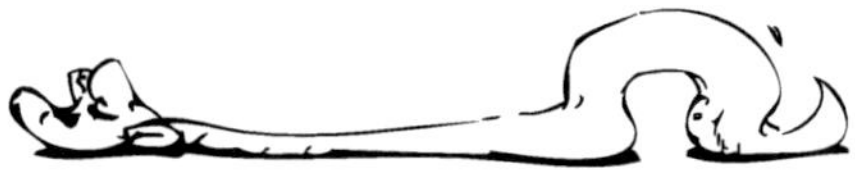

g- Slow Pulse - "Chí"

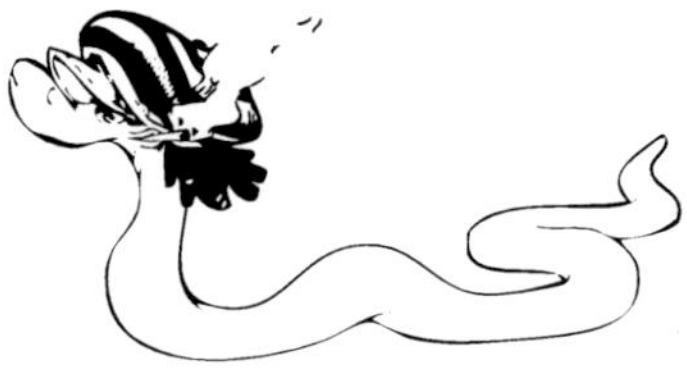

h-Relaxed/ Moderate Pulse - Huan

Figure 14.14 The pulse illustrations inspired by Dr. B. Chmielnicki (I), extracted from "Pulsqualitäten der chinesischen Medizin auf einen Blick".

Dài ≈ Intermittent Pulse 代 (Yin)

- Description: Weak and slow, stops as though it could not start again, at regular intervals. (▶ Fig. 14.19.b)
- Significance:
  - Exhaustion of the 5 Zang//organs; Yuan Qi Xu//vacuity
  - 100th day of pregnancy
  - Pain, fear, convulsions
- Differential Diagnosis:
  - *Cu* ≈ Hasty pulse also stops but starts right away
  - *Jie* ≈ Knotted pulse stops at irregular intervals

Fast pulse categories

Shùo ≈ Rapid, Fast Pulse 數 (Yang)

- Description: over 5 beats/ breath: over 80 beats/ minute (▶ Fig. 14.19.c)
- Significance:
  - Normal in infants, during effort or emotions
  - Rapid and Full: Heat repletion
  - Rapid and Thin: Heat from *Yin* deficiency
- Differential Diagnosis:
  - *Hua* ≈ Slippery is round and rolls under the finger
  - *Cu* ≈ Hasty has irregular stops
  - *Dong* ≈ Moving pulse is erratic, with no head or tail

Cù ≈ Hasty Pulse 促 (Yang)

- Description: Fast with intermittent irregular stops (arrhythmia). (▶ Fig. 14.19.d)
- Significance:
  - Yang-Shi ≈ Repletion; stagnant Qi
  - Blood or Phlegm stasis
- Differential Diagnosis: *Jie* ≈ Knotted is slower and softer with irregular stops.

Slippery pulse categories

Huá ≈ Slippery Pulse 滑 (Yin in Yang)

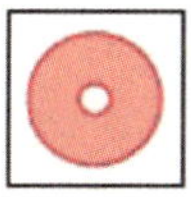

Figure 14.16: Slippery pulse

- Description: Round, firm, smooth, slides and rolls under the finger like a pearl in water. (▶ Fig. 14.16, ▶ Fig. 14.19.e)
- Significance:
  - In a healthy person: abundant *Ying* ≈ Nourishing and *Wei* ≈ Defensive *Qi*
  - In women: an abundance of Blood; or on the Spleen position: menses
  - In women in all 6 positions: signifies pregnancy
  - In a sick person: accumulation of Dampness, Phlegm or food
- Differential Diagnosis:
  - *Shi* ≈ Full pulse is strong and hard

- *Jin* ≈ Tight pulse s like a twisted rope untwisting
- *Dong* ≈ Moving pulse is less slippery, more erratic, felt in one zone only

Dòng ≈ Moving Pulse 動 (Yang)

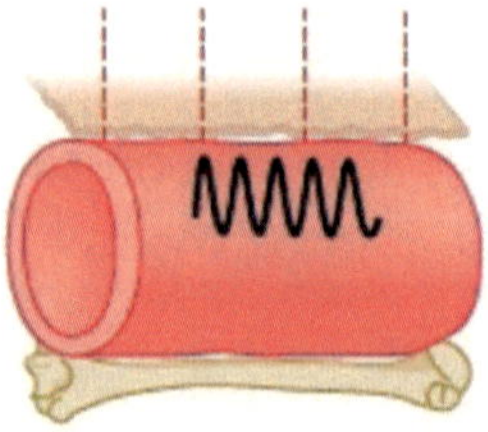

Figure 14.17: Moving pulse

- Description: Fast, and slippery, moves up and down like a bean and is usually felt only at the *Guan* ≈ Bar zone. (▶ Fig. 14.17, and ▶ Fig. 14.19.e)
- Significance:
  - Pain or great fear, shock
  - In women in the Kidney position: pregnancy
- Differential Diagnosis:
  - *Duan* ≈ Short pulse is neither fast nor slippery
  - *Hua* ≈ Slippery is more calm, flowing and smooth

Choppy pulse categories

Sè ≈ Choppy Pulse 澀 (Yin)

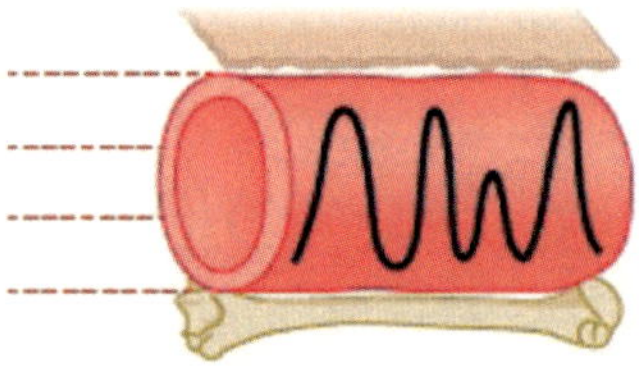

Figure 14.18: Choppy pulse: irregular in strength

- Description: Slow and thin, irregular in strength, it's movement is difficult and does not return when the pressure is released, rough like touching bamboo knots (▶ Fig. 14.18, and ▶ Fig. 14.19.g).
- Significance:
  - Blood and *Qi* stasis from Cold
  - Blood and *Qi Xu; Jing Xu*
- Differential Diagnosis:
  - *Chi* ≈ Slow pulse is slower
  - *Ru* ≈ Soft pulse is more floating and soft
  - *Ruo* ≈ Weak pulse is deeper and weaker
  - *Wei* ≈ Minute pulse is soft, tiny and vague

Empty pulse categories

Xū ≈ Empty Pulse 虛 (Yin)

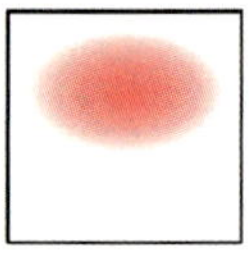

Figure 14.20: Empty pulse

- Description: Slow and big, with indistinct edges, it is superficial and becomes weak and soft under pressure. (▶ Fig. 14.19.h, ▶ Fig. 14.20)
- Significance: Vacuity of *Qi* and/or Blood
- Differential Diagnosis:
  - *Ru* ≈ Soft pulse is fine and weak
  - *Kou* ≈ Hollow pulse is empty in the middle but with clear edges (described as an onion stem)
  - *Se* ≈ Choppy pulse does not return when the pressure is released
  - *San* ≈ Scattered pulse is irregular in strength and rhythm and disappears under pressure

Rú ≈ Soft, Soggy 濡 (Yin)

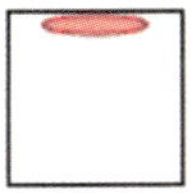

Figure 14.21: Soft (soggy) pulse

- Description: Superficial and fine, like cotton soaked in water, disappears with pressure. (▶ Fig. 14.21, ▶ Fig. 14.29.a)
- Significance:
  - Dampness
  - Exhaustion of Blood, *Qi*, and *Jing*
- Differential Diagnosis:
  - *Xu* ≈ Empty pulse is larger
  - *Wei* ≈ Minute pulse is very fine and vague
  - *Ruo* ≈ Weak pulse is very similar but is only felt in deeper levels

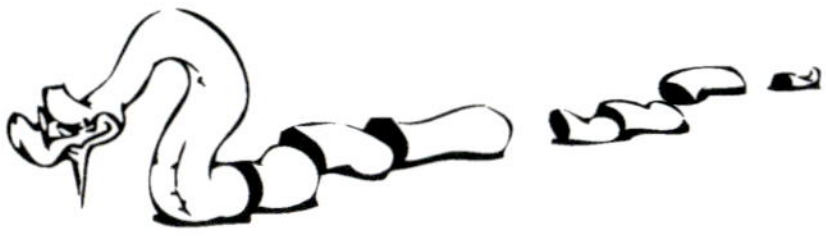

a- Knotted Pulse - Jié

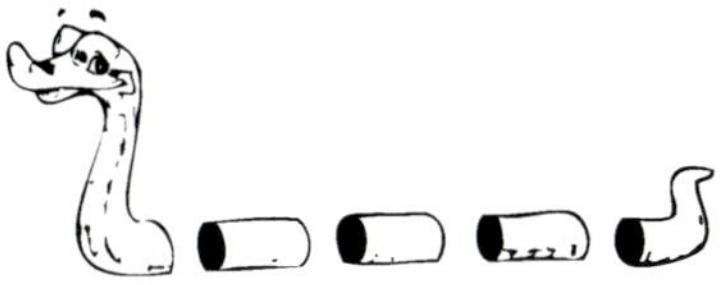

b- Intermittent Pulse - Dài

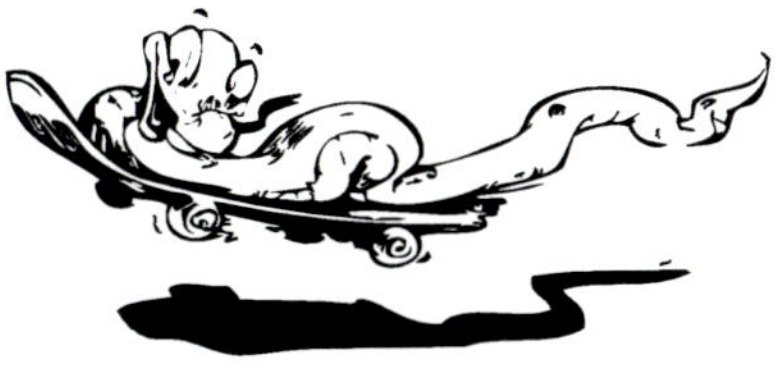

c- Rapid/ Fast Pulse - Shùo

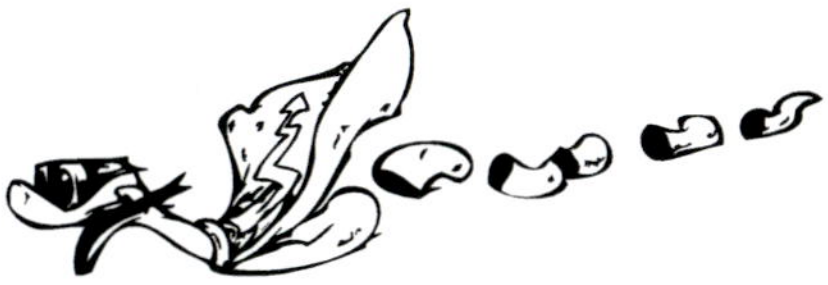

d- Hasty Pulse - Cù

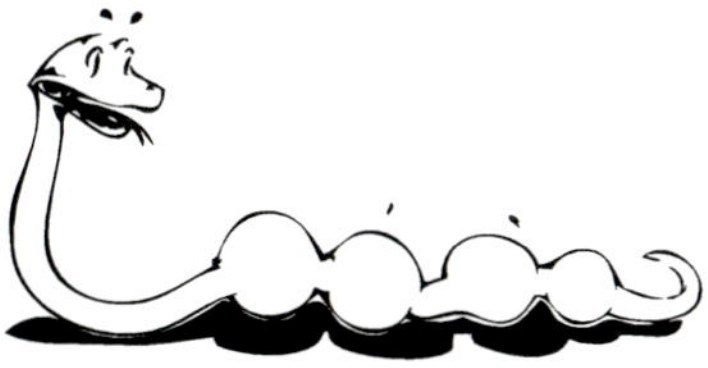

e- Slippery Pulse - Huá

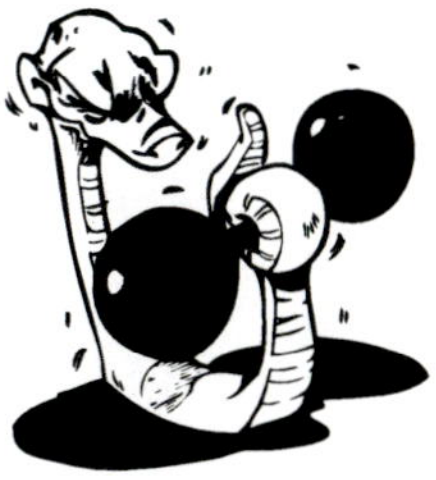

f- Moving Pulse - Dòng

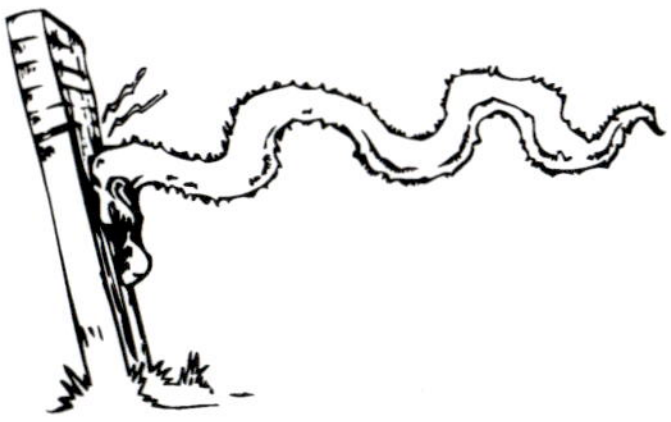

g- Choppy Pulse - Sè

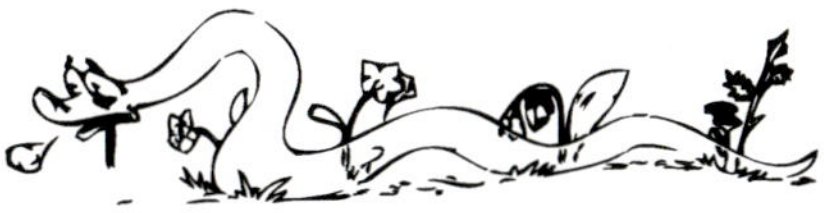

h- Empty Pulse - Xū

Figure 14.19 : The pulse illustrations inspired by Dr. B. Chmielnicki (II), extracted from "Pulsqualitäten der chinesischen Medizin auf einen Blick.

Wēi ≈ Minute 微 (Yin)

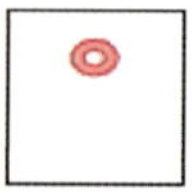

Figure 14.22: Minute pulse

- Description: Very fine and soft and vague under pressure, seems to fade out. (▶ Fig. 14.22, ▶ Fig. 14.29.b)
- Significance:
  - In acute conditions: Collapse of *Yang*
  - In chronic conditions: Heart and Kidney-*Yang Xu*, fatigue
- Differential Diagnosis:
  - *Ruo* ≈ Weak pulse is soft and deep but is clearly felt
  - *Xi* ≈ Fine pulse is thin like a silk string but is felt clearly

Sàn ≈ Scattered Pulse 散 (Yin)

- Description: Superficial and irregular rhythm and strength, disappears under pressure. (▶ Fig. 14.23, ▶ Fig. 14.29.c)
- Significance: Exhaustion of *Yin*, *Yang*, and Blood
- Differential Diagnosis: *Xu* ≈ Empty pulse is larger and more regular

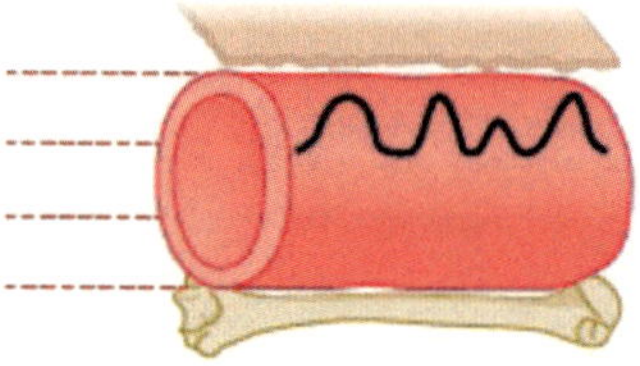

Figure 14.23: Scattered pulse

Ruò ≈ Weak Pulse 弱 (Yin)

- Description: Soft, fine, thin felt only in deeper levels. (▶ Fig. 14.24, and ▶ Fig. 14.29.d)
- Significance:
  - The vacuity of Blood and *Qi*, in a chronic disease
  - Constant anxiety
- Differential Diagnosis:
  - *Wei* ≈ Minute pulse is finer and very blurred
  - *Ru* ≈ Soft pulse is very similar but can also be felt on the surface
  - *Xi* ≈ Fine pulse is like a silk thread at all levels

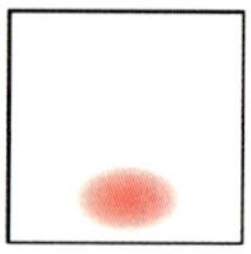

Figure 14.24: Weak pulse

Xì ≈ Fine (Thin) Pulse 細 (Yin)

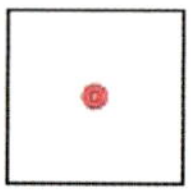

Figure 14.25: Fine (thin) pulse

- Description: Discrete and very fine like a silk thread (all levels), but distinct. (▶ Fig. 14.25, and ▶ Fig. 14.29.e)
- Significance:
  - Thin and Fast *Yin* and Blood *Xu*
  - Thin and Empty: Chronic Blood and *Qi Xu*
- Differential Diagnosis: *Wei* ≈ Minute pulse is fine but blurs under pressure

Duǎn ≈ Short Pulse 短 (Yin)

- Description: Seems not to quite make it to its normal location, is often felt in the Inch or Cubit. (▶ Fig. 14.26, and ▶ Fig. 14.29.f)

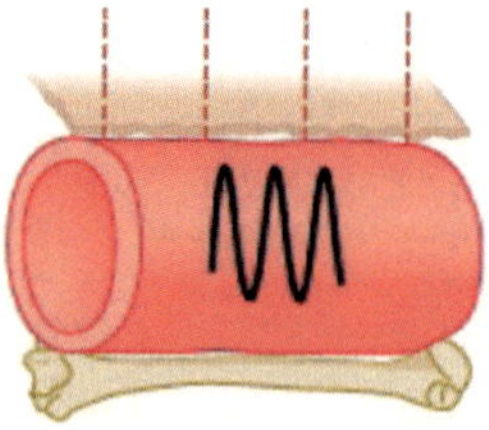

Figure 14.26: Short pulse

- Significance: Severe *Qi Xu* (especially of the Stomach)
- Differential Diagnosis:
  - *Fu* ≈ Hidden pulse is found under the tendons
  - *Dong* ≈ Moving pulse is only felt at the Bar and is fast and slippery

Full pulse categories

Shí ≈ Full Pulse 實 (Yang)

- Description: Big, strong and large and firm at all three levels. (▶ Fig. 14.27, and ▶ Fig. 14.29.g)

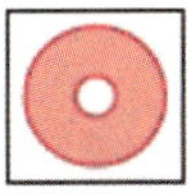

Figure 14.27: Full pulse

- Significance:
  - Repletion/ Excess
  - Full and Fast: Heat repletion
  - Full and Tight and Slow: Cold repletion
  - Full and Slippery: Damp accumulation
- Differential Diagnosis:
  - *Xian* ≈ Wiry pulse is harder like a guitar string
  - *Hua* ≈ Slippery is less large, more round and rolling
  - *Hong* ≈ Overflowing pulse is still larger but diminishes under pressure

Hóng ≈ Overflowing, Flooding Pulse 洪 (Yang)

- Description: Very large but gets weaker under pressure. Like a wave, comes strong and then fades away. (▶ Fig. 14.28, and ▶ Fig. 14.29.h)
- Significance: Normal in summer or for the Heart pulse.
  - Flooding and Full and Fast: Fire repletion, internal Heat
  - Flooding less large and Slow: *Qi Xu* ≈ Vacuity; Heart-*Yin Xu*
- Differential Diagnosis:
  - *Shi* ≈ Full pulse is harder and does not fade out.
  - *Hua* ≈ Slippery is rounder and smoother and rolls like a pearl.
  - *Da* ≈ Big pulse is not as strong.

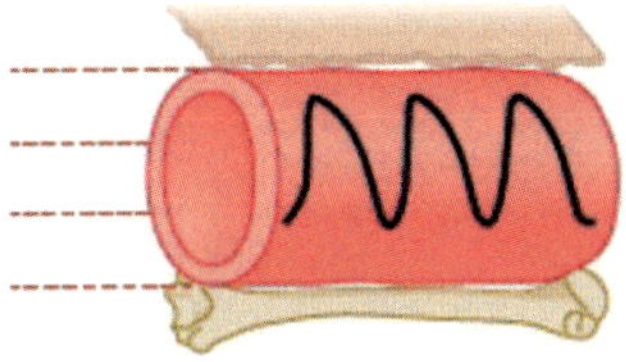

Figure 14.28: Overflowing (flooding) pulse

Dà ≈ Big, Wide Pulse 大 (Yang)

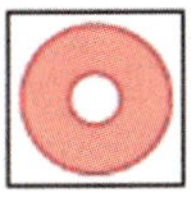

Figure 14.30: Big (wide) pulse

- Description: is big and very broad and long. (▶ Fig. 14.30, ▶ Fig. 14.34.a)
- Significance:
  - Repletion; repletion of *Yang*
  - Big and Empty: *Qi-Xu*// vacuity
  - Differential Diagnosis:
  - *Chang* ≈ Long pulse is longer.
  - *Hong* ≈ Overflowing pulse is larger and stronger.

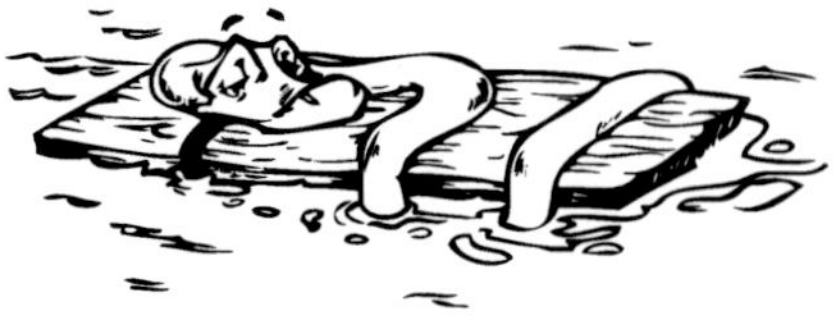

a- Soft/ Soggy - Rú

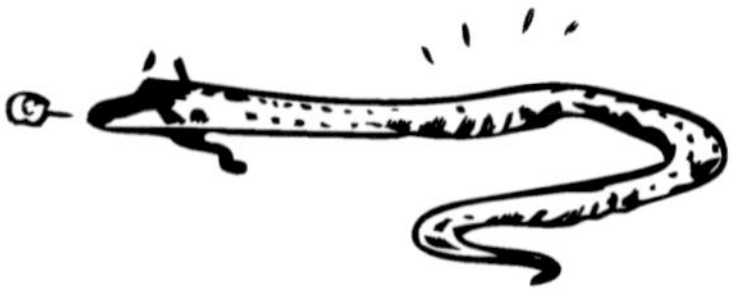

b- Minute - Wēi

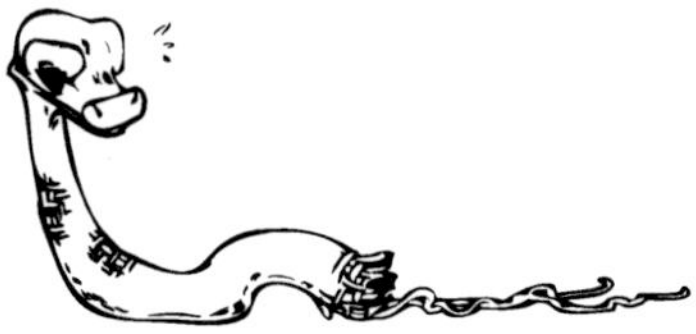

c- Scattered Pulse - Sàn

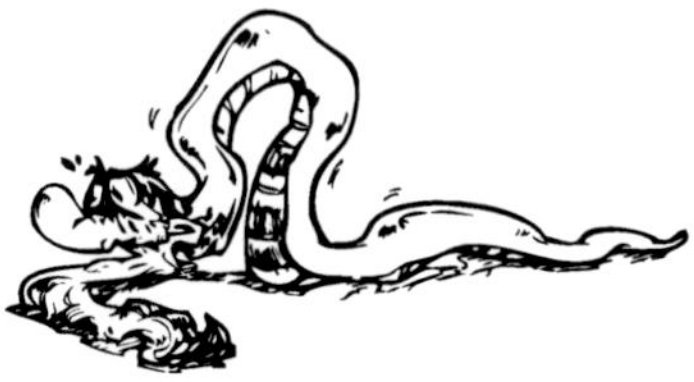

d- Weak Pulse - Ruò

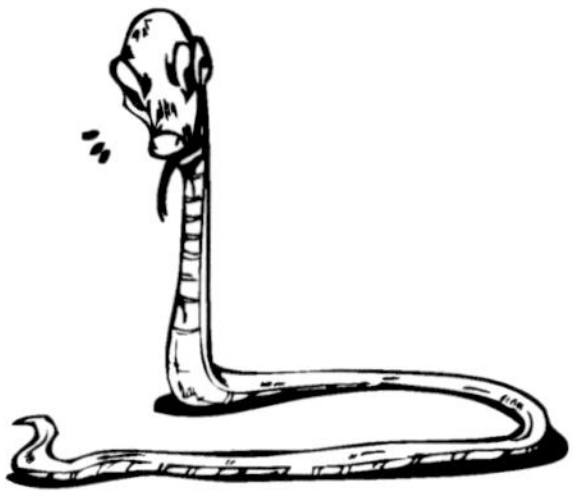

e- Fine (Thin) Pulse - Xì

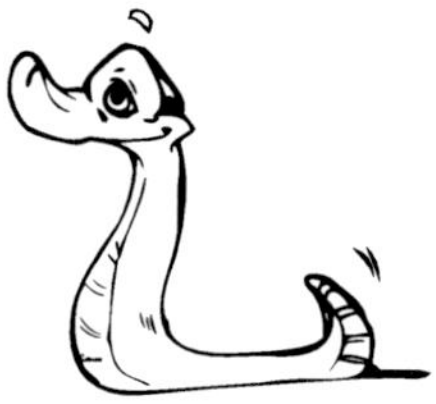

f- Short Pulse - Duan

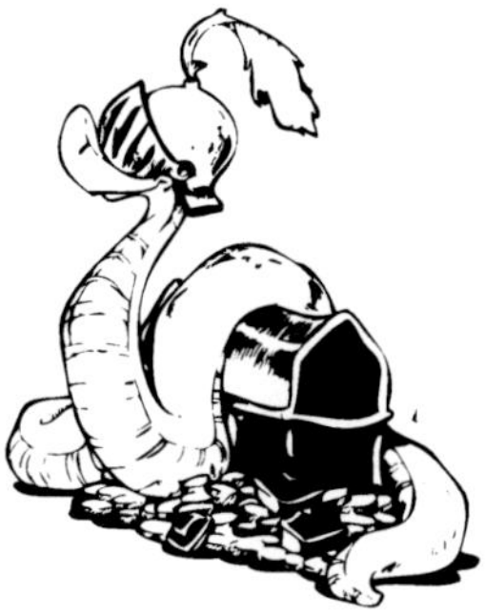

g- Full Pulse - Shí

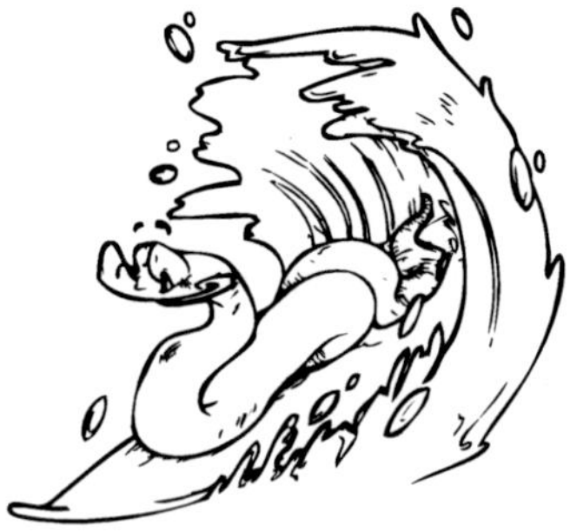

h- Overflowing/Flooding Pulse - Hóng

Figure 14.29: The pulse illustrations inspired by Dr. B. Chmielnicki (III), extracted from "Pulsqualitäten der chinesischen Medizin auf einen Blick

Xián ≈ Wiry Pulse 弦 (Yang of Yin)

- Description: Straight and long and hard like the lower (thin) strings of a guitar, hits hard and evenly, does not vibrate much. (► Fig. 14.31, and ► Fig. 14.34.b)

- Significance:
  - Normal in Spring
  - In pathology: Liver-*Qi* or Blood stasis; Liver-Wind; pain
  - Wiry and Empty: *Qi* stasis and *Qi Xu*
  - Wiry and Choppy: Blood stasis and Blood *Xu*

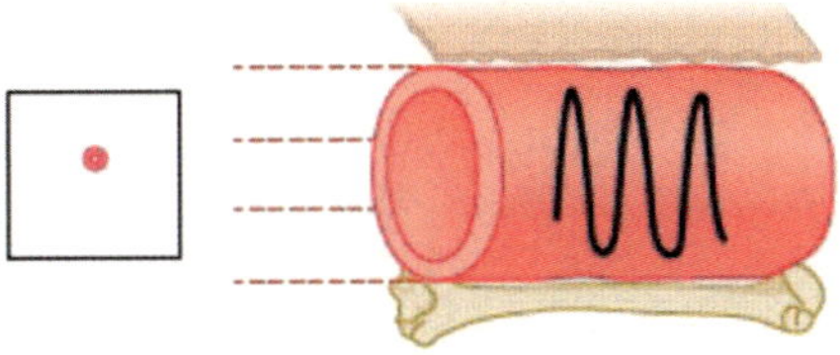

Figure 14.31: Wiry Pulse

- Differential Diagnosis:
  - *Jin* ≈ Tight pulse is thicker and moves about like an unwinding rope
  - Ge ≈ Leathery pulse is tight outside but soft inside

Jǐn ≈ Tight Pulse 緊 (Yang)

- Description: Hard, moving with force but not consistent; vibrates like a twisted rope that is untwisting. Or the thicker strings of the guitar. (► Fig. 14.32, and ► Fig. 14.34.c)
- Significance: Internal or external Cold

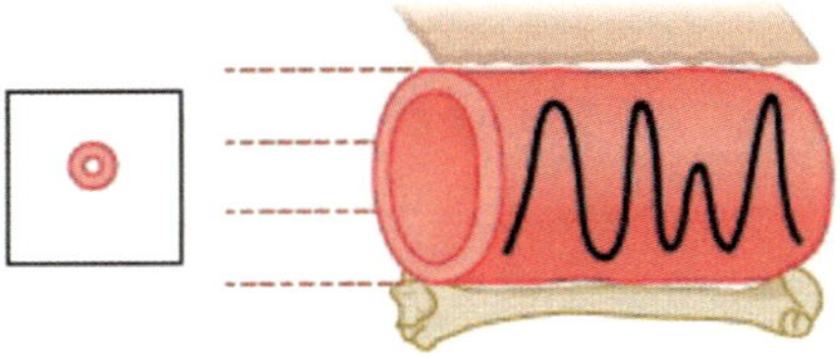

Figure 14.32: Tight pulse

- Differential Diagnosis:
  - *Xian* ≈ Wiry pulse is harder like a violin cord but not vibrating
  - *Ge* ≈ Leathery pulse is more resistant on the surface but empty inside

Cháng ≈ Long Pulse 長 (Yang)

- Description: Neither big nor small but felt beyond its normal position. (► Fig. 14.33, and ► Fig. 14.34.d)
- Significance:
  - Normal in a healthy person.
  - Long and Wiry: Repletion; Heat in the *Yang Ming*
- Differential Diagnosis:
  - *Da* ≈ Big pulse is larger but not longer
  - *Hong* ≈ Overflowing pulse is larger but gets weaker under pressure
  -

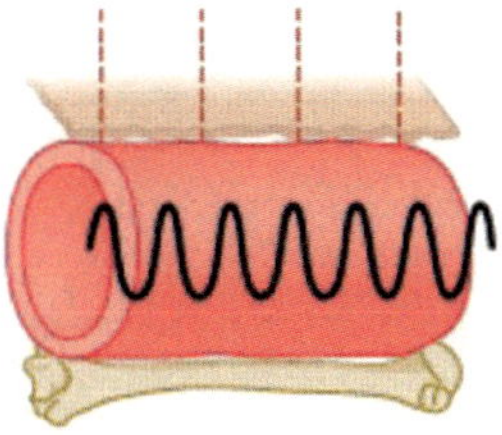

Figure 14.33: Long pulse

Dangerous Pulse Signs

The following pulses are considered to represent dangerous conditions:

- Intermittent pulse with loss of weight, no other symptoms
- Knotted pulse with *Qi* and Blood stasis
- Soft pulse with night-sweats: exhaustion of Blood and *Jing*
- Minute pulse: severe exhaustion
- Scattered pulse: *Qi* and Blood vacuity
- Leathery pulse in chronic diseases.
- Fast:
  - 5-6 beats per breath, hard and big

  - 9 beats hasty and strong or small, hollow, irregular
- Slow:
  - 2 beats, without consistency, irregular
  - 1-3 beats, arriving fast, leaving slow
- Complex forms:
  - Overflowing and Weak: exhaustion of body fluids.
  - Short, hard, found in the bar zone: separation of *Yin* and *Yang*
  - Slippery and Full: coagulation of Phlegm
  - Slippery and Weak
  - Jumpy formless pulse

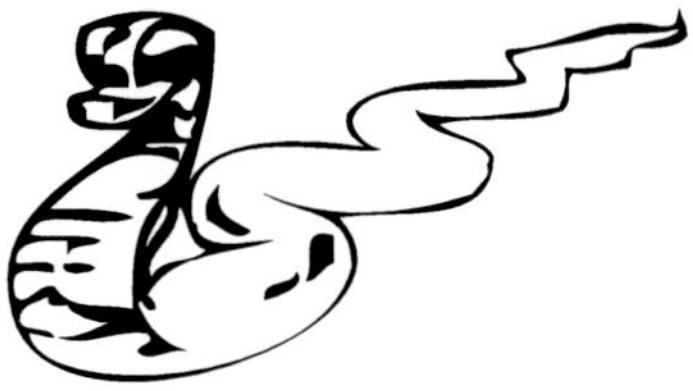

a- Big (Wide) Pulse - Dà

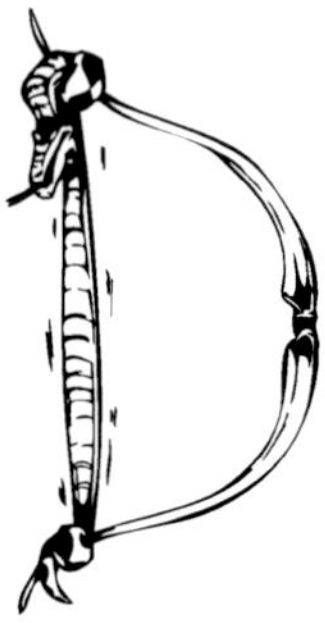

b- Wiry Pulse - Xián

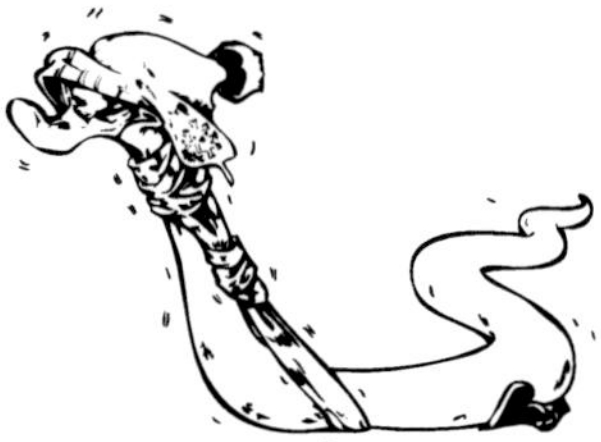

c- Tight Pulse - Jin

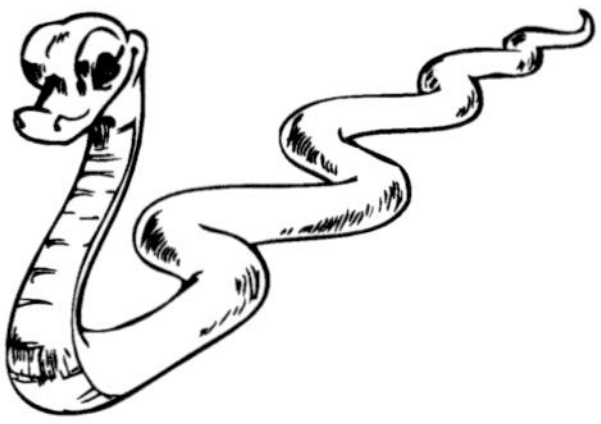

d- Long Pulse - Cháng

Figure 14.34 : The pulse illustrations inspired by Dr. B. Chmielnicki (IV), extracted from "Pulsqualitäten der chinesischen Medizin auf einen Blick"

Seasonal and Daily changes of the pulses

- Spring: The general pulse is *Xian* ≈ Wiry, with predominance on the Liver pulse. If there is too much external wind the pulses become Fu ≈ Floating and Wiry.
- Summer: The pulses are *Hong* ≈ Overflowing, with predominance on the Heart pulse; if there is too much external heat it becomes *Da* ≈ Big.
- Fifth Season: The pulse is *Jin* ≈ Tight if there is too much humidity the pulse becomes *Ru* ≈ Soft.
- Fall: The pulse is *Fu* ≈ Floating or *Ru* ≈ Soft if there is too much climatic dryness, the pulse becomes *Dai* ≈ Intermittent.
- Winter: The pulse is *Chen* ≈ Deep and *Lao* ≈ Firm, if the weather is too cold, the pulse becomes *Shuo* ≈ Rapid, especially in the *Chi* ≈ Cubit/ proximal zone.

- Daily, the pulses show an energy tide during their corresponding time, reflecting the flow of energy to the respective organs.

Pulse changes during Pregnancy

The pulse is *Hua* ≈ Slippery in all 6 levels. Furthermore, in normal conditions, the stage of the pregnancy may be determined:

- *Hua* ≈ Slippery and *Jin* ≈ Tight: 3 months
- *Jin* ≈ Tight pulse with no pathology: 5 months
- A *Se* ≈ Choppy pulse in a pregnant woman announces complications.
- Evaluation of the sex of the fetus:
  - Male fetus: *Cun* ≈ Inch (distal) pulses are stronger than *Chi* ≈ Cubit (proximal) and left Kidney stronger than the right Kidney and in general left pulses stronger than the right pulses.
  - Female fetus: *Chi* ≈ Cubit (proximal) stronger than *Cun* ≈ Inch (distal), right Kidney stronger than the left; in general right pulses stronger than the left.

Pulses for the 8 Extraordinary vessels according to Li Shi Zhen

Certain pulse qualities may also reveal the disturbances of the Extraordinary vessels:

Chong Mai	Deep, Wiry, Tight and Firm
Du Mai	Floating, Wiry and Long
Ren Mai	Deep, Long, Tight and Thin especially in the *Guan* and *Cun* positions
Yin Wei Mai	Deep, Big, Full that rolls to the thumbor to *Cun* (distal) position
Yang Wei Mai	Floating, Big, Full that rolls to *Chi* (proximal) position
Yin Qiao Mai	Left-right vibration and Tight on the *Chi* (proximal) position
Yang Qiao Mai	Left-right vibration and Tight on the *Cun* (distal) position
Dai Mai	Left-right vibration and Tight on the *Guan* (Barrier)

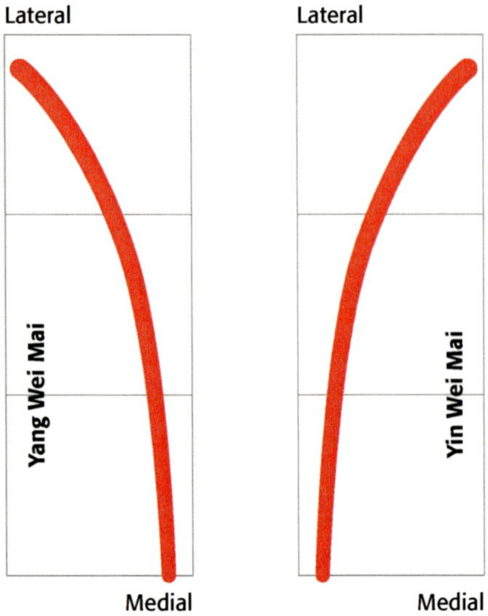

Figure 14.35: Pulses of *Yin* and *Yang Wei Mai* according to Li Shi Zhen

Pulses of the 8 Extraordinary vessels according to Master J. Yuen

Chong Mai	Deep, Wiry, Tight and Floating on the Chi ≈ Cubit position
Du Mai	Empty, Wiry, Tight and also Floating on the Chi position
Ren Mai	Moving (Bean) or Soft and Choppy, or Hollow and Tight
Yin Wei Mai	Thready, Choppy and Rapid
Yang Wei Mai	Floating, Slippery and Rapid
Yin Qiao Mai	Left-right vibration and Weak and Empty
Yang Qiao Mai	Left-right vibration and Full
Dai Mai	Left-right vibration and Tight and Slippery

15. A Comprehensive Approach to Diagnosis

Quite often to perform a complete and proper diagnostic investigation is not compatible with our Western medical structures as it definitely takes too much time. It is quite unfortunate that most practitioners of acupuncture and TCM, revert to the symptomatic treatment of a complaint, and find it unnecessary or even wasteful to explore the patient's history or other signs and symptoms. Furthermore, some of the diagnostic skills require certain talents, such as the capacity to observe, being able to smell, the taking of pulses or the palpational dexterity, do not come naturally to every person. The ability to observe, at a mere glance, has the great advantage of informing the practitioner on the patient's constitution and temperament, as well as giving valuable information about the condition of the disease and possibly the organs involved. The advantage of olfactory acuity is to inform the therapist in a fraction of a second about certain conditions such as a Liver *Qi* stasis or Kidney *Qi* deficiency, or even certain emotional states of a patient. Taking the pulses can proffer a wealth of information, but it takes years of practice to master. The Western physicians are much more trained in the gathering of information through anamnesis. Still, this interrogation needs to be done in a systematic and comprehensive manner. It has to be stressed that there are no conditions minor enough to justify dispensing with a proper diagnosis. Of course our main concern, as therapists, is to respond primarily to a patient's chief complaint. But as often as not, there are related or unrelated factors in the life of a person that might need even more attention.

The following check-list that can easily be modified to personal preferences.

Patient information	• Name and Date of birth (useful for stems and branches calculation) • Particulars/ profession
Chief Complaint	• Since when; frequency and timing; outer circumstances • The 8 Diagnostic principles; for pain: a scale of 0 to 10
Medical History	• Birth and early childhood conditions; vaccinations • In order: Disease; operations; accidents; hospitalizations
Anamnesis	
Head and Neck	• Headaches; migraines • Ears: Otitis; deafness; tinnitus; vertigo ... • Nose: rhinitis; hay-fever; frequent colds; sinusitis; anosmia • Eyes: vision problems; conjunctivitis; other ... • Mouth: stomatitis; halitosis, teeth, and Gums

	• Throat: angina; loss of voice; plum-pit; Thyroid problems...
Sleep	• Duration; hypersomnia; insomnia, disturbed sleep section (initial – middle – end); General state upon waking (rested or tired) • Parasomnia: hunger or thirst; restless legs; hot flashes; Night sweating; Palpitation; pruritis; bruxism, sleep apnea • Dreams: nightmares; emotional state when waking from a dream (worry, fear, frustration and anger ...)
Heart & Lungs	• Chest pains; palpitations; oppression; circulation problems • Blood pressure • Bronchitis; asthma; shortness of breath • Smoking
Digestive System	• Appetite; indigestion; gastritis; ulcers,; nausea and vomiting • Food intolerance: fats, dairy, alcohol, eggs, gluten ... • Hypoglycemia; diabetes • Abdominal pains; bloating; tired after meals • Bowel movement: constipation, diarrhea (frequency), alternating stools • Stools: soft stools; hard stools; goat pellets; undigested food; mucous or blood • Hemorrhoids
Genital System	• Cycles: regular, irregular, duration • Periods: duration; amount; aspect (color, consistency); clots • Premenstrual syndrome: pelvic cramps; lumbar pains; breast distension; migraines; moods ... • Endometriosis; ovarian cyst; myoma; discharge; infections • Breasts • Pregnancy or infertility/ Contraception • Menopause: symptoms • Sexual energy; libido; sexual difficulties • In men: prostatic problems / erectile problems
Urinary System	• Urinary frequency, amount, color, night urination, incontinence • Cystitis; nephritis; kidney stones; prostatitis
Osteo-articular System	• Dorsal pains: lumbar spine/ Thoracic spine/ Cervical spine • Shoulders (trapezius area) • Upper limbs: Shoulders, Elbow, Wrist, Hand, and fingers • Lower limbs: Hip; knee; ankle; foot and toes
Skin, Hair,	• Dermatitis: eczema; psoriasis; acne ; pruritis; heat; redness;

Nails	swelling; Hair-loss; dandruff; dermatitis of the scalp • Shape and quality of nails; color
Sweating and Body Tempera-ture	• Sweating: absent; spontaneous, night-time; hands; feet; head; chest; armpits • A feeling of Heat; hot extremities; hot head • Felling of Cold; cold feet; cold hands
Neurological System	• Neuralgia; hyperesthesia; hypoesthesia; paresthesia • Paralysis: flaccid or spastic; area • Uncontrolled movements: tremors; epilepsy ... • Speech impediments • Muscle cramps or muscle weakness
Mental Functions	• Memory; concentration; excessive mental activity; • Obsessive worry; fixations ...
Psycho-emotional Profile	• Depression; sadness; stress; anger; moodiness; anxiety; nervousness; obsession ... • Fear and phobias • Evaluation of the Temperament
Energy	• Tiredness after effort, heaviness/ after mental effort or eating, • Habitual energy drop at a certain time ...
Observation	
5 Element Correspon-dence System	• Body shape and constitution • Temperament and behavior (constitution and temperament are important in understanding the root of the disease and further help to orient the best therapeutic strategy and acupuncture point selections) • Preferences and dislikes: climates, colors, tastes, foods, smells, emotions • Seasonal manifestations
General Facial diagnosis	• Facial shape and contours • Colors, moles, wrinkles ...
Body and Mobility	• Particular deformities; chest; spine; knees; feet ...; posture (relation of the "Bony structures" and the spinal curvatures; the balance of the muscles and sinews) • Disturbed (hampered) mobility • Presence of scars (establishing if a scar is active : causing a local stagnation of Qi and Blood or disturbing the corresponding Channel flow with distal manifestations)

Physical Examination	
Tongue	• Color; shape, coating ...
Pulse	• General speed, rhythm; quality; the 3 zones and the 3 levels .
Abdominal Palpation	• Organic zones and Aortic pulsations • *Mu* points
Point Palpation	• Back Shu, Mu, Special Mu, Sian (emotional), *Luo, Xi, Yuan* • Lower *He*, Master points, Meeting points, Barrier points, … • *Ah Shi* points and tension areas

PART V- Tools and Treatment Modalities in Chinese Medicine

16. Scope of treatment

The "Branch-Knot and Root" principles applied in diagnosis, will have defined the site, cause, and condition of a disease. In all logic, the treatment also aims at relieving the manifested symptoms, the site of the disturbance, followed by eradicating the causative factor, as well as treating the root condition in the patient. The latter is the deeper root of the disease having permitted the pathological process to evolve. This is one of the great strengths of Chinese medicine, even in the absence of symptoms, by balancing the basic energetic structure of a person; it may prevent the occurrence of disease, a veritable preventative medicine.

The importance of this concept was so salient in the Chinese way of thinking that during a certain period, physicians employed for treating affluent families, only received payment when the whole household was healthy, their stipend would stop when any member of the family got sick. This could possibly explain the fact that *Hoa To*, as early as the 2nd century, attempted a rudimentary method of vaccination, by diluting a drop of urine or sweat from the sick person in 100 drops of water and administering it to the whole household. This primitive approach to inoculation was abandoned a few centuries later, as it was further understood that supporting the *Zheng* ≈ Upright energy of a person was paramount to preventing disease.

It is unfortunate that today, most practitioners of Chinese medicine, are simply treating the manifestations and relieving symptoms, rather than aiming at the deeper roots of disease.

> *[...] a good physician cures a disease,*
> *but the superior physician prevents it from occuring [...].*

Chinese medicine offers a wide range of tools and methods that could be very roughly classified as external, such as acupuncture, moxibustion, and *Tuina/ Anmo*-massage. The common denominator to the external therapies is the fundamental concept of the *Jing-Luo*, the rivers, and channels that constitute the pathways of *Qi* and the energetic structure of the body. By stimulating certain points, the circulation of *Qi* in the channels can be influenced, hence having an effect on the deeper organs and their functions. Other methods are classified as internal, including herbal remedies and diet. These methods act directly on the energetics of the inner organs. But be it external or internal, the treatment and healing depend on the intervention of another person, and hence are in the domain of the *Wai Dan* ≈ Outer elixir (path). The true healing, transformation, and salvation can only come from within, the *Nei Dan* ≈ Inner elixir (path), and this through practices such as *Qi Gong* or *Tai Ji*, as well as the cultivation of the mind and meditation.

17. External Therapies

17.1 Acupuncture (Zhen Jiu 针灸)

History

Although acupuncture is the best known of the Chinese healing methods, historically it seems to have possibly originated from Korea. In fact, the oldest Chinese medical texts the Mawangdui silk scrolls (circa 250 B.C.), discovered in the 1970s, cover various aspects of therapy, lifestyle, health exercises, herbal treatments, and cauterization but not acupuncture. Whatever its origin, acupuncture greatly developed in China, and many of the acupuncture techniques of stimulation, as practiced today, find their origin in the manual techniques of *Tuina* massage. The use of iron needles appeared around the second century, prior to that it would seem that acupuncture might have been performed using slivers of stone or bamboo.

With the development and refining of the use of iron, the needles became thinner and less aggressive.

Acupuncture reached France as early as the 19th century, but was popularized only in the early period of the 20th century by Soulié de Morant and his extensive writings, and further propagated in Europe by his student Dr. de la Fuye. Although acupuncture is based on exactly the same principles as acupressure massage or moxibustion, it has been the subject of extensive debate in Europe as to who is authorized to practice it. The penetration of the skin by a needle is considered a medical act and is argued to be reserved to medical personnel only. Strangely the same debate does not concern tattoo artists, who also penetrate the skin! Another concern, involving the needles, was the fear of infection; especially of viral infections such as HIV or hepatitis C. In Europe, this risk is presently being avoided by the use of disposable and single-use needles.

During the last Chinese dynasty, acupuncture fell into disfavor with the emperor, who disliked needles and encouraged herbalism as a therapeutic modality. Chinese herbal medicine, became even more popular during the earlier years of the Chinese Republic, as it resembled more the Western, scientific and allopathic medicine. In 1914, there was even an attempt by the Marxist regime, to abolish Chinese medicine as accumulated "garbage" of centuries. Although later, *Mao Tse Tung* declared Chinese medicine a "Great Treasure House", and hence Chinese medicine was called Traditional as opposed to Western medicine. But the newly labeled Traditional Chinese medicine (TCM) had lost all its classical roots and dimensions. Acupuncture was considered to be a mere form of reflex therapy. The acupuncture points were assigned simple properties, similar to those of herbal remedies, and point combinations were constructed exactly as herbal prescriptions would be structured. Fortunately, while the Chinese regime was struggling with their new identity, classical acupuncture had already spread and taken root, not only in neighboring countries, such as Japan and Vietnam but especially in France and Europe. Many classical texts were translated, and a European tradition was already well established. Would it, therefore, be too presumptuous to state that the expansion of "Classical" Chinese medicine in Europe, especially in France, may have been an inspiration for the Chinese practitioners to take a deeper look into the classical texts and the oral traditions that had been forced underground for almost a century?

Needles

Historically the ancient acupuncturists carried a pouch containing the "Nine Traditional" needles, having very specific shapes and length based on chapter 1 of the *Ling Shu* (▶ Fig. 17.1).

Chan needle, arrow-shaped	For superficial and external diseases
Yuan needle, rounded tip	For superficial massage
Di needle, rounded tip	Not for needling, superficial conditions
Feng needle, sharp	For bleeding
Pi needle, sword-shaped	For lancing an abscess
Yuan Li , thick, rounded	For acute conditions
Hao needle, fine and sharp	For *Qi* obstruction, the common needle used in acupuncture
Chang needle, fine, long and sharp	For Bi-obstruction and Wei-atrophy
Da needle, round, pointed	For articular swellings

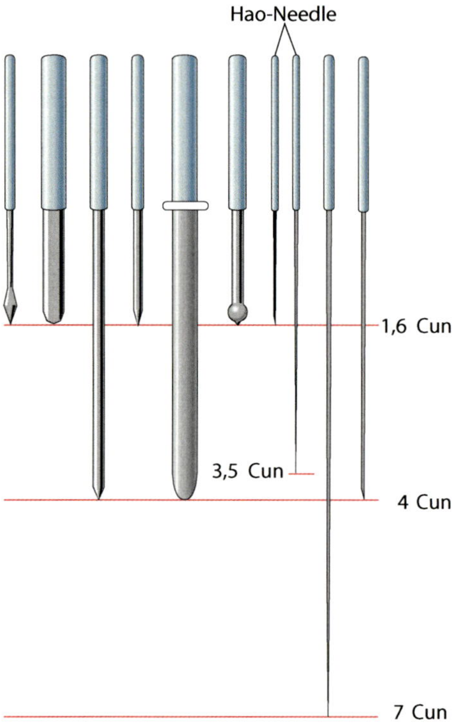

Figure 17.1: The Nine Traditional Needles according to *Ling Shu Jing*

Today only the *Hao Zhen* ≈ *Filiform* needle, a fine, hair-like, and sharp needle is used in daily practice. Even the *Feng* needle, is replaced by disposable lancets for the purpose of blood-letting. The *Hao* needles may be made of gold, silver, alloys or steel. The gold and silver needles are costly and difficult to manipulate, and their traditional use is not really justified. The most common needles are made of stainless steel, quite flexible, resisting heat and corrosion.

In the West, acupuncturists are currently using disposable stainless steel needles, pre-sterilised and vacuum packed, with a large choice of diameters and lengths. There are even choices of needle handles ranging from steel to copper or even plastic. Some newer generation needles are silicone coated to facilitate the penetration into the skin. When the needles are very thin, many Western practitioners favor using a tube to insert the needle. The guide tube has the double advantage of being more comfortable both for the patient and the practitioner as well as offering a more sterile manipulation by eliminating the need to touch the body of the needle (▶ Fig. 17.2).

The length of the needle is given in *Cun* ≈ Body inch or millimeters, the most commonly used lengths being 0.5 to 3 *Cun*. The diameter is often described in millimeters or in gage, the higher gauge representing thinner needles.

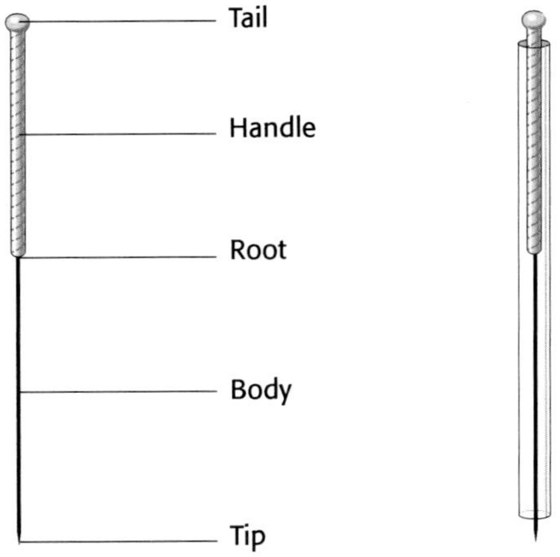

Figure 17.2: Filiform needle and guide tube.

Table 17.1: Thickness of the needle

Gauge	26	28	30	32
Diameter (mm)	0.45	0.38	0.32	0.26

Methods and Techniques

There are numerous varieties of acupuncture methods and techniques, from the superficial needling of the Japanese acupuncture to the deeper needling of the Chinese method, attempting to reach the proper channel depth and obtain a needle sensation, termed *De Qi* ≈ Obtaining the *Qi* (▶ Fig. 17.3).

The concept of *De Qi* is a subjective sensation, mostly felt by the patient, but at times by the practitioner as well, and might include one or a combination of the following sensations: numbness, itching, tightness, swelling, radiating sensation felt along the channel pathway. Please note that a stronger pain is not considered *De Qi* and could result from the puncture of a nerve, a vein or the contraction of a muscle resulting from an improper manipulation of the needle. An electric sensation along the channel is the ideal sensation of *Qi*, again not to be confused with the electric shock-like sensation produced when a nerve is punctured, the latter is quite painful and unpleasant, appears immediately and fast, and quite often the sensation will persist for several days. Once the *De Qi* is obtained, certain manipulation techniques would then aim at producing a further sensation of heat, of cold or the, sought after radiating electric sensation along the desired portion of the channel. For example, when treating an eye pathology, if the *Fengchi* GB-20 is needled, the desired sensation should propagate to the eye area: or when treating a gynecological problem, the *Sanyinjiao* SP-6 point is punctured, the needle is manipulated in order to have the sensation travel up to the pelvic area. Some practitioners insist on obtaining this sensation and would remove the needle after obtaining the *De Qi*. In general, more than 80% of the patients would feel this sensation. It is believed that a strong *De Qi* reflects an accumulation or repletion of *Qi* at that point, this could be the case with *Ah-Shi* (pain) points or major *Jia* ≈ Crossing points. An absence of *De Qi*, in spite of the correct localization of the point,

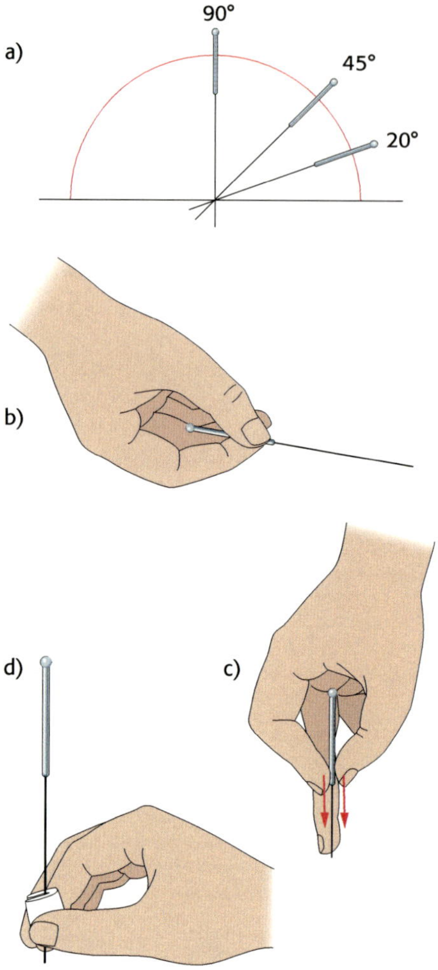

Figure 17.3: Various angles and techniques of needle insertion:
a) the insertion angle mainly depends on the anatomical structure,
b) holding the needle firmly between thumb and index at the root,
c) perpendicular insertion, the middle finger is used as an axis, the thumb and index push the needle in a piston-like movement,
d) insertion of a long needle by holding it at the tip, using a sterile gauze.

could signify a *Xu* ≈ Vacuity/ deficiency condition and would require a supplementing treatment. Quite often the patient would feel the *De Qi* in the subsequent sessions.

Between the single point-treatment of some traditions to the insertion of multiple needles, which constitutes the most common modality, there are as many schools of thought and technique, as there are practitioners around the world. Although some practitioners may treat one point at a time, removing them before treating the next point, in general, it is agreed that the combined and simultaneous action of the needles is preferable. Six to twelve points are treated in one session, the needle insertion is not painful and the manipulation of the needle, the direction, depth, strength and vibration, all depend on the desired effect, simply resumed as:

Supplementing, "Tonification"	"*Bu*" (补)
Reduction, "Dispersion"	"*Xie*" (泻)
Harmonization, stimulation	"*Ping Bu Ping Xie*" (平补平泻)

The treatment time is variable and in general, depends on the age of the patient, and the site and nature of the disease, as well as the channels, treated. The needles may be left between five minutes when treating an acute condition, involving the superficial *Jing Jin* ≈ Sinew channels, to up to thirty minutes for diseases of the interior and when treating the Extraordinary vessels or the *Jing Bie*≈ Divergent channels. Intradermic or permanent needles, in the shape of a wheat grain or thumbtack, may also be applied for on-going stimulation, and are often used in Auriculotherapy.

The body permanent needles are much less utilized today because of the risk of infection; it is advised to use gold or silver needles, less likely to cause irritations (▶ Fig. 17.4).

Another dermal stimulation may be obtained by the tapping of a hammer like instrument with small needle points at the tip, called the "plum blossom" needle or the "seven-star" hammer. This instrument is ideal for treating larger zones; the strength of tapping could be adapted to the patient and type of disease. Today, we dispose of hammers with disposable heads that guarantee safe use (► Fig. 17.5).

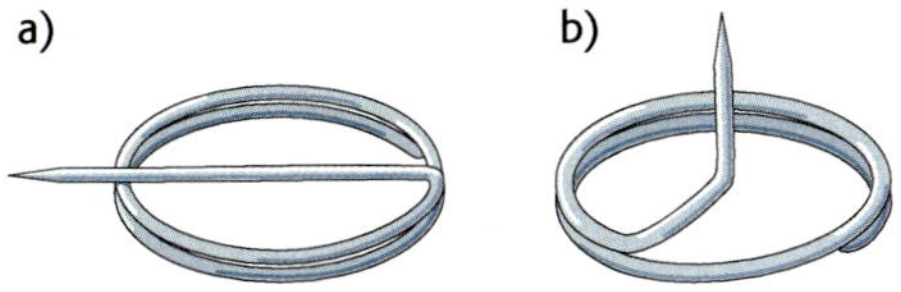

Figure 17.4: Intradermal needles: a) wheat grain or b) thumbtack

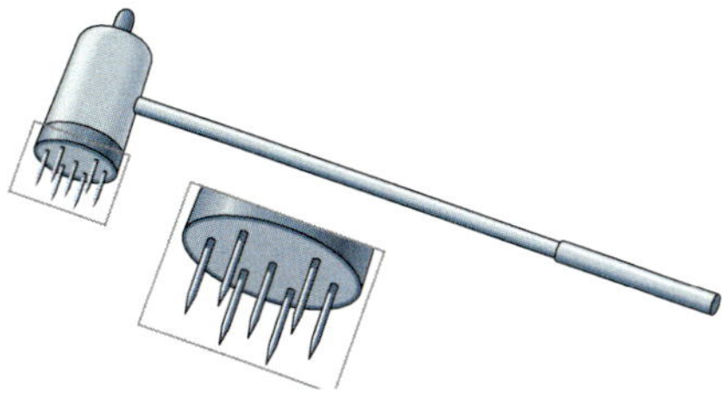

Figure 17.5: Plum-blossom needle also called the Seven-star hammer

Usually, children are not needled under the age of seven. Special care is taken when treating exhausted patients as to number and choice of points, lesser needles are used in children and the elderly, and certain points are avoided in pregnancy. Otherwise, there are no contraindications to needling providing proper hygiene is respected.

Besides using heat, pressure or cupping, a number of modern-day stimulation methods of the acupuncture points may replace the traditional needles:

- Electro-stimulation, originally developed in China for the purpose of analgesia during surgery;
- Laser therapy, commonly with a mid-laser infrared, which has a superior penetrating capacity to the older Helium-neon lasers used in Auriculotherapy. This method constitutes the ideal stimulation mode for small children or persons who are afraid of needles, although in my experience it is less effective than needles in adults;
- Chromotherapy: the use of color filters to stimulate a point with a colored light;
- Certain non-invasive therapies, based on the Chinese channel concepts have been integrated into acupuncture practice, such as Electro-acupuncture according to Dr. Voll (EAV). The original EAV was later complemented with homeopathic remedies for balancing the channels. The addition of the computer technology has even allowed for digitalized vibrations to replace the homeopathic information.
- Other techniques are derived from point-stimulation without keeping the original Chinese concepts, such as Point injection therapy, Trigger points, and Dry Needling, as well as Mesotherapy which consists of multiple injections of various types of substances into the subcutaneous tissues.

17.2 Microsystems

Based on the principle that each body part reflects the whole, in the image of a hologram, several therapeutic systems have been developed, generally referred to as Microsystems:

Auriculo-therapy

History

The whole body is represented on the ear. The *Neijing* already mentioned the connection of the Six *Yang* channels directly with the ear auricle and of the Six *Yin* channels via the Divergent *Yang* channels. During the Tang Dynasty, the first ear points are mentioned in treatment protocols. It is not before the 60's that some systematic research was conducted in China, to verify the action of the ear points. Over the years more than 220 points have been described on the two sides of the ear. In France in the '50s, a similar tradition initiated by Dr. Nogier was named Auriculo-medicine. Dr. Nogier devoted his life to Auriculotherapy and developed the main somatotopic map of the "inverted fetus" on the ear. His work has been expanded by many researchers, not least of all the Chinese, who took his findings to the test on vast numbers of treatment subjects. Thus, Dr. Nogier is rightly known as the “Father of Auriculotherapy”. The Chinese research had the great advantage of being more adapted to the principles of Chinese medicine, whereas Nogier’s Auriculo-medicine is more geared to the Western medical concept.

Method

The ear points are selected based on classical indications and point reactivity, by pressing on the point or by modern point-detectors, which measure the skin’s electrical resistance. A reduced resistance signifying a disturbance of the related organ, body part or function.

There are three categories of ear points:

- Local points: are ear points associated with a specific body area or organ. Points on the left ear relate to the left side of the body; right ear to the right side of the body.
- Masterpoints: these points complement most treatment protocols. All have a wide-ranging effect. Most have more than one name to describe the same point by different sources (Chinese, German, French, and English). Masterpoints are divided into 2 sub-sets: Primary and Secondary. They are mainly used on the dominant ear
- Functional points are mainly used on the dominant ear; there are two types:
- Chinese Functional points are based on the Five Phase correspondence system; for example, the Liver point would be used for eye problems...
- French and Chinese Empirical points: usually their name describes their use, for example. Libido point, Aggressivity point, etc. (▶ Fig. 17.6).

Treatment protocols usually consist of at least 2 of the 3 categories of points. Typically, the local points are applied first, followed by one or two Master points, followed by one or two functional points.

The ear-point stimulation may be achieved through needling, blood-letting, moxibustion, electro-stimulation, laser or color filters, and even massage.

The ear also offers the added advantage of being used for on-going stimulation with seeds, magnets or intra-dermal permanent needles. In this case, the patient is instructed to press or massage the point several times a day for the duration of the treatment.

The precautions and contraindications of ear acupuncture are the same as for general body acupuncture.

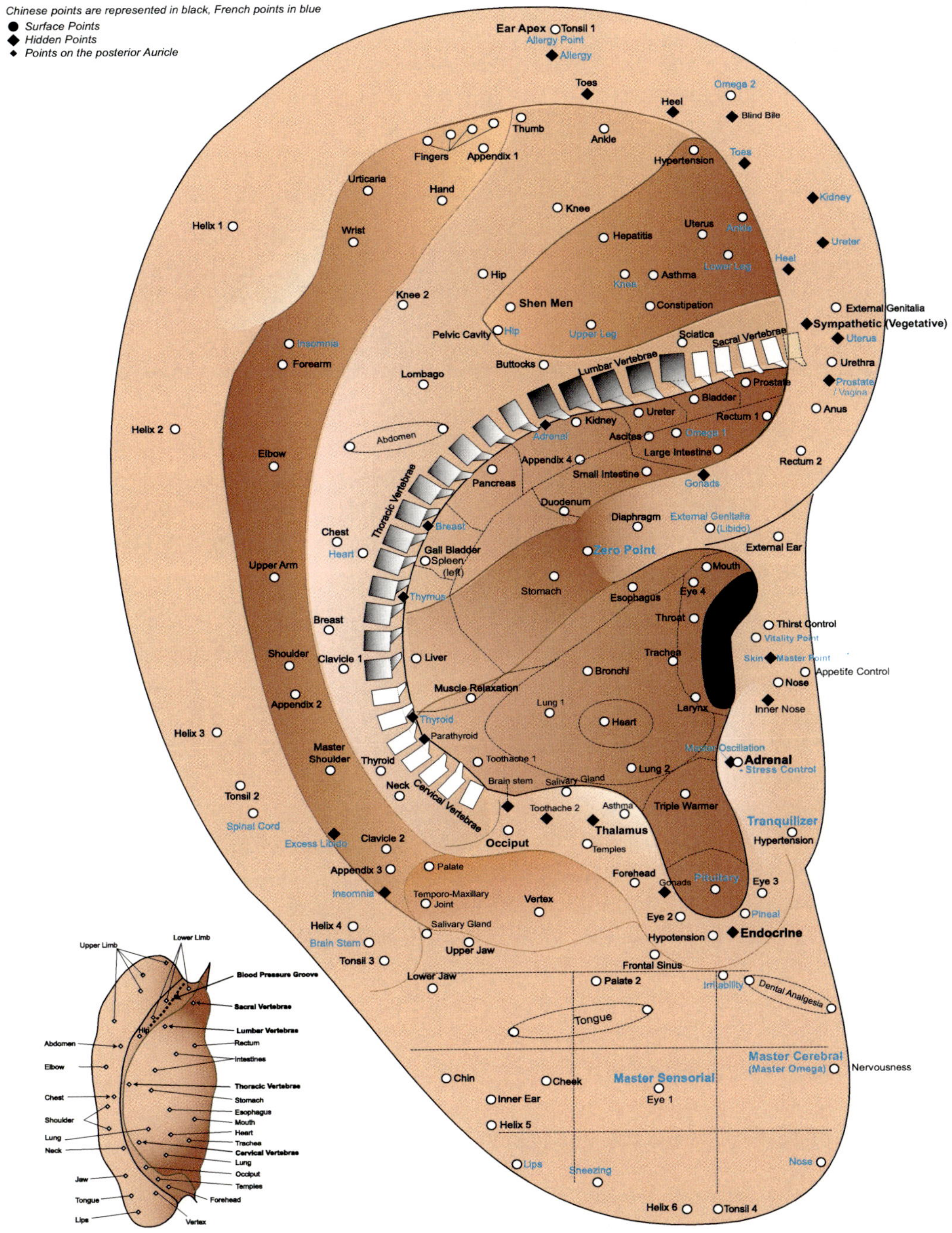

Figure 17.6: Ear points according to the Chinese system, with the addition of French functional points

Scalp Acupuncture

History

Originally started as a method for treating cerebral and neurological conditions, but extended to include the whole body and other pathologies. Scalp needling is a combination of traditional acupuncture with modern knowledge of the representative areas of the brain cortex. Much of the pioneering work in this field was conducted during the Cultural Revolution at the Jishan County Peoples' Hospital of Shanxi province, where excellent results were obtained in treating certain diseases of the central nervous system.

Method

- For a disease affecting a local anatomical structure, the contra-lateral head site is treated.
- For diseases affecting the limbs bilaterally, or the internal organs or systemic diseases, both sides are treated.
- Generally, a principal site is selected corresponding directly to the representative area on the cerebral cortex with an additional supplementary site, which is less directly related. For instance, when treating paralysis of the lower limb, the principal site is the lower limb and trunk area in the Motor zone; a supplementary site could be the leg motor and sensory area.
- Usually thicker gauge needles are utilized and are inserted almost horizontally; stimulation is achieved by a rapid twirling with wide rotation amplitude until the *De Qi* is obtained. Twirling may then be continued for 3–4 minutes after which the needle is left in place for 5–10 minutes, and then twirled again. After repeating this procedure 2–3 times, the needle is withdrawn. The most common response to needling is a hot sensation on the limb opposite the needling site. Less frequently, this sensation will be perceived over the entire body, or only at a single joint or muscle. Other responses include numbness and a tightening sensation, rarely a sensation of cold and pain; however, these sensations usually disappear as needling continues. Generally, if these responses accompany the needling, the result will be good, although in some cases treatment is effective despite their absence.

The original location of the points as described below has evolved over the years (► Fig. 17.7). There are different correspondences of scalp points particularly described by the Japanese Yamamoto school.

Face, Nose, Hand and Foot Acupuncture

- Hand Acupuncture was mainly developed in Korea, where again the whole body is projected on the two sides of the hands. The charting of the points varies greatly between the Korean and the Chinese schools.
- The principle of the Microsystems is also present in Foot reflexology, mainly used for diagnosis and pressure massage.

- Face acupuncture is much less practiced; the facial projection of the organs was described in Chapter 10.1 (▶ Figures 10.4 and 10.5).
- Nose acupuncture is again not a very commonly practiced method.
- Iridology, a diagnostic modality developed in the West, is also applying the same concept of the holographic projection of the body on the iris.

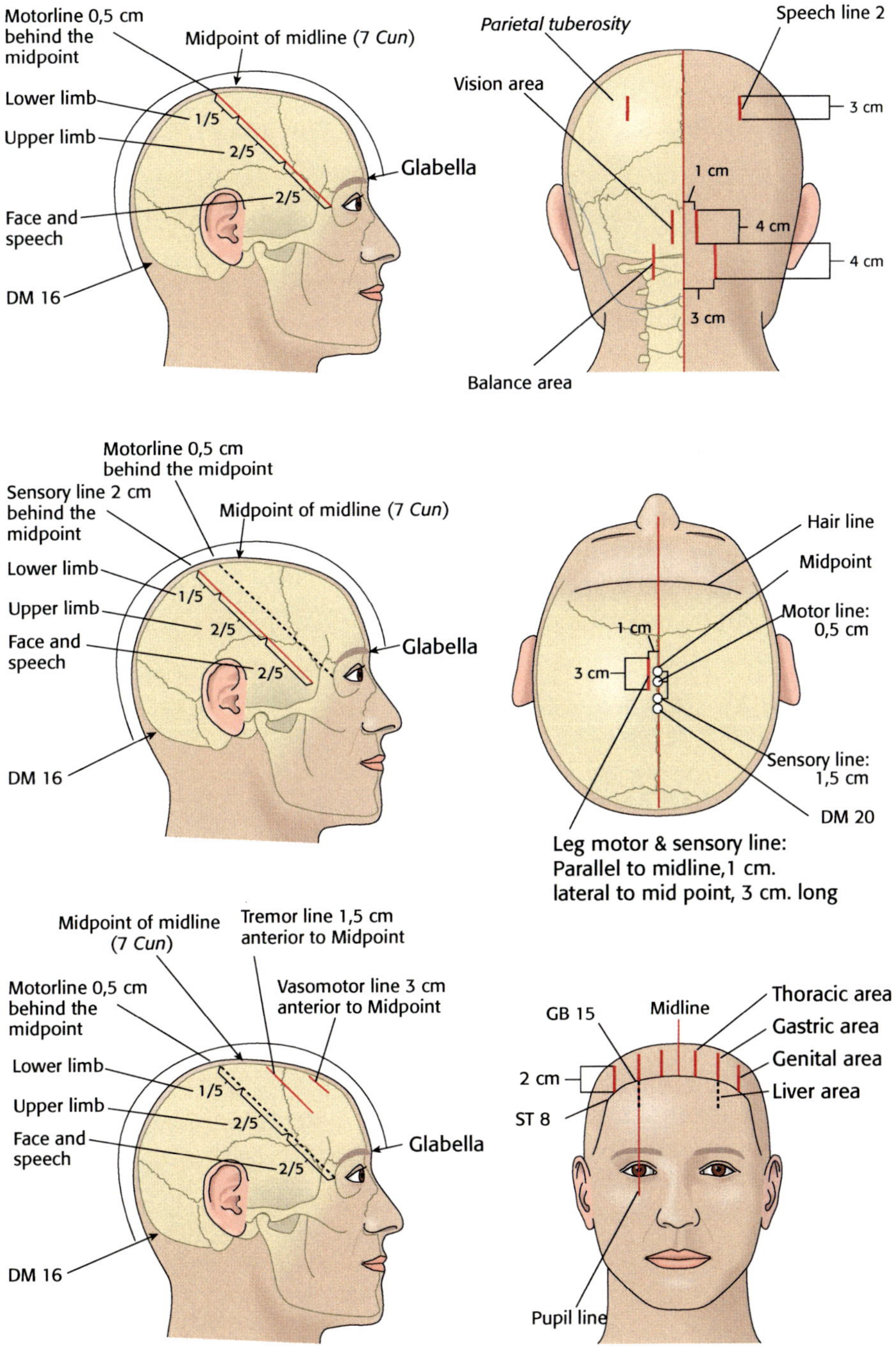

Figure 17.7: Scalp Acupuncture zones

17.3 Moxibustion-Jiu Fa 灸法

[...] what can be treated by needles, may also be treated by Moxa.

Ling Shu, chap. 73

History

The term Moxa appeared in the west for the first time around 1677, deriving either from the Portuguese word mechia (wick) or Japanese mogusa (a variety of mugwort). *Jiu Fa* ≈ Moxibustion is one of the oldest of the Chinese treatment modalities, as evidenced by the extensive descriptions in the Mawangdui silk scrolls (250 B.C.).

Application

The main principle in Moxibustion is to stimulate an acupuncture point by the application of heat, usually obtained by the combustion of a substance. Since the third century A.D., Mugwort, *Ai Ye* ≈ Artemisia vulgaris or Artemisia argyi, has been the herb of choice. *Ai Ye* ≈ Artemisia is a spicy and bitter herb, its nature is considered hot, and it has an affinity for the Lung, Liver, Spleen, and Kidney channels. Very often other herbs with warming, or blood moving nature may be added.

In general, the Moxa application is divided into three groups (▶ Fig. 17.8):

- Direct Moxa: small cone-shaped moxa punk is applied directly onto the skin
  - Non-scarring method: the cone is removed before it reaches the skin;
  - Scarring technique: the cone is allowed to burn the skin, producing a blister, which will continue stimulating the acupuncture point. This method is less and less used in the West today.
- Indirect Moxa: a moxa cone is placed on a slice of garlic, ginger, aconite, pepper paste or salt,

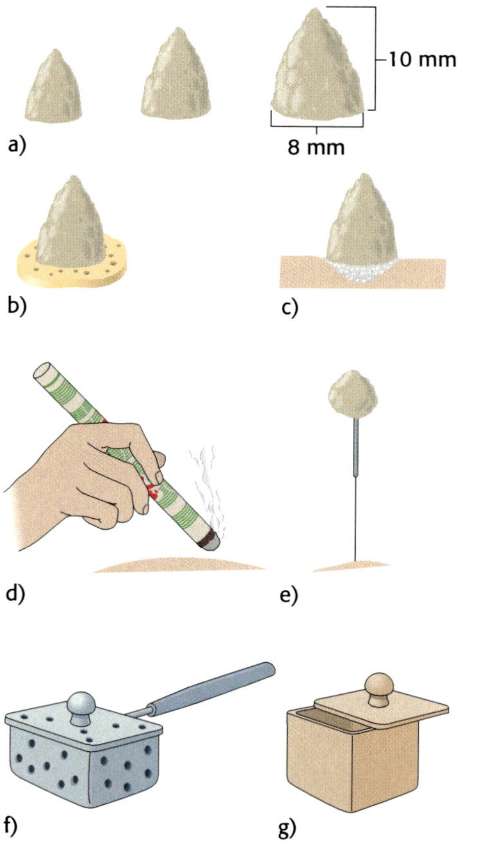

Figure 17.8: Direct and indirect Moxibustion: a) Moxa cones for direct Moxa, b) indirect Moxa using a perforated slice of ginger or garlic, c) indirect Moxa on the navel using kitchen salt, d) indirect Moxibustion with a Moxa roll, e) indirect Moxa on the needle, f) Moxa pan, g) Moxa box.

depending on the desired effects and body parts.

- Moxa on the needle: a small ball of Moxa punk is attached to the top of the needle handle, the heat progressively penetrates inside.
- Moxa stick: The use of Moxa rolls started in the 17th century. The stick is constructed from the Moxa punk pure or mixed with other herbs and rolled into a cigar shape of different sizes or diameters, and may then be used suspended above a point, close or away from the skin, through a needle, in a fixed position or moving in a circular, longitudinal or tapping manner.

The length of time or the number of Moxa cones have been traditionally indicated in the classical texts in relation to the nature of the disease and the point to be treated. In practice, Moxibustion is applied until the skin is red or if the person starts reacting to the heat.

Indications

- Dispel external and internal Cold and alleviate pain
- Warm channels and stop bleeding
- Supplement deficiency, especially of *Qi* and *Yang*
- Dissipate Dampness and dissolve Phlegm and stop cough and Asthma
- Contra-indications
- Hot type diseases, Full-Heat or Empty-Heat
- "Closed type" apoplectic shock
- Dehydration from loss of fluids or from blood loss
- Moxa on fragile skin, the face or near the portals and mucous membranes
- Certain points have been empirically contraindicated to Moxibustion

The relative facility of Moxibustion makes it an ideal complement to acupuncture treatments. Quite often I propose a Moxa stick, or even an incense stick, to my patients, indicating to them the points to be warmed. For example, the supplementing property of Moxa is excellent in strengthening the production of *Wei Qi* in children who are prone to frequent exogenous infections, when applied for seven days around the new moon on *Zusanli* ST-36. Moxibustion on *Qihai* RM-6 and *Zusanli* ST-36, two or three times a week, help build up the *Qi* in convalescent patients. Or again for heavy and abundant bleeding during the periods, the Moxibustion of *Yinbai* SP-1 and *Dadun* LR-1 helps reduce or stop the bleeding.

17.4 Cupping-Ba Guan 拔罐

Well known to the West, the original cupping method in China using animal horns was later replaced by bamboo cups. Today mostly glass and plastic cups are used to create a vacuum, either by fire consuming the air within the glass cup or simply by a vacuum pump. Different sized cups allow the treatment of different parts of the body.

Methods

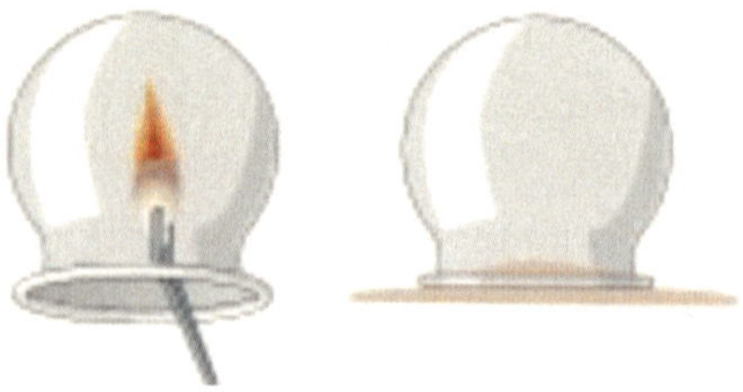

Figure 17.9: Fire Cupping, using an ignited paper to create a vacuum

- Fire cupping: with an ignited cotton or paper. The cupping is removed once the skin has become purplish, this usually is achieved after 5-10 minutes of application. Longer cupping often results in petechiae that may last a few days (▶ Fig. 17.9).
- Hot water cupping, using bamboo cups heated in boiling water, and medicinal cupping in which herbal remedies are added to the boiling water.
- Mechanical vacuum pumps (hand pumps or electric pumps)
- Moving cupping: the cup is slid over the area to be treated
- Cupping over a needle
- Cupping with bleeding, often to draw blood from a point or in case of chronic stagnant blood.

17.5 Blood-letting-Fang Xie 放血

Blood-letting consists of letting out a few drops of blood from an acupuncture point or from a congested capillary. Traditionally a triangular needle was used, replaced today by disposable lancets for distal points, or even hypodermic needles for deeper bleeding.

Indications

- Reducing Heat
- Releasing pathogenic Heat or Cold from the capillary *Luo*≈ Connecting channels
- Bleeding of the *Jing*≈ Well points for acute febrile conditions
- Bleeding the *Shixuan* (Extra) at the tips of the fingers for coma and convulsions
- Cooling Blood, especially with *Weizhong* BL-40, for dermatological conditions
- Moving stagnant Blood especially after trauma
- In Auriculotherapy, for reducing high blood pressure

Precautions

- In hemophilic patients or patients under anti-coagulants, care should be taken to ensure that proper hemostasis has been obtained before releasing the patient.
- In systemic infections and contagious diseases, proper aseptic measures have to be respected against contamination.

17.6 Friction- Gua Sha 刮痧

Gua Sha is a releasing-dispersing method mainly indicated for acute *Biao* ≈ Surface conditions as well as stagnant *Qi* and Blood on the surface. *Gua Sha* is quite popular and widely used due to its simplicity and relative safety. *Sha*, which actually signifies sand, refers to retained Heat causing obstruction of Blood.

Method

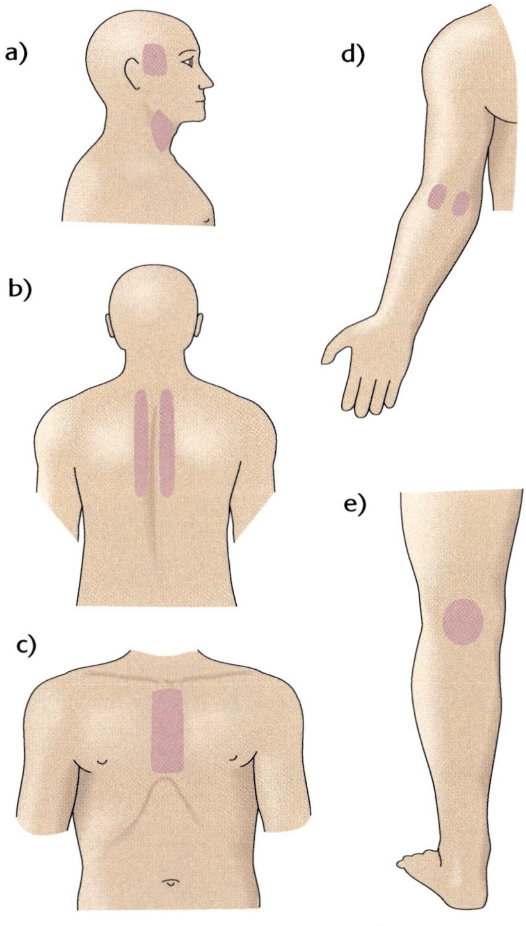

Figure 17.10: Most common *Gua Sha* areas: a) *Tai Yang* (temple) and ST-9 (throat) areas, b) upper back area, c) chest-sternum, d) elbow (LU-5, PE-3), e) knee (BL-40).

- First, the area is checked for the presence of *Sha* by pressing with several fingers then rapidly pulling away. If the blanching caused by the fingers is slow to disappear this confirms the presence of *Sha*.
- The skin area is lubricated with sesame oil or some other oil or jells or even water.
- The edge of a ceramic spoon, a rice bowl, even a coin or the lid of a jar may be used. Professionals use special scraping tools made from buffalo horn (*Fu Ju*). Using a moderate amount of pressure (painless), strokes are applied from above to below.
  - "*Gua Fa*": Even strokes are repeated until a rash appears
  - "*Che Sha Fa*" or the stretching method consists of maintaining with one hand the above area, while with the other hand using the second and third fingers bent into a hook shape rubbing the area using water. First small red petechiae will appear, which gradually blend into areas of ecchymosis. Lighter color rash indicates a more recent *Sha*, darker color, bluish, purple or black rash indicates a longer standing Blood stagnation. An intense color indicates a *Shi* ≈ Replete, condition. A weak response with a lighter color indicates a *Xu* ≈ Vacuity condition.
- Frequency: follow-up sessions are applied only after the disappearance of *Sha*, which usually occurs after 2-3 days. If the *Sha* fades slower, this indicates a poor circulation of *Qi* and Blood or *Yang Xu* ≈ Vacuity.

Areas

Mostly but not exclusively on the back (▶ Fig. 17.10).

Temple	Tai *Yang* area
Throat	ST-9 area
Back	the upper zone of the medial branch of the BL channel
Chest	sternal area
Elbow	anterior area of the crease: LU-5, PE-3
Knee	popliteal crease: BL-40

Indications

Mostly acute conditions:

- Acute conditions, Damp-Heat, acute gastroenteritis: ST-9; elbow; BL-40
- Sunstroke: *Tai Yang*; elbow
- External *Biao* diseases: *Tai Yang*; upper back
- Acute skin conditions: Upper back; BL-40
- Headaches: *Tai Yang*
- Cough; asthma: Upper back; LU-5
- Sore throat: ST-9
- Stomach pains, Gastritis: elbow; ST-9; BL-40
- Abdominal pains: ST-9; BL-40
- Chronic and persistent pains: treat locally

Contraindications

- Skin ulcers, injuries; infected areas, cancer area; burns; varicose veins, moles and pimples
- Abdominal areas in pregnant women.
- Caution in old and weak patients.

17.8 Tuina/ Anmo Massage 推拿/按摩

by Philipp Haas

History

The basis of *Tuina* goes back to 2600 BC, when Yu Fu described the "Eight Methods of Massage", but its theory only appears in the *Huangdi Neijing*, many centuries later, in which two techniques are described: *An* ≈ Pressing and *Mo* ≈ Rubbing. In the Qin- and Han-Dynasties (221 BC until 220 AD) *Anmo* became an important part of the traditional Chinese medicine, particularly specializing in orthopedics and traumatology. At that time, due to the development of economy, politics, and transportation, *Anmo* spread to other countries like Korea, India, and Japan. Shiatsu developed out of these techniques in Japan.

It was not until the Ming Dynasty (1368–1644) that the term *Tuina* (*Tui* ≈ Pushing; *Na* ≈ Grasping) appeared with specific clinical applications, whereas the notion of *Anmo* continues to designate massage in general. After the Ming Dynasty, *Tuina* started being used for pediatric and gynecological problems and even became an integral part of Chinese Medicine. During the Qing Dynasty (1644-1911), *Tuina* became more popularised and its practice was not reserved for doctors only. Nevertheless, during this time a few books about *Tuina* were published.

During the period of the Guomindang (1912–1949), as Chinese Medicine was partly prohibited, *Tuina* was considered as antediluvian and was not developed further.

Mao Tse Tung re-established Chinese Medicine and the government opened the first Technical School of *Tuina* in 1958 in Shanghai. Later in the '70s, the first *Tuina* department was attached to a TCM-college, further inspiring other colleges in Beijing, Nanjing, Fujian, and Anhui.

Today most TCM-hospitals in China have their *Tuina* department where manual therapies are combined with acupuncture, herbal medicine along with modern diagnostic and therapeutic techniques. In these hospitals, *Tuina* is widely used to treat traumatology and orthopedic conditions, as it offers numerous techniques to treat the *Jing Jin* ≈ Sinew channels concerning affections of the muscles, the tendons, and the sinews.

Prior to treating with *Tuina*, the doctors establish a full Chinese diagnosis, including the medical history, anamnesis, tongue and pulse examination and the palpation of the muscles and their related acupuncture points.

Indications and Techniques

Musculo-skeletal diseases

Example of a typical Tuina session

A middle-aged man presenting lower-back pains, but also as the anamnesis reveals, a feeling of coldness in spite of the warm weather and he feels exhausted. His tongue is pale and the pulse is slow. The therapist first will examine the lower back to exclude a possible discus hernia. He will then palpate the various muscle groups and examine the patient's posture. Based on the symptoms and the examination, the diagnosis is established as a *Yang Xu* ≈ Vacuity of the Kidneys being the cause of the back pain. The treatment's aim would be to strengthen the Kidney-*Yang* and to relieve the symptoms in the lower back area.

- First, a warming ointment is applied, rubbing the skin smoothly in circles with fingers stretched, steadily increasing the speed of the rotation. This technique, called *Mo Fa*, looks like a spinning top on the surface of the body. It disperses cold and opens the vessels.
- Next, the muscles are softened, by using a rolling technique called *Gun Fa*. This is a dynamic movement in which the practitioner rolls his fisted hand from the ulnar side over to the backhand. *Gun Fa* has the property of relaxing the mussels as well as of warming them.
- Finally, *Rou Fa* is applied. This consists of a kneading technique with the palm of the hand allowing for deeper penetration into the tissues in order to eliminate the pain.
- These techniques always go along with specific acupuncture points, which relax the lower back and supplement the Kidney-*Yang*. With the thumb, the doctor kneads and presses points like *Shenshu* BL-23, *Mingmen* DM-4, *Weizhong* BL-40, and *Taxi*. KI-3
- To relax the vertebral joints and increase the space between them, the practitioner uses the technique *Ba Shen Fa*, stretching the muscles of the lower back. By grasping the patients' anterior

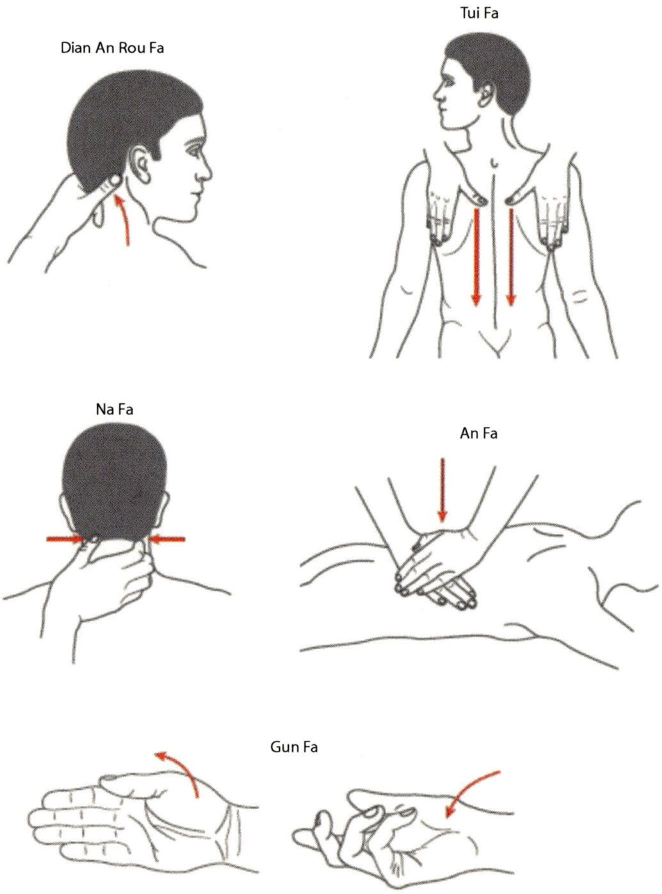

Figure 17.11: Some Tuina hand techniques

iliac crest, he lifts the body gently and usually combines it with a smooth shaking, which the Chinese call *Dou Fa*. Another frequently used technique is even more spectacular. The doctor puts a long towel under the patient's anterior iliac crest, climbs on the table and lifts the pelvic area to stretch the lower back, similar to a coachman conducting his carriage.

- In case of malposition of the vertebrae or of the ilio-sacral joints, the Chinese doctors apply *Ban Fa*. By pulling the joints, the practitioner adjusts and balances the skeletal system as chiropractors do. Although *Ban Fa* is currently practiced in China, in the West, these techniques are often prohibited for *Tuina* therapists and reserved for Doctors of Chiropractic and Osteopathic medicines.

Some other musculoskeletal diseases that can be treated with *Tuina* are epicondylitis, carpal tunnel syndrome, stiff neck, cervical spondylopathy, just to name a few.

Although *Tuina* seems to be a Chinese version of physiotherapy or chiropractic medicine, this is only partly true. Besides the treatment of the musculoskeletal system, *Tuina* excels in moving *Qi* and *Xue* ≈ Blood. In other words, the *Tuina* practitioner can also affect the body on the level of the *Zang-Fu* ≈ Organs and Bowels. By rubbing "*Mo Fa*" the channels and pressing "*An Fa*" the acupuncture points, *Tuina* moves, disperses and even supplements (tonifies) *Qi* and Blood (▶ Fig. 17.11).

- To supplement a point, the practitioner applies the *Mo Fa* or *An Fa* techniques softly, slowly and not too deep.
- To reduce or disperse a point or to move the *Qi*, the channels and points are treated more forcefully and faster.

Other indications

Hence *Tuina* can be used to treat internal diseases, as was evidenced as early as the 14th century when doctors treated gynecological and pediatric problems with *Tuina*. *Tuina* is a method of choice for the treatment of Children. In fact, the *Qi* of children is not as stable as the *Qi* of adults, therefore they react much faster to the treatments. As the channel system in children is not yet fully developed before the age of twelve, *Tuina* therapists focus their work on the children's hands and fingers mainly.

Treatment of Children

For example, a five-year-old girl suffering from weak digestion with belly aches and loose stools. The anamnesis first eliminated the possibility of an infectious or another more serious condition. The diagnosis established a Spleen *Xu* ≈ Vacuity. The treatment, besides the dietary advice, included *Tuina*:

- *Tui Fa* is applied on the child's thenar eminence towards the thumb for several minutes
- *Mo Fa* is applied on the belly in an anticlockwise movement
- In order to fortify the Spleen-*Qi*, *Nie Fa* is practiced on the back, consisting of gently pinching the skin on the back, from below towards the head.

The mother was instructed to apply these techniques on a daily basis. The involvement of the parents is one of the great advantages of *Tuina* therapy for children. Most parents are happy to be able to help their children and increase the effectiveness of the therapy. The mother and child are scheduled the for the following week to observe the improvement and to possibly adjust the treatment.

Nowadays a lot of traditional hospitals in China have a pediatric *Tuina* clinic where doctors treat digestive disorders, enuresis, allergies and respiratory diseases amongst many others.

Treatment of Adults

In adults, very good results may be achieved by applying *Tuina* for digestive, gynecological, respiratory and mental disorders, especially when the condition involves *Qi*-stagnation.

Another example of a 50-year-old male patient suffering from insomnia. Having difficulty in falling asleep, and feeling stressed and tense, with a weak digestion. The pulses show a Wiry quality in the Liver and an Empty quality in the Heart positions. The diagnosis is *Qi*-stagnation in the liver leading to a Heart-*Qi Xu* ≈ Vacuity. The treatment principle would be to supplement the Heart-*Qi* and to move the Liver-*Qi*. The *Tuina* treatment consists of:

- *Mo Fa*: a soft rubbing of the abdomen clockwise.
- *Tui Fa*: applied to the liver area, consisting of pushing with the palm of the hand deeper into the tissues and helping to relax the liver.
- *An Fa*: pressing on the point *Shaohai* HE-3, to supplement the Heart-*Qi*, followed by *Tui Fa* (pushing) with the thumb from HE-3 towards *Shenmen* HE-7, and ending by *An Fa* (pressing) on HE-7. This procedure is repeated for several minutes.
- Finally the extra-point *Yintang* is kneaded to help relax the mind.
- Tension points are searched on the patient's back and shoulders and relaxed, as well as the muscles in the area around *Ganshu* BL-18, related to the Liver. Some general exercises to relax are further suggested.
- *Tuina* is particularly beneficial for patients who are stressed or suffer from emotional problems. The touch itself relaxes the body and the mind and has a healing effect. Specific *Tuina* techniques to stretch the channels greatly improve these conditions through daily practice.

As *Tuina* needs a lot of energy, practitioners often strengthen their *Qi* by exercising martial arts. Furthermore, *Tuina* techniques often have similar movements as in *Kong Fu*, *Tai Chi* or *Qi Gong*.

Tuina could be even considered as a type of martial arts applied on the body of the patient with healing as its goal.

18. Chinese Herbal Medicine; Pharmacopeia

by Stefan Englert and Simon Becker

Even though in the West "Chinese medicine" or "TCM" is most commonly associated with acupuncture, in China the treatment with herbal medicine plays a much more important role than acupuncture. About 75% of all patients treated with Chinese medicine in Chinese Hospital outpatient departments are treated with herbal medicine.

Therefore, Chinese herbal medicine is sometimes called the "heart" of Chinese medicine. It is the center around which Chinese medicine developed. Over the course of the millennia, thousands of books on herbal medicine have been written by hundreds of authors.

Chinese herbal medicine belongs to the most sophisticated traditional herbal medicine in the world. Besides its very large materia medica including not only plant but also animal and mineral material, it combines single substances into highly complex poly-pharmacy prescriptions, which traditionally were prepared as decoctions, pills, syrups, medicinal wines and more.

This introductory chapter, gives an overview of this fascinating pillar of Chinese Medicine, the classification system of the individual substances, the art of formula composition and the practical application in modern day clinics.

18.1 Herbal Medicine in the East and the West

Chinese herbal medicine differs in quite a few points from the herbal medicine known in the West. In Europe, herbal medicine describes the application of herbal teas prepared as infusions or herbal extracts for which one or a small number of dried herbs are used. In Chinese herbal medicine, many more aspects are taken into account.

Processing of herbs: herbal substances are not only dried but are often processed in different ways, traditionally called *Paozhi*. For example, dried *Gan Cao* ≈ Licorice can be fried with honey to yield a sweeter and therefore more supplementing/ tonifying substance called *Zhi Gan Cao*. *Di Huang* ≈ Rehmannia is stripped of its blood cooling properties and turned into *Jing* ≈ Essence supplementing substance by way of cooking it. Highly toxic Aconite root is detoxified with heat and water to become the medicinal substance *Fu Zi*. The processing of the Chinese medicinals serves primarily two goals: changing properties and therefore medicinal action and detoxification. For example, adding honey makes herbs more supplementing and strengthening and emphasizes their tonifying potential. It also directs them more to the Spleen. On the other hand, the processing of Aconite transforms highly toxic alkaloids into non-toxic ones and makes it possible to use this substance medicinally. The processing of individual substances demonstrate the profound century-old pharmacological insights in finding the ideal form for clinical practice.

Chinese herbal medicine uses always only a specific part of a plant for a certain function. Sometimes, two parts from the same plant have different functions. For example, the herb of *Ma Huang* ≈ Ephedra is strongly diaphoretic, when the root of the same plant is used to astringe and stop sweating. The plant parts that are used are: root, bark, fruits, seeds, leaves, twigs, stems, bulbs and fruit-peel. Furthermore, even though the Chinese Pharmacopea is called *herbal*, it does not only use plants but also animal and mineral substances. For example, *Di Long* ≈ Earthworm is an efficacious substance employed for asthma and wheezing, *Chan Tui* ≈ Cicada moultings extinguish wind and can be employed in the treatment of itchy eyes, or *Shi Gao* ≈ Gypsum, which clears heat and is used in the treatment of "Hot" type skin conditions or in certain types of fevers. Overall, about 95% of the materia medica are plant substances.

Application of prescriptions: Even though each Chinese medicinal substance is described in great detail, these substances are never used on their own. They are almost always combined into sophisticated prescriptions, called "formulas." In Chinese medicine, *the therapeutic unit is the formula*, not the single medicinal substance. A large body of texts describe the thousands of traditional formulas that were developed by famous scholar physicians over the course of many centuries. Herbal formulas are not composed to address a specific symptom. Rather, they are precisely designed to treat specific energetic disharmonies. Their composition is such that the individual herbs support each other in various ways. Therefore, for herbal formulas the saying *the whole is greater than the sum of its parts* holds true.

18.2 Classification and description of the individual herbs

The first question that must be posed is: why is a Chinese herb "Chinese"? It is not that Chinese medicinal substances only grow in China. On the contrary, quite a few were actually imported into China. Chinese herbs are Chinese because they are classified and described according to the theoretical framework of Chinese medicine. Every single medicinal substance listed in the Chinese materia medica – and there are some modern collections describing more than 6000 substances – list the characteristic properties and actions required for the Chinese practitioner to select the correct herb. The main properties are temperature, taste, and location.

- The temperature defines how an herb affects the body temperature of the patient after its digestion.
- The taste is responsible for the effect.
- The location defines where the herb will primarily act.

Temperature

The temperature has nothing to do with the temperature of ingestion. So an herb can be cooling even though it is administered as a hot tea. The temperature reveals what will be the herb's thermic effect on the body after its administration. Cooling herbs are able to clear heat from the body. They are used if there is excessive heat, such as in fevers or in patients complaining of a feeling of inner heat. Warming herbs will heat the body up. They are employed if patients feel cold and lack inner warmth. There are five grades of temperature: Hot, Warm, Neutral, Cool and Cold. Furthermore, the classifier "very" can be added. A "very Hot" herb is therefore intensively heating; a very Cold one strongly cooling. For example:

- Hot herbs are prepared Aconite root (*fu zi*), Cinnamon bark (*rou gui*) or dried Ginger rhizome (*gan jiang*).
- Cold herbs are: mineral Gypsum (*shi gao*) and Coptis rhizome (*huang lian*).

Taste

Each taste has a certain effect and focuses its action on a certain part of the body. An herb can have several tastes (▶ Table 18.1).

Table 18.1 Herb Tastes

Tastes	Actions
Acrid	Releases the surface, opens up and regulates
Sweet	Replenishes, builds up, nourishing and sedating
Neutral	Eliminates dampness, diuretic promotes urination
Sour	Holds back, astringes and prevents energy loss
Bitter	Eliminates directs downwards, detoxifies
Salty	Nourishes and softens hardness

Acrid taste

- Effect: Acrid guides up and out and brings to the surface. It opens the pores and can induce sweating which can be used to expel pathogenic factors from the outer layers of the body. Furthermore, the acrid taste frees and unblocks and is used for all kinds of blockages.
- Clinical use: Acrid medicinals are used if the body has been invaded by external wind-cold or wind-heat (i.e. viral infections of the upper respiratory tract). Acrid herbs can also be used for all kinds of pain.

Sweet taste

- Effect: Most grains have a sweet taste. After prolonged chewing, they develop a distinctive sweet taste. Sweetness supplements strengthens and tonifies. All supplementing medicinals, regardless if they supplement *Qi*, Blood, *Yin* or *Yang* have a sweet taste.
- Clinical use: For all types of vacuity/ deficiency, such as Spleen *Qi* vacuity, Fluid vacuity, and blood vacuity. Such patterns often appear after a prolonged illness or after birth. They can also develop from continuous overwork and too little rest.

Neutral taste

- Effect: the neutral taste regulates the fluid metabolism and promotes urination. It eliminates accumulated watery fluids (dampness).
- Clinical use: Neutral medicinals are commonly used if the Spleen cannot effectively transform fluids anymore, the common consequences of such fluid accumulation are dampness, edema, diarrhea or disturbed urination.
- Sour taste
- Effect: The sour taste astringes and holds back. This action saves the body fluids and other precious substances such as essence, *Qi* and Blood. The sour taste also generates fluids.
- Clinical use: Sour medicinals are used for all kinds of loss of bodily fluids and other vital substances, i.e., diarrhea, bleeding, spontaneous sweating and night sweating. Furthermore, sour medicinals can be used to relieve thirst and dryness.

Salty taste

- Effect: The salty taste corresponds to the Water phase and therefore to the Kidneys. For this reason, salty medicinals have a supplementing effect on the Kidneys. Furthermore, the salty taste softens hardness and dissolves nodules and harnesses and stabilizes the Spirit.
- Clinical use: Because of the Kidney supplementing action, salty medicinals are used in Kidney vacuity. As a matter of fact, some medicinals are processed with salt in order to make them more Kidney-supplementing. Salty medicinals are often products of the sea such as algae or seashells, which are also used for nodulations and lumps, such as swollen glands.

Bitter taste

- Effect: the bitter taste eliminates, drains, leads out through the intestine and detoxifies. Bitterness also dries dampness.
- Clinical use: Bitter medicinals are also often Cold in temperature. Bitter and Cold medicinals are very potent Damp-Heat or even toxin clearing substances with strong antibiotic properties. Furthermore, bitter medicinals are employed to drain accumulations in the intestines, such as in constipation.

Location of Action

All medicinals act on or “enter” one or several channel systems (▶ Table 18.2). The place of action describes where the medicinal unfolds its effect and is important for herbal selection and combination. The place of action is generally described in terms of *Zang-Fu*≈ Organ-Bowel systems. To such systems belong to the respective channels and its traversed area, related tissues, sense organs, and emotions. In addition, some herbs have an affinity to certain bodily regions such as the head, the lower extremities, the shoulder, etc.

For example, *Xu Duan* ≈ Dipsacus Radix acts on the Organ-system of the Kidneys. However, it particularly strengthens bones, so is useful to support the healing of broken bones, as it strengthens the tissue related to the Kidneys. Furthermore, it is a commonly used medicinal for lumbar pain as the lumbar area corresponds to the Kidney organ system.

Table 18.2: Area of action

Acting on	Examples
Organ (*Zang-Fu*)	Lung, Liver, Stomach
Acupuncture channel area	Area traversed by *Shou Tai Yin*-LU, *Zu Jue Yin*-LR or *Zu Yang Ming*-ST channels
Body area	Head, neck
Sensory organs	Eyes, Ears
Tissue	Skin, Muscles, Tendons

18.3 Illustrative examples from the Chinese Materia Medica

In order to demonstrate the profound descriptions of individual Chinese medicinals, examples of some of the most commonly used and most widely known Chinese herbal substances are listed below.

Ginseng root (*Ren Shen*)

Pharmaceutical name	Ginseng radix
Taste	Sweet, slightly bitter
Temperature	Slightly warm
Area of action	Spleen, Lung
Actions	Supplements *Qi*
Indications	*Qi Xu* ≈ Vacuity presenting with fatigue, exhaustion, lack of vitality, lack of concentration

Special Note: If Ginseng root is steamed, it turns reddish and is called *Hong Shen* ≈ Ginseng radix rubra. Red Ginseng is more Heating and is used in Cold conditions with *Qi* Vacuity.

Zizyphi seeds (Sour Jujube seed) (Suan Zao Ren)

Pharmaceutical name	Zizyphi spinosae Semen
Taste	Sweet and sour
Temperature	Neutral
Area of action	Gallbladder, Heart, Liver, Spleen
Actions	Nourishing and spirit calming
Indications	Spirit restlessness with blood deficiency presenting insomnia, dreams, and restlessness. Because of its sour taste, it is also astringent and is particularly suitable for insomnia with night sweats.

Fresh Ginger (Sheng Jiang)

Pharmaceutical name	Zingiberis Officinalis Recens Rhizoma
Taste	Acrid
Temperature	Warm
Area of action	Lungs, Spleen, Stomach
Actions	Releases the surface, moves *Qi* outward,

	regulates Stomach *Qi*
Indications	Acute Wind-Cold external illness presenting with fever and chills, headache and body pains. Also for rebellious Stomach *Qi* with nausea and vomiting.

Carthamus flower (Safflower) (Hong Hua)

Pharmaceutical name	Carthami tinctorii Flos
Taste	Acrid
Temperature	Warm
Area of action	Heart, Liver
Actions	Activates and moves the blood circulation
Indications	For all kinds of Blood stasis; particularly in gynecology: painful menstruation, endometriosis, infertility.

Lycium berries (Goji berries) (Gou Qi Zi)

Pharmaceutical name	Lycii Fructus
Taste	Sweet
Temperature	Neutral to Cool
Area of action	Kidney, Liver
Actions	Nourishes *Yin* and blood and brightens the eyes
Indications	All types of eye problems due to liver blood vacuity: dry eyes, night blindness, decreasing vision. In combination with *Yang* descending medicinals, such as *Ju Hua* ≈ Chrysanthemum flower, can also be used for ascending *Yang* conditions with photophobia, migraines, and red eyes. By nourishing Liver Blood and *Yin*, Lycium berries also "relax" the Liver and thereby promote inner calmness.

Cornus fruits (Asiatic Cornelian cherry) (Shan Zhu Yu)

Pharmaceutical name	Corni Officinalis Fructus
Taste	Sour and astringent
Temperature	Neutral, slightly Warm
Area of action	Kidney, Liver
Actions	Astringes and holds Body fluids and Blood
Indications	Loss of Body fluids and Blood with night sweats, enuresis, or gynecological bleeding. Because Cornus fruits also nourish *Yin* and *Jing* ≈ Essence, they are particularly indicated if such symptoms appear in combination with *Yin* or Essence deficiency. This is common during menopause or in children.

Astragalus root (Milk-vetch root) (Huang Qi)

Pharmaceutical name	Astragali membranacei Radix
Taste	Sweet
Temperature	Slightly warm
Area of action	Spleen and Lung
Actions	Supplements *Qi*, raises *Yang* into the upper part of the body
Indications	*Qi* vacuity and sinking *Yang Qi* with fatigue, dizziness, and prolapse. Astragalus is one of the most powerful *Qi* tonics. It can also be used in athletes to promote recovery or in burnout patients. As Astragalus also regulates the immune system and promotes healing, it is also used during chemotherapy and for poorly healing wounds.

Chinese Angelica root (Tangkuei root) (Dang Gui)

Pharmaceutical name	Angelica Sinensis Radix
Taste	Acrid, sweet, bitter
Temperature	Warm
Area of action	Liver, Spleen, Heart
Actions	Nourishes and regulates blood
Indications	All types of systemic blood deficiency presenting with pale lips, pale face, dizziness, hair loss, dry skin. Angelica root is particularly useful in the treatment of gynecological and menstrual problems due to Blood Vacuity, as it not only nourishes but also gently activates the blood. As an important medicinal tonic, it is commonly combined with Astragalus root in the treatment of postpartum exhaustion or exhaustion after operations or prolonged diseases.

Prepared Rehmannia root (Cooked Earth Yellow) (Shu Di Huang)

Pharmaceutical name	Rehmanniae praeparata Radix
Taste	Sweet
Temperature	Neutral to warm
Area of action	Kidney, Liver, and Heart
Actions	Nourishes blood and essence
Indications	Prepared Rehmannia root is a classic *Yin*, Essence, and Blood Tonic. It moistens and nourishes the body and is used for constipation, slow and poor development, hair loss and early aging.

Special Note: *Sheng Di* ≈ Unprepared Rehmannia root is also a commonly used medicinal. However, as it is unprepared, its temperature is Cold. It is used to Cool the Blood and treats dermatitis, bleeding and fevers.

Scutellaria root (Baical Skullcap root) (Huang Qin)

Pharmaceutical name	Scutellaria baicalensis Radix
Taste	Bitter
Temperature	Cold
Area of action	Gallbladder, Large intestine, Lungs, Stomach
Actions	Clears Damp-Heat
Indications	This very bitter medicinal is an effective herbal antibiotic which clears Dampness and Heat especially from the Upper Burner (TW). It is used in the treatment of a cough with yellow phlegm, sinusitis, fevers and ear infections.

Special Note: *Huang* means yellow. In the Chinese pharmacopeia, there are three "*Huang* ≈ Yellow" medicinals: *Huang Qin*, *Huang Lian*, and *Huang Bai*. All of them are Bitter and Cold and have strong antibiotic properties. However, each focuses on one of the three Burners. As explained above, *Huang Qin* ≈ Scutellaria focuses on the Upper Burner. *Huang Lian* ≈ Coptis Rhizoma focuses on the Middle Burner and *Huang Bai* ≈ Phellodendri Cortex treats Damp-Heat in the lower burner.

Forsythia fruit (Lian Qiao)

Pharmaceutical name	Forsythia Fructus
Taste	Bitter, slightly Acrid
Temperature	Cool
Area of action	Lung, Heart, Gallbladder
Actions	Clears heat, resolves toxins and dissolves nodulation
Indications	Forsythia fruit resolves all types of toxins and clears Heat. It can be used for all kinds of "Hot" diseases, such as fever, sore throat, boils, dermatitis, hot type, and urinary tract infections.

Prescriptions – Bundling the power of individual medicinals

The study of Chinese Medicine does not end with the study of the individual medicinal. Rather, the individual medicinals are only the building blocks of the actually prescribed "unit" of medicine, the prescriptions. Throughout the long tradition of Chinese medicine, many thousands of prescriptions have been recorded and passed on. These are today recognized as the so-called "classical prescriptions". For example, in the 2000-year-old *Shang Han Lun* (On Cold Damage), one of the earliest texts on Chinese herbal medicine, around 100 different prescriptions have been recorded. Many are still in frequent use today. Modern collections of classical prescription list many thousands. However, modern formula textbooks generally discuss between 250 to 300 classical prescriptions. The combinations are often similar and certain combinations of herbs appear over and over in the classical prescriptions and can be regarded as general building blocks. An experienced practitioner recognizes the function and indications of a prescription immediately by looking at its ingredients.

One key characteristic of Chinese prescriptions is that they are not simply a collection of medicinal substances with a certain similar aim, for example, a collection of stop coughing herbs. Chinese prescriptions are composed according to certain rules of composition in which each medicinal substance has its function and position.

- The main medicinal, the Emperor or Chief, addresses the main aspect of the presenting pathology and therefore rules the entire prescription.
- The second most important medicinal is called the Minister which supports and complements the Emperor medicinal in its function. Furthermore, the "Minister" may address a secondary pathology itself.
- The Assistant medicinals – often several – have three functions. First, they support the Emperor or the Minister or address a minor aspect of pathology by themselves. Next, the "Assistants" may be used to reduce the toxicity or moderate the harshness of the Emperor or Minister. Last, the Assistant can counteract the Minister's functions. This strategy is employed in complex disease mechanisms where opposing pathological events take place at the same time.
- The "Envoy" is added to focus the action of a prescription on a certain part or channel of the body (see above *Location of Action*). Furthermore, the "Envoy" generally has the function to harmonize all the ingredients and their actions and to make the prescription well-rounded and harmonious.

Structure of a Chinese prescription

Medicinal Position	Function
Emperor (King)	• Focus on the main pathology
Minister	• Supports the Emperor

	• Focuses on the main secondary pathology
Assistant	• Focuses on minor secondary pathologies • Counteracts a toxic medicinal • Moderates the harshness of other medicinals
Adjuvant, Envoy	• Harmonizes and regulates • Leads the prescription to the right location of an action

Even though the basic structure for the prescription only describes four roles, most Chinese prescriptions contain more than four ingredients. Hence, each role can be occupied by several medicinals. This is particularly true for the Assistants. As a matter of fact, prescriptions can be composed of several Emperors, several ministers, quite a few Assistants, and one or two Envoys. Thus, they can contain 10, 12 or even more ingredients.

This poly-pharmaceutic approach is one of the key characteristics of Chinese Herbal Medicine.

Classical prescriptions: three examples

Four Gentlemen Decoction (Si Jun Zi Tang)

This famous classic prescription is employed in the treatment of all types of fatigue and exhaustion as long as the Chinese pattern differentiation corresponds to Spleen-*Qi* vacuity. Hence, it can be used for low blood pressure, depressive states, weakness after surgery or chronic illness, etc.

Medicinal	Dose	Function
Radix Ginseng (*Ren Shen*)	3 g	**Emperor:** Supplements Spleen-*Qi*
Rhizoma Atractylodis macrocephalae (*Bai Zhu*)	9 g	**Minister** • Supplements Spleen-*Qi*; • Dries dampness
Poria (*Fu Ling*)	6 g	**Assistant:** Eliminates dampness by promoting urination. Gently supports the Spleen-*Qi*
Radix Glycyrrhizae (*Gan Cao*)	3 g	**Envoy:** Harmonizes the prescription. Gently supports the Spleen-*Qi*

Application Spleen-*Qi* Vacuity

Body Type Spleen-*Qi* deficient patients are generally tired and have little energy. *Qi* is the engine for our motivation and our drive to move. Spleen-deficient patients are therefore fatigued and have an aversion to movement and sport. Over time, a weak Spleen can cause accumulation of Dampness and Phlegm and lead to weight gain. Casually put "couch-Potato".

Symptoms Fatigue, lack of drive, listlessness, pallor, cold extremities, loose stools, bloating, no thirst, lack of appetite, heaviness, puffiness, edema, swelling

Mental-emotional The same process of separation of clear from turbid that takes place after the intake of food also takes place on a mental-emotional level. Important information is separated from less important information by the Spleen's mental function *Yi*, the intellect. If the Spleen is weak, the efficient separation process turns in circles and leads to brooding and procrastination. The patient is unable to make decisions and has a tendency to worry excessively.

Four Substances Decoction (Si Wu Tang)

This prescription is the classic counterpart to the above *Si Jun Zi Tang* prescription and is also used in case of exhaustion. However, it focuses on nourishing the Blood. It is used after childbirth or during the recovery from long illness. *Si Wu Tang* is commonly used in female problems such as weak menstruation or lack of breast milk after childbirth. It is the basic prescription for regulating the Blood and can be used in any condition that presents with a Chinese medicine pattern of Blood vacuity.

Medicinal	Dose	Function
Radix Rehmanniae Praeparata (*Shu Di Huang*)	6–12 g	• Nourishes Blood of the Liver • Nourishes Essence of the Kidneys
Radix Angelicae Sinensis (*Dang Gui*)	6–9 g	• Nourishes and slightly activates Blood • Regulates the menstruation
Radix Paeoniae lactiflorae (*Bai Shao*)	6–9 g	• Nourishes Blood • Gently astringes with its sour taste • Smoothens and "softens" the Liver
Rhizoma Ligustici (*Chuan Xiong*)	6 g	• Activates and regulates Blood and *Qi*

Application Blood Vacuity

Body Type Blood vacuity leads to a lack of nourishment of the body. The skin, as well as the complexion, is sallow, lustreless and withered.

Symptoms Fatigue, pallor, pale, lacking luster and slightly yellowish complexion, restlessness, nervousness, dry skin, brittle nails, hair loss, a tendency to constipation, muscle cramps, paresthesia, blurred vision, loss of visual acuity, particularly at dawn or at night, night-blindness. Gynecological disorders such as weak menstruation, amenorrhea or irregular cycles.

Mental-emotional Whereas *Qi* is the drive for activity and motivation, Blood is the nourishment which provides us with self-confidence. Sufficient Blood lets us accept ourselves the way we are without having to prove anything. Hence, if Blood is weak, patients present with decreased self-confidence, nagging self-doubt and exhaustion that is coupled with anxiety and restlessness.

Rehmannia Six Flavour Pill (Liu Wei Di Huang Wan)

This most famous prescription is commonly employed in the elderly with a deficiency of Kidney-*Yin*, presenting such symptoms as fatigue with anxiety, lumbar pain and weakness, tinnitus or dizziness. This is the primary and most famous prescription to fill-up the *Yin* of the Kidneys without being cloying and heavy.

Medicinal	Dose	Function
Radix Rehmanniae Praeparata (*Shu Di Huang*)	12 g	• Nourishes *Yin* and Essence of the Kidneys • Nourishes Blood
Fructus Corni (*Shan Zhu Yu*)	6 g	• Astringes the Kidneys and holds *Yin* • Nourishes *Yin* and Essence
Rhizoma Dioscoreae (*Shan Yao*)	6 g	• Supplements the Spleen-*Qi* • Nourishes the Fluids and *Yin* • Astringes the Kidneys
Rhizoma Alismatis (*Ze Xie*)	6 g	• Eliminates dampness by promoting diuresis • Clears empty Heat from the Kidneys
Cortex Moutan (*Mu Dan Pi*)	6 g	• Clears Heat, especially Liver-Heat • Gently activates Blood
Poria (*Fu Ling*)	6 g	• Eliminates Dampness by promoting diuresis • Gently supports the Spleen

Application Kidney-*Yin* Vacuity

Body type Kidney-*Yin* is the basis of all *Yin* of the body. If Kidney-*Yin* is deficient, an imbalance of *Yin* and *Yang* of the entire body arises. *Yang* rises up to the upper and outer body. *Yin* fails to nourish and moisten and dryness and lack of substance develop. Patients, therefore, present with skinny or even emaciated bodies. The skin is dry and wrinkled.

Symptoms Exhaustion, restlessness, weak willpower, red face and cheeks, flushing, night sweats, hot extremities, dry skin and mucous membranes, constipation, lumbar aching and pain, osteoporosis, hair loss, loose teeth, deafness, tinnitus

Mental-emotional The inner Heat that develops from the imbalance with weak *Yin* leads to agitation and restlessness. There is a lack of inner peace and because the Kidneys store *Zhi*≈ Willpower, patients may become more fearful and anxious or present with an excessive fixation on a specific goal.

18.4 Administration of Chinese medicinal herbs

Chinese medicines are prepared in various classical forms of application. The most traditional and most important is certainly the soup, the so-called decoction (*Tang*).

However, Chinese medicine is also administered in the form of pills, powders, and drops or externally as soaks or poultices. More recently, several modern forms of administration have become available:

- Granules
- Tablets
- Hydrophilic concentrates
- Alcoholic tinctures
- Ointments, creams, lotions

Decoctions

A decoction is an aqueous extract, much like a tea. However, different from normal tea, the herbal mixture is boiled for prolonged periods of time, often even twice. This is also the reason why *Tang* is often translated as soup. Generally, patients prepare their own decoction at home. Although in recent years, it is becoming more and more popular for pharmacies to offer this service to the patients.

The decoction is still the most widely used form of administration in China. In the West, it has been replaced with the more modern forms that overcome some of the main problems of Chinese medicinal decoctions: quantity and taste. Because the decoction is simply a soup of the herbs, the amount that has to be ingested is considerable. Furthermore, the taste of Chinese herbs is not particularly pleasant. Although freshly prepared decoctions are highly effective, fewer and fewer people are willing to take them. The most commonly used modern forms of administration are dry extracts (granules) and concentrated liquid extracts (hydrophilic drops and tinctures).

Modern forms: Granules and tinctures

Granules *(San)* became popular in Taiwan during the fifties. Granules are basically a concentrated dried form of decoctions. After the herbs have been cooked just like a traditional decoction, the liquid is concentrated by spraying it upon a carrier substance. This coarse powder is then dried and ground into even-sized, fine granules. The patient dissolves the granules in a small amount of water and takes this. The granular powder can be stamped into tablets or filled into capsules. These forms of administration further improve ease of ingestion.

Tinctures *(Jiu)* are liquid extracts prepared by using an alcohol-water mixture as the solvent. Tinctures generally have high alcohol content. However, some forms are available where the alcohol is replaced with glycerine after the extraction process. This form is called “hydrophilic concentrate”. Liquid extracts are either taken straight or added to warm water before ingestion.

Clearly, granules and tinctures are advantageous when it comes to ease of preparation and ingestion. They are more fitting to the fast-lived modern lifestyle. Furthermore, because single herbs are prepared into granules or tinctures, these forms can be handled just like raw herbs. This means one can prescribe individually tailored prescriptions made up of individual herb granules or tinctures. Similarly, classical formulas can be modified by the practitioner, by adding other single herbs. For both granules and tinctures, the entire line of 350 to 400 single medicinals as well as many classical prescriptions, are available.

Why then do patients still prepare decoctions and why do more and more pharmacies in China and the West offer the service of cooking the medicinal prescriptions into ready-to-use decoctions? Regardless of the many advantages the tinctures and granules may have, the decoctions are so far still the most powerful way of administering Chinese medicinals. A freshly prepared raw herb decoction is equal to none in strength and potency. One reason for this is the fact that all the substances are cooked together for almost an hour. The interactions and symbiotic events taking place during this cooking process are estimated to be a very important factor in raw herb decoction efficacy. These interactions and symbiotic events are lost in many modern forms of medicinal administration.

18.5 Safety and Quality of Chinese Medicine

Is Chinese herbal medicine safe?

Chinese medicinals have been used for thousands of years and are all natural substances; these two facts should not lead to the hasty and erroneous conclusion that Chinese medicine is inherently safe. Among the hundreds of Chinese medicinals are some very strong acting and toxic substances. The safe prescription of Chinese medicine is directly linked to an understanding of the medicine as a whole and the individual substances within this system. Furthermore, individual herbal toxicities and interactions with modern Western drugs need to be taken into consideration. Still, Chinese medicine can be regarded as a safe and side-effect-free medicine if – and only if – prescribed by a properly trained practitioner.

A word about Quality

The quality of Chinese medicinals concerns primarily two important issues: correct identification and contamination. Both of these issues can be sufficiently and reliably addressed through serious quality control management. This means that all medicinals are tested for various environmental contaminants and that all medicinals undergo strict identification controls. In more and more countries, such quality control measures are adhered to by pharmacies or are enforced by the government. If such quality control systems are in place, there is generally no need for any worries about the quality of the Chinese medicinal substances.

19. Chinese Dietetics – Healing with Foods

by Stefan Englert, Christine Dam

According to the immutable pillars of Western dietetics, dairy products are recommended for strong bones, whole-meal bread for perfect digestion, plenty of raw fruit, vegetables and salads to supply the body with enough vitamins. However, why do we still deal with so many digestive problems in our practice? Why do chronic diseases not improve although we do our best with acupuncture and Chinese herbs? The answer often lies in the eating habits of our patient, which does not fit his or her constitution. In contrast to most common Western ideas about healthy food and healthy eating, the Chinese dietary system is very flexible and relies on an individualized system of nutrition which tailors the diet according to the pattern of disharmony and the patient's constitution.

The extent to which dietary therapy and healing foods can be included in the treatment depends largely on the willingness of the patient. A change in dietary habits has more far-reaching effects than simply taking Chinese herbal medicine or going once weekly for an acupuncture treatment. It truly means a life-adjustment and change of established habits, which begins with conscious and purposeful shopping for food. However, a health-supporting diet often lies at the center of health and healing: this applies to all types of digestive disorders, skin problems, deficiency and excess diseases, and other chronic illnesses.

An easy way to detect "bad" eating habits is to ask the patient to write down what he or she eats and drinks and at what times, over a period of three days. By doing so, in general patients realize the potential for change by themselves.

19.1 Foods and their properties

Similar to Chinese herbal medicine, all foods have three main properties:

- Temperature: effect on the body; Hot, Warm, Neutral, Cool or Cold
- Taste: sweet, sour, bitter, salty and acrid. The taste influences the direction of action; i.e, sour foods, such as lemon, astringe and move inward.
- The area of action determines which Chinese organ system the food will influence and effect.

Based on the combination of these properties, each food has a specific action. For example, Hot type foods can be employed in the treatment of Cold diseases Acrid foods can be employed to open and release the pores. The combination of individual foods is similar to an individualized herbal prescription and can help to correct bodily disharmonies.

Change of established habits

For example, a young woman is freezing even during the summer, with cold extremities, loose stools and low energy. Her diet consists of a yogurt and some raw fruit for breakfast. Some salad for lunch. In the afternoon, she is so hungry that she eats a whole bar of chocolate and some cookies. For dinner she has bread with cheese. In order to improve her situation, she should eat mostly cooked meals. Here are some ideas about how she could change her diet:

- Warm oat porridge in the morning with apple sauce and roasted walnuts
- Beef curry with cooked vegetables and rice for lunch
- Pumpkin soup with some toasted spelt bread in the evening

Oat gives energy in the morning. Beef as meat supports the *Yang*, together with the curry and its warm spices like pepper, chili, curcuma, cardamom, cumin etc. It warms up the cold constitution of the young woman. Pumpkin is warm and supports the spleen and the stomach. If bread is toasted it is much more digestible than fresh bread. Spelt is warmer than wheat.

On the other hand, a businessman who is sweating day and night and who does not come to rest in the evening can also benefit from a change in his diet. Looking at his eating pattern, he drinks 6 to 7 cups of coffee a day. No breakfast, sandwich for lunch (which is also a business meeting) and dinner with clients late at night. Here are some recommendations for his diet:

- Breakfast: Cooked rice with grapefruit and almonds
- Lunch: Fish, e.g. trout with spinach and potatoes
- Dinner: Polenta with vegetables
- 1-2 coffees a day (or green tea instead), for the rest: herbal tea or hot water

The rice and grapefruit Cool the tense Liver of this man. Almonds nourish the *Yin*. Freshwater fish, such as trout nourish the Kidney-*Yin*. Spinach Cools and nourishes *Yin* and Blood. The reduction of coffee or replacement by green tea will bring more calmness to his restless heart.

In general, foods are less potent than herbal substances. However, because we eat much more of it and because the daily meals represent the base on which the body functions, a healthy change in dietary habits can have a very powerful effect on health and disease.

Properties of Foods

A few examples of foods and their properties.

Pear

Temperature	Cool
Taste	Sweet and sour
Area of action	Lung, Stomach
Action	Transforms Hot Phlegm clears Heat and moistens
Indications	Cough with yellow phlegm; constipation

Rice (e.g. Basmati)

Temperature	Neutral
Taste	Sweet
Area of action	Spleen, Stomach
Action	Supplements the Middle Burner, supplements Spleen-*Qi* and Stomach-*Qi*, regulates *Qi*, eliminates Dampness
Indications	Diarrhea, nausea, reduced appetite, stress Example: cooked together with mung-beans (equal parts) as a cleansing meal

Oat

Temperature	Neutral
Taste	Sweet
Area of action	Spleen, Stomach, Heart
Action	Regulates the middle burner, descends *Qi*, supplements the Heart, astringes sweat and eliminates Dampness
Indications	Fatigue and exhaustion, reduced appetite, spontaneous sweating

Corn

Temperature	Neutral
Taste	Sweet
Area of action	Spleen, Stomach, Bladder
Action	Regulates the middle burner, supplements Stomach-*Qi*, eliminates Dampness
Indications	Reduced appetite, edema, general water retention

Wheat

Temperature	Cool
Taste	Sweet
Area of action	Heart, Kidney, Spleen
Action	Nourishes the heart, calms the *Shen*, supplements the Spleen and enriches Kidney-*Yin*
Indications	Night-sweats, palpitations, restlessness, insomnia, depression
Caution	Due to its cool and moistening property, wheat must be used cautiously in people with dampness and phlegm

Tomato

Temperature	Cold
Taste	Sweet and Sour
Area of action	Stomach
Action	Clears Heat, nourishes Body fluids, cools the Blood and nourishes *Yin*
Indications	Thirst, restlessness, dry eyes, reduced appetite, bleeding gums
Caution	Due to its cold property, tomatoes must be used with caution in people with deficiency and coldness of the Spleen

Leek

Temperature	Warm
Taste	Acrid, sweet
Area of action	Liver, Lung, Stomach, Kidneys
Action	Warms the Spleen and Stomach, descends rebellious *Qi* of Lung and Stomach, warms Kidney-*Yang*, regulates *Qi* and Blood and clears toxins
Indications	Reduced appetite, belching, weakness of hips and lumbar area, frequent urination, pain in the chest secondary to *Qi* and Blood stagnation
Caution	Due to its warm temperature, leek must be used cautiously in people with *Yin* deficiency and heat signs

Onion

Temperature	Slightly warm
Taste	Acrid and Sweet
Area of action	Stomach, Lung
Action	Fortifies the Stomach, increases appetite, regulates *Qi*
Indications	Reduced appetite, epigastric fullness and bloating, enduring diarrhea

Radish

Temperature	Warm (cooked); Cool (raw)
Taste	Sweet, slightly Acrid; raw radish is Acrid
Area of action	Lung and Stomach
Action	Clears heat, transforms Phlegm, stops a cough, generates Body fluids, cools the Blood, eliminates Dampness and clears toxins
Indications	Cough with thick Phlegm, hoarseness, sore throat, nose bleeding, fullness and bloating of the abdomen, belching, nausea, and vomiting

Beef

Temperature	Slightly warm
Taste	Sweet
Area of action	Spleen and Stomach
Action	Supplements the Spleen and Stomach, nourishes Blood and strengthens tendons and bones.
Indications	Fatigue and exhaustion, diarrhea, lumbar pain

Pork

Temperature	Cool
Taste	Sweet and Salty
Area of action	Spleen, Stomach, Lung, Liver, and Kidney
Action	Nourishes Blood and *Yin*, moistens Dryness
Indications	Exhaustions, constipation

Chicken

Temperature	Warm
Taste	Sweet
Area of action	Spleen and Stomach
Action	Supplements Spleen and Stomach nourishes Blood and fortifies Kidney and *Jing*≈Essence
Indications	Exhaustion and fatigue, for example after childbirth

Sesame

Temperature	Neutral
Taste	Sweet
Area of action	Kidney, Liver, Lung, Heart, Spleen
Action	Supplements *Jing*, Blood, *Yin*, and *Qi*, moistens the Intestines
Indications	Osteoporosis, tinnitus, infertility, early grey hair

Coffee

Temperature	Warm
Taste	Bitter and sour
Area of action	Pericardium, Heart, Lung, Liver, Kidney
Action	Regulates Liver-*Qi* drains, resolves food stagnation, supplements *Qi*, transforms Dampness
Indications	Stress, poor digestion, edema, tiredness
Caution	Due to its draining and warm property, coffee must be used cautiously in people with *Yin* and Blood deficiency and Heat signs.

19.2 General Chinese medical guidelines for eating

- Eat in a quiet and pleasant atmosphere and focus your consciousness on what you eat. Do not work, read or watch television during meals. Eat in a sitting position. Eat at the same times every day, preferably in a balanced and relaxed mood.
- Eat neither too fast nor too slow. Eat only to about ¾ of your satiation amount and leave the table neither hungry nor too full.
- Do not eat before having digested the previous meal (approximately 3 to 6 hours in between means).
- With your meals, drink small amounts of water or tea. Preferably, avoid cold drinks with your meals, as this will cool your digestive fire.
- In general, meals should be balanced and contain all five tastes. Variations are made according to individual constitutions and to the seasons.
- In the evening, the intake of excessive animal protein should be avoided (yogurt, milk, cheese or heavy meat dishes).
- Avoid ice-cold foods and drinks (ice cream, iced water, etc.) as this will weaken the digestive system.
- After meals, take a few minutes to sit quietly before going back to work or becoming active.

Yin and Yang in eating

The nervous system is mainly controlled by the sympathetic and the parasympathetic functions. They also represent the *Yang* and *Yin* of body activities and in constant interchange; they reign over the entire life process. The sympathetic fight or flight reaction is active during work, in traffic or in hectic daily life. The parasympathetic ensures recovery and regeneration. Detoxification, repair and tissue construction and renewal take place in this *Yin* phase. This happens primarily at night and at quiet moments during the day.

The balance of this *Yin* and *Yang*, of sympathetic and parasympathetic systems, can be supported by the right diet: in the morning (and to some extent at noon) a lot of fuel within a relatively small amount of food, i.e. high energy density food, is required whereas In the evening, in order to be able to relax and to activate the parasympathetic system, a low energy density is necessary so as not to excessively stimulate the body. An bit old advice: eat like an emperor in the morning, like a prince for lunch and like a beggar in the evening.

Breakfast like an emperor

According to the Chinese organ clock, our digestive organs are most active in the morning (► Fig. 4.18). In addition, because the digestive process corresponds to a form of "cooking process" in the Middle Burner (TW), warm and cooked meals are preferable. In China, the standard breakfast is congee, which is rice porridge. Other types of porridge, such as oat porridge, provide the necessary energy and are easy to digest. Of course, porridge can be modified according to taste, a pattern of disharmony and constitution. For example, for a *Yang* deficiency constitution, the congee can be warmed up by adding warm spices such as cinnamon, cardamom, and ginger. Nuts, various fruits, and honey or butter can be added according to taste. A breakfast consisting of animal protein, like eggs or even meat or fish combined with vegetables and rice or millet supports the *Yang* in the morning even more than the usual "sweet" breakfast. Vegetarians benefit from dishes with lentils or beans.

Dinner like a beggar

With the family coming together in the evening and having – at last – enough time to enjoy a good meal, this recommendation is not easy to put into practice for many people. However, the digestive system generally needs only a small amount of energy at night.

Meals should be light and easy to digest. In Chinese medicine, this refers to cooked light foods. This includes especially vegetables and soups. Excessive amounts of carbohydrates (bread and pasta), as well as animal proteins, should be avoided. Slowly cooked vegetable soups, possibly with small amounts of meat in the soup (beef, pork, chicken) are ideal. Or even sweet meals with cereals like cooked millet, rice or polenta combined with cooked fruits and nuts help to calm us down in the evening. Cold and uncooked foods such as yogurt from the fridge, cheese, and bread and big plates of salad should be avoided.

Important for in between meals: Hot water

The digestive system in Chinese medicine runs on Spleen-*Yang* and hence likes warmth and heat and loathes cold and ice. A very simple measure to support the digestive system is to regularly drink hot water – either cooked for ten minutes or boiled in the water boiler. It can then be stored in a thermos and drank over the course of the day in small sips. This stimulates the Spleen energy and the metabolism and aids in eliminating dampness and phlegm. This measure can be used by most anyone and for all conditions. As it optimizes the digestion, it helps to support long-term health.

Conclusion: Acupuncture and Chinese herbs are mighty tools in helping the patient to overcome his health problems. If this process is supported by an individually tailored diet the success of the treatment will have a lasting effect.

20. Qi Gong – Cultivating the Healing Energies

by Christine Reist

History

What is known today as *Qi Gong* has its roots in the very beginning of the Chinese culture and religion. Already, the founder of the *Shang* Dynasty (1766–1122 B.C.), a famous shaman himself, is quoted in the *Lushiqunqiu* with a detailed concept of cultivating the energies in order to live longer. According to the Chinese historian Guo Mu Rou, there were records of breathing exercises in the *Jin Wen* (writings on bronze) of the *Zhou* Dynasty (1200–221B.C.). Since then, the concepts of nourishing life *(Yang Sheng)*, long living *(Chang Shou)* and supporting health (*Jian Kang*), have been major concerns in the Chinese culture. Various ways to cultivate the inner energies were developed mainly by the Daoist and Buddhist schools of pre-modern China. The belief that certain techniques would help to maintain physical and mental health was merely common sense for the members of the educated society, and even Mengzi (372–289 B.C.) Confucian teacher stated:

> *The Will is the director of Qi, and Qi is something that permeates the body. So the Will is primary and Qi is secondary. Therefore, it is said: "Hold on to your Will; do not scatter your Qi." [...] And further: The Will influences Qi and Qi influences the Will. For instance, jumping and running, though mostly concerned with the Qi, also have an effect on the mind [...]*
>
> *Mengzi (3^00. BC)*

Breathing exercises, the intake of cosmic energies, diet, sexual techniques, consuming certain pharmaceuticals as well as gymnastic exercises, called *Dao Yin* at the time, contributed to the life-nourishing concept "*Yang Sheng*", which seems to be at the basis of modern *Qi Gong* (► Fig. 20.1). In spite of the efforts of the Chinese government after the Big Cultural Revolution (BCR) to classify, simplify and standardize energetic exercises, today we still find innumerable methods being taught. Some of them are offering "Traditional practicing methods" which derive directly from the "Original sources" of famous Daoist teachers. Others point out their medical background or just promise some wellness and relaxing experience.

In all these fields there are serious teachers with the appropriate background – and others. In order to make it easier to find a good teacher and a suitable method, this chapter proposes to discuss some very basic and important questions that are frequently asked by beginners. This should support the readers on their way to exploring one of the most beautiful and rich treasures of Chinese culture.

20.1 What kind of exercise is Qi Gong?

Qi Gong is usually translated with "Energetic *Qi* exercises":

.*Qi* has been explained earlier in this book. *Gong,* has the notion of merit, result, effect, ability, and skill. In Chinese it is said, that a person has *Gong Fu,* meaning that he or she has already done a lot of work in a certain field and therefore achieved a degree of skill that is outstanding. With regular practice, the *Gong Fu* of a person will grow. With internal methods (see below) the growing of *Gong Fu* also means the progressing of the energetic and spiritual cultivation.

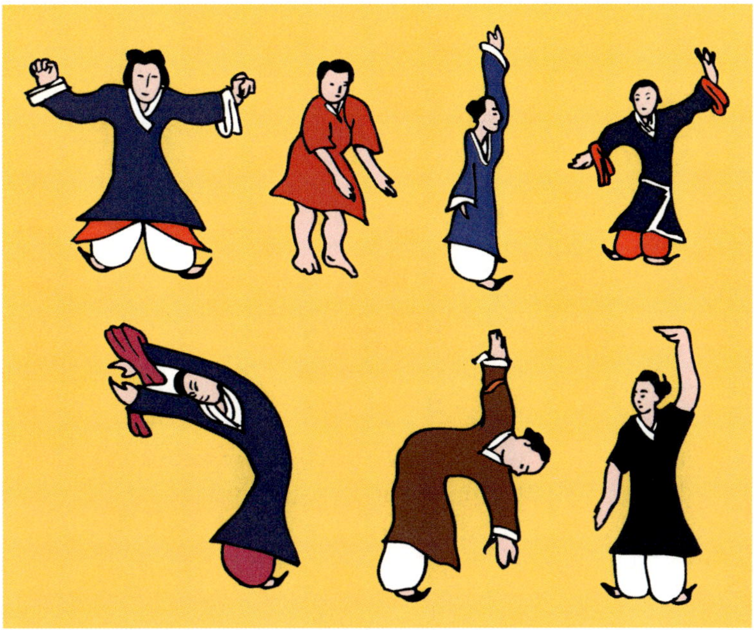

Figure 20.1: Reproduction of Silk roll *Daoyin Tu* (guiding and stretching chart) from Mawangdui-tombs (circa 168 B.C.)

"What kind of *Gong* do you practice?" may be a question that you are asked when meeting Chinese friends practicing *Qi Gong* or martial arts. The simplest distinction that can be made in the jungle of *Gong* is between *Jing* ≈ Still and *Dong* ≈ Moving *Qi Gong*. Beginner classes usually start with a set of movement exercises. The most traditional and famous ones are: The *Ba Duan Jin* ≈ Eight Brocades*, Yi Jin Jing* ≈ Sinew transforming method and *Wu Qin Xi* ≈ Five Animal *Qi Gong* These exercises have been changed and adapted throughout the centuries and have reached us under numerous variations in the present day practice. They all have in common the primary purpose of harmonizing *Shen* ≈ Body, *Qi* ≈ Energy, *Xi* ≈ Breath, *Yi* ≈ Awareness and *Shen* ≈ Spirit, according to the fundamental rules of Chinese Energetics. The "5 Harmonizations" demonstrate that *Qi Gong* exercises are truly holistic. Their value as a body and mind integrated training method cannot be overestimated in contemporary physical and psychological health care.

In different schools, the teacher will have a different focus: As a good basis, all will emphasize the correct posture and movement of the body. In some schools breathing techniques are very important. Concerning the energetics, the focus depends on the method: some *Qi Gong* styles put more emphasis on the intake of *Cai Qi* ≈ Good energy from the surrounding, other schools emphasize the method of *Tu Gu Na Xin* ≈ Expelling the old (bad) energy and the intake of the new (good) energy. Some, like the *Nei Yang Gong* ≈ Nourishing the Internal, mainly want to strengthen and harmonize the internal energy. No matter what method one chooses, it is essential to learn step by step, i.e. the exercises need to be adapted to the student's ability and health. There are schools offering classes in *Jing Gong* ≈ Still *Qi Gong,* referring to meditation (harmonization of the spirits) and the internal movements of *Qi* while not moving the body externally i.e. in a sitting position. Although *Jing Gong* is extremely effective and most important for the understanding of the internal arts, often the students start this method a little later in the training schedule and only after a good basic training in moving *Qi Gong*. In this manner, the body and mind are well prepared for the *Jing Gong*, thus no unwanted effects may appear. It is said, that advanced students should practice both, *Jing Gong* and *Dong Gong*, for equal periods of time.

20.2 Medical Qi Gong

Historically the development of modern *Qi Gong* started at the beginning of the 20th century with the ending of imperial China. In pre-modern China, the various methods of Self-cultivation were practiced and passed on within a lineage, in family clans or in religious contexts of Buddhist and Daoist communities. As these rather strict social structures had started to erode, the access to self-cultivation methods opened up to a broader range of people. In 1914 the Buddhist Philosopher Jiang Weiqiao (1873–1958), author of the article "*Yin Shi Zi Jing Zuo Fa*" (Yinshizi's method of quiet sitting), was one of the first modern *Qi Gong* experts and teachers. He reported that he had cured himself of tuberculosis by practicing a certain style of *Jing Gong* ≈ Still *Qi Gong.*

After the communist revolution, Hu Yao Zhen (1897–1973), a well-known doctor and martial artist who had been trained in Daoist, Confucian and Buddhist philosophy, had started to apply his method of *Jing Gong Qi Gong* in a clinical setting and wrote down his procedure and experience. As the first chairman of Beijing's Outpatient *Qi Gong* clinic, he successfully instructed patients suffering from various internal diseases, such as diabetes, high blood pressure, liver, and heart diseases.

In Japan, Hu is still admired and considered the "father of modern *Qi Gong*." One of his well-known followers in Europe was Jiao Guo Rui, founder of the German "Gesellschaft für *Qi Gong Yang Sheng*" and author of several standards for medical *Qi Gong*.

In the 1940's Liu Gui Zhen reported, that he had been cured of his stomach ulcer by a method that was taught within his family. Liu then decided, not to follow the tradition of teaching only one person of the next generation, but to make this method, called "*Nei Yang Gong*", available to all those who were interested. Until recently, his method was taught in Bei Dai He *Qi Gong* hospital in the Hunan province.

Although a lot of the material written down in the fifties, including all except one of Hu Yao Zhen's books, were lost or destroyed during the Big Cultural Revolution (BCR), still, the seed, which had been planted in the early years of communism had survived. After the end of the BCR in 1976, the interest in Chinese self-cultivating arts was growing again in China as well as in the West.

What is meant by medical *Qi Gong*? All of the methods mentioned above may have the potential to harmonize the energetic body as understood by Chinese physiology and may be called "medical" because practicing it will harmonize the energetic system of the practitioner and thereby support or even restore health. Some contemporary methods of *Qi Gong* literally address a certain disease (cancer) or concern a particular organ (Heart, Kidney etc.). This may be helpful as it obviously fits into our Western way of thinking. However, it is contradictory to the holistic view of traditional medicine that considers the human being as a living, circulating organism and avoids dividing it up. In spite of this, the Chinese government is actively supporting the development and dissemination of these methods.

Curing disease with Qi Gong practice

Hu Yao Zhen used to distinguish two kinds of exercises:

- *Zhi Liao Gong* ≈ Therapeutic exercises, and
- *Bao Jian Gong* ≈ Health preserving exercises

Before applying *Qi Gong* a proper Chinese diagnosis should be established. The exercises must be chosen to be appropriate to the patient's condition and skill, and the patient must be instructed very carefully.

If for instance one chooses one of the *Liu Zi Jue* ≈ Six Healing Sounds as a therapeutic method for a patient with chronic lung disease, it has to be established first whether the disease is of a *Shi* ≈ Repletion or a *Xu* ≈ Vacuity condition, in order to choose the correct breathing rhythm. Practicing the exercise regularly and in a way that is well adapted to the patient, the progress will be fast and the disease may disappear. Wrong exercises can make a patient feel worse. All in all a lot of research is still needed before *Qi Gong* can be established as a recognized therapeutic tool in the West.

When asked by a patient as to what exercise they should choose to cure a particular disease, the correct answer is: "regular exercise". In fact, the daily practice is mandatory if *Qi Gong* is chosen as a therapeutic modality. In the Chinese *Qi Gong* clinics, the patients were hospitalized for a certain number of days or weeks. During that time, besides acupuncture, herbal medicine, they were trained for several hours a day in class settings. When they left the clinic, they had gained a solid knowledge of the exercises as well as dietary advice and other useful information concerning their lifestyle. *Qi Gong* can do miracles but in fact, you need to practice it. It is like the sage's answer to the man pleading to be made a lottery-millionaire: "Go and buy a ticket!"

Although less specific, the practice of health preserving exercises often have fast and lasting results: blood pressure is lowered, insomnia gets better, digestion problems are resolved and back pains disappear within weeks or months. Of course, a severe disease would also require medical treatment. When applied correctly, *Qi Gong* can play a major role in our personal as well as medical life.

Transferring Healing Energy with Qi Gong

Western and Chinese people are often fascinated by demonstrations of so-called *Fa Qi*≈ Sending out energy. The practitioner is sending out *Qi* through their *Lao Gong* PE-8 points on the palm of the hands without touching the patient. The patient is standing with his back towards the practitioner while getting treated, and his body may undergo involuntary movements under the influence of the practitioner's *Qi*. It is not easy to work on one's own internal *Qi*, but the sending out of harmonizing *Qi* to others is even more difficult. In addition, "transferring" energy to another person on a regular basis may deplete the donor's energy and therefore endanger his/her health. Demonstrations of *Fa Qi* should, therefore, be looked at with a critical eye.

For a practitioner of Chinese medicine, regular practice of *Qi Gong* can be of invaluable support, as they can learn more about the flow of *Qi* through the direct insight of the energetic system within themselves which will enhance their diagnostic and therapeutic skills. As today's acupuncture training is often very intellectual a *Qi Gong* class will make it possible to experience first hand and help the understanding at a different level.

Harmonizing one's inner energy by a daily exercise routine, makes one not only more sensitive towards the energy of the patient but also helps the therapist recognize and respect the natural border between one's own and the patient's energy. Getting in touch with a patient adequately requires a lot of awareness. In the long run, *Qi Gong* exercises enable the practitioner to be "right here and now" and to be able to better meet the patient's needs. In the presence of a harmonious practitioner, the patient will feel at ease, this being the most helpful premise for a good treatment with any applied method.

A therapist may apply *Qi Gong* while doing *Tui Na* or acupuncture.

Qi Gong side effects

Qi Gong may produce unwanted side effects. I experienced this with a method that was taught by someone who obviously did not know about the natural flow of *Qi* in the body. After practicing the method for some weeks I developed severe vertigo and circulation problems. I was told by the teacher that this was the manifestation of "intense cleansing" and a sign of a "spiritual crisis". However, I only regained my health after stopping the exercises and getting help from an excellent Chinese doctor.

Today we have access to a lot more background information about a particular teacher, their lineage and their style. Many Western countries already have guidelines for the education of teachers. Usually, the graduation from an established school provides professional teaching of a particular method. What is often missing though is the Chinese medical background.

There is a basic guideline to all *Qi Gong* exercises: their practice should be relaxed (*Fang Song*), quiet (*Jing*) and natural (*Zi Ran).*

However, when starting *Qi Gong* practice, one may expect some "side effects“ though. Some are considered positive and some may signal a wrong or an ill-adapted practice. It is common that when intensely practicing any "energy" technique, some old or unresolved issues, be it physical or psychological, may surface. This should not be confused with pain appearing in a knee that had surgery, simply signaling a wrong body posture that needs to be corrected by the teacher. In another person, the knee pain could reflect the activation of the flow of *Qi* and the initiation of a healing process. Only constant exchange and collaboration between student and teacher can shed light on the appearance of any given side effect. I recommend to all beginners not to hesitate to inform their teacher about their experiences so that the teacher may better adapt the exercise to the student's capacity and need. The same exchange is necessary for psychological issues; in general, it is sometimes good to go through some emotions when practicing *Qi Gong*. It is then important not to linger on the emotion but to simply let it pass and to continue with the practice. If however, the same reaction appears over and over again, or if a heavy suppressed trauma suddenly emerges to the surface, professional help is needed, as a *Qi Gong* class is not the adequate place for resolving problems such as these.

Contra-indications of Qi Gong

Qi Gong is adaptable to nearly all-physical conditions. The exercises may be practiced in standing, sitting or lying postures. With a little imagination, a fitting exercise may be found for whatever handicap the person has. If somebody is very weak, they should, of course, practice very carefully in order not to deplete their energy further. In the presence of a terminal disease, the person can go on practicing a "still method" in order to prepare for death and a peaceful departure.

According to Hu Yao Zhen, the only real contraindication to energy work is severe mental illness. This is easy to understand. The first stage of any *Qi Gong* exercise is called *Ru Jing* ≈ Entering the silence which entitles the relaxing of the mind (calming of the *Xin* ≈ Heart). If the mind is relaxed, the body will follow and the *Qi* starts to move through the body. A calm Heart is needed for a harmonious flow of *Qi*, which then moves the body (*Shen* 身). The *Qi* serves as a medium between the Spirit and the body. If a person's mind is disturbed it may be impossible to "enter the silence" and their mental condition may worsen.

However, in mild depression, anxiety, insomnia or other less severe mental problems it may be very helpful to practice *Qi Gong* or *Tai Ji* because both methods help to reintegrate the person's mind & body.

The meditative aspect of Qi Gong

Very often *Qi Gong* and *Tai Ji Quan* are also called "meditation in motion" or "contemplative movements" – expressions that are very much to the point. The difference between a simple gymnastic exercise and a "meditation in motion" lies in the fact that the latter includes relaxation and calming of the mind. The practice of slow flowing exercises has itself a relaxing influence on the mind. If one really wants to enter into silence, some appropriate instructions have to be given by the teacher.

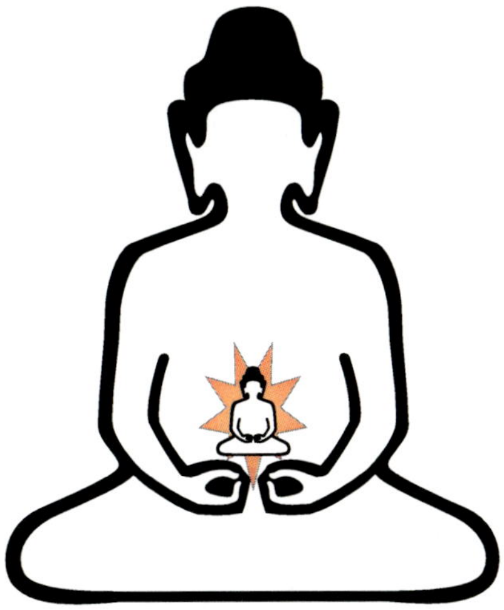

Figure 20.2: *Qi* Gong-Meditation: Calm the mind and bring the attention back to the center of the body

Some students may have prior experience with meditation in the tradition of *Vipassana*, *Zazen* etc. This is a good preparation for the moving exercises. The Buddhist and Daoist martial arts have their own meditation techniques, but for practitioners of Chinese medicine "still *Qi Gong*" is the method of choice. It is further advisable that the "still" and "moving" exercises be of the same tradition in order to complement each other better.

The first step in meditation is to bring one's attention back to only one subject in order to calm down the chaos of thoughts and feelings that the untrained mind is busy with. It is important to follow one technique and not to get scattered. For example, if one still method focuses on breathing while another method brings the attention on the energetic center in the lower belly (*Dan Tian),* then applying both methods will not calm the mind, and on the long term, progress will be slow and hampered (▶ Fig. 20.2).

If the exercises are practiced within a spiritual context, an internal transformation may be achieved. As described in the ancient writings on *Tai Ji Quan*, a well-trained teacher may guide the advanced student into the process of transforming the *Jing* ≈ Essence into *Qi* ≈ Energy, *Qi* into *Shen* ≈ Spirit and the Spirit into *Xu* ≈ Emptiness.

20.3 The difference between Qi Gong and Tai Ji Quan

Qi Gong is an exercise that is usually practiced alone or in a group, but without an actual training partner. Hence it is called a self-cultivating method. The *Qi* that is trained in this way may be applied to others in two ways: for a medical purpose or in martial arts. Chinese martial arts (*Wu Shu),* has so-called internal and external styles. The famous Cheng Man Ch'ing *(1901 - 1975),* one of the first teachers of traditional *Tai Ji Quan* in the US, explains the two styles.

- External styles came down from the Buddhist monastery of *Shaolin,* and because Boddhidarma was not a Chinese, these styles are called external i.e. coming from abroad. The kind of *Qi Gong* that is practiced by these impressive and acrobatic styles is called hard *Qi Gong* (*Ying Gong*) (▶ Fig. 20.3). Martial artists practice the hard exercises in order to make the body invulnerable and to concentrate the *Qi* in certain areas of the body at will. The result of this kind of *Gong* can be admired in the stunning skills of the shows of *Shaolin* fighters. Of course, it needs a lot of *Gong Fu* to get a simple needle flying through a piece of glass and hitting the water balloon behind it!
- The soft *Qi Gong* (*Rua Gong*) is at the basis of the martial arts that Chinese call "internal",

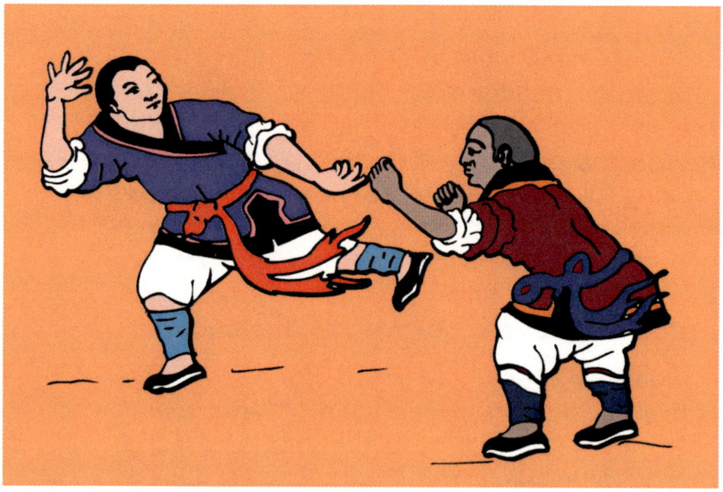

Figure 20.3: Shaolin Boxing belongs to the hard forms *Ying Gong*

like *Tai Ji Quan, Xin Yi Quan*, *Ba Gua Zhang*, *Liu He Ba Fa*, *Tong Bei Quan etc.* Their roots lie in the sacred mountains of Wu Dang and they have been developed in Daoist schools and family clans (i.e. are "originally" Chinese). Internal martial arts are based on the concept of "the soft overcoming the hard". People who are trained in *Tai Ji Quan* will move like water, hence if opponents attack, they won't find a single hard place to apply their strength.

The legend says, that the Daoist sage Zhang San Feng roaming the forests of sacred Wudang mountain, was inspired to create *Tai Ji Quan* when he watched a snake fighting a crane. Historically the first traces of *Tai Ji Quan* can be found in the 17th century in the valley of Chen Jia Gou, where *Chen*-style *Tai Ji Quan* originated from. Other family clans developed different styles, the most famous ones being *Yang-*, double *Wu-*, and *Sun*-styles. A *Tai Ji* form is a sequence of self-defensive techniques that have been created for the practice of the 13 movements (*Shi San Shi*) of *Tai Ji Quan* i.e. five steps and eight hand techniques. No matter how different their performance might look – it is always grounded in the same basic principles of movements that will appear in variations with different interpretations.

Classical training in *Tai Ji Quan* consists of a form, application, partner-exercise, for example, *Tuishou* ≈ Pushing-hands *Qi Gong*-meditation. The first form to be taught is usually a hand form. Later on the various traditional weapons like the sword (*Jian*), saber (*Dao*), spear (*Qian*) and halbard (*Da Dao*) will follow. Although these movements are actually techniques of self-defense, they are based on the same energetic principles as *Qi Gong*. So today *Tai Ji* often misses the boxing-part (*Quan)* and is practiced as a self-cultivating method like *Qi Gong*. In fact, it is a fantastic health preserving exercise as well!

Benefits of practicing Qi Gong

Cheng Man Ch'ing, one of the first teachers of traditional *Tai Ji Quan* who came to the US in 1964 was asked by a student, why he was practicing *Tai Ji Quan*, his answered: "So that when you finally get to know about life, there will be some health left to enjoy it". Practising *Qi Gong* or *Tai Ji* is good for your health, but if you really get into it, it turns out to be a way to look at life itself.

Those students who prefer a short-term class in *Qi Gong* or *Tai Ji Quan* will have a short-term effect of relaxation (body and mind) and a superficial idea of the Chinese self-cultivating arts. Students, who visit a class for one year or longer, will have regular input to their energetic system and therefore a longer lasting benefit for their physical and mental balance. However, only students who practice alone at home will get the full benefit of the exercise. Why is that? In daily life "the ten thousand things" that are more important than our practice will come to our minds: Getting another coffee, driving the kids to school, cleaning the cat's litter or finishing a very important piece of work, seems to keep us away from practicing. And at the end of that busy day, we are, of course, too tired to practice! To cut this pattern it often takes effort for the beginner. But when they've started to practice on their own, major changes start taking place, not only is their progress faster but they also start to really care about themselves. Regular practice at home means taking time for oneself every day, no matter how one feels, or what is going on around us, or where we actually are. I remember a *Qi Gong* student who had just come back from her holidays, sitting in the changing room, crying sadly; during her holiday she had lost half of her family in a natural disaster. In spite of the horrible experience she had just gone through, she went on practicing and reported that the exercises gave her hope and confidence. She showed me, how strong a person's spirit can be and that *Qi Gong* can be more than a health-preserving exercise.

Qi Gong and religious beliefs

There has been some controversy concerning *Qi Gong* practice and certain religious movements. Trying to cut off Chinese medicine, martial arts, and *Qi Gong* from their philosophical and spiritual roots is likely to deprive these methods of their genuine power. The concepts of *Yin, Yang*, and *Qi* are deeply holistic and they must be understood properly to practice these methods successfully. Without getting involved in the political ramifications in a modern world, it makes sense, to put a lot of emphasis on the health benefits of *Qi Gong*. No one should be afraid of any kind of religious indoctrination when participating in a *Qi Gong*-class! *Qi Gong* exercises finally may be a way to get in touch not only with ourselves but also with what the Chinese call Heaven, Earth and the *Dao*. In the words of the Daoist master Zhuang Zi (400 BC):

> *[...] To pant, to puff, to hail, to sip, to spit out the old breath and draw in the new, practicing bear-hangings and bird-stretching, longevity his only concern, such is the life favored by the scholar who practices Induction, the man who nourishes his body, who hopes to live to be as old as P'eng-Tsu. But to attain loftiness without constraining the will; to achieve moral training without benevolence and righteousness, good order without accomplishments and fame, leisure without rivers and seas, long life without Induction; to lose everything and yet possess everything, at ease in the illimitable, where all good things come to attend - this is the Way of Heaven and earth, the Virtue of the sage.*

20.4 Qi Gong Self-massage

Practice daily, early in the morning or at any convenient time.

Chest and Trunk (► Fig. 20.4)

- Put both palms of the hands (*Lao Gong* PE-8) on the navel.
- Bring your attention inside to the middle of the belly between the navel (*Shen Que* RM-8) and the lower back (*Ming Men* DM-4). Calm your mind.
- For women put the right hand on the chest (*Shan Zhong* RM-17), the upper sea of *Qi*, and the left hand on top. For men put the left hand on the chest and the right hand on top of the left hand. Now massage with regular strokes down to the pubic symphysis (*Qu Gu* RM-2)

Repeat 36 times. If you are excited or suffering from any discomfort in the chest you can do up to 100 strokes, or repeat the exercise until you feel better. Counting is important as it helps to calm the mind. Important: Do not try to push the energy down, just follow the hands with your attention. Qi will follow naturally

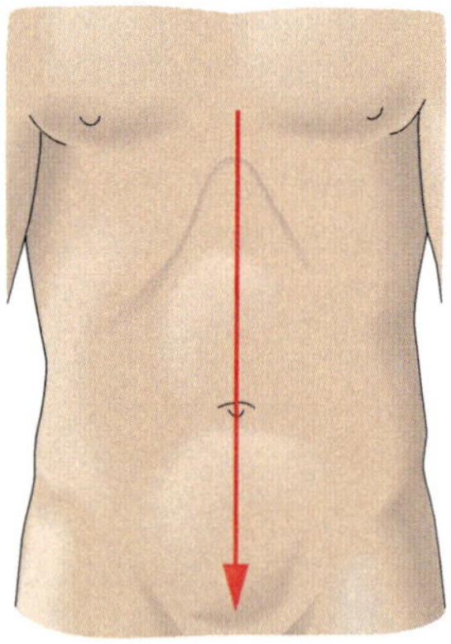

Figure 20.4 : Chest and trunk massage

Abdomen (▶ Fig. 20.5)

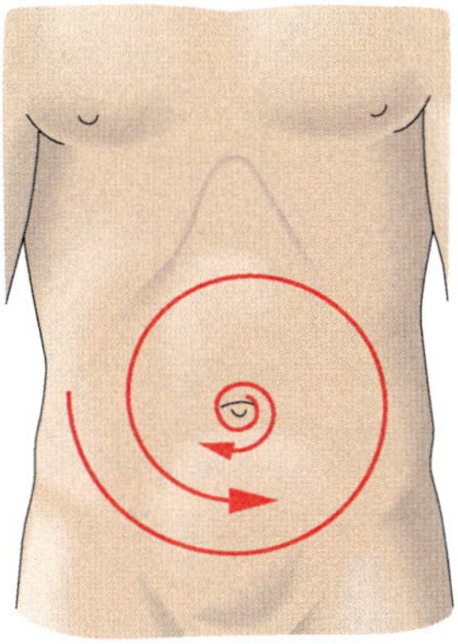

Figure 20.5 : Abdomen

- Put your hands on the navel (*Shen Que* RM-8) and wait until the belly and the hands get warm and comfortable.
- Women should massage in clockwise circles around the navel (from smaller to bigger circles) 36 times. Then change the direction and again massage in circles (from bigger to smaller) 24 times.
- Men should start massaging counter-clockwise 36 times from smaller to bigger, then 24 times clockwise from bigger to smaller.

Lower back and abdomen (▶ Fig. 20.6)

- The hands lay again on the navel and the lower belly, waiting until the belly and the hands get warm and comfortable.
- Bring your attention from the navel (*Shen Que* RM-8)) to the lower back (*Ming Men* DM-4).
- For men as well as for women after menopause, the attention should be kept at the lumbar area (*Ming Men* DM-4) for a while.
- For women before menopause the attention and the hands move from the lower back (*Ming Men* DM-4) to the lower belly (*Qi Hai* RM-6 and *Guan Yuan* RM-4), staying there for a while.

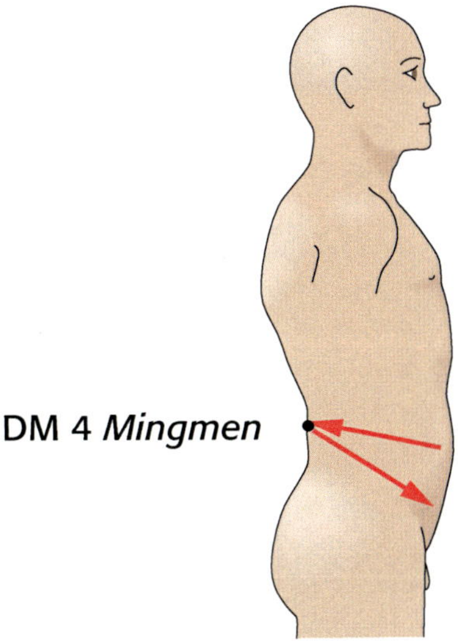

Figure 20.6: Lumbar and abdominal massage

Face and head (▶ Fig. 20.7)

Rub your hands until they are warm. Put the palms of your hands (*Lao Gong* PE-8) on the eyes and let the warmth flow into them. Gently rub your face with both hands up and down, with the middle finger next to the nose, the index at the outer canthus of the eye and the thumb in front of the ear. Then put the tips of your fingers to the frontline of the hair and "comb" your hair to the base of the skull 3 times (along *Du Mai*, Bladder and Gallbladder channels). Rub the base of the skull (*Feng Chi* GB-20). Grab your ear between index finger and thumb and gently massage it from top to bottom (ear lobe) 3 times.

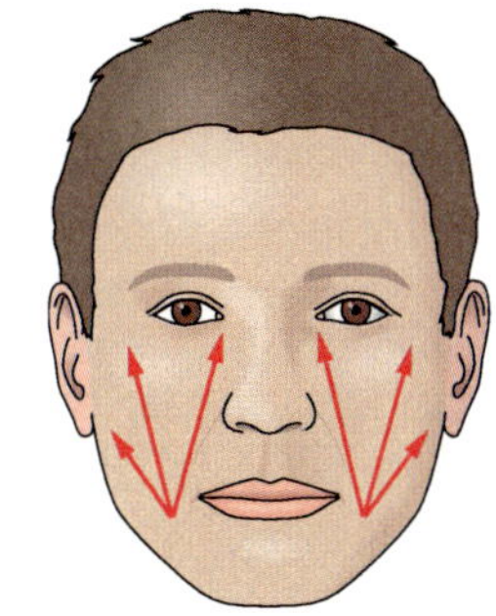

Figure 20.7: Face and head massage

Hands and Arms (▶ Fig. 20.8)

- Hands: With your right hand first rub the thumb-side of the left hand, thereby stimulating Large Intestine, Lung and

Pericardium channels. Then change to the small finger-side and carefully rub Small Intestine, Heart and Triple Warmer channels. Make sure your rub from fingertip towards the wrist. Then change hands.

- Arms: Put your right hand on the thumb side of the left wrist and gently rub towards the elbow back and forth, including both joints and the Large Intestine, Lung and Pericardium channels. Then rub the small finger side the same way, thereby stimulating Small Intestine, Heart and Triple Warmer channels. Change sides.

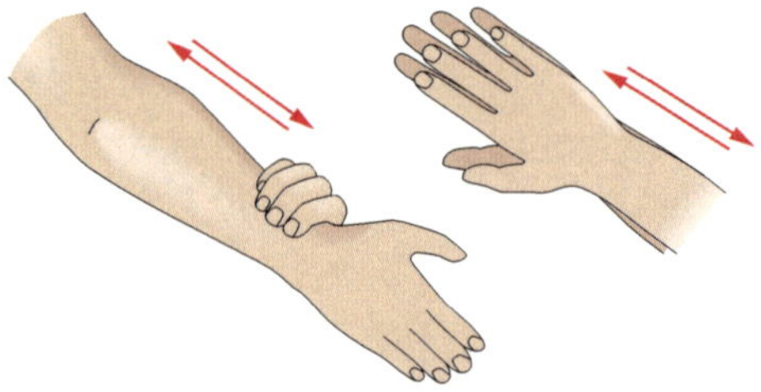

Figure 20.8: Hands and arms

Feet (► Fig. 20.9)

Put the palm of your right hand (*Lao Gong* PE-8) on the sole of the left foot (*Yong Quan* KI-1) and do 100 small circles towards you. Change hand and foot and repeat the exercise.

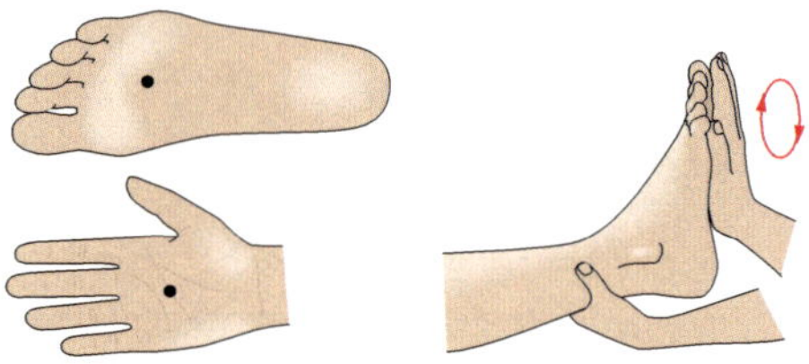

Figure 20.9: Massage of the feet

Legs (► Fig. 20.10)

- Put the palm of your right hand on the inside ankle of the left leg. Rub from ankle to knee up and down, thereby stimulating Spleen, Liver, and Kidney channels. Change to the outside and stimulate Stomach, Gallbladder and Bladder channels. Make sure you include the ankle and knee joints. Change hand and leg and repeat the exercise.
- Lift one leg, bending the knee and drawing an inward circle, the sole of the foot (*Yong Quan* KI-1) and the energy in the center of the belly thereby get connected and gather in the lower belly. Then flex the foot and make a heel-kick forward. Repeat 9 times with each foot.

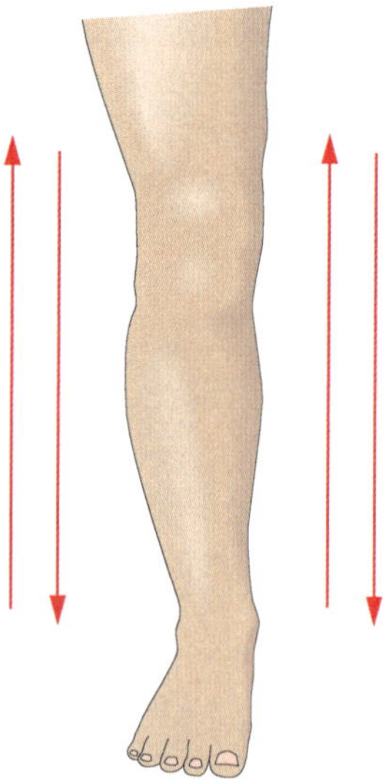

Figure 20.10 Leg

Final Exercise

Put your hands back on the navel and gather your attention in the area behind it. Feel the energy flow

Qi Gong self-massage is a safe and simple exercise that can be practiced by everyone. No matter if one is healthy or suffers from any kind of disease, this massage technique will help to harmonize the energy of organs and channels. As the exercise enhances the production and distribution of defensive energy/ *Wei Qi*, the quality of the skin, as well as the immune system, will profit from regular practice. For the same reason, it is important not to take a shower directly after the massage, water may disrupt the energy-circulation that has just been induced. Parts 1 (chest and trunk) and 2 (Abdomen) may be practiced alone at any time during the day. They help to calm the mind, promote sleep and harmonize digestion.

21. Cultivation of the Mind Psycho-energetics

by Solange Montakab-Pont

[...] what disturbs and alarms us are not the things, rather our opinion about the things [...]. Epictetus (Greek philosopher)

21.1 The Hidden Causes of Dis-ease

Historically, Chinese medicine has emphasized the continuity of the physical, emotional and spiritual dimensions of the human being. Furthermore, in the causative factors of disease, categorized as external, internal and mixed, the internal causes, the emotions, and mental attitudes, hold prime importance. The Chinese premise of "the body holds the mind and the mind contains the body" demonstrates this belief clearly. The arrival of Buddhism in China further reinforced the concept that the source of all suffering was to be found in the mind, specifically in the manner in which we perceive reality.

We are shaped by our thoughts, we become what we think. The Buddha

Unfortunately, modern TCM, has reduced the practice of Chinese medicine to the treatment of *Zang-Fu* organs and the Five Substances, disregarding the ancient emphasis on the inner causes of disease, human emotions.

On the opposite end of the spectrum, the 20th-century Western theories about the psyche and the consequent development of numerous therapeutic approaches are offering extremely effective methods for shedding light and helping to resolve psycho-emotional issues and to liberate the hidden roots of dis-ease.

The Eastern models of the psyche give us a veritable insight into the three fundamental mechanisms of suffering and dis-ease:

- The illusion of separation;
- The illusion of what is reality;
- The identification with this so-called reality.

The true source of suffering is the illusion of separation and of duality: me versus the other, ego versus unity, attachment versus rejection, health versus disease...

Identification with what we believe to be the reality, which in truth is an illusion created by our habitual fixation. These fixations are the guiding fictions that we repeat to ourselves so often and with such conviction, that we forget that they are simply scenarios we have written at some point in the past, and we act as if they are the reality. Just as when we watch a movie, we might become so emotionally involved and identified with the drama, that we forget that this is just "a movie".

We do not see things as "they" are, rather we see things as "we" are.

In fact, it is our projections and emotions, which make this scenario we call our “lives” appear to be so real. The notion of “reality” is very personal. Hence the same movie has a very different meaning and impact, depending on who is watching it.

Obviously, the choices we make with our minds and the actions that follow these choices will shape and affect our world and also affect the feedback the world has on us. This notion joins the oriental concept of *Karma*. *Karma* refers to an action, which causes an entire cycle of cause and effect, actively shaping past, present and future experiences. In the Daoist belief, certain actions may even have consequences on the descendants, transmitted via the *Zong* ≈ Ancestral *Qi* and hence beyond the reach of therapy. Sun Si Miao, the 7th-century Chinese physician, maintained that acupuncture may be effective in removing the pain or karmic imprint of a person, by working on the Eight Extraordinary channels.

In a nutshell, the mind affects the body, and one’s beliefs and attitudes shape the world and the experiences and hence create one’s reality. Any fixation or identification on pain or disease will create more suffering and a stronger imprint, further giving "density" to the disease. But if one can modulate the physical fixation into a mere sensation that comes and goes, and in fact is modified and is changing when one breathes in and out, the related physical or emotional fixation turns into a living experience. For example, a pain that has been diagnosed as osteoarticular arthrosis, confirmed by X-rays, has a "fixed" reality, as defined by medical science. The patient either has the choice to submit to this fixation and identify with it, hence surrender to the inevitable evolution of the disease. Or consider the condition as a moving and changing phenomenon, attempting to express deeper aspects of the psyche. Just watching physical pain and its mental emotional links can help us deal with the anger, sadness or fear behind the pain. On the other hand, just talking about emotional issues without attending to the expression of those emotions in the body would cause even further emotional unrest and physical symptoms. Both body and mind have to be integrated into treatment. Today, psychosomatic medicine is taken much more seriously. Many approaches to healing and recovery utilize techniques like meditation, guided imagery, visualization, hypnosis and so on. Furthermore, it is important to let the body talk and the mind listen, establishing a dialogue between the two so that true healing may happen in the physical, emotional and spiritual dimensions of the human being.

When appropriate, I like to help establish a dialogue between the body and mind of the patient during an acupuncture session. In fact, by activating the points and channels of acupuncture, a modulation of the energetic vibration takes place and resonates not only in the material body but also in the subtle body, thus affecting the body, emotion, and mind. I believe the most important stage in healing is to be able to make a connection between the physical, emotional and spiritual dimensions of the human being. Hence with a little support from the therapist, the acupuncture session could constitute the ideal moment for the patient to discover the links and connections between their body and their mental attitudes.

The Dissolution of Mass – Concept of the Void

The Tao is like a well: used but never used up.

It is like the eternal void: filled with infinite possibilities. It is hidden but always present: .... *Lao Zu, Taotejing ch.4*

According to the Daoist concepts the origin of the universe is considered to be "Nothingness", the void (▶ Fig. 21.1). The best analogy to describe the void is to consider the concept of space. There are no points of reference in space, as there is no center in the universe, no up or down or in and out, in fact, no boundaries, it is limitless. Yet, space contains all the possibilities as everything in creation contains space. Today, Quantum physics has demonstrated that the fundamental particles of matter are not so solid after all. They are made of 99.999% of emptiness or space. The Daoist vision that at the beginning there was nothingness and that also all disappears into this nothingness or space, is being supported by modern physics. So, it can be resumed that matter appears out of nothingness and dissolves back into this nothingness. Furthermore, it has been demonstrated that at the sub-atomic level, particles behave either as mass or a wave. In simple words, this means that matter can become vibration and vice versa.

In the pursuit of healing, the aim would be to find this inner space in to which a materialized mass could dissolve and out of which a new creation could emerge.

Let us explore further, what this concept actually means.

Again in Quantum physics, which is the study of tiny sub-microscopic particles, very recently scientists at the CERN institute in Geneva (Switzerland) have discovered a particle that was named the Higgs boson also called the "God particle". This discovery gives more credence to the existence of elementary particles and forces that give rise to the world around us. The theory that there has to have been something that bound together protons, electrons, and neutrons after the "Big Bang" had never been proven. This particle is the answer to the questions of what gives mass to matter and how the universe was formed. After the Big Bang, some 13.7 billion years ago, the early universe was filled with electrons, protons, and neutrons floating around by themselves. The Higgs boson particle would be the element that supplied the glue that shaped and gave the objects matter and is holding the physical fabric of the universe together. The theory further states that the more they attract, the bigger their mass will be.

Let us apply these concepts to our previous case. The more there is a fixation on disease and on its symptoms, the stronger the attractive forces, hence, the bigger the mass. In practice, the more the mind believes and concentrates on the "physical" reality of a disease, the truer the disease becomes. In this case all the allopathic and surgical measures make sense. Acupuncture, a vibratory medicine, attempts to move the matter back towards a more fluid and vibratory state and could go a step deeper in the healing process. But it is not until the mind establishes a connection with the dis-ease, and can put a definition or a "name" on it, that the pathological process can reverse itself and resolution be achieved.

When we are no longer preoccupied with self-centered pursuits based on the insecurities of the illusory self and its desires and aversions, the mind becomes spacious.

The fundamental premise in all of the oriental philosophies is that beneath sensation and feeling, the reality is of a vibratory nature, and at its core is the "Void". Out of this fundamental wholeness or void, sensation and feeling arise, and back into this void, they dissolve. When we identify with these sensations and feelings we identify with our suffering. When we un-identify with our pain, that is, when we cease to grasp and reject, we spontaneously dissolve the delusions of dualism. Now wholeness and healing may happen.

> *Free from desire, you realize the mystery. Caught in desire, you see only the manifestation. Yet mystery and manifestation arise from the same source. This source is called darkness [...].* *Lao Tzu,* Tao Te Jing, *chap. 1*

The pain that once hurt us now enriches our lives with greater meaning, purpose, and insight. We have followed a raging river until it emptied into a serene sea. Healing is the gift of being at one with suffering and giving space in one's heart for it to let go.

Taking either view of ancient wisdom or modern thought, we come to the same conclusion: "Fundamental reality is not a mass of separate entities; it is a ground of vibratory wholeness". Compassion seeks this space for healing. Compassion is a quality of the *Xin* ≈ Heart and of the *Shen* ≈ Spirit. It is fundamental to distinguish the difference between "love" and "compassion". Love, as is commonly understood, refers to sentimental and emotional love, which is totally conditional and relates to human interactions and is delegated to the *Xin Bao* ≈ Pericardium, the Heart-minister. Compassion is defined as unconditional, non-judgmental and non-possessive love, and is the quality emanating from the Heart-Emperor as one of the attributes of *Shen*≈ *S*pirit. Compassion is a condition through which healing and recovery may happen regardless of the nature of the pain. Thus, compassion is to be able to see the current difficulty through the eyes of the Heart with a loving and an expanded view. It is also to be able to unite the rejected, suffering part of the self. Because when we are in the Heart, we are above judgments and only then can we start seeing the bigger picture. From this viewpoint we understand how both the negative and positive sides of ourselves are valid, each having their necessary purposes. Only then can we start to let go, forge, accept and not be in denial and judgment. In this manner, suffering is neither ignored nor rejected; we do not try to resist it, we go deeper towards what the Daoists call the "Empty Heart". The empty Heart is the necessary condition and the space in which healing and recovery can take place. Emptying the Heart signifies getting rid of not only mundane thoughts but also of all judgments, preconceived notions and values, thus making space for the *Shen*, the sacred and spiritual healer within us.

Quantum physics by itself is not complete and the "God particle" does not explain God; "*Shen*", consciousness, the spirit or the mind, the observer is necessary to complete it.

> *The Tao can't be perceived. Smaller than an electron, it contains uncountable galaxies [...].* *Lao Tzu,* Tao Te Jing, *chap. 32*

Dealing with the source of suffering

As it was defined, suffering originates from a compulsive state of agitation leading to mental-emotional fixation, which then causes physical transformation and disease. So a true healing process has to address all these issues.

Here is the case of a patient suffering from tinnitus, which started after a period of stress at work. He also had hypertension and recent insomnia caused by the ringing in his ears. He was getting more and more stressed and fixated on the tinnitus. With acupuncture, I treated his “Internal Wind” and his “Liver-*Yang* rising" and also used the technique of "Dialogue with the Body" (see below). He realized the direct relation between his fixation on the noises and the increase in the sound volume of the ringing. With his mental attitude and meditation, he could change his way of being and establish a new relationship with the sounds in his ears. He could use it as a feedback signal for his stress. The sounds diminished and at times completely disappeared. He could sleep and be generally more at ease.

A story, coming from the east, about a man and a horse. The horse is galloping quickly, and it appears that the man and the horse are going somewhere important. Another man, standing alongside the road, shouts, “where are you going?” and the first man replies, “I don’t know, ask the horse!”.

This parable is referring to the state of humanity today. The horse represents our inborn human tendencies, our impulses towards particular behaviors. Because we respond with grasping (attachment or desire) or aversion (rejection or dislike), we give away our free will and become powerless. We are asleep during the day and having the illusion of being in control of our lives and we are always running and in stress, hence we cannot stop. And of course, as our nights reflect our days, at night we are often struggling in our dreams as well.

Many ancient philosophies and religions have indicated ways of dealing with this state of agitation and suffering. The eastern traditions have proposed a way for gaining self-knowledge, of separating the world of illusion “Maya” from reality, in order to liberate us from this state of confusion.

The proposed method is the practice of "Mindfulness Meditation" (▶ chap. 20.).

The Healing Process

True and complete healing has to address not only the manifested stagnation but also the underlying causative factor, the emotion, which itself is the result of how the mind perceives the world. The healing process could be, very schematically, broken down into the following stages:

- Helping the patient identify the true source of their disease
- Exploring with the patient, the ramifications, links, beliefs, projections, and judgments, involving their condition,
- Releasing the mental attitudes, which could be:
  - Either a grasping or compulsive fixation
  - Or in the form of an aversion, a rejection, a resistance, or even an aggression
  - Or complete ignorance and denial of the true issue

    Ideas that are prominent in our thoughts quickly appear as images in the energy field. If the energy field is the blueprint that guides and molds the body, it may be that by imaging an illness, even unconsciously, and

> *repeatedly reinforcing its presence in the field, we are in effect programming the body to manifest the illness [...].* Michael Talbot

The new-age approach to self-development can be an obstacle to a real self-liberation. There is a growing fascination with psychotherapy, archetypes, astrology, relationships, channeling, angels, past lives, dream work, and many others. All of these methods reflect our inherent desire to grow and to become perfect. To consider this kind of self-examination, as the ultimate journey, is to risk becoming very narcissistic, even a kind of "self-developing new age addict".

On the other hand, there is the opposite tendency, in many of us, not only with patients but even with practitioners and students, to avoid self-questioning, looking for quick solutions and recipes. There is a trend today towards a compulsive accumulation of knowledge, a veritable "learning munchies"! Rather than real involvement with the patient, the application of acquired techniques is very tempting.

> *Let the healers train themselves to know the inner stage of thought or desire of the one who seeks help. They can thereby know the source from which the trouble comes.* Diwhal Khul

In my opinion, in order to respond to basic human needs, we should first address and understand our own unresolved issues before we can help our patients face their emotional problems. Our fear of our own pain and suffering prevents us from developing a "Healing Heart" attitude. Denial is not compatible with healing. Especially, deep down we know that everything we do not deal with is a burden we will have to carry.

A compassionate healing approach involves openness without judgment. By putting our heart into what we do, the world around us begins to change and so do we. We can become co-creators in our next step of evolution. The narcissistic attitude of thinking that we are separate from each other is obsolete. Understanding the law of interdependence and realizing that we are not separate from each other and from existence is opening the mind. Whatever we put out will very soon come back to us, multiplied. Out of this realization, we will have the readiness to take responsibility for the creation of our own suffering. When this responsibility is understood and accepted, respect and healing can take place on this planet.

21.2 Self-Cultivation for the Practitioner

Sun Si Miao (7th century AD), one of the most illustrious figures in the Chinese Medical history, states in *Da Yi Jing Chen* on the "Sincerity and Devotion of Great Doctors": ..."When great doctors treat a patient, they must concentrate, calm down, and be free of desires and pursuits. Above all, they need to have a compassionate heart and be devoted to freeing the patient from the suffering of illnesses.

In this passage Sun Si Miao stresses the fundamental importance of compassion and advises the healers to remain at the service of their patients irrespective of rank and race, to treat them with equality, remaining non-judgmental and kind.

The cultivation of ethics was already emphasized by the Greek Hippocrates a thousand years earlier and remains true even today. To become a true healer certain qualities need to be integrated, what Sun Si Miao names "Self-Cultivation".

Therapists in Relation to themselves

In order to treat a patient, the first and foremost requirement for the therapist is inner stability. I call this the "Central Axis", referring to the ability of standing, rooted like a tree in the ground, head raised up to the open sky thus able to deal with the reality at hand. The Chinese concept of “Heaven, Human and Earth” represents this idea very clearly.

Our nature includes Earth and Heaven, symbolizing form-structure and space-emptiness. When we connect with the earth we interact with the horizontal plane of solidity and when we connect with the sky we meet the vertical plane of space and emptiness. In the ancient Chinese system of thought, Humanity (Man), as placed between Heaven and Earth, is characterized by the capacity of sensitivity and feeling, represented by the “Heart”.

The axis represents the universal principle of change and stability. Daoist philosophy states that change is successful when both, “the great rooted tree”, by the “flowing river” are combined within a natural setting. This Oriental nature metaphor is a reminder that during times of change it is necessary to incorporate in equal proportions, the qualities of quietude (the great rooted tree), with activity (the flowing river).

When one is in this "Central Axis", one is automatically connected to the universal energies. In this manner, healing happens *through* the therapist and not *because* of him or her. When, as therapists, we are not in connection with this universal energy, there is the tendency of using our own energies with the risk of either depleting ourselves or the danger of absorbing the patient’s problems.

Sun Si Miao further emphasizes clearing the mind and concentrating. This infers maintaining a clear intention. The mental attitude of the therapist during the healing process is a major key element in the benefits that a patient might get from a session.

The "Central Axis", reminds us that through choice we have the ability to select fortunate, positive, and abundant changes for ourselves as well as for our patients. In other words, when one is rooted in one's "Central Axis", one has access to all possibilities and choices, without being limited by mental or emotional fixations that are the source of attachment or rejection. Successful change requires that we follow what is meaningful and has Heart and *Shen* ≈ Spirit. The fusion in the Heart center reminds us that change is an opportunity for creating new realities that expand and deepen our healing Heart and our essence.

Exercise to develop the "Central Axis" (▶ Fig. 21.2)

Keep in mind that throughout the exercise the axis should remain firm and yet flexible, solid without being rigid.

- Starting position: feet parallel, placing them at shoulder width. Knees slightly bent, arms hanging on the sides, hands open and relaxed. Back and head are held straight in the axis.
- The "Central Axis" has 2 poles, Heaven and Earth.

- From the sole of the foot (*Yong Quan* KI-1), visualize roots growing and reaching to the center of the earth. Connect with the fire at the center of the earth and visualize a red spiral moving anti-clockwise upwards and through your feet, surrounding the bones and the sinews in the legs. Then moving further up to the inside of the trunk to wrap around the internal organs and further up to reach the top of the head (*Bai Hui* DM-20). Visualize this red spiral shooting out of the head towards the sky. Imagine this energy moving effortlessly upwards with an uplifting, supportive, and nourishing quality.

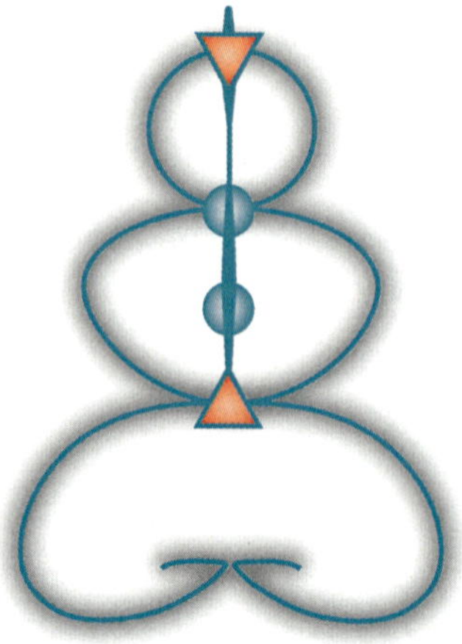

Figure 21.2: The central Axis

- This upward movement of Earth improves the stability, rooting, incarnation, and nourishes and supports the vitality of the physical body. (Supplementing the *Ying* ≈ Nourishing energy)
- Now connect to the vast sky, the pure luminous white light taking the shape of a white spiral moving clockwise downwards to surround the outside of the body and further down, all the way into the earth (► Fig. 22.1). This downward white spiral movement, like a white waterfall from Heaven, enhances evolution and change. It cleanses and clears the subtle energetic body as well as protecting it from external aggressions. (Fortifying the *Wei* ≈ Defensive energy)
- Now concentrate on the Heart center and the chest. Visualize the red and white spirals meeting in the Heart, where the colors are mixing together creating the shape of a beautiful pink rose or lotus.
- This fusion of the celestial "Heaven" energy and the Earth movement, meeting in the Heart center, stimulates the "Healing *Shen*" with its capacity to unify, to understand, to love and to respect life.
  Sample affirmations to help integrate the qualities of the "Central Axis":

- I enjoy the combination of remaining centered while in movement.
- I accomplish things easily and well.
- I am responsible for what I cause.
- I am balanced and centered.
- I trust and have faith in the deep essence of who I am.
- I enjoy making important decisions.
- Through choice, I can change my experience.

Therapists in Relation to their patients

In relating to patients the following points need to be respected:

- Adopting a receptive rather than a directive attitude and remaining non-judgemental at all times. To truly heal, one needs to resonate with their clients and to develop "empathy". This means, to be receptive, capable of listening to the patient with an open mind, avoiding assumptions of what the client should be feeling, or making any projections, or evaluations.

- Remaining compassionate without becoming emotionally involved. Not getting fixated on the specific problem allows the therapist to see the context from the patient's point of view. The therapist should be focused on what the patient is actually experiencing and feeling rather than the objective facts and general considerations.
- Respect the patient with authenticity and understanding, without prejudice, solutions, and manipulations. The journey of life is not always a simple one, as clinicians, we cannot predict the patient's path. We can respect their choices and give them opportunities to learn through cause and effect and support the healing process rather than the disease process. Supporting the healing process means focusing in the direction of what is life-giving, even while something or someone is in the process of being negative, sick or even dying. It is about being willing to face every new moment, any circumstance as it unfolds, with the capacity of compassion toward oneself and others, and the strength to deal with all that is occurring. To understand the meaning of our illnesses is to honestly look at aspects of our lives that need healing and to have the courage to face all that is present. We should particularly give attention to the hidden parts, the masked areas of our existence. The true positive attitude is learning to accept what is, simply trusting the process. Healing does not come through denying the reality of our experiences, but through affirming our power as the creator of those experiences, and that includes the power to change our thoughts, and therefore our experiences, from negative and life-denying to positive and life-affirming. We can never know what strength, courage, and insight might lie on the other side of our illness until we face it and feel it all the way through. Changing our vision towards disease is the real key, pathology does not have to be considered as a bad thing that has to be fought, rather we should consider that health and illness, life and death, are complementary and part of a larger movement of life. Illness is a way by which the body attempts to initiate a change in our lives. It could be seen as a challenge rather than an obstacle. We can begin to see all the negative experiences and individuals in our life as teachers and helpers, rather than as obstacles and enemies. Our illness gives us an opportunity to make healing changes in our life, to get back on the path of health and wholeness.
- Clear communication should be facilitated. This means that the therapist should be helping the patients to understand the messages of their unconscious rather than interpreting them or providing ready-made solutions and advice. Patients know better than anyone else what their problems are, and they can find their own way to what they actually need and to heal. The main mistake in trying to help patients is to believe that we understand what another person is telling us, when in fact we are interpreting or projecting our own ideas onto the situation. As therapists, we have to keep in mind that patients have all the resources they need for doing just that. Heart-to-Heart communication is essential for keeping the atmosphere of equality that is fundamental between two persons, even though one is directing the healing and the other is receiving it.
- Finally, as therapists, we evaluate our success by the disappearance of the patient's complaints. We take pride when the symptoms disappear, or we feel a failure if the treatment has not been successful. These are the moments to

remember the advice of the ancient masters, to remain humble, to always keep in mind that the patients' disease or suffering, is their own life challenge and path. For some the cessation of their symptoms, is the conclusion of their experience, for others, their pain is the means through which they need to learn. We, as therapists, are merely accompanying them, lending a helping hand and a compassionate presence. The transformation and alchemy that one is challenged to go through during illness may not be for everyone. Hence the limits that a patient might set have to be respected.

Treatment or healing is a sharing experience between two human beings who are searching and suffering. One of them plays the role of the giver, and the other the role of the receiver and vice versa. Healing provides us with opportunities to teach others our knowledge about balance and the laws of cause and effect, but also to learn from them. To remember that we are together in this process of healing and that we are doing the best we can. Each patient is unique, and in his or her own way may also be a teacher for us. The transformations that patients achieve will not only affect and change their own lives but also the lives of those that are in contact with them.

> *is true power [.[...] Knowing others is intelligence; knowing yourself is true wisdom;*
> *Mastering others is strength; mastering yourself..].*
>
> Lao Tzu, *Tao Te Jing*, chap. 33

An Example of how to work with a patient combining visualization and acupuncture

A 45-year-old woman, married, mother of 3 children, whose husband has been unemployed for 6 months, is suffering from chest oppression with shoulder and neck pains, and pre-menstrual migraine headaches. She also has lumbar pains and cold feet. Her tongue is purplish with red sides. Her pulse is wiry, with a weak Kidney-*Yang*. I had treated her four times with acupuncture for Liver-*Qi* stagnation and Kidney-*Yang Xu* ≈ Vacuity over six weeks. She reported getting better but then the symptoms would recur. She also mentioned that she had been having recurrent dreams of stress. In a dream, she saw herself driving a heavy truck with a very heavy load. The truck could hardly move and she was worried not to be able to reach her destination. She also realized in her dream that she was very worried because she did not have a license to drive a truck.

So I took the opportunity this time to treat her only with "mind-body dialogue". I explained briefly the process to the patient that she should mainly be aware of her bodily sensations and welcome any thoughts, feelings, or images connected to the body impressions. The treatment session was structured to devote 20 to 30 minutes for the dream exploration, and a further 10 to 15 minutes to talk about the experience and bring the process to a conclusion. I usually take the pulses at the start and at the end of the session.

. I started by suggesting to her to become aware of the most predominant feeling, or of any thought or issue that was present in her dream or in her life now. I asked her to put words on these feelings.

Patient: It just feels too much pressure on me to carry the whole family and the

insecurity of my husband's situation.
I asked her to scan the body and relate this feeling to a place in her body. And to let me know what is going on in the concerned area, in terms of sensations, shape, color, landscape, quality.
. Patient: I feel like a huge stone on my shoulders and neck, it weighs a ton. I feel like I could just collapse and be smashed by it. The setting is in a place where trucks go to discharge their loads, close to the evening with a sort of heavy atmosphere like before a rain. No one is there, and I feel a bit frightened. A strong wind is blowing and scattering the objects around.
. Question: what are you experiencing in your neck and shoulder area now?
. Patient: I feel shaky and moved. My shoulders and neck are very tight.
. If your shoulders and neck could speak and express what would they say?
. Patient: My shoulder and neck say: I have enough of this pressure, my arms are restless and they feel like pushing the pressure away. They feel angry.
. Just be with it and recognize and accept that anger is there. Now, open up to the fact that your shoulder and neck feel pressure, and would like to push it away. What is happening now in your body?
. Patient: As I focus on my neck and shoulders I am aware of some pain in my lower back and feel tired, cold and sort of empty there.
. Question: If this area in your body could talk what would it say?
. Patient: I am feeling sad and lonely as if my throat is tight and my lower back is missing something to warm it, to support it.
. Question: Just be with it and acknowledge the sadness and loneliness, the lack of support and warmth. Now could you ask this area what qualities, colors, and sensations it would need?
. Patient: I just see myself floating in a hot spring in a beautiful natural area with wildflowers and big trees. Nearby there is a powerful river with a sort of milky water that sends me a lot of vitality.
. Are there any messages that you could receive from this environment?
. Patient: The River is whispering in my ear: You can let me carry you to the sea; you can drink from my milky waters. I drink and feel the power coming into me. My whole body receives the warm and soothing waters.
. If there is any other message or healing that you need to receive? And later, I asked her: how are her neck and shoulders and the lower back pain now?
. Patient: I just feel very good, relaxed and without pain.
. Question: Is it all right if we finish the process now?
. Patient: I feel fine and we can end now.
. I said: Gently open your eyes and bring your awareness back to your breathing, stretch if you need to.

After concluding this process I took some time with the patient to evaluate her pulses and speak about the experience. This helps the person to integrate. I also asked the patient to later write or paint some of the scenes of the story at home, and I would see her again the next week. In the following session, the main focus was on the integration process of the mind-body dialogue into everyday life.

During the next session, the patient reported having had some new realizations. That she had re-sourced herself by going to a spa and also for a walk near a particular river that she liked. She had shared her dream with her husband, who had offered to take up some of the household tasks. She had also realized that she enjoyed painting and she would like to take up art classes. We talked together about her compulsion to be needed and her tendency to overwork. Through our discussion, it became clear to her that she had issues about loneliness and fear of being abandoned. That would be the next topic to work with. I saw her occasionally after that, she had been free of her physical symptoms and had made some constructive changes in her life.

Approach to work with meditation and healing

My personal approach to working with meditation and healing is a blend of modern psychotherapy, Daoist principles, but modeled mainly on the Buddhist approach for self-liberation. The latter emphasizes openness, non-judgment, acceptance, and insight. This approach concerns not only the patient but also the therapist, willing to explore his or her own deeper cores. The various steps include:

- Intention: willingness to help or ask for help. This on the part of the therapist requires the art of openness and compassion. On the part of the patient, the sincere involvement with the process and the willingness to face the suppressed aspects, to define and recognize the problem. The Daoists say, to deal with a problem, you have to own it, in order to own it you have to name it.
- Central Axis: this is an obligatory condition for the therapist to maintain. It is equally important to bring the patient into their axis as well.
- Compassion: the development of a compassionate non-judgemental Heart is another prerequisite of a good therapist. Only then can one bring the patient into a non-judgemental attitude, a necessary step towards acceptance.
- Acceptance: of the duality, of the suffering and pain. To understand, to work with, and to accept the dualistic nature of life, is a whole process in itself. I have developed a workshop, the "Duality Process", to explore our dualistic mind, the source of our judgments, attachments, and sufferings. Understanding this, we attain freedom of choice and the capacity to create our own reality.
- Insight: this stage may only happen with the realization that the source of all creation and the dissolution of all pain is the "Central Void". In a nutshell, we create our own so-called realities. Therefore we also have the power of creating our own healing.
- The strategy of reconstruction: after the dissolution of a harmful attitude, it is important to replace it with supportive beliefs, and to empower the patient to re-create their own lives. I explore these steps through two approaches: the "Healing Heart" and the "Central Axis".

21.3 Meditation a Self-cultivation tool

The most important and major tool for the cultivation of the self and the inner alchemy is Meditation. More often than not, the Western concept of meditation is defined wrongly and is often misleading. Although there are many types of meditation, the common denominator could be said to be a state of contemplation. Meditation is called *Dhyana* in Sanskrit or *Chan* in modern Chinese, *Zen* in Japanese, *Seon* in Korean, *Thien* in Vietnamese, and *Samten* in Tibetan. In various types of Chinese martial arts, the meditative part is referred to as "Still *Qi Gong*", and is considered as important as the dynamic part. (► Chap. 20.2)

In the Buddhist tradition, the two poles of meditation are *Vipassana* or insight into the nature of reality, and *Samatha*, consisting of focusing, pacifying and calming. The latter is used as a preparation for *Vipassana*. In Tibetan, *Samatha* is called *Shine*, in which *Shi* refers to the pacification of the mind, the thoughts and the obsessive concerns with past and future, and *Ne* signifies to remain with stability in this state (► Fig. 21.3).

Thich Nhat Hanh a Buddhist monk in his book: “The four foundations of mindfulness” (Boston; Wisdom 1990), explains very clearly about the practice of *Shamatha*, the art of stopping, calming, resting and healing by practicing mindfulness with meditation.

- The first step of *Shamatha/ Shine* is to stop the mental processes.
- The second step is the art of calming the mind, this involves:
  - Recognition: If we are angry, we say, “I know that anger is in me”
  - Acceptance: When we are angry, we do not deny it
  - Embracing: We hold our anger in our arms like a mother holding her crying child
  - Looking deeply: When we are calm enough, we can look deeply to understand our anger
  - Insight: The fruit of looking deeply, is understanding the cause and the cessation of our suffering (anger)
- The third step of *Shine* is *Ne* the art of resting. In meditation we allow our body and mind to rest so our wounds may heal.
- Stopping, calming and resting are the preconditions for the art of healing. If we cannot stop, the course of our destruction will just continue. The world, as well as individuals, communities, nations and our earth, need healing. This is a very compassionate and respectful attitude towards our suffering. Compassion is essential for bringing the body and our being into healing and recovery. It is as much an attitude as a practice of meditation. It may be integrated into our daily lives and be developed, as a skill, to bring about recovery and healing, living in compassion towards oneself and towards others.

Compassion, as related to the art of healing, is the total acceptance of the disease, as opposed to the rejection and the denial of the condition. In practice, this means to embrace and to become one with our suffering! This might seem quite a strange idea, to welcome our pain and disease! Yet this is exactly what is asked of us on our journey to recovery. We do not ignore the pain, nor try to resist it, but we embrace it, looking deeper until we reach a point where that suffering opens into a much larger experience. The origin of the pain, as well as the dissolution of it, is to be found in this "Central emptiness".

Tao Te Jing (King), starts by emphasizing this point:

> *Empty your mind of all thoughts; let your Heart be at peace.*
> *Watch the turmoil of beings, but contemplate their return.*
> *Each separate being in the universe returns to the common source.*
> *Returning to the source is serenity.* Lao Tzu, *Tao Te Jing*, chap. 16

Meditation has energetic and physiological effects

While we meditate, our body undergoes noticeable changes: adrenaline levels, blood pressure, and heartbeat decreases, as well as other biochemical changes, take place. In this manner, meditation and visualization help repair the body.

Meditation, visualization, hypnosis, and biofeedback, produce electrochemical responses in the body. Physiology researcher, Dr. Candace Pert, in the mid-'80s, discovered the chemical interrelation between the mind, behavior, the neuroendocrine and the immune systems, in the form of neuropeptides. These discoveries are the base of the science of psycho-neuro-immunology or PNI. In her book "Molecules of emotion", she explains that this mind-body relation is primarily an emotion-body communication. Our physiology is connected to our emotions. She works with dreams and believes that "dreams are direct messages from our body-mind, giving us valuable information about what is going on physiologically as well as emotionally".

One of the important functions of visualization seems to be emotional processing. Ideally, the best way to bring about a state of change and balance would be by consciously directing one's dream or visualization. But other methods, such as hypnosis, biofeedback, various body-oriented therapies, acupuncture, and guided imagery seem to have the same psycho-physiological responses in a patient as dreams. Wendy Pannier, in her presentation on "Dreams: A creative Portal to Healing" in Minneapolis in 2006, states: "The limbic system speaks in the language of symbolic imagery. Working with guided imagery in the waking state can help change perceptions and resolve conflicts, which are critical keys for mind-body healing."

A vast amount of research has been done in recent decades on the mind-body connection.

Meditation not only calms down an agitated mind but also causes structural changes in the brain that can improve several functions, as found by a new research study conducted in Boston, Massachusetts. (Psychiatry Research: Neuro-imaging; January 30, 2011). Results showed that the meditating group had increased density of grey matter in their brain's hippocampus and other structures related to such functions as memory, self-awareness, empathy, and learning. Accordingly, meditation decreases anxiety and stress, as reported by the subjects.

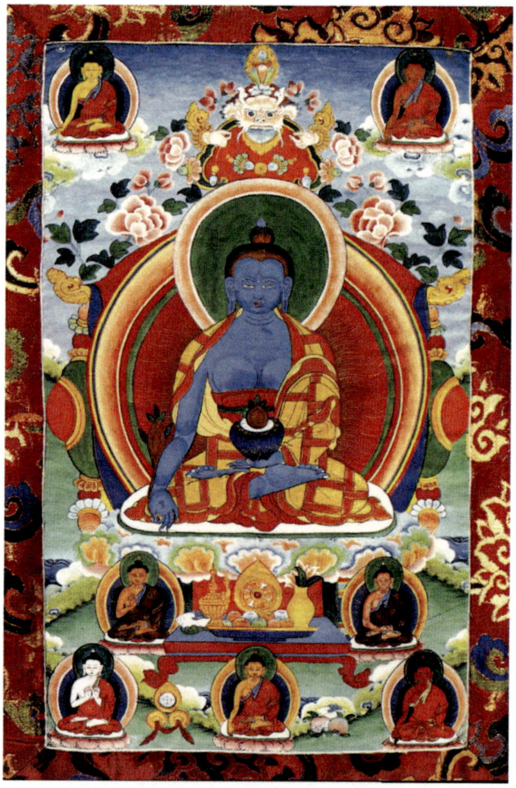

Figure 21.: The Medicine Buddha: *Yao Shi Fo* (Chinese) or Sangye Menla (Tibetan)

Other research has demonstrated that imagery and visualization may have beneficial effects:

- Increase in the number of circulating white blood cells as well as levels of a hormone used by T helper cells. (Nicholas Hall, neuropsychologist, at George Washington Medical Centre)
- Affect the functioning of neutrophils, the first line of defense against infectious agents or "non-self" substances in very specific ways. (Dr. Frank Lawlis et al., University of Texas)
- Reduce aversion responses to chemotherapy. (Jeanne Lyles et al., Vanderbilt University)
- Lower surgical stress and speed up post-surgical healing. (Carole Holden-Lund at Southeastern Louisiana University School of Nursing)

How does visualization work? Here are three operating principles of imagery, as described by Belleruth Naparstek, author of “Staying well with guided imagery" (Warner Books) and "Your Sixth Sense", (Harper):

- Our bodies don’t discriminate between sensory images in the mind and what we call reality, mainly due to the Amygdala and “Limbic logic”.
- In a relaxed, meditative state, we are capable of more rapid and intense healing, growth, learning, and change.
- Imagery and visualization work helps participants feel better about themselves because they have a sense of mastery over what is happening to them. Patients who have an enhanced belief in their coping abilities tend to have better treatment outcomes.

However, the visualization practices have some limitations:

- If the subject is unable to relate to the imagery or to visualize
- The subject is lacking focus and concentration
- The subject is fixed on how things are, i.e. the disease, rather than the desired outcome
- The subject is not able to involve all their senses
- The person cannot feel the visualization in their body
- More credibility is given to the external reality rather than the internal healing powers
- Resistance

22. Which Medicine, which Method?

In the more affluent societies, the biggest dilemma facing a patient today is which medicine to choose from. In the past century, allopathic medicine with its great leaps of progress in surgery and synthetic pharmacology has been saving lives where older traditional methods were incapable of doing so. However, the price to pay for this rapid evolution is high. The dangers, inherent to side effects and combined toxicity of chemicals, are taking their toll. Massive immunizations and antibiotic therapy, is weakening the natural resources of the population, the *Jing-Qi* while strengthening the infectious agents. I believe the problem should be looked at differently, not as one approach versus another, but rather, which medicine or method for a specific person and their condition in a given context. To put it simply, the question should be, who is it we are treating, rather than what are we treating. A particular infection presently treated with a specific antibiotic, may be handled differently depending on whether we are treating a child, a robust adult, an elderly person or a pregnant mother. The debate is very limited when the only tools we have at our disposal are chemical compounds that are matched to a particular diagnostic label. As the famous saying goes, "when the only tool I have is a hammer, everything looks like a nail!"

For the sake of simplification, we could group all existing therapeutic modalities into three groups (► Fig. 23.1):

- Allopathic medicine, including pharmacology, surgery and radiation therapy.
- Mechanical medicine, including osteopathy, the variety of chiropractic methods, physical therapy, and the more traditional "bone setting" modalities.
- Vibrational medicine, which covers, acupuncture, traditional herbal medicine, homeopathy, Ayurveda, shamanic healing, sound therapy, chromotherapy, and scores of more recent methods.

Each of these groups of medicines has its specific sphere of action, overlapping with the other two. The question then would be: which is the most appropriate approach for the patient at that particular moment? It is obvious that when we break a leg, we seek a surgeon, not an acupuncturist or a bone-setter. But in the presence of a bacterial infection, are antibiotics the only solution?

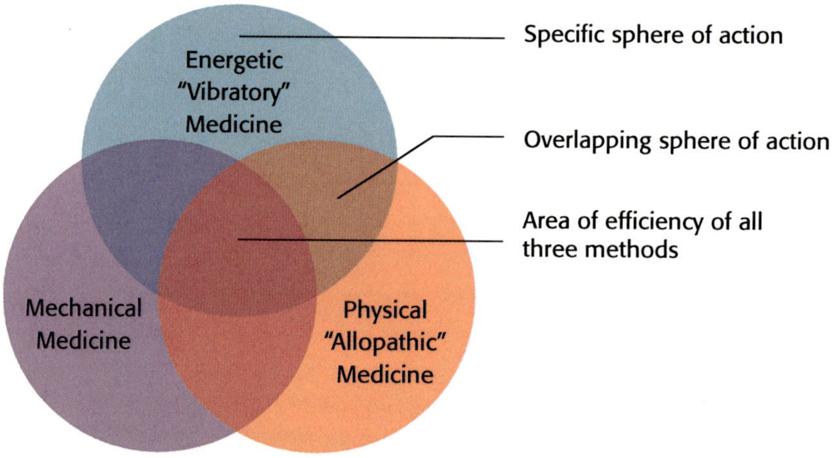

Figure 23.1: The three spheres of therapy

What are the consequences of an infection treated by softer methods that support the immune system of the person, versus the side effects a particular chemical compound that eradicates the infectious agent but decimates the intestinal flora, and further damages the liver and the kidneys? A particular infection might have catastrophic consequences in a small child or an elderly person, and greatly outweigh the side effects of the chemical drug; therefore the allopathic treatment should be administered. The same infection in a robust and healthy adult could be treated quite differently, supporting the constitution to fight the pathogenic invasion. Understanding the reasons that allowed for the infectious agent to invade the system in the first place and correcting them, would be a more intelligent approach. I believe that in a better health system, patients should have access to all therapeutic modalities, and especially that the practitioners of each of the three medicines should be aware of the other two and may thus better advise the patient as to the best therapeutic modality to choose. For best results, two or even three approaches may be combined.

Every so often, there is the odd unfortunate case, usually greatly publicized, pleading against the use of alternative methods and in favor of allopathic medicine. For example the case of a patient consulting in alternative medicine for symptoms that were caused by cancer, or a patient who may have supposedly contracted HIV through acupuncture, or wrong herbal treatments resulting in kidney or liver failures; or a whip-lash patient, becoming tetraplegic after an osteopathic manipulation. In most cases, these accidents may have been avoided had there been better collaboration between institutional medicine and the alternative or complementary methods. Here are a few cases of how allopathic medicine working isolated from the others could be more harmful:

- A patient who had rapidly developed incapacitating vertigo consulted an MD, who conducted all the proper investigations, including X-rays and brain scans, with no results. The patient was referred to an ENT specialist with suspicion of Meniere's disease, again not confirmed. She was given 10 sessions of physiotherapy twice, which did not help. After 7 months off work due to her illness, she was labeled "psychosomatic" and referred to a psychiatrist. Eventually, she consulted me as a last resort. The general anamnesis and pulse diagnosis did not reveal any evidence of "Internal Wind", the physical examination revealed a C2 vertebrae lateral dislocation. When I asked her, she told me that none of her doctors had touched her neck! I explained to her that although with acupuncture we could unblock the "occipital barrier", she would save time by consulting an osteopath, as the C2 sub-luxation was secondary to a spinal misalignment further down. I asked her to call me 10 days later. She reported that after the acupuncture, her symptoms had lessened by 50%, that she had been treated by an osteopath 2 days later and was free of vertigo since then. This case is a good example of a pathology that is in the domain of mechanical medicine but can also be helped by energetic medicine.

- Another case concerned a woman who consulted her GP for a burning sensation of her palms and chest with no apparent lesion; she was referred to a dermatologist, who diagnosed her as having Psoriasis that had not yet manifested, and gave her cortisone. After 3 months of treatment, there was no improvement of her symptoms, the prescription was changed to another steroid.

Six months later she was presenting with generalized edema, a weight gain of 15kg and she started to have bleeding ulcers; fortunately, her gastroenterologist stopped her steroids. She consulted me with all the above symptoms; the heat in the palms and chest was diagnosed as a classical "five heart heat", confirmed by the pulse and tongue findings, due to an empty heat from Kidney and Heart-*Yin-Xu*. Two sessions and a course of "*Zhi Bai Di Huang Wan*" to supplement *Yin* and reduce Heat, resolved the original symptoms, the Stomach-Fire also responded rapidly; it took longer, however, to reverse the water retention and weight gain which had been caused by the allopathic drug treatment. This patient's initial symptoms fall into the realm of energetic medicine for which allopathic medicine has no definition or solution.

- Another case that may demonstrate the possibility of combining allopathic medicine with Chinese medicine: a 6 year-old child who received a course of antibiotics for an infectious and febrile otitis a year ago, has been presenting all the classical symptoms of Spleen-*Qi Xu*, fatigue, loss of appetite, soft stools and a propensity to catching colds, with frequent clear nasal discharge, the interrogation reveals that he sweats easily, especially when sleeping, a further confirmation of *Wei-Qi Xu*. Fortunately, his pediatrician had not prescribed any further courses of antibiotics. In fact, antibiotics, which are "Cold" in nature, had successfully treated the "Heat" factor in the original Damp-Heat condition of the otitis but had simply aggravated the Dampness and further damaged the Spleen *Qi*. Incidentally, the Spleen-*Qi* is quite delicate in infants and small children and may easily be disturbed by wrong diet and cold. The treatment aimed at supplementing the Spleen-*Qi* and harmonizing the center to support the production of *Wei-Qi*. I used a 40 milli-watt infrared laser to stimulate the points. The mother was instructed to moxa *Zu San Li* ST-36, with an incense stick, 7 consecutive days around the new moon every month. Dairy products and cold foods were restricted for a month to help the digestive fire to recover. He was seen one month later, and once again three months later in autumn to consolidate the treatment before the cold season. He passed the winter without any further infectious episodes.

22.1 What can Chinese Medicine treat?

This is a question that we are frequently asked. My answer is invariably the same: that Chinese medicine can "Treat" any condition but not "Cure" everything. I further explain that holistic medicines, such as Chinese medicine, treat the person, not the disease, hence anybody may benefit from the range of therapeutic modalities offered by Chinese medicine. Pathological processes, before getting to the organic and physical stage, have a period during which the symptoms described by the patient do not yet have a physical manifestation. Various medical explorations such as X-rays, scans and laboratory tests may remain inconclusive, while symptoms may be falling into clear TCM patterns. At this stage Chinese medicine may cure a disease, providing the causative factors and the deeper roots of the disease are eradicated. Once the disease has become organic, that is, the physical damage has become apparent with the presence of arterial plaques and stenosis, joint deformities, wearing of cartilage and bone, or the development of tumors or cancer, the pathology is much harder to reverse. At this stage, a prognosis of cure is much harder to make, although the person can always be treated and symptoms may still be alleviated.

The following case may demonstrate this point:

- A 38-year old man, strong and robust, with a taxing job requiring heavy lifting, presented with cervicobrachial neuralgia (neck-arm and hand syndrome), with pain in the neck and upper arm area, weakening, and numbness in the hand. The neurosurgeon diagnosed a cervical discus hernia and proposed immediate surgery. The patient was scared of the surgical prospect, as he had a friend who had experienced the same symptoms and continued to suffer after surgery. I explained that if his condition was a true discus hernia and the disc membrane ruptured with the nucleus pressing on the nerve, it had to be surgically removed. However if the condition was just a protrusion simply due to the excessive tension of the local muscles, it may be treated without surgery. From a Chinese diagnostic perspective, this condition may be seen as an accumulation of *Yang* in the neck area, possibly due to Liver-*Qi* stasis and local blockage of "barrier" points. I saw him twice. After the first session, the symptoms were reduced by 60%. He did not show up for his third session and I presumed that he had gone for surgery. A year later he consulted me again and told me that his symptoms had entirely disappeared after the second session and that he had canceled the surgery. He was consulting me again as he was experiencing the recurrence of some very mild symptoms, which were resolved with one session of acupuncture.

22.2 Which Chinese Method to choose

The question of what is the best Chinese modality, acupuncture, herbs, diet or *Tui Na* massage, is another interesting debate.

Acupuncturists pretend to treat everything with needles, moxa, and cupping; herbalist would contend that all is treatable with herbs, whereas manual therapists, only swear by the magic of the fingertips. I believe that ultimately it is not the method but the degree of training, experience, and talent of the therapist that makes the difference.

Without getting involved in controversial discussions, there are some general guidelines that may be helpful:

- Acupuncture and its panoply of complementary methods, moxa, cupping, *Gua Sha*, bleeding, is best suited for conditions involving peripheral pain and consequences of channel blockages. Skilled acupuncturists can also reach the deeper energetic layers and affect the organic functions, the psyche and the mind and even the constitutional levels.

- Herbal medicine has the great advantage of supplying "substance", and finds its main indication in the treatment of the "Vital Substance" deficiencies, but it is also quite effective in resolving accumulations, especially of Dampness and Phlegm.
- Diet, was not traditionally classified as a Chinese therapeutic tool. I personally believe that diet is not medicine, but that wrong diet can cause disease, and that inappropriate diet can prevent a cure from happening. Dietary advice should, therefore, be part of all Chinese modalities.
- *Tui Na/ An Mo* massage, based on the same principles as acupuncture, finds its indications in musculoskeletal conditions and is an ideal tool for patients or children who may not want to be needled, or the elderly, or as a complement to acupuncture. A skilled *Tui Na* therapist can access the same depths as a good acupuncturist.
- *Qi Gong* is primarily practiced as a lifestyle modality, to maintain health, quiet the mind and prevent disease. With the practice of *Qi Gong*, the patient is empowered to take into their own hands their disease and healing. *Qi Gong* practice affects the deepest energy structures of the person, the *Jing* level, and can produce changes where all the other therapeutic modalities may fail. Hence it may show good results observed in pathologies which have damaged the *Jing* level, such as cancer, post-traumatic stress disorders or childhood abuse.
- Psycho-energetic work, although entirely based on classical Chinese concepts, is not, in reality, an individualized method of Chinese medicine. The inner causes of disease, the emotions, have been historically recognized; in fact, the Confucian principles of "Cultivation of the mind", or the Daoist or Buddhist concepts of emotional transformation, underline their importance. Yet no systematic approach has been offered in the texts, in spite of the psycho-emotional indications of many of the acupuncture points. I strongly believe that today we have not only access to the wisdom of the ancient traditions but also to many modern-day therapy methods, and should use both to help our patients deal with and resolve their deeper conflicts and sources of their pathologies.

Part VI- Additional Methods Applied in Chinese Medicine

23. Yi Jing (I Ching) Book of Change, and its application to Chinese Medicine

by Peter Firebrace

Behind the traditional medicine of China is a perspective that is deeply rooted in *Yin-Yang* thinking. It provided a foundation for the "*Yin Yang* Five Phases" school (*Yin Yang Wu Xing* 陰陽五行) that divides all natural phenomena into associated resonant groups, from the world outside to the organs and body parts within, and it also later created a clear structure for the Pattern Identification school (*Bian Zheng* 辨證) that uses the eight principles (*Ba Gang* 八剛) of internal/external, hot/cold, empty/full and *Yin/Yang* in their differentiation. But long before these important systems evolved, the Chinese were studying, observing and recording the notion and the nature of change.

The *Yi Jing* 易經, The Book of Change is a book of divination and transformation and of trend-spotting, a book far older than the *Huangdi Neijing*, a link back to shamanic times when the power was invested in the ancestral lines of shaman kings. The *Yi Jing* is also a link to the future and the unravelling of the genetic code (see chapter 2.8). At its heart is a study of cycles in patterns of change and to understand nature from the movement of the heavenly bodies above to the inner workings of our earthly bodies below and to find the best course of action to take in any given situation.

Embedded in the culture of China, the *Yi Jing* is a book for all of humanity, where its tell-tale signs and symbols are not actually written in Chinese, but in their own unique coded language of lines ⚊ ⚋, bigrams ⚍ ⚎, trigrams ☳ ☵ and hexagrams ䷴ ䷄, much like the universal terms used in mathematical formulae.

There are many ways to use the *Yi Jing* in medical practice. Some take the elements of the upper and lower trigrams to assess their interaction. Others take the organ resonances or the parts of the body. Some use the links with the extraordinary channels (for which there are several systems) for example ☰ *Qian* with *Du Mai* and ☷ *Kun* with *Ren Mai.* Some look at the associations with the heavenly stems and earthly branches and the cycles of time. Others take the text of the *Yi Jing* itself and give its general instruction a medical meaning. Some see in the position of the changing line an indication of the location of the disorder, for example the top line 6 indicates the head, lines 3, 4 and 5 indicate the lower, middle and upper heater respectively.

The topic is too complex to be addressed here, please refer to the specialized literature

24. Chinese Astrology (Ba Zi) 八字

Ba Zi or the "8 Terms or Words" refers to the ancient Chinese Astrology, and would be the origin of the *Yi Jing* or *I Ching*. It is attributed to three personalities: *Huang Di* the Yellow Emperor, *Wen Wang* or King Wen and *Kong Zi* or Confucius. Since the ancient times until today the Chinese Horoscope has been used in all the domains of life, from the prediction of life events, carrier, wealth and health to the relationship with parents and the choice of spouse and work associates. So much emphasis is put into *Ba Zi* that couples would plan on having a child on a specific date to ensure a harmonious relationship with the parents.

The Chinese had very detailed knowledge of Astronomy as so did the Babylonians, the Greeks, the Hebrews, the Romans, and the Muslims. Most calendars devised by these cultures were lunar and needed to be adjusted in relation to the Earth's rotation around the sun.

The Chinese calendar has 12 lunar months and 13 months in a leap year, but distributed according to the Solar solstices and equinoxes, hence the term "Soli-lunar". The Chinese new-year starts on the second new moon after the winter solstice and at times is referred to as the "Lunar" new-year.

24.1 The Energies of Earth and Heaven

In the heavens as on earth, the *Yang* principle is represented by unity and by odd numbers: 1-3-5-7-9; *Yin* represents duality, hence even numbers: 2-4-6-8-10. In this symbolism, the middle numbers 5 and 6 symbolize respectively *Yang* and *Yin* and are considered the "generators" of the decimal "10" and duodecimal "12" series. The heavenly energies are referred to as the "10 Heavenly Stems", 10 being the *Yang* principle in its duality (5 x 2). The Earthly energies are named the "12 Terrestrial Branches", the *Yin* principle in its duality (6 x 2).

The combined influences of Heaven and Earth will define the energetics of each year, hence each Chinese year is characterized by the name of a stem and a branch, for example, 1950 is a *Geng* (stem 7) and Metal element, with *Yin* (branch 3) and *Tai Yin* energy (see further).

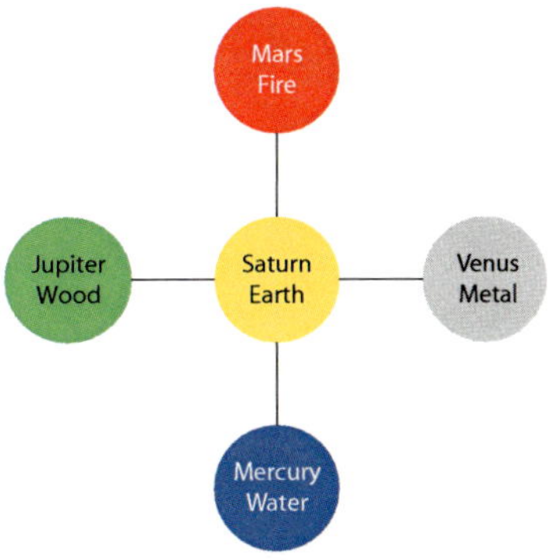

Figure 24.1: The Five Planets and the Five Elements

As it takes a cycle of 60 years for the first combination of the first Stem and the first Branch to repeat itself, in the Chinese calendar, the lapses of time are measured by periods of 60 years, equivalent to the Western concept of a century.

The ancient Chinese had observed that besides the two main stellar bodies, the sun and the moon, that defined the rhythms of the day and the year, there existed five other bright points in the heavens that seemed to change positions, hence the notion of the Five Elements (▶ Fig. 24.1).

From astronomical observations and the positions of these planets, the astrologers would predict events and climates and make divinations of the political situations and particularly configurations concerning health, as described in the *Nei Jing* chapter 69.

Please note that in the above figure the Earth Element is not the planet Earth, but rather a particular type of movement (▶ chap. 2.4). In this representation, the Earth Element is the link and the intermediary between the energies of Heaven and Earth, hence its pivotal position.

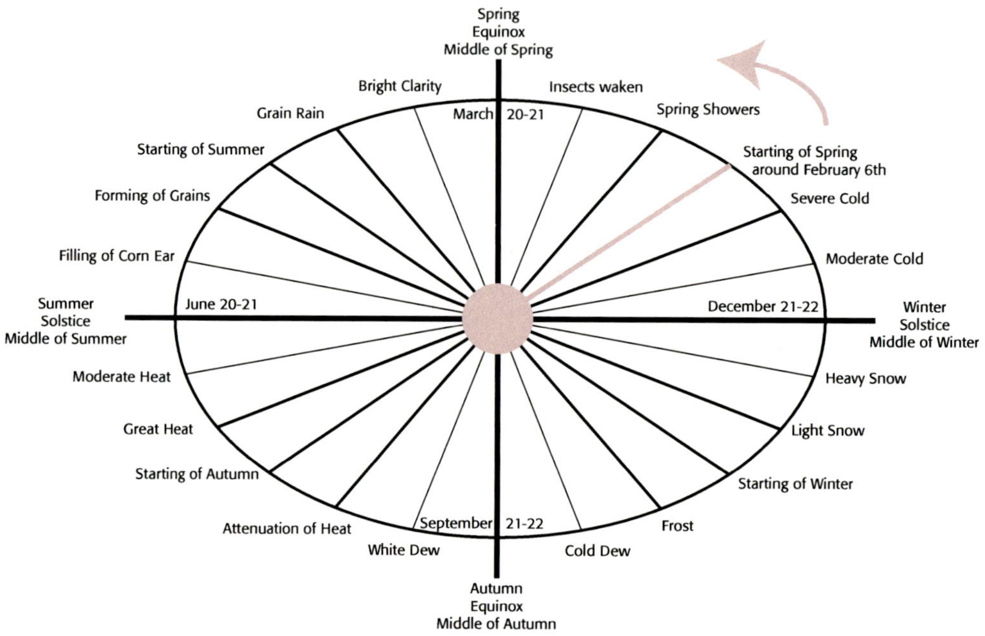

Figure 24.2 : The composition of the Chinese Solar year and the lunar months: Soli-lunar system. The Chinese new-year starts on the second new moon after the Winter Solstice, around February 6th.

The relation between the Five Elements and the Seasons

The elliptical rotation of the Earth around the sun defines the four seasons. The Chinese year is made of 12 segments of 30 days, subdivided into periods of 15 days. (▶ Fig. 24.2)

Each season is bisected by an equinox or a solstice and presents a period of waxing and waning. Hence the 21st of March is not the beginning of spring, as it is erroneously and commonly considered, but the middle of spring.

Each season is influenced by two Heavenly Stems:

Jia and *Yi*	Influence the Wood Element
Bing and *Ding*	Influence the Fire Element
Wu and *Ji*	Influence the Earth Element
Geng and *Xin*	Influence the Metal Element
Ren and *Gui*	Influence the Water Element

The first half of the season corresponds to a concentration of energy and is *Yang*. During the second half of the season, the energy declines and is considered *Yin*. As each organ corresponds to an Element and a season, the same can be observed about the rising and declining of organic energy, which according to the *Su Wen* only concerns the *Zang* organs: "... the *Zang* conserve jealously their energy, only to let go of it at the end of each season". This also explains the seasonal variations observed in the radial pulses.

- Liver corresponding to the Wood element
- Heart related to the Fire element
- Lung related to the Metal element
- Kidney corresponding to the Water element

In this manner, each organ finds itself in a state of strength (*Yang*) in the first half of the season and weakness (*Yin*) in the second half (▶ Fig. 24.3).

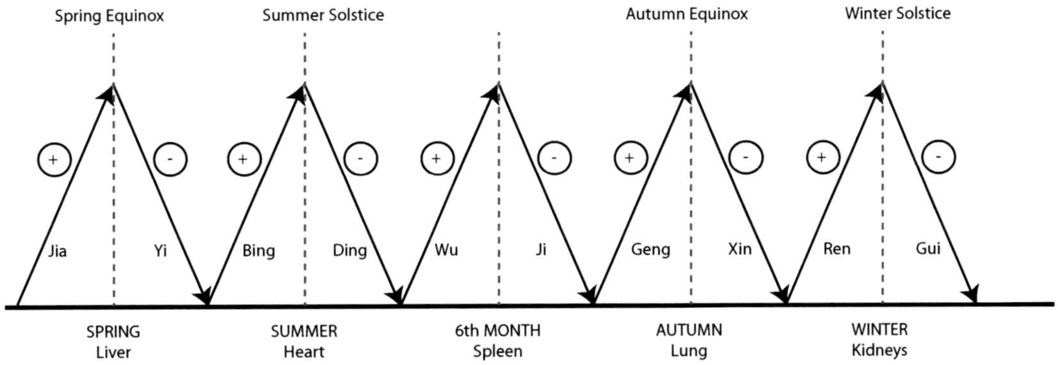

Figure 24.3: The 10 Heavenly Stems and the periods of concentration and decline for each *Zang*-organ system.

For example, in the case of Liver *Xu* ≈ Vacuity, the Liver cannot be attacked by the Lung in the first half of the season, but in the second half, as its energy is being channeled towards its son, the Heart (*Sheng* ≈ Nourishing cycle), it finds itself in a state of depletion and now can be attacked by the Lung (*Ke* ≈ Destruction cycle). In the opposite case, when the Liver is in a state of repletion, it will have a tendency to attack the Spleen (*Ke* ≈ Destruction cycle) in the first half of the season.

In practice, for the above case, a weak Liver would be supplemented by its seasonal supplementing point in the second half of Spring. Whereas in the case of a Liver in repletion, the Spleen would be supported during the first half of Spring.

Furthermore, as the 10 Heavenly stems define the main characteristics of each Chinese year, the strength of the corresponding element would depend on the polarity of the *Gan*≈ Stem. For example, a person born in a year with *Jia* (stem 1), which has a strong Wood element, would enjoy a strong Liver, whereas the year with *Yi* (stem 2), a weak Wood, might present with a delicate Liver.

The Earth Element and the Fifth season

The position of the Five Elements based on the model of the cosmos places the Earth element in the center. In this position, the Spleen is the intermediary between Heaven and Earth and distributes to the four directions and the other four organs impartially.

Although from the perspective of seasons and the calendar, this position has no significance, hence it is stated in the *Su Wen* that the four organs delegate to the Earth the 18 last days of their respective seasons.

From an energetic perspective, the Spleen has its own activity during the 6th month. (▶ Fig. 24.4) Hence, the two models of the Five Elements, the cosmic or cosmogenic model with Earth/ Spleen in the center and the energetic model with Earth/ Spleen between the Fire and Metal elements. The latter, as it relates to the organic activities, is termed *Wu Xing* ≈ Five movements or "Five Moving Forces".

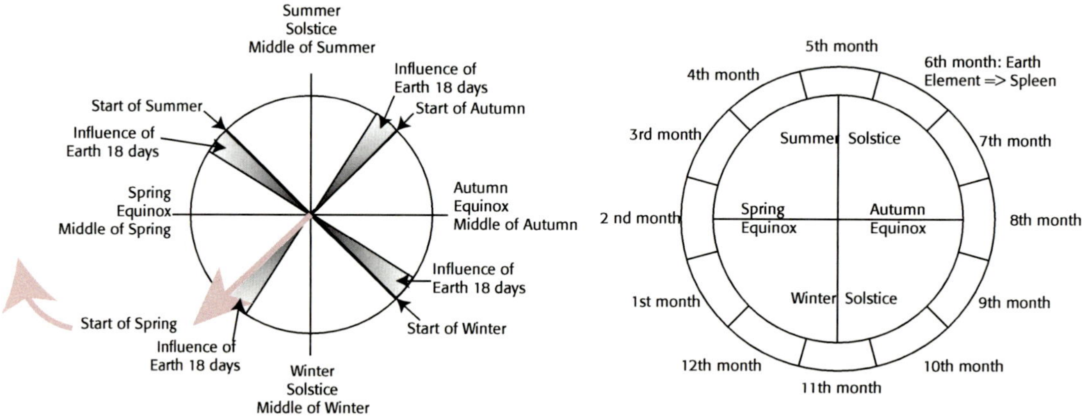

Figure 24.4: The two influences of the Earth Element on the seasons: 18 last days of each season and the 6th month.

24.2 Gan ≈ Heavenly Stems and Zhi ≈ Earthly Branches (干支)

The 10 Heavenly stems describe the waxing and waning of the five seasons and reflect the activity of the Five Planets as described above.

The *Gan* ≈ Stem defines the year. The 10 stems correspond to the Five Elements, the order starting with the Earth element, as intermediary between Heaven and Earth:

Heavenly Stem	Number	Element	Polarity	Direction	Influencing	Zang-Fu
Jia	1	Earth	*Yang* (+)	East	Wood phase & Spring	Gall Bladder
Yi	2	Metal	*Yin* (-)			Liver
Bing	3	Water	*Yang* (+)	South	Fire phase & Summer	Small Intestine
Ding	4	Wood	*Yin* (-)			Heart
Wu	5	Fire	*Yang* (+)	Center	Earth phase & 5th season	Stomach
Ji	6	Earth	*Yin* (-)			Spleen
Geng	7	Metal	*Yang* (+)	West	Metal phase & Autumn	Large Intestine
Xin	8	Water	*Yin* (-)			Lung
Ren	9	Wood	*Yang* (+)	North	Water phase & Winter	Bladder
Gui	10	Fire	*Yin* (-)			Kidney

Please note the following point of confusion: although the years *Jia* or *Yi,* both are Wood years, the *Jia* (stem 1) actually corresponds to the Earth and the Yi (stem 2), corresponds to Metal and so on. The difference being that in the *Jia* year, the stem is of a *Yang* nature and will confer a strong character to the Wood, whereas the *Yi* year (*Yin*) will define a weak Wood.

The 10 heavenly stems define and direct the energies of the year. The stem of the year is used to define the 大運 *Da Yun* ≈ Great Movement (see below).

The 12 Earthly branches correspond to the planet earth's rotation around the sun, the 12 months, and its rotation around itself: 12 Chinese hours (▶ Fig. 24.5).

The Earthly branches, also present *Yin* and *Yang* polarities, the odd branches being *Yang* and the *Yin* branches are *Yin*. Furthermore, each Earthly branch will correspond with a channel system, according to the horary system. Please note that there is a discrepancy between the *Yin-Yang* polarity of the channels and the Earthly branches, the former being an anatomical classification and the latter referring to astronomical considerations.

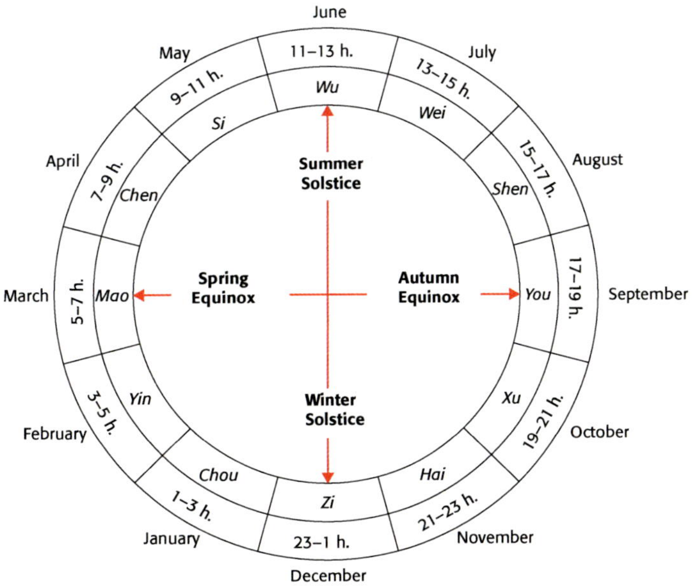

Figure 24.5: Earthly Branches, the 12 months and the 12 Chinese hours.

Furthermore, each Earthly Branch also corresponds to a "Celestial Guest Energy", in the following order as defined in the *Suwen* chapter 66: *Shao Yin–Tai Yin–Shao Yang–Yang Ming–Tai Yang–Jue Yin.* Again there is an apparent discrepancy as to the relation of *Zhi* ≈ Branch, the corresponding channel system and the Celestial Energy. For example, the *Zi* (Branch 1) corresponds to *Zu Shao Yang*- GB channel and yet the Celestial /Heavenly Energy is the *Shao Yin*. Unfortunately, I have not been able to find a clear and satisfying explanation for this, as there seems to even exist a debate on this point amongst experts themselves.

Earthly Branch	Number	Polarity	Channel system	Animal	Time Month	Guest Energy Climate	Organs
Zi	I	*Yang*	*Zu Shao Yang*-GB	Rat	11 pm–1 am December	*Shao Yin* Heat	Kidney, spine, liquids
Chou	II	*Yin*	*Zu Jue Yin*-LR	Ox	1–3 am January	*Tai Yin* Dampness	Spleen, abdomen, limbs, stool
Yin	III	*Yang*	*Shou Tai Yin*-LU	Tiger	3–5 am February	*Shao Yang* Fire	Gallbladder, veins, arteries, hair
Mao	IV	*Yin*	*Shou Yang Ming*-LI	Rabbit	5 –7 am March	*Yang Ming* Dryness	Liver, blood, eyes
Chen	V	*Yang*	*Zu Yang Ming*-ST	Dragon	7 am–9 am April	*Tai Yang* Cold	Skin, neck shoulders.
Si	VI	*Yin*	*Zu Tai Yin*-SP	Snake	9 am–11 am May	*Jue Yin* Wind	Triple Warmer, Small Intestine, face, teeth
Wu	VII	*Yang*	*Shou Shao Yin*-HE	Horse	11 am–1 pm June	*Shao Yin* Heat	Heart, tongue
Wei	VIII	*Yin*	*Shou Tai Yang*-SI	Goat	1 –3 pm July	*Tai Yin* Dampness	Stomach, mouth, lips
Shen	IX	*Yang*	*Zu Tai Yang*-BL	Monkey	3 –5 pm August	*Shao Yang* Fire	Large Intestine, bones
You	X	*Yin*	*Zu Shao Yin*-KI	Rooster	5 –7 pm September	*Yang Ming* Dryness	Lungs, nose, voice
Xu	XI	*Yang*	*Shou Jue Yin*-PE	Dog	7 –9 pm October	*Tai Yang* Cold	Knees, *Ming Men*
Hai	XII	*Yin*	*Shou Shao Yang*-TW	Pig	9 –11 pm November	*Jue Yin* Wind	Bladder, anus urethra, head

The relation of *Gan* and *Zhi* can be summarised as the 10 heavenly stems (5X2) representing "Space" when the 12 Earthly branches represent "Time", and the combination of the two defining the present moment.

The relation between the Gan-Zhi and climates

As mentioned, there are Five Earthly Elements and Six Heavenly energies. The 10 Stems (*Gan*) correspond to the Earthly Five Elements, the 12 Branches (*Zhi*) represent the Heaven.

The Five Elements govern the five directions and engender the five climates, which could be seen as a "materialization" of the more subtle heavenly energies:

- Wood corresponds to Wind, a materialization of *Jue Yin* energy
- Fire corresponds to Heat, the concretization of *Shao Yin*

- Earth relates to Dampness, condensation of *Tai Yin* energy
- Metal responds to Dryness, a materialization of *Yang Ming*
- Water corresponds to Cold, a consolidation of *Tai Yang*
- The sixth energy, *Shao Yang*, corresponds to the Fire element (Fire-minister)

The main characteristics of the year are defined by its Heavenly stem, the main climate of the year will then be defined by its Earthly branch; for example, years with branch *Chen* (V) or *Xu* (XI) correspond to *Tai Yang*, hence they will have a Cold tendency. For example, the year 2012 is characterized by *Ren* a strong Water-year (stem 9), and *Chen* (branch V= *Tai Yang*), both suggest a year with a cold tendency.

The Great Movement (Da Yun 大運)

Is defined by the *Gan* ≈ Stem of the year. The Great Movement dominates the year's energetic tendencies: the year 2013: *Gui* (10)-*Si* (VI), is a Water year due to *Gui*, the 10th stem corresponding to the Water element, although the 10th stem itself is a *Yin* (weak) Fire, this suggests that the seasons will be delayed and lacking in heat. The year 2014 *Jia-Wu* is a Wood year with a strong Wood, whereas 2015 *Yi-Wei,* which is also a Wood year, has a weak stem. In general, when the stem has a strong (*Yang*) nature, the seasons will be in advance. When the stem has a weak (*Yin*) denomination, the seasons will be delayed.

The Host Movement

These are the normal and constant evolutions of the seasons, starting from the day of the *Dai Han* ≈ Great cold around the 21st of January for a period of 73 days, following the five phases: Wood–Fire–Earth–Metal–Water. These movements describe the normal climates in relation to the seasons, that is wind–heat–dampness–dryness–cold. These climates are constant from one year to the next.

The Guest Movements

These movements explain the individual variations from one year to another. For example in a *Jia* (stem 1) or *Ji* (stem 6) year, the stems correspond to Earth, therefore the Guest movement will start with Earth, following the *Sheng* ≈ Creation cycle: Earth–Metal–Water–Wood–Fire. The Guest Movements explain, for example, the abnormal presence of Dampness (Earth) during the first phase of the year, spring.

The Six Energies/Climates

The actual climates of the seasons are designated by the six terms in the following order:

Jue Yin (Wind-Spring)–*Shao Yin* (Heat-Summer)–*Shao Yang* (Fire-Summer)–*Tai Yin* (Dampness-5th season)–*Yang Ming* (Dryness-Autumn)–*Tai Yang* (Cold-Winter)

The Host Energy

Same as for the Host Movement, the Host energy will describe the dominant and natural climate of each season, following the *Sheng*- creation cycle of the Five Movements.

Here, the 24 climatic divisions of the year are taken in to account (▶ Fig. 24.2). Each of the six sections of the year (60 days), referred to as a "Step" will include four climatic divisions (15 days).

Step	**1**	**2**	**3**	**4**	**5**	**6**
Energy	*Jue Yin* Wind	*Shao Yin* Heat	*Shao Yang* Fire	*Tai Yin* Dampness	*Yang Ming* Dryness	*Tai Yang* Cold
Divisions	1-2-3-4	5-6-7-8	9-10-11-12	13-14-15-16	17-18-19-20	21-22-23-24

The Guest Energy

Explains the abnormality for each season. The relations are given in the *Suwen* chapter 66 (table below). For each "Guest Energy", the Earth responds by another, compensating energy in the following manner:

Earthly Branches	**Heaven's Energy "Guest Energy"**	**Earth's response**
Zi (I) and *Wu* (VII)	*Shao Yin*	*Yang Ming*
Chou (II) and *Wei* (VIII)	*Tai Yin*	*Tai Yang*
Yin (III) and *Shen* (IX)	*Shao Yang*	*Jue Yin*
Mao (IV) and *You* (X)	*Yang Ming*	*Shao Yin*
Chen (V) and *Xu* (XI)	*Tai Yang*	*Tai Yin*
Si (VI) and *Hai* (XII)	*Jue Yin*	*Shao Yang*

The actual climate of a particular season will depend on the Guest Energy, presiding over the first half of the year, and the Earth's response to it, which is influential during the second half of the year. Here the calculations become much more complicated, as the relation between the Host and Guest Movements and Celestial energies have to be integrated. There could be five possibilities:

- Favorable: the Energy produces/ engenders the Movement (according to the *Sheng* ≈ Nourishing cycle), i.e. the Energy corresponds to Wood and the Movement corresponds to Fire (Wood nourishes Fire).
- Celestial form: the Energy is destroying the Movement (according to the *Ke* ≈ Control cycle); i.e Water destroys Fire
- Small vexation: The Movement produces/ engenders the Energy
- Disagreement: The Movement destroys the Energy
- Concordance: Both, Movement and Energy are of the same nature

25. Stems-Branches Acupuncture

by Bernhard Nessensohn

The concept of Stems and Branches appears in chapters 66 and 74 of the *Nei Jing Su Wen* where they are described as the *Wu Yun Liu Qi* 五運六氣 or the "Five Movements and the Six Energies". These chapters were added to the *Su Wen* around 762 AD by a Daoist named Wang Bing, who claims that this material was from a copy of the *Su Wen* which his teacher held in secret possession.

The Stems and Branches acupuncture *Wu Yun Liu Qi* is based on the Five Movements (Wood, Fire, Earth, Metal, Water) and the Six Energies (*Jue Yin, Shao Yin, Shao Yang, Tai Yin, Yang Ming,* and *Tai Yang*). Together they create the Ten Heavenly Stems *Shi Tian Gan* 十天干and the Twelve Earthly Branches *Shi Er Di Zhi* 十二地支. The Stems and Branches - *Gan Zhi* - are mostly known because of the Chinese calendar and Chinese Astrology, but the *Gan Zhi* method as an acupuncture technique to work with the constitution is rare. This approach was mainly propagated in Europe by the late Dr. J.D van Buren, who studied under Dr. Jaques Lavier and Dr. Wu Wei Ping, and later with the Korean Doctor Chang Bin Lee who introduced him to the principles of Stems and Branche's acupuncture.

The most common application of *Gan-Zhi* in acupuncture is the use of the "Open Hourly Clock" system. This technique combines the concept of the "Ten Stems" with the notion of the cyclic ebb and flow of *Qi* in the channels. The open hourly clock system appears in a book called *Zi Wu Liu Zhen Jing*, giving the points that have the highest level of energy on a certain day and at a certain time. A similar system, called the *Ling Gui Ba Fa*, describes the active opening points of the *Qi Jing Ba Mai* ≈ Eight Extraordinary Vessels.

The ancient method of Stems and Branche's acupuncture aims at treating people according to their constitution "Personal *Qi*", as well as the changes in the year "Universal *Qi*".

- The "Personal *Qi*" is related to the time of birth of a person, which in turn reflects a certain aspect of the Moon and the Sun. The particular configuration of the Stems and Branches of the time of birth will confer very specific energy to the person. These energetic aspects are evaluated as strong or weak and are taken into account not only to describe the characteristics of a person but also to understanding the imbalances and therefore offer excellent guidance for the treatment.
- The "Universal *Qi*" is related to the obvious changes occurring throughout the year, and is calculated based on the "Four Pillars", which are, the year, the month, the day and the hour.

The calculation of the years, describing the Chinese calendar, started in the time of the legendary emperor *Huang Di* 黃帝 more than 4500 years ago. In fact, the tradition has it that in the year 2637 BC the five main planets Mercury, Venus, Mars,

Jupiter, and Saturn could be seen aligned with the Sun and the Moon (▶ Fig. 25.1). This was the beginning of the counting of the Chinese calendar.

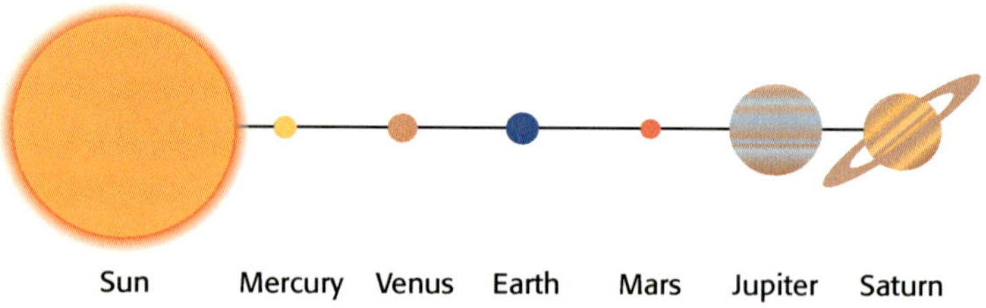

Figure 25.1: The start of the Chinese Calendar: 2637 BC alignment of Mercury, Venus, Mars, Jupiter, and Saturn with the sun and the Moon.

Based on the concept of the Microcosm being in the image of the Macrocosm, the "Heaven" is reflected here on "Earth" and therefore also within mankind.

Heaven has five aspects, as on Earth there are five continents with five populations and two polarities, women and men (*Yin* and *Yang*). Everything in Heaven seems to turn around a central axis and creates, as seen from the center, in each direction another Heaven. The Five Heavens or skies are depicted as animals. The central Heaven of the Yellow Dragon contains the big dipper, *Bei Dou* 北斗. Around it there are the other four heavens, each containing a seven-star constellation, forming together the twenty-eight-star constellations that are used in the Chinese horoscopes. Each of the Heavens has its own ruler in the form of a planet, which represents the motive force of the Five Movements (▶ Fig. 25.2).

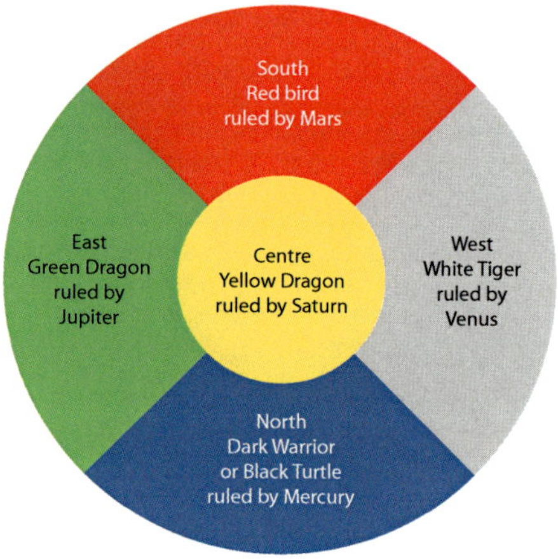

Figure 25.2: The Five Heavens and their symbolic animals

This principle of the “Five Heavens” is based on the archetypes of the Four Emanations with *Qian* at the Centre and its emanation *Yuan* in the East, *Heng* in the South, *Li* in the West and *Zhen* in the North. *Yuan* gives rise to the Wood Element, *Heng* gives rise to the Fire Element, *Li* engenders the Metal Element, *Zhen* produces the Water Element and *Qian* the Earth Element (▶ Fig. 25.3).

The Stems and Branche's acupuncture consits of is calculating the person's birth chart and selecting the acupuncture points according to the *Gan-Zhi* of the year and of the person and their pathology.

For a more detailed explanation please refer to the appropriate specialized texts.

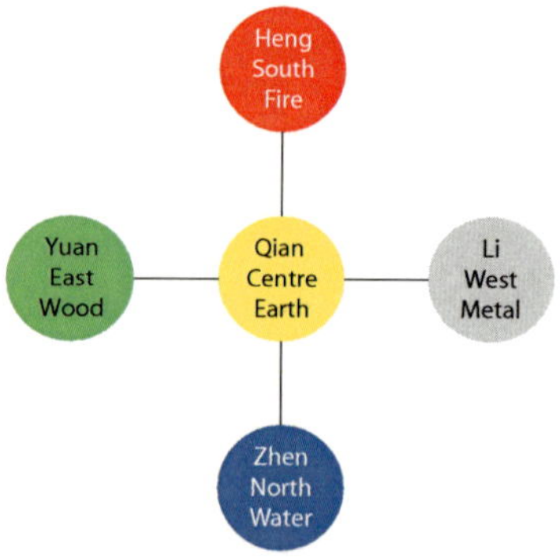

Figure 25.3: The Five emanations

26. Feng Shui (風水) in Medical practice

History

Feng Shui literally means Wind and Water and is based on ancient Chinese beliefs about nature and the human being's place within it. It is the equivalent of Western Geomancy.

Historically, some authors consider Yang Yun Sang (9th century AD), of the Tang Dynasty to be the founder of this method, although Qing Wuzi of the Han dynasty (circa 200 BC) described it in relation to burial sites, and there are numerous further archaeological proofs of the application of the principles of *Feng Shui*, dating as far back as 3000-3500 BC. The practice and teaching of *Feng Shui* suffered greatly under the Chinese Cultural revolution, considered a "feudalistic superstitious practice" and banned. However today the official attitude has become more tolerant and *Fen Shui* is even applied in the design and building of some public sites and universities in China.

Basically, the primary purpose of *Feng Shui* is to harmonize and align the human existence with the surrounding environment to maximize health and well being. The theoretical and philosophical principles of this system are the same as the fundamental principles applied in Chinese medicine. Besides these principles, there are many notions based on astronomy and astrology, as well as simple popular common sense and life experience, as well as a body of superstition. Once the superstitious aspect is ignored, the metaphysical and rational aspects of *Feng Shui* have proven quite effective in their impact on people's lives and health, explaining the present day *Feng Shui's* popularity both in the East and the West.

The main principles of *Feng Shui*, as in Chinese medicine are, the notion of *Qi* ≈ Energy, polarity, *Yin* and *Yang*, the *Bagua* ≈ Eight trigrams, the Five Elements, and their correspondences, the *Wu Xing* ≈ Five moving forces and especially their inter-relations of *Sheng* ≈ Nourishment and *Ke* ≈ Control/ destruction cycles.

As it was established that the environment has a beneficial or detrimental effect on the person's state of physical and psychological health, it becomes quite logical to apply the *Feng Shui* principles and techniques in the evaluation and even treatment of some types of ailments, hence the concept of "Medical *Feng Shui*". When individuals are suffering from poor health or disease, it is extremely important to evaluate the conditions of their homes and working places, in particular where they spend a greater proportion of their time. Making changes in the flow of *Qi,* eliminating disturbing influences, adding appropriate colors and forms and incorporating personal symbolism, can all improve an individual's emotional, psychological and physical health. It is also vital for practitioners to become aware of the *Feng Shui* of their clinics and treatment rooms to facilitate the healing process. For this purpose, a simplified style of *Feng Shui* could be adopted, without going into the complicated aspects of the Compass school and the calculations of *Gan-Zhi* ≈ Stems and Branches.

Centuries of tradition have given birth to numerous methods of *Feng Shui*, but two schools dominate the practice:

- Form School: originally concerned with the location and orientation of tombs (*Yin* House *Feng Shui*), it later included the consideration of homes and buildings (*Yang* House *Feng Shui*). The Form School studies the shape of the environment, such as mountains, rivers, and general surroundings in relation to the five celestial animals the Red Bird (South), Green Dragon (East), White Tiger (West), Black Turtle (North), and the Yellow Ox (Centre). The concept of *Wu Xing* ≈ Five moving forces: Wood, Fire, Earth, Metal, and Water, play an important role. In this manner, the Form School analyses the shape of the land and flow of the wind and water to find a place with ideal *Qi*.
- The Compass School is more recent, based on the eight cardinal directions, as well as introducing the concept of "Time", the person's date of birth. It uses the *Loshu* ≈ Magic square and is less concerned with the shape of the landscape. The use of a magnetic compass the *Luopan*, a disc marked with formulas in concentric rings, characterizes this school. The Compass School includes techniques such as Flying Star and Eight Mansions.
  Contemporary *Feng Shui*, incorporates notions from both schools.

26.1 Basic Premises

The basic premises in *Feng Shui* are the following:

- *Qi*-≈ Energy, is defined as the Cosmic Breath or Vital Breath. The main emphasis in the *Feng Shui* practice, very similar to the practice of Chinese medicine or *Qi Gong*, is to capture and contain vital energy and to avoid damaging or dispersing *Qi* or letting it go stagnant.
- The belief of the Form School, at times called the landscape *Feng Shui*, is that the Cosmic breath of the Green Dragon is the source of peace, prosperity, and health. Therefore the aim is to build and live in areas plentiful of *Qi*, avoiding windy areas where the *Qi* can disperse, favoring the presence of water, such as lakes, that help contain the *Qi*, but again avoiding fast flowing straight rivers that can carry the *Qi* away, or stagnant waters. The Green Dragon, in this context, refers to natural landscapes such as hills, mountains, waterways, or can even be man-made monuments or towers. The art of *Feng Shui* practice lies in finding this Dragon Breath and harnessing and preserving *Qi*.
- It is understood that *Qi* travels in a spiral manner; therefore any *Qi* traveling in a straight line, similar to an arrow, is considered aggressive (poison arrow), causing damage to the Vital *Qi*. In general, places under cliff-sides or ridges are avoided. The same applies to furniture placed in a room with its angles directed towards the working or sleeping places. Natural or manmade objects, the line of a building or a roof, that point at a dwelling have also the same negative influence. Roads or rivers and other waterways bring *Qi* or carry it away. Any straight road leading

to a dwelling or its main entrance brings aggressive *Qi* and has to be blocked out by a bush or a hedge. Inside the house, the front door should not directly face the back door or a large window as the *Qi* will just go through and out, this may be corrected using wind chimes or screens, to slow the *Qi* down. Inside the dwelling, the presence of plants with sharp pointy leaves, like needles, has the same effect as an arrow.

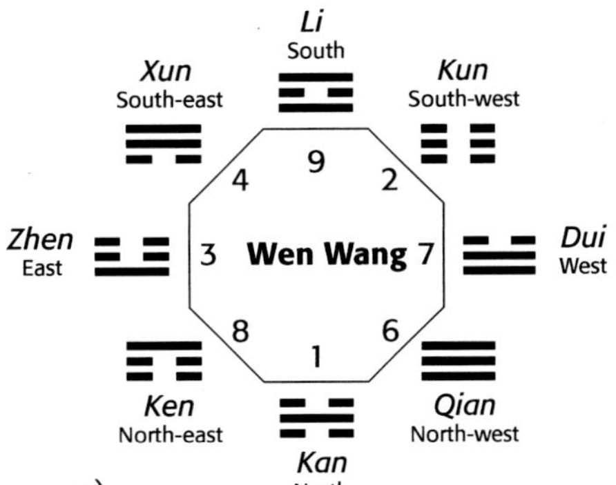

a)

4	9	2
3	5	7
8	1	6

b)

Figure 26.1: The Posterior-Heaven *Pa Gua* ≈ Eight Trigrams and the *Lo Shu* ≈ Magic square

- In the landscape, *Yin* and *Yang* are represented by, either very flat areas *(Yin)* or very rocky and hilly areas with no trees or rivers *(Yang)*. For houses built in this kind of landscape, the *Yin* or *Yang* has to be balanced by introducing plants, ponds or rocks in a controlled and harmonious manner. Hilltops or houses built on the edge of a steep incline tend to drain the *Qi* away.
- The Five-element correspondence system, particularly the colors and directions, as well as their inter-relations, play an essential role in the *Feng Shui* practice. For example, decorating with red colors and objects the South section of a dwelling, or placing candles, will supplement the Fire and its attributes, which are fame and reputation (see below). If a particular influence is too strong, it may be attenuated by the controlling cycle.
- The *Pa Gua* ≈ Eight Trigrams has a central position in the practice of *Feng Shui* and constitutes an important balancing "Talisman". As discussed in chapter 2.8, the Eight Trigrams are represented in two ways, referred to as Anterior-Heaven, related to Fu Xi, and Posterior-Heaven attributed to King Wen. (▶Fig. Fig. 26.1a).
- *Lo Shu* ≈ Magic square is actually the Posterior Heaven disposition of the Trigrams, also called the *Kan* ≈ Water and *Li* ≈ Fire disposition. The magic square consists of 9 squares designating the 8 compass points with Earth at the center (▶Fig. 26.1b). Each square has a number attributed to it, the sum of which always adds up to 15, no matter which line is selected. The *Lo Shu* is used as a pattern to superimpose over the house, the apartment or the room, which is being studied. Each square has its specific symbolism .

26.2 Feng Shui Practice

Without the complexity of considering the gender and birth-dates of the inhabitants and adapting the dwelling place for each, there is an easier way of using the *Lo Shu* ≈ Magic square by simply superimposing the below grid onto the house, apartment, working place or even each room.

Each section of the *Loshu* is assigned to a Trigram and has its particular characteristics (▶Fig. 26.2):

Figure 26.2: The Magic Square in Feng Shui

Wealth Prosperity, Abundance Self-worth	Reputation Social-life **Fire**	**Relationship** Marriage Partnership
Family Parents, Ancestors Health (together with Earth) **Wood**	**Nurturing** Health (together with Wood) **Earth**	**Creativity** Children Spirituality **Metal**
Wisdom Self-Knowledge Education, Study Rest and Peace	**Career** Opportunities Life-path/ Individuality **Water**	**Friends** Mentors, Helpful people Supportive Energies

Again there are two ways of placing the *Lo Shu* or the *Ba Gua* on the map of the house or the room:

- In traditional practice, the *Lo Shu* or the *Ba Gua* is placed with *Li* ≈ Fire always oriented towards the South.
- In the Black Hat sect, the bottom row of the *Lo Shu* or the *Ba Gua* is placed towards the main entrance of the dwelling or the room. In this manner, the entrance door will either fall in the *Ken* (North-East: education and study), or *Kan* (North: opportunities and career), or *Qian* (North-West: helpful mentors and friends).

In both cases, if the shape of the dwelling is not square, there will be some areas of the *Lo Shu* that will be more supported and some areas might be weaker or even non-existent. For example in an L-shaped space, if the missing part falls on *Xun* (South-East), the Prosperity corner, and if the family is having financial difficulties, it is advisable to add a section to the house, when this is possible, or else to increase the missing space by the placing of mirrors and appropriate objects and colours. (see table below). Fortunately, *Feng Shui* has a cure for all situations, using mirrors, plants, screens, wind chimes,etc...

For example, a patient having health issues should be advised to particularly pay attention to the East/Wood section, representing Health and Family. By nurturing this area, adding green plants and colors, avoiding stagnancy produced by closed spaces, storerooms, or the loss of *Qi* through drains or toilets, in this case, to hold and preserve the *Qi,* hollow objects, such as bowls or vases could be used. Additionally, the outer form of the body may be drawn on the floor map of the home or room, with the head located at the main entrance door. Narrow passages, protruding corners or other disturbances would be identified in relation to the patient's area of manifested pathology. The structural anomalies of the room are then corrected, mainly by using mirrors or other cures.

A person having financial problems will need to nurture the South-East corner, by adding symbols of wealth, coins, bills, or a money plant.

In the bedroom, where we spend a good third of our life, particular care has to be taken in the placing of furniture and objects. It is not recommended to have mirrors facing the bed, as it would disturb the *Hun* ≈ Ethereal soul and cause bad dreams. Sharp objects and protruding corners should not be directed towards the bed, if unavoidable, then the sharpness has to be somehow attenuated by a cloth or a plant.

In general, it is advisable not to have too many plants in the bedroom.

Visible roof beams crossing the sleeping area are also blocking the energy of that particular area of the body; simply corrected by covering the beams.

The presence of TV or computer screens in the bedroom has scientifically verified disturbing effects on sleep, especially for children, even if the TV screen is placed in an adjacent room, as long as the bed happens to be in the radiation field of the screen. Although classical *Feng Shui* does not mention this point, it should definitely be added to disturbing factors.

The same attention should be given to the professional working area, in the placing of the treatment bed and the choice of colors and objects (see below). Additionally, as the treatment rooms absorb a lot of pathogenic *Qi*, they need to be regularly cleaned and purified, utilizing such methods as Essential oils, fumigation by Sage or special incenses, or again clearing by burning Epsom salt with alcohol.

The following table offers some simple ways, by adding colors or objects, to help and affect various areas of the home (▶Table 26.3):

Table 26.3: Additional objects and colors to improve each section of the home

To improve prosperity: Money plant; Wind chimes; Coins, round objects Valuable items; Aquarium (fish) Gold, Green, Purple, Red, Blue	**To improve fame and reputation:** Fireplace; Candles Light source; Diplomas, trophies; Triangular shapes Red	**To affect relationships:** Pairs of candles; Doves Paired objects; Love symbols (hearts, photos); Romantic or erotic art Pink, Red, White, Ochre
To affect family and health: Plants; Flowers; Wooden objects, pillars; Family photos Family souvenirs; Painting or images of healthy bodies Green, Blue	**To balance the entire home and improve unity:** Sunshine; Open space Square objects; Fruit bowl Meditation area Yellow, Orange, Brown, Ochre, Red	**To affect creativity and spirituality and help finish projects:** Metallic objects; Bells Wind chimes; Photos of children Naïve art; Round objects White, Silver, Pastel colors
To improve self-awareness: Books; Learning materials Images of wise people; Rock garden; Area of contemplation Blue, Green, Turquoise, Black	**To improve the career:** Water fountain; Aquarium Mirrors, glass-work; Paintings or photos of water Smooth, shapeless objects Black, Dark blue, Grey	**To affect supportive friends and benefactors and travel:** Spiritual symbols, altar; Angels Spiritual guides; Photos of exotic places; Ideal travel destinations Grey, Silver, Black

Although *Feng Shui* remains mostly an empirical and non-scientific practice, many of its principles rely on solid common sense, and most of all quite often the observable results speak for themselves.

Appendix

App. 1. Evidence of Acupuncture

When Acupuncture reached France, doctors attempted to demonstrate the anatomical substratum of the acupuncture channels and points. As such a correlation was never found, the term "Meridian" was chosen to designate the concept of the *Jing Luo*, channels and collaterals. Meridians being imaginary lines on the surface of the earth, was considered an appropriate term to signify an "invisible" path believed by the Chinese only, through which the energy flowed. For decades the Western hard-core materialistic medicine would not admit acupuncture as scientific, relegating its well established and proven efficacy to mere "psychosomatic" effects. In the 1940's, S. Kirlian in the Soviet Union accidentally placed his hand between a photographic plate and a high-tension electric spark, and found a picture upon developing the plate. The picture was unusual in that it showed an aura as well as several bright spots on the skin. Similar points were equally found on other parts of the body, as well as in plants and animals. A chance comparison with Chinese charts of acupuncture points revealed that the bright points observed by Kirlian and the acupuncture points were identical. Nevertheless the Kirlian effect remained in the domain of parapsychology and pseudoscience. In the 1960's it was discovered that the acupuncture points could be detected by using a galvanometer to measure the electrical resistance of the skin, which proved to be lower than the surrounding skin prompting Voll to develop "Electroacupuncture".

Recently years, several microscopic studies of the fascia have shown significant differences with the surrounding structures. In 1966, Prof Heine from the University Witten Herdecke discovered the anatomical correlation of the acupuncture point. In 80% of the cases, the acupuncture point corresponded to a vascular nerve bundle passing through the outer fascia. Acupuncture points presented with a two-fold receptor-density compared to surrounding tissues (Kellner, 1966), with 3.4 times as much electrical activity, also the acupuncture points were embedded in adventitia high in fluids (water) and Paccini bodies.

In a recent publication, Dr. D. Keown develops further the theory of the acupuncture channels being in fact the spaces between the fascia,

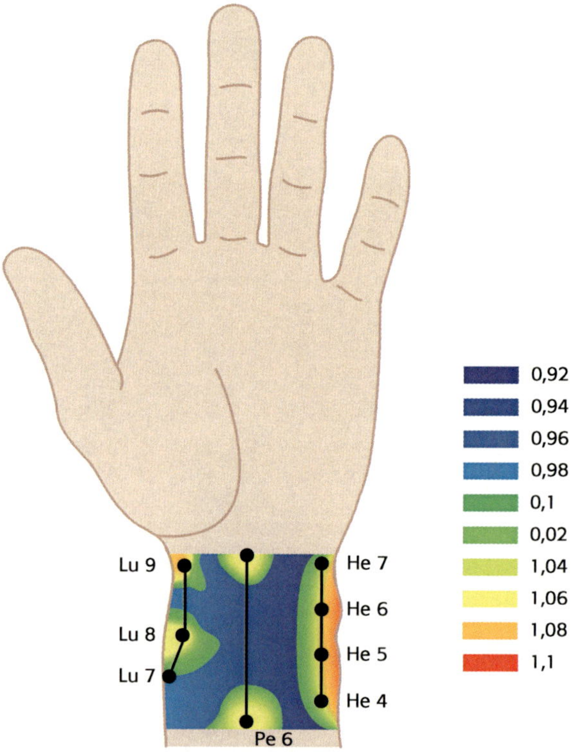

Figure A1: Partial oxygen pressure measured by amperometric oxygen microsensors.

exploring the embryological relation between the development of the organs and their related channel systems. According to him, the fascia would be the areas of least resistance for the electrical currents produced in the organs, to propagate to the extremities. These theories would further link the previous dicoveries concerning the electrical and anatomical properties of the channels. Could this then explain the Chinese mysterious concept of the *Huang* membranes (*Gao Huang* 膏肓)?

The contributions of CT (computerized tomography) scans, have further revealed the acupuncture point's anatomical structures. The CT exploration of points ST-36 Zusanli & ST-37 Shangjuxu demonstrated a very distinct structural difference from the surrounding areas in the form of microvascular densities with bifurcations around thick blood vessels. Acupuncture points contained fine structures with high density vascularization of vessels 15-50 micrometers in size, not found in non-acupuncture areas.

Another study, using an amperometric oxygen microsensor to detect partial oxygen pressure variations at different locations on the anterior aspect of the wrist, showed an oxygen pressure significantly higher at acupuncture points, clearly visualizing the points and channels (▶ Fig. A1)

References
- Chenglin, Liu, Wang Xiaohu, Xu Hua, Liu Fang, Dang Ruishan, Zhang Dongming, Zhang Xinyi, Xie Honglan, and Xiao Tiqiao. "X-ray phase-contrast CT imaging of the acupoints based on synchrotron radiation." Journal of Electron Spectroscopy and Related Phenomena (2013).
- Minyoung Hong, Sarah S. Park, Yejin Ha, et al., "Heterogeneity of Skin Surface Oxygen Level of Wrist in Relation to Acupuncture Point," Evidence-Based Complementary and Alternative Medicine, vol. 2012, Article ID 106762, 7 pages, 2012. doi:10.1155/2012/10a6762.
- Yan X H, Zhang X Y, et al. Do acupuncture points exist? Phys. in Med. & Biology, 54 (2009):N143–N150.
- Zhang Y, Yan X H, Liu C L, et al. Photoluminescence of acupuncture points "Waiqiu" in human superficial fascia [J]. J Lumin. 2006, 119-120:96-99.
- Julia J. Tsuei, Scientific Evidence in Support of Acupuncture and Meridian Theory: I. Introduction. IEEE Engineering in Medicine and Biology Magazine. 1996, 15(3):58-63.
- Li Lei, Yau To, Yau C.H.. What Is the Origin of Acupoint. J. Acupunct. Tuina. Sci. 2012, 10 (2):125-127
- Song X J, Zhang D. Study on the manifestation of facial infrared thermography induced by acupuncturing Guangming (GB 37) and Hegu (LI 4) [J]. Chinese Acupuncture & Moxibustion. 2010, 30(1):51-54.
- Liu P, Zhou G Y, Zhang Y, et al. The hybrid GLM– ICA investigation on the neural mechanism of acupoint ST36: An fMRI study [J]. Neuroscience Letters, 2010, 479: 267-271.
- Fei L, Cheng H S, et al. The experimental exploration and the research prospects about the material basis and the functional characteristics of the meridian [J]. Chinese Science Bulletin, 1998, 439(6):658-672.
- http://www.healthcmi.com/Acupuncture-Continuing-Education-News/1230-new-ct-scans-reveal-acupuncture-points#sthash.baMfBhpi.dpuf

My colleague Dr. Bartosz Chmielnicki has been greatly contributing to this study by creating a Metabase of all the pertinent research conducted in the field of Chinese Medicine and Acupuncture:

Please refer to **"Evidence Based Acupuncture. Effectiveness and mechanisms of action of acupuncture"** showing the current state of knowledge about acupuncture, using the language understood by Western scholars – the language of science

https://www.evidencebasedacupuncture.org/dt_testimonials/15363/

I sincerely hope that these studies and their results would further contribute to the full acceptance of Acupuncture as a therapeutic modality in the Western medical arena.

App. 2. Historical Background of Chinese and French Acupuncture

Dynasty	Author, Physician	Text, Treatise	Medical land-marks
Legendary period: Xia (3000–1500 BC)	Fu Xi	Ba Gua and Yi Jing	Cosmology
	Shen Nong	Shen Nong Ben Cao	Herbal medicine
Shang (1600-105) Zhou (1027-770)	Huang Di	Nei Jing, Su Wen/ Ling Shu/ Tai Shu and Ming Tang (lost)	Stone acupuncture, Moxa, notion of Gui ≈ Spirits and Feng ≈ Wind
Waring states: 2nd Zhou (770–222 BC)	Confucius	–	Conficianism and Daoism influence medicine
	Lao Tzu	Dao De Jing	
	Chuang Tzu	–	
	–	–	Yin-Yang / 5 Movements/ Wei Qi versus Xie Qi/ Iron needles/ Mawangdui scrolls
Qin (221–207 BC)	Bian Que	Nan Jing	Commentaries on the Ling Shu
Western Han (206BC–24AD)	–	Shen Nong Ben Cao	Herbal matria medica
	Hua Tuo (140-208)		Anesthesia; immunization
Three Kingdoms (220–280)	Wang Shu He	Mai Jing	Pulse diagnosis
Sui (581-618) Tang (618–907)	Cao Yuan Fang	Zhu Bing Yuan Hou Lun	Disease etiology and symptoms
	Sun Si Miao	Qiang Jin Yao Fang, Dan Jing Yao Yue	Alchemy/ Ethics/ Gynecology/ Extraordinary Vessels/ Ah Shi points
	Wang Tao	Wai Tai Mi Yao	Formulas and receipts
Five Dynasties (618–960) Song (960–1279)	Wang Wei Yi Liu	Shu Xue Zhen Jiu Tu Jing	Bronze statue
	Liu Wan Su	Han Liang Pai	6 pathogens; Heat: Cooling school
	Zhang Congzheng	Gong Xie Pai	Purging methods: Purging school
	Chen Wu Ze (Yen)	San Yin Ji Yi Bing Zheng Fang Lun	3 causes of disease
	Chen Zi Ming	Wai Ke Jing Yao/ Fu Liang Fang	Surgery, Gynecology
	Li Dong Yuen	Pi Wei Lun	Earth school: Spleen & Stomach
	Dou Han Qing	–	Extra Vessel points/ De Qi/ Antic Shu points

	Yang Jie	Xun Zhen Tu	Anatomy / Patho-cosmology
	–	Sheng Ji Zong Lu	Imperial encyclopedia of medicine/ medical examinations
Yuan (1280–1368)	Zhu Dan Xi	Dan Xi Xin Fa	Yin tonification school
	Du Ben	Ao Shi Quan Lu	Tongue diagnosis in typhoid
Ming (1368–1644)	Li Shi Zhen	Ben Cao Gang Mu	Pharmacopea
		Qi Jing Ba Mai Kao	The 8 Extraordinary Vessels
		Bin Hu Mai Xue	Pulse diagnosis
	Yang Ji Zhou	Zhen Jiu Da Cheng	Acupuncture and moxibustion
	Zhang Jie Bing	Jing Yue Quan Shu	
	Gao Wu	Zhen Jiu Ju Ying	Compilation of ancient texts
	Li Yan	–	Tonification-sedation points
	Wang Ken Tang	Zheng Zhi Zhun Sheng	Male-female and left-right Therapeutic encyclopedia
Qing (1644–1911)	Fu Qing Zhu	Fu Qing Zhu Nu Ke	Gynecology and urology
	Ye Tian Shi	Wen Bing Lun	Feverish diseases; 4 stages
	Wu Ju Tong	Wen Bing Tiao Pien	Differentiation of feverish diseases
	Cheng Zhong Ling	–	–
	Wu Qian	Yi Zong Jin Jian	8 Diagnostic principles/ Zang-Fu
	Wang Qing Ren	Yun Lin Gai Cuo	Errors of medicine
	Zhou Xue Hai	–	Tongue diagnosis
	(1822)		Acupuncture loses stature
Chinese Republic (1911–1949)	Tang Rong Chuan	Xue Zheng Lun	Blood and bleeding conditions
	Zhang Xi Chun	Yi Xue Zhongzhong Canxi Lu	Chinese and Western medicine
	(1914)	–	Chinese Medicine is official
Communist China (1945–1963)	1958: Mao declares Chinese Medicine to be a “Great Treasure House”		The term “TCM” is coined around 1955

Acupuncture in Europe

Date	Author, Physician	Text, Treatise	Medical land-marks
16th century	(Portuguese)	–	Testimony on Chinese Medicine
17th century	(Jesuit)	–	Texts and references
18th century	De Halde	–	Description on Chinese Medicine
	Father J. Amiot	–	–
	Dr. C.J. Saillant	–	Exchanges on pulse diagnosis
	Dr. Abel Rémusat	*on tongue diagnosis*	–
	Dr. F.A. Lepage	*on Pharmacopea*	–
	Louis Berlioz	–	–
1826–1898	Dabry de Thiersant	–	–
1878–1955	G. Soulié de Morant	*Acuponcture Chinoise (1939)* *Wrote over 20 books on acupuncture*	Influence of Chinese, Vietnamese and Japanese acupuncture
Students of Soulié de Morant	Dr. Ferreyroles	*Acupuncture Chinoise (1951)*	Acupuncture practice in hospitals
	Dr. R. De la Füye	*Traité d'Acupuncture (1947)*	1945 French Acup. Society (SIA) / numerisation of channels
		Acupuncture Moderne Pratique (1947)	
	Dr. J. Lavier	*Acupuncture Chinoise*	Studied also with Wu Wei Ping; developed 5 Element acupuncture
		Médecine chinoise médecine totale (73)	
	Dr. J.E.H Niboyet	*Essai sur L'acupuncture Pratique (51)*	–
	Dr. A. Chamfrault	*Traité de Méd. Chinoise, 6 vol. (54–96)*	Associat. Française d'Acupuncture (AFA)
Students of Dr. De la Füye	Dr. J. Bischko (A)	–	Austrian school
	Dr. Felix Mann (GB)	*Acupuncture series (>1962)*	Founder of British Medical Acupuncture Society
	Dr. Stefvater (D)	*Acupuncture as Neural Therapy (1955)*	German school
	Dr. G. Bachmann (D)	–	German school
	Dr. H. Schmidt (D)	*Acupuncture Journal in Germany (> 52)*	–
	Dr. Lawson Wood (GB)	*Chinese System of Healing (1959)*	–
Students of Dr. Lavier	Worsley	Also influenced by Wu Wei Ping and Lon Kok Yuen, as well as the Japanese school	Five Element Acupuncture school
	Roysten Low	–	British Acupuncture

			Association
	Van Buren	–	Int. College of Oriental Medicine
French School since 1960	Dr. J. Lavier	*Médecine chinoise médecine totale (73)*	–
	Dr. A. Chamfrault	*Traité de Médecine Chinoise (54–96)*	Founder of Associat. Française d'Acupuncture (AFA) in 1945
	Dr. Nguyen Van Nghi with Chamfrault	*Pathogénie et pathologie energétique en médecine Chinoise (77)*	Hon. President AFA
		L' Energétique Humaine en Médecine Chinoise (69)	
	Dr. Dr. Ch. Laville Mery and Dr. A. Duron	*Bioénergétique et Médecine Chinoise*	–
	Dr. J. Borsarello	*Acupuncture Pratique (98)*	–
	A. Faubert	*Traité didactique d'Acup. Traditionnelle*	–
	Père C. Larre and E. Rochat de la Vallée	*Translation of Chinese medical texts*	Ecole Européenne d'Acupuncture
		Cahiers préparatoires	
	Dr. J.M. Kespi	*Acupuncture (1982)*	AFA
	Dr. C. Roustan	*Traité d'Acupuncture (1979)*	AFA
	Dr. M. Mussat	*Physique de l'Acupuncture (1972)*	AFA
	Dr. G. Andres et. al	*Les méridiens extraordinaires (1997)*	AFA

App.3. Glossary of Chinese terms used in the book

Pinyin	English	Chinese
Ān	Calm, quiet	安
Àn	Press/*An Mo massage*	按
Ān Mián	Peaceful sleep	安眠
Bā	Eight	八
Bā Gāng	Eight (diagnostic) principles	八纲
Bā Guà	Eight trigrams	八卦
Bā Zì	Eight words, terms (astrology)	八字
Bá Guàn	Cupping	拔罐
Bái, Bái Hǔ	White (*Bai Hu* ≈ White tiger)	白, 白虎
Bāo	Uterus (*Bao Mai* ≈ Uterine vessel)	胞
Bēi, Āi	Sadness	悲, 哀
Běi	North	北
Bēn Tún	Running piglet (syndrome): panic attack	奔豚
Bí	Nose	鼻
Bì	Impediment, obstruction (painful obstruction of *Qi* and Blood mainly due to External Wind, Damp, or Cold)	痹
Biàn Zhèng	Pattern differentiation, identification	辨證
Biǎo	Exterior, surface	表
Biǎo-Lǐ	Exterior-interior	表里
Bǔ	Supplement, tonify	补
Cái	Agent, expert, gifted (3 *Cai*: active agents of the universe)	才
Chán	Meditation (*Zen* in Japanese)	禅
Cháng	Long	長
Cháo Rè	Tidal fever (recurring afternoon or evenings)	潮熱
Chén	Deep, sinking	沉
Chéng	Over-act (Xiang Cheng/ over-acting)	乘
Chí	Slow, late	遲
Chǐ	Cubit (*Chi-Guan-Cun:* cubit-bar-inch, the 3 radial pulse positions)	尺 (关-寸)
Chōng Mài	Penetrating vessel	沖 (衝) 脉
Còu Lǐ	Interstice (space between skin & sinew)	腠理
Cù	Hasty, agitated	促
Cùn	Body inch (*Chi-Guan-Cun:* cubit-bar-inch, the three radial pulse positions)	寸
Dà	Big, large, wide	大
Dà Cháng	Large intestine	大肠
Dà Yùn	Great movement (of the year)	大運
Dài	Intermittent, interrupted, regular replacement (of generation)	代
Dài Mài	Belt, girdle vessel	带脉
Dân	Gallbladder	胆
Dān, Dān Tián	Cinnabar, elixir (*Dantian* ≈ Cinnabar chamber)	丹, 丹田
Dào	Road, path, way, circuit, doctrine, method, principle	道
Dì	Earth, soil (*Tian-Ren-Di* ≈ heaven-human-earth)	地
Dé Qì	Obtaining *Qi* (needling sensation)	得气
Diān	To withdraw, depression	癲
Diān Kuáng	Depression mania	癲狂
Dìng	Settle, stabilize (*Ding Chuan* ≈ Settle wheezing)	定
Dōng	East	东

Dòng	Moving	動
Dòng Qì	Moving *Qi* (between the kidneys)	動气
Dū Mài	Governing vessel	督脉
Duǎn	Short, brief	短
Èr	Two	二
Ěr	Ear	耳
Fán	Agitation, restlessness, vexation	烦
Fán Zào	Agitation and restlessness (mental agitation and physical restlessness/fidgetiness)	烦躁
Fèi	Lung	肺
Fēng	Wind	风
Fēng Shuǐ	Wind and water; Chinese geomancy	风水
Fú	Hidden	伏
Fú	Superficial, to float	浮
Fù	Abdomen	腹
Fǔ	Bowel (*Zang-fu* ≈ Organs and bowels)	腑
Fú	Floating, superficial	浮
Fú Luò	Superficial connecting - network vessels	浮络
Gān	Liver	肝
Gān Zhī	Stem and branch (Chinese astrology)	干支
Gāo	Fatty tissue, protective membrane (*Gao Huang* ≈ Protective and Vital/Nourishing membranes)	膏
Gé	Leathery (drum-skin)	革
Gēn	Root	根
Gēn-Jié-Zhī	Root, Knot and Branch	根-结-支
Gōng	Power, merit, result, ability, skill	功
Gù	Consolidate, secure, strengthen	固
Gǔ	Bone	骨
Gǔ Qì	Food energy (Essence of food)	谷气
Guā Shā	Scraping	刮痧
Guān	Pass; bar (*Chi-Guan-Cun*: cubit-bar-inch, the three radial pulse positions)	关（尺-寸）
Guǐ	Ghost, unnamed spirit, demonic	鬼
Guī	turtle (*Xuan Gui* ≈ Black Turtle)	龟 (玄龟)
Hǎi	Sea, ocean	海
Hán	Cold	寒
Hàn	Sweat	汗
Háo Zhēn	Filiform acupuncture needle	毫针
Hé	Harmonize (*He Zhong*≈ Harmonize the centre)	和
Hé	Sea; join, combine	合
Hóng	Overflowing, flooding	洪
Hòu Tiān	Later, post-heaven, post-natal	后天
Hǔ	Tiger	虎
Huá	Slippery	滑
Huà	Transform (*Hua Duo* ≈ Transform turbidity)	化
Huǎn	Retarded, slowed-down	緩
Huāng	Vital membranes	肓
Huì	Meeting (*Hui Xue* ≈ Meeting points)	会
Hún	Ethereal soul	魂
Huó	Invigorate	活
Huǒ	Fire phase	火
Huò Luàn	Sudden turmoil disorder (sudden, severe diarrhoea, vomiting and abdominal pain; gastro-enteritis)	霍亂
Jī	Accumulation, clumping (*Ji Re* ≈ accumulated Heat)	积
Jī	Muscle, flesh	肌
Jiàn	Strengthen, fortify (*Jian Pi* ≈ Fortify the Spleen)	健
Jiān	Shoulder	肩
Jiàng	Descend, down-bear (*Jiang Ni* ≈ Down-bear counter-flow)	降
Jiāo	Exchange, confluence, intersection	交
Jiǎo Qì	Foot *Qi* (leg and foot	脚气

	numbness, pain and weakness)	
Jiě	Release, resolve (*Jie Biao* ≈ Resolve the exterior)	解
Jié	Knotted	结
Jié	Knot (*Gen-Jie-Zhi* ≈ Root, knot, branch)	结（根–支）
Jìng	Quiet, still	静
Jīn	Sinews, muscles	筋
Jīn	Metal phase	金
Jǐn	Tight, tense	緊
Jīn Yè	Body fluids	津液
Jǐng	Well	井
Jīng	River, channel	经
Jīng	Shock, fright	驚
Jīng Qì	Channel energy	经气
Jīng Bié	Divergent channels	经别
Jīng Jīn	Sinew/ tendino-muscular channels	经筋
Jīng, Jīng Qì	Essence, essential qi	精气
Jǐng Shén	Alertness	警神
Jiǔ	Nine	九
Jiǔ	Liquor; tincture; extract	酒
Jiǔ Fǎ	Moxibustion	灸法
Jù	Concentration, gathering (mass)	聚
Jué Yīn	Terminal yin	厥陰
Jué Zhèng	Reversal/collapse syndrome (coma with coldness)	厥证
Kè	control (*Xiang Ke* ≈ Controlling cycle)	克
Kǒng, Kǒng Jù	Fear	恐, 恐惧
Kǒu	Mouth	口
Kōu	Hollow (scallion stalk)	芤
Kuān	Loosen, unbind (*Kuan Xiong* ≈ Unbind the chest)	宽
Kuáng	Mania (*Dian Kuang* ≈ Depression-madness)	狂
Kuáng Zǒu	Mad walking	狂走

Láo	taxation, consumption (*Wu Lao* ≈ 5 taxations)	勞（劳）
Láo	Firm, confined	牢
Lǎo	Old	老
Lè, Xǐ Lè	Elation (music), happiness, joy	乐(樂), 喜乐
Lì	Pestilence; scrofulous lumps or swellings	沥, 疬
Lǐ	Interior (*Biao-Li* ≈ Exterior-interior)	裏（里）
Lǐ	Chinese mile, village	裏（里）
Lǐ	Rectify	理
Lǐ Jí	Abdominal urgency (cramping pain, urgency; dysentery)	裡(里)急
Liáng	Cool	凉
Lìn	Strangury (painful urination syndrome)	淋
Líng	Soul, spirit	靈
Liù	Six	六
Liù Yín	Six excesses	六淫
Lóng	Dragon	龍（龙）
Luàn	Mental confusion	乱
Luò	Connecting	絡
Lǔo Lì	Small and large nodules/scofula (neck, axillary or inguinal nodules)	瘰疬
Luò Mài	Connecting/ Network channels/ vessels	絡脉 / 脈
Mài	Vessel	脉 /脈
Máo	Body hair, wool	毛
Méi Hé	Plum-pit (feeling of a lump in the throat)	梅核
Mìng	Destiny, life, mandate (*Ming Yun*≈ Fate 命运)	命
Mìng Mén	Life, vitality gate	命门
Mó	Rub (*An Mo* massage)	摩
Mù (Mo)	Collecting point	募
Mù	Wood phase	木
Ná	Grasp, hold (*Tui Na* massage)	拿
Nǎo	Brain	脑

Nán	South	南
Nèi	Internal	内
Nèi Dān	Inner elexir (alchemy)	内丹
Nì Qì	Counterflow/rebellious/inverse *Qi* (abnormal *Qi* flow)	逆气
Nù	Anger	怒
Nüè	Malaria	疟
Páng Guāng	Bladder	膀胱
Pí	Spleen	脾
Pí	Skin	皮
Pǐ	Glomus, focal distension	痞
Pí Bù	Skin, cutaneous regions	皮部
Píng Bǔ Píng Xiè	Reinforcing-reducing; harmonisation	平补平泻
Pò	Corporeal/ animal soul	魄
Qì	Energy	气（氣）
Qī	Seven	七
Qì Gōng	Energy cultivation (exercise)	气功
Qī Qíng	Seven passions	七情
Qí Jīng Bā Mài	8 extraordinary vessels	奇经八脉
Qiào	Orifice, portal, opening	窍
Qiāo	Springing, stepping (*Qiao Mai* ≈ Stepping Vessel)	跷
Qíng	Emotion	情
Qīng	Green-blue (*Qing Long* ≈ Green dragon)	青（青龙）
Qīng	Clear, quiet (*Qing Re* ≈ Clear Heat)	清
Qīng Qì	Clear, pure energy	清气
Rè	Heat	热
Rén	Human, human being, man (*Tian-Ren-Di* ≈ heaven-human-earth)	人（天人地）
Rèn Mài	Conception (controlling) vessel	任脉
Ròu	Flesh	肉
Rú	Soft, soggy, immersed	濡
Rùn	Moisten (*Run Fei* ≈ Moisten the Lung)	润
Ruò	Weak, frail	弱

Sàn	Dissipate, dispersed, scattered	散
Sān	Three	三
Sǎn	Powder	散
Sān Bǎo	Three treasures	三宝
Sān Bù	Three regions	三部
Sān Jiāo	Triple warmer/burner/heater	三焦
Sè	Choppy, rough	澀
Shàn	Hernia (accumulations); acute urinary and bowel retention; disease of the external genitalia	疝
Shān Zhōng	Chest centre	膻中
Shào Yáng	Lesser *Yang*	少陽
Shào Yīn	Lesser *Yin*	少陰
Shé	Tongue	舌
Shén	Spirit, consciousness, intelligence, mind, emotions	神
Shèn	Kidney	肾
Shēn	Body	身
Shēng	Generate (*Xiang Sheng* ≈ Generating cycle)	生
Shí	Repletion, excess, solid, real	实（實）
Shí	Season, fixed time (*Si Shi* ≈ Four phases)	時
Shǐ	Discharge, release	泄
Shī	Dampness	湿
Shǒu	Hand, arm	手
Shū	Course, relax (*Shu Gan* ≈ Course the Liver)	疏
Shū	Stream	輸
Shù, Bèi Shù	Transport point, back transport	俞，背俞
Shuǐ	Water phase	水
Shùn	Normalize, favourable (*Shun Qi* ≈ Normalize *Qi*)	顺
Shùo	Rapid, fast	數
Sì	Four	四
Sī	Pensiveness (thought), worry	思

Suǐ	Marrow	髓
Sūn Luò	Deep connecting/ network vessels	孙絡
Tài Yáng	Supreme Yang	太陽
Tài Yīn	Supreme Yin	太陰
Tài Jí	Supreme ridge or great pole	太極
Tán	Phlegm	痰
Tāng	Soup, decoction	汤
Tí	Raise, lift	提
Tiān	Heaven	天
Tiān Chu-āng	Window of heaven/ sky	天窗
Tiān Gŭi	Growth promoting and reproductive substance; menstruation	天癸
Tiān-Rén-Dì	Heaven-human-earth	天人地
Tiáo	Regulate	调
Tòng	Pain	痛
Tōng	Free, open, unstop	通
Tóu	Head	頭
Tóu Fēng	Head-Wind: severe recurrent headaches; or External PF headache with vertigo and facial paralysis	頭风
Tŭ	Earth phase	土
Tuī	Push	推
Tuī Ná	Massage	推拿
Wáng	Emperor, king	王
Wài	External	外
Wài Dān	Outer elexir	外丹
Wèi	Stomach	胃
Wēi	Minute, faint	微
Wěi	Wilting, atrophy	痿
Wèi Qì	Defensive energy	卫气
Wěi Zhèng	Wilting syndrome: atrophy, flaccidity and weakness	痿症
Wēn	Warm (*Wen Bing* ≈ Warm disease)	温
Wŭ	Insult (*Xiang Wu* ≈ Insulting cycle)	侮
Wŭ	Five	五
Wŭ Zhì	Five emotions (minds)	五志
Wŭ Xíng	Five moving forces/ phases	五行
Wŭ Jī	Five accumulations (five types of mass)	五积
Wú Jí	Primordial chaos	無極
Wŭ Láo	Five taxations (excessive use of the eyes = Blood, sitting = flesh, standing = bones, walking = sinews, lying = Qi)	五劳
Wŭ Shù	Martial arts	武术
Xì	Fine, thin, minute	細
Xí	Extinguish, pacify	熄
Xĭ	Joy	喜
Xī	Cleft, accumulation	郗（郄）
Xī	Knee	膝
Xī	West	西
Xī	Breath	息
Xián	Wiry, bowstring, chord	弦
Xiān	Immortal	仙
Xiān Tiān	Pre-heaven, earlier heaven, pre-natal	先天
Xiàng	Likeness, similarity (*Si Xiang* ≈ 4 symbols)	象
Xiāo	Wheezing (*Re Xiao* ≈ Heat wheezing)	哮
Xiāo	Disperse, regulate	消
Xiăo Cháng	Small intestine	小肠
Xiāo Kě	Dispersion/wasting and thirsting (thirst, hunger, polyuria and loss of weight; diabetes mellitus)	消渴
Xiè	Discharge, reduce, drain, vent	泄
Xié Qì	Pathogenic, perverse, aggressive energy (External Wind, Heat, Damp, Dryness or Cold, causing disease)	邪气
Xīn	Heart	心
Xīn Bāo	Pericardium	心包
Xū	Vacuity, deficiency, empty	虛
Xuān	Diffuse, effuse (*Xuan Fei* ≈ Diffuse the lung)	宣

Xuán	Dark; mysterious	玄
Xuè	Blood	血
Yǎn	Eyes	眼
Yáng	"Yang" active, mobilising principle	陽（阳）
Yáng Míng	Yang brightness	陽明
Yáng Qiāo Mài	Yang motility/ Stepping Vessel	陽蹻脉
Yǎng Shēng	Nourish, cultivate, support life (vitality)	养生
Yáng Wéi Mài	Yang binding/ Linking Vessel	陽維脉
Yè	Thick fluids, humor	液
Yì	Intellect, thought, reflection, intention, awareness	意
Yī	One	一
Yì Jīng	Book of changes	易經
Yīn	"Yin" passive principle	陰（阴）
Yīn Qiāo Mài	Yin motility/ Stepping Vessel	陰蹻脉
Yīn Wéi Mài	Yin binding/ Linking Vessel	陰維脉
Yíng	Spring	滎
Yíng (Róng) Qì	Nourishing/ constructive energy	營(榮)气
Yōu, Chóu Yōu	Oppression, worry	憂，愁憂
Yù	Jade	玉
Yuán Qì	Source, original energy	元(原)气
Zàng-Fǔ	viscera & bowels/ Yin & Yang organs	脏腑
Zào	Mental agitation, irritability	躁
Zào	Dryness	燥
Zhēn Qì	True/ authentic energy	真气
Zhēn Jiǔ	Acupuncture	针灸
Zhèng	Syndrome, pattern	证（證）
Zhèng	Symptome	症
Zhēng Gǔ	Steaming bone syndrome (tidal fever, from Yin-Xu with night sweats)	蒸骨
Zhèng	Primary channels	正经

Jīng		
Zhèng Qì	Upright/ correct energy	正气
Zhēng-Jiǎ-Jī-Jù	Concretions and gatherings: masses; *Zheng* and Ji ≈ hard masse with fixed pain; *Jia* and *Ju* ≈ mobile masse	癥瘕积聚
Zhì	Will power (mind)	志
Zhǐ	Suppress, relieve (*Zhi Tong* ≈ Relieve pain)	止
Zhǐ Zhǐ	Foot, toe	趾趾
Zhī	Branch; limb (*Gen-Jie-Zhi* ≈ Root, knot and branch)	支 (根-结-支)
Zhōng Guó	Central empire, China	中國(国)
Zhōng Qì	Central/ middle energy	中气
Zhōng Zhèng	Central rectitude; righteousness	中正
Zhōng Jí	Central ridge/ polar star	中極
Zhú	Expel, dispel (*Zhu Tan* ≈ Expel Phlegm)	逐
Zhū	Red; Cinnabar	朱
Zhū Què	Red bird; Phoenix	朱雀
Zhuàng	Invigorate (*Zhuang Yang* ≈ Invigorate Yang)	壮
Zī	Nourish	滋
Zǐ Gōng, Bāo	Uterus	子宫/胞
Zōng Qì	Ancestral/ Gathering Energy	宗气
Zú	Foot	足

Bibliography

Classical Chinese Texts

In chronological order

Huang Di Nei Jing Su Wen (黄帝内经素问) *Yellow Emperor's Classic of Internal Medicine*: The oldest text on Chinese Medicine, attributed to Huang Di, compiled around 100 BC from medical texts dating between 400-200 BC. It is composed of two parts: *Su Wen- Simple Questions*, covering the fundamentals of Chinese medical concepts, and *Ling Shu* (灵枢) *Spiritual Axis (Pivot)*, concerning more specifically the practice of acupuncture. Tradition has it that two other books also existed, but have been lost since: Tai Shu, describing the Mu-accumulation and Xi-cleft points, and the Ming Tang, on the location of the acupuncture points.

Nan Jing Jiao Shi (难经校释) *(Explanation of) Classic of difficulties*: published around 1st-2nd century AD and generally attributed to Bian Que. Contains 81 chapters attempting to explain the difficulties of the Nei Jing.

Zhong Zang Jing (中藏经) *Classic of the Central Organ*, by Hoa To circa 198 AD, discusses mainly pulse diagnosis and warming herbal remedies.

Shang Han Lun (伤寒论) *Cold-induced Diseases*, by Zhang Zhong Jing 220 AD, one of the four most important classics, discussing the diagnosis and herbal treatment of feverish diseases from external cold, as well as prognosis and medical errors.

Jin Gui Yao Lue Fang Lun- 金匱要略方論 – Prescriptions of the Golden Cabinet by Zhang Zhong Jing, circa 220 AD, later modified by Wang Shu He, indicating herbal prescriptions for internal, surgical and gynecological conditions

Zhen Jiu Jia Yi Jing (针灸甲乙经) *Systemic Classic*: ABC of Acupuncture and Moxibustion, by Huang Fumi (215–281), published in 282 AD, discussing and complementing the Su Wen, the Ling Shu as well as the Ming Tang (the lost text). It remains the reference book for acupuncturists covering the treatment of various diseases.

Mai Jing (脉经) *The Classic of the Pulse* by Wang Shu He (210–286); describing 24 pulse qualities and their significance. This text had a great influence later on Asian and middle-eastern medicine.

Zhou Hou Bei Ji Fang (肘後備急方) *Emergency Prescriptions* by Ge Hong (284–364), offering herbal prescriptions and moxa for emergencies.

Qian Jin Yao Fang (千金要方) *Prescriptions Worth a Thousand Ducats* by Sun Si Miao (581-682), published around 652, it is a compilation of herbal, acupuncture and moxibustion treatments for external, internal, gynecological and pediatric conditions. He also covers the 13 Gui-ghost points, previously cited by Bian Que, for the treatment of 100 diseases.

Qian Jin Yi Fang (千金翼方) *Supplement to the Thousand Ducats*, in which Sun Si Miao complements the previous text.

Zhen Jiu Zi Sheng Jin (針灸資生經) *Supplementing life with Acupuncture and Moxibustion* by Wang Zhi Zhong, (1220). Elaborating on acupuncture points, methods of treatment for various diseases.

Biao You Fu (標幽賦) *Ode to Elucidate mysteries* attributed to Dou Mai (1196–1280)

Ma Dan Yang Tian Xing Shi Er Xue Ge (馬丹陽天星十二穴歌) *Song of Ma Dan Yang's Twelve Celestial Star points*, cited in the Zhen Jiu Da Quan by Xu Feng, 15th century; describes the coupling of the main 12 acupuncture points: LU-7, LI-11, LI-4, ST-36, ST-44, HE-5, BL-40, BL-57, BL-60, GB-30, GB-34 and LR-3.

Yu Long Jing (玉龍經) *Classic of the Jade Dragon*: Bian Que's Spiritual Guide to cupuncture and Moxibustion by Wan Guo Rui, 1329; includes the Yu Long Ge

Yu Long Ge (玉龍歌) - Song of the Jade dragon by Wang Guo Rui, 1329, included in the You Long Jing, on 120 acupuncture points.

Zhen Jiu Da Quan (鍼灸大全) *Complete Collection of Acupuncture and Moxibustion* in six volumes by Xu Feng (1439); describing more over needling techniques and choice of points according to the Stems and Branches.

Ling Guang Fu (靈光賦) Ode of Spiritual Brightness, cited in the Zhen Jiu Da Quan by Xu Feng (1439)

Xi Hong Fu (席弘賦) *Ode of Xihong*, cited in the Zhen Jiu Da Quan by Xu Feng (1439)

Zhen Jiu Ju Ying (针灸聚英) *Glorious Anthology of Acupuncture and Moxibustion*, by Gao Wu (1529). This is a compilation of ancient texts by eminent acupuncturists, commented and complemented by Gao Wu.

Bai Zheng Fu (百症賦) *Ode of One Hundred symptoms*; by an unknown author, cited in the Zhen Jiu Ju Ying by Gao Wu (1529).

Yu Long Fu (玉龍賦) *Ode of the Jade Dragon*, cited in the Zhen Jiu Ju Ying by Gao Wu (1529), is a digest of the main points of the earlier Yu Long Ge.

Za Bing Xue Fa Ge (雜病穴法歌) *Song of Points for Miscellaneous Diseases*, recorded in the Zhen Jiu Ju Ying by Gao Wu (1529).

Yi Xue Gang Mu (醫學綱目) *Outline of Medicine* by Lou Ying (1565); a compilation and commentaries of ancient texts.

Zhen Jiu Da Cheng (針灸大成) *Great Compendium of Acupuncture and Moxibustion* by Yang Ji Zhou (1601); is the most complete text on acupuncture, compiling over 30 ancient texts with commentaries and additions.

Sheng Yu Ge (胜玉歌) *Song more precious than Jade*, cited in the Zhen Jiu Da Cheng by Yang Ji Zhou (1601).

Xun Jing Kao Xue Bian (循經考穴編) *Investigation into Points of the Channels*, attributed to Yan Zhen, referring to Ming Wan Li (1573–1620), with commentaries on the points of the 14 channels.

Dong Yi Bao Jian (東醫寶鑑) *Precious Mirror of Oriental Medicine*, by the Korean author Xu Sun (1611).

Jing Yue Quan Sh (景岳全書) *Complete Works of Jing Yue*; Zhang Jie Bin (1624); in which he analyses various diagnostic and therapeutic methods, states that there is no *Yang* exuberance but only *Yin* vacuity, and moreover indicates supplementing and warming techniques.

Lei Jing Tu Yi (類經圖翼) *Illustrated Supplement to the Classic of Categories*, by Zhang Jie Bin (1624), is an illustrated adaptation of the Nei Jing.

Shen Jiu Jing Lu (神灸经論) *Divine Moxibustion*; Wu Yang Cheng (1853). He states that during his time only about 2 out of 100 doctors practice acupuncture and only 1 out of 10 use Moxibustion.

Zhen Jiu Ji Cheng (針灸集成) *Compilation of Acupuncture and Moxibustion* by Liao Run Hong (1874)

Shi Si Jing Yao Xue Zhu Zhi Ge (十四經要穴主治歌) S*ong of the Points of the Primary Fourteen Channels*, unknown author.

Yi Zong Jin Jian (醫宗金鑑) *Golden Mirror of Medicine*, by Wu Qian (1742), on methods of Acupuncture and Moxibustion.

Zhen Jiu Feng Yuan (針灸逢源) by Li Xue Chan, 1815, in 4 volumes, discusses the principles of acupuncture with a description of 361 main and 96 extra points.

Classical Chinese texts in *Pin Yin* alphabetical order

Bai Zheng Fu (百症賦) *Ode of One Hundred symptoms*; by Gao Wu (1529).

Biao You Fu (標幽賦) *Ode to Elucidate mysteries* attributed to Dou Mai (1196–1280)

Dong Yi Bao Jian (東醫寶鑑) *Precious Mirror of Oriental Medicine*, by Xu Sun (1611).

Huang Di Nei Jing Su Wen (黄帝内经素问) *Yellow Emperor's Classic of Internal Medicine*:

Jin Gui Yao Lue Fang Lun- 金匱要略方論 – Prescriptions of the Golden Cabinet by Zhang Zhong Jing, circa 220 AD

Jing Yue Quan Sh (景岳全書) *Complete Works of Jing Yue*; Zhang Jie Bin (1624

Lei Jing Tu Yi (類經圖翼) *Illustrated Supplement to the Classic of Categories*, by Zhang Jie Bin (1624)

Ling Guang Fu (靈光賦) Ode of Spiritual Brightness, cited in the Zhen Jiu Da Quan by Xu Feng (1439)

Ma Dan Yang Tian Xing Shi Er Xue Ge (馬丹陽天星十二穴歌) *Song of Ma Dan Yang's Twelve Celestial Star points*, cited in the Zhen Jiu Da Quan by Xu Feng, 15th century;

Mai Jing (脉经) *The Classic of the Pulse* by Wang Shu He (210–286)

Nan Jing Jiao Shi (难经校释) *(Explanation of) Classic of difficulties*: published around 1st-2nd century AD and generally attributed to Bian Que

Qian Jin Yao Fang (千金要方) *Prescriptions Worth a Thousand Ducats* by Sun Si Miao (581-682), published around 652

Qian Jin Yi Fang (千金翼方) *Supplement to the Thousand Ducats*, by Sun Si Miao.

Shang Han Lun (伤寒论) *Cold-induced Diseases*, by Zhang Zhong Jing 220 AD

Shen Jiu Jing Lu (神灸经論) *Divine Moxibustion*; Wu Yang Cheng (1853)

Sheng Yu Ge (胜玉歌) *Song more precious than Jade*, cited in the Zhen Jiu Da Cheng by Yang Ji Zhou (1601).

Shi Si Jing Yao Xue Zhu Zhi Ge (十四經要穴主治歌) *Song of the Points of the Primary Fourteen Channels*, unknown author.

Xi Hong Fu (席弘賦) *Ode of Xihong*, cited in the Zhen Jiu Da Quan by Xu Feng (1439)

Xun Jing Kao Xue Bian (循經考穴編) *Investigation into Points of the Channels*, attributed to Yan Zhen, referring to Ming Wan Li (1573–1620)

Yi Xue Gang Mu (醫學綱目) *Outline of Medicine* by Lou Ying (1565)

Yi Zong Jin Jian (醫宗金鑑) *Golden Mirror of Medicine*, by Wu Qian (1742)

Yu Long Fu (玉龍賦) *Ode of the Jade Dragon*, cited in the Zhen Jiu Ju Ying by Gao Wu (1529)

Yu Long Ge (玉龍歌) - Song of the Jade dragon by Wang Guo Rui, 1329

Yu Long Jing (玉龍經) *Classic of the Jade Dragon*: Bian Que's Spiritual Guide to cupuncture and Moxibustion by Wan Guo Rui, 1329

Za Bing Xue Fa Ge (雜病穴法歌) *Song of Points for Miscellaneous Diseases*, recorded in the Zhen Jiu Ju Ying by Gao Wu (1529).

Zhen Jiu Da Cheng (針灸大成) *Great Compendium of Acupuncture and Moxibustion* by Yang Ji Zhou (1601)

Zhen Jiu Da Quan (鍼灸大全) *Complete Collection of Acupuncture and Moxibustion* in six volumes by Xu Feng (1439)

Zhen Jiu Feng Yuan (針灸逢源) by Li Xue Chan, 1815

Zhen Jiu Ji Cheng (針灸集成) *Compilation of Acupuncture and Moxibustion* by Liao Run Hong (1874)

Zhen Jiu Jia Yi Jing (针灸甲乙经) *Systemic Classic*: ABC of Acupuncture and Moxibustion, written by Huang Fumi (215–281), published in 282 AD

Zhen Jiu Ju Ying (针灸聚英) *Glorious Anthology of Acupuncture and Moxibustion*, by Gao Wu (1529)

Zhen Jiu Zi Sheng Jin (針灸資生經) *Supplementing life with Acupuncture and Moxibustion* by Wang Zhi Zhong, published in 1220

Zhong Zang Jing (中藏经) *Classic of the Central Organ*, by Hoa To circa 198 AD

Zhou Hou Bei Ji Fang (肘後備急方) *Emergency Prescriptions* by Ge Hong (284–364)

Modern Chinese References

Xin Zhen Jiu Xue (新针灸学) *New Acupuncture and Moxibustion*, by Zhu Lian (1951), relates acupuncture to the nervous system.

Zhong Hua Zhen Jiu Xue (中華鍼灸學) *Contemporary Acupuncture*, by Zhao Erkang (1953).

Zhen Jiu Xue Shou Ce (針灸學手册) *Origin and Development of Acupuncture and Moxibustion*, edited by Wang Xue Tai (1956).

Zhen Jiu Xue Jian Bian (針灸學簡編) edited by the TCM Institute of research in 1957, covers methods and pathologies as well as acupuncture analgesia.

Shanghai Zhen Jiu Xue (上海针灸学) *A Study of Acupuncture*, edited by TCM Institute of Shanghai in 1974

Zhong Guo Zhen Xue Jiu Gai Yao (中國針灸學) edited by Qi Ye in Taipei (1979).

Western References

Andrès Gilles : *Proposition pour une méthodologie d'étude des points d'acupuncture*. Revue Française d'acupuncture, No55, 1988, pp.5-11

Andrès Gilles, J. B., G. Berger, G. GuillaumeJ.M. Kespi, Chieu Mach, B. Teboul-Wang: *Les méridiens extraordinaires*; (1997), La Tisserande, Paris

Autroche B., Navailh P.: *Le Diagnostic en Médecine Chinoise*; (1983) Maloine

Autroche B. et al: *Pratique des Aiguilles et de la Moxibustion;* (1989) Maloine

Barrey J-F., Deporte P.: *Vivre en Cinq Mouvements;* (1994) Ed. du Prieuré

Beinfield H., Korngold E.: *Between Heaven and Earth;* (1991); Bllantine Books

Bensky D., O'Connor J. (1996). *Acupuncture A Comprehensive Text Shanghai College of Traditional Medicine*. Eastland Press.

Bertschinger R., *Golden Needle; Yang Jizhou's Great Compendium*. (1991). Churchill Livingston.

Bertschinger R., *The Great Intent* (2013); Singing Dragon

Borsarello J.F.: *Cahiers d'Acupuncture* (1987), Masson, Paris.

Borsarello J.F.: *Acupuncture Pratique* (1998), Masson, Paris.

Borsarello J.F.: *Les Pouls en Médecine Chinoise* (1981), Masson, Paris.

Bossy J., Maurel J.C.: *Acupuncture*; (1976), Masson Paris

Bridges, L.: *Face Reading in Chinese Medicine;* (2004); Churchill Livingston

Brown S.G.: *The Practical art of Face Reading*; (2000); Carroll & Brown limited

Campbell, J.: *Acupuncture Channels and Points; (2008)*By (author) Joan Campbell, Churchill Livingston

Chamfrault A.: Editions Coquemard; Angoulème, France:

- Tome 1 : *Traité de médecine chinoise. Acupuncture, moxas, massages, saignées* (1954)
- *Tome 2 : Traité de médecine chinoise d'après les textes chinois anciens et modernes.*
- *Tome 3 : Traité de médecine chinoise. Pharmacopée* (1959)
- *Tome 4 : Traité de médecine chinoise d'après les textes anciens et modernes, formules magistrales* (1961)
- *Tome 5 : Traité de médecine chinoise - de l'astronomie à la médecine chinoise*
- *Tome 6 : Traité de médecine chinoise - l´énergétique humaine en médecine chinoise* (1996)

Chang Po-Tuan: *The Inner Tachings of Daoism;* (1986); Shambhala

Chmielnicki B.: *Pulse Qualities;* Compleo

Clavey S.: *Fluid Physiology and Pathology in TCM;* (1995); Churchill Livingstone

Coste M., Paugam J.Y.: *Acupuncture, Tradition et Recherche Moderne* (2006); FLETC, PALAJA.

Darras J.C.: *Zhen Jiu Da Cheng*, translated by Leung Kwok Po; 1981, Darras editions, Paris (F)

Deadman, P., Al-Khafaji, M., & Baker, K. *A Manual of Acupuncture.* (2007). Journal of Chinese Medicine pub., East Sussex (GB).

Deng T.: *Practical Diagnosis in TCM;* (1999); Churchill Livingston

Desoutter, B. *Merveilleux Vaisseaux*.: (1996); Sauramps medical, Montpellier

Ding, L. *Acupuncture, Meridian Theory and Acupuncture Points.* (1991). Foreign Languages Press.

Di Villadorata M, Côté B.: *Acupuncture en Médecine Clinique*; (1989); Maloine, Paris.

Duron A., Laville-Mery Ch., Borsarello J.: *Bioénergétique et médecine chinoise*; 1973, Maisonneuve, Paris

Eckman, P.: *In the Footsteps of the Yellow Emperor*, (1996); Cypress Book, San Francisco.

Ellis, A., Wiseman, N., & Boss, K. *Fundamentals of Chinese Acupuncture (Paradigm Title).* (1991). Paradigm Publications (MA).

Eyssalet J-M: *Shen ou l'Instant Créateur;* (1990); Guy Trédaniel

Eyssalet J-M: *Le Secret de la Maison des Ancêtres;* (1990); Guy Trédaniel

Farrell Y., Chan D.: *Psycho-Emotional Pain and the Eight Extraordinary Vessels* (2016) Singing Dragon

Faubert, A.: *Traité didactique d'Acupuncture Traditionnelle* (1977);. Guy Tredaniel.

Faubert, A. *Le Sceau du Destin*;(1988). Guy Tredaniel.

Faubert G., Crepon P.: *La Chronobiologie Chinoise*; (1983) Albin Michel

Fisch G. : *La Médecine Traditionelle Chinoise*; (1993); LEP

Frey M.: *l'Acupuncture, comprendre cette médecine*; (2007); You Feng

Füye de la R. *Traité d'acupuncture* (1956). Editions Le François, Paris.

Gardner-Abbate S.: *Palpatory Diagnosis in Oriental Medicine*; (2001); Churchill Livingston

Gaurier T.: *Acupuncture Traditionelle*; (1985); Encre

Gaurier T.: *Bioclimatopathologie en Acupuncture*; (1980); T. Gaurier

Geng J. & Su Z. *Acupuncture and Moxibustion* (Practical Traditional Chinese Medicine & Pharmacology). (1998). New World Library.

Hammer L. I.: *Chinese Pulse Diagnosis*; (2001); Eastland Press

Harper D.: *Early Chinese Medical Literature*, (1998), KPI London

Helms J.M.: *Acupuncture Energetics: Clinical Approach for Physicians* (1995); Thieme

Hempen C.H.: *dtv-Atlas Akupunktur*, (1995); Deutschert Taschenbuch Verlag, München.

Hseuh, C. C. *Acupuncture: A Comprehensive Text. (*1981). Eastland Press.

Hua-Ching Ni: *I Ching* (1983). Tao of Wellness

Keown D. *The Spark in the* Machine (2014); Singing Dragon, London UK & PA, USA

Kespi, J.-M. *Acupuncture* (1982). Maisonneuve, Moulin-les-Metz, France.

Kespi, J.-M. *Cliniques: Acupuncture* (1995). De la Tisserande, Paris.

Kirschbaum, B.: *Atlas of Chinese Tongue Diagnosis*; (1998). Eastland press

Lade, A. *Acypuncture Points: Images & Functions* (1989). Eastland Press.

Larre C.: *Les Chinois*; 1981, Lidis-Brepols, Paris

Larre C., Schatz J, Rochat de la Vallée E.*: Survey of Traditional Chinese Medicine* (1976); Institut Ricci, Paris

Larre C., Rochat de la Vallée E.: *The Seven Emotions;* (1996); Monkey Press

Larre C., Rochat de la Vallée E.: *Les Mouvements du Coeur;* (1992), Desclée de Brouwer, Paris

Laurent Ph. *L'esprit des points : étude des trajets des méridiens et de la signification du nom des points.* (2000). Librairie You-Feng.

Lavier, J. A. *Médecine chinoise médecine totale.* (1973); Grasset.

Lawson-Wood O. & J.: *Acupuncture Vitality and Revival Points*, (1960); Health Science Press, Devon.

Leung Kwok-Po: *Points d'acupuncture*; Revue Française d'acupuncture, No12, 1977, pp. 7-17

Legge D. *Acupuncture Points and Meridians*, (1999); Sydney College Press, Australia

Li Ding: *Acupuncture, Meridian Theory and Acupuncture Points*, (1991); Foreign Language Press, Beijing.

Li Shi Zhen: *Pulse Diagnosis;* (1985) Paradigm

Li Tian, Lachner A.: *Wortschatz Chinesische Medizin*,;(2005); Elsevier, München

Li X., Zhao, J. Acupuncture Patterns & Practice; (1993); Eastland Press

Low R. : *The Celestial Stems;* (1985); Thorsons

Lu H. C.: *Tongue Diagnosis in Color;* (1977) The Academy of Oriental Heritage, Canada

Maciocia, G.: *Tongue Diagnosis in Chinese Medicine;* (1987); Eastland Press

Maciocia, G.: *The Foundations of Chinese Medicine;* (1989) Churchill Livingstone.

Maciocia, G.: *Diagnosis in Chinese Medicine;* (2004); Churchill Livingstone.

Maciocia, G.: *The Channels of Acupuncture: Clinical Use of the Secondary Channels and Eight Extraordinary Vessels;* (2006)*;* Churchill Livingstone.

Maciocia, G.: *The Psyche in Chinese Medicine;* Churchill Livingstone

Matsumoto, K. & Birch, S.: *Extraordinary Vessels (Paradigm Title).* (1993). Churchill Livingstone.

Matsumoto, K. & Birch, S.: *Hara Diagnosis;* (197887); Paradigm

Medicine, T. A. o. T. C. *An Outline of Chinese Acupuncture.* (1975). Foreign Languages Press.

Mi, H. *Zhenjiu jiayi jing (2 Volumes).* (2004). Editeur Guy Tredaniel.

Mitchel, S. *Tao Te Ching*, (1943). Harper & Row

Montakab H.: *Acupuncture for Insomnia* (2012); Thieme

Montakab H.: *Acupuncture Point and Channel Energetics* (2014). Kiener

Montakab H.: *Acupuncture for Headaches, Eyes and other ENT Pathologies* (2019), Singing Dragon

Mussat M.: *Physique de l'Acupuncture*: Hypotheses et Approches. Experimentales. 1972: Librairie le Francois, Paris, France

Nguyen Van Nghi: *Pathognie et pathologie énergtiques en médecine chinoise: Traitement par acupuncture et massages,* (1971). Impr. Ecole techniques Don Bosco. Marseille

Nguyen Van Nghi *Topography énergtiques en médecine chinoise,* (1971); Impr. Ecole techniques Don Bosco. Marseille

Nguyen Van Nghi, Tran Viet Dzung, Recours Nguyen C.: *Lingshu.* (1972); NVN. Marseille

Nguyen Van Nghi *Zhen Jiu Da Cheng.* (1982); NVN Marseille

Niboyet J. E.H. *Essai sur l'Acupuncture Chinoise Pratique,* (1951); Dominique Wapler. Paris

Niboyet, J. E.H. *Traitement des algies par l'acupuncture et certains massages chinois* (1959). Jacques Lafitte. Paris.

Niboyet. J. E. H.: *Pratique de la médecine manuelle* (1968). Maisonneuve et Larose.

Niboyet, J. E. H. *Nouveau traité d'acupuncture* (1998). Maisonneuve et Larose.

O'Conner J., Bensky D. *Acupuncture – A Comprehensive Text* (1981); Eastland Press, Chicago

Oury C. : *Les Points fenêtres du Ciel*; Institut Ricci, Paris

Pan, A. *Océan d'énergie: étymologie des noms des points d'acupuncture* (1998). Maloine, Paris.

Paugam J-Y, Coste M. (2006). *Acupuncture Tradition et Recherche Moderne - Compendium de Recherche.* Fletc.

Quaglia-Senta A.: *Système Sympathique en Acupuncture Chinoise*; (1976), Maisonneuve, Ste-Ruffine

Quirico P. E., Pedrali T.: *Teaching Atlas of Acupuncture* (2007); Thieme Stuttgart.

Reuben A., Babey-Brooke A.M.: *The Pulse in Occident and Orient;* (1966) Aurora

Réquéna, Y.: (1996), Maloine, Paris.

- *Terrains et pathologie en acupuncture -I*
- *Terrains et pathologie en acupuncture-II*
- *Terrains et pathologie en acupuncture-III*

Réquéna Y.: *Acupuncture et Psychologie;* (1982), Maloine, Paris.

Réquéna Y.: *Morphotypological Hand Diagnosis in Acupuncture;* (1986); Solal

Rochat de la Vallée E.: *Cahiers préparatoires à une meilleure comprehension des points d'acupuncture Tome-1.* Paris: Institut Ricci

Rochat de la Vallée E. et al: *Jing Shen (Huainzi chapter 7)*; (2010) Monkey Press

Ross J.: *Acupuncture Point Combinations: the Key to Clinical Success.* (1995). Churchill Livingstone.

Ross J.: *Zang Fu, The Organ System of TCM;* (1994) Churchill Livingstone

Rossbach S.: *INterior Design with Feng Shui;* (1987) Rider

Roustan C. : *Traité d'Acupuncture, Médecine Traditionelle Chinoise*, 3 vol. (1979); Editions, Masson, France

Rozeg J.: *Vaisseaux Merveilleux* (1983); Maisonneuve, Moulin-lès-Metz

Schatz J., Larre C., Rochat de la Vallée E.: *Apérçus de médecine traditionelle chinoise* (1979), éd Maisonneuve, Paris.

Shima, M. & Chace, C.: *The Channel Divergences: Deeper Pathways of the Web* (2000). Blue Poppy Press.

Shima M.: *The Medical I Ching;* (1992); Blue Poppy Press

Sionneau, P. *Acupuncture : Les points essentiels* (2000). Guy Trédaniel, Paris.

Simons R.: *Feng Shui step by step;* (1996); Rider

Song T.B.: *Atlas of Tongues and Lingual Coating in Chinese Medicine;* (1986); Sinomedic

Soulié de Morant, G.: *l'Acuponcture Chinoise, Atlas.* (1972); Maloine Paris

Soulié de Morant, G.: *l'Acuponcture Chinoise, Texte.* (1972); Maloine Paris

Spears J. A.: *Meridian Circuit Systems*, (2010); Integrative Healing Society

Stercks P., Jun C.: *Diagnostic des Symptomes;* (2002), Presses Universitaires Guang Ming

Stercks P., Jun C.: *Diagnostic des Syndromes;* (2002), Presses Universitaires Guang Ming

Stercks P., Jun C.: *Organes et Entrailles;* (2002), Presses Universitaires Guang Ming

Taylor K.: *Chinese Medicine in Early Communist China* (2005); Routledge Curzon, Oxon.

Tchao Ming-Te: *l'Acupuncture et la Moxibustion.* (1967); Tcha Ming Te, Paris

Twicken D. *Eight Extraordinary Channels*; (2013); Singing Dragon

Veith, I. *The Yellow Emperor's classic of internal medicine;* chapters 1-34 translated from the Chinese with an introductory study by Ilza Veith. (1966). *New ed. Uni Cal press, Berkley*

Wang D. *Manual of International Standardization of Acupuncture Point Names.* (1987).

Wang Ju-Yi & Robertson J.: *Applied Channel Theory* (2008); Eastland Press, WA, USA

Walters D.: *Chinese Astrology;* (1992); Aquarian

Walters D.: *Feng Shui handbook;* (1991); Aquarian

Wilhelm R., Perrot, E.: *Tao Te King (Lao Tseu)*; (1974) Librairie de Médicis

Wiseman, N. *Glossary of Chinese Medical Terms and Acupuncture Points.* (1991). Paradigm Publications (MA).

Wiseman, N. & Feng, Y.: *A Practical Dictionary of Chinese Medicine*(1998); Paradigm Publications

Wu Wei Ping: *Chinese Acupuncture.* (1962). Health Sci. P.

Wühr E.: *Chinesische Syndromdiagnostik*; (2010) Verlag für Ganzheitliche Medizin

Yan, L. *New Chinese-English Dictionary of Traditional Chinese Medicine.* (2003). China Medical Science and Technology Press.

Yan Zhenguo: *Anatomical Atlas of Acupuncture Points* (2003); Donnica publishing

Yu Lin Lian, Chen C.-Y., Hammes, M. *Seirin- Bildatlas der Akupunktur. Darstellung der Akupunkturpunkte.* (1999); Könemann, Köln

Yuan-Kuang: *Méthode Pratique de Divination Chinoise par le Yi-King;* (1977) Guy Trédaniel

Yuen J. C.: *Extract of lectures between 2000 and 2013*, Academy of Chinese Healing Arts, Winterthur

Zhenguo, Y. (2003). *Anatomical Atlas of Acupucture Points.* Donica Publishing.

Guide to Pinyin pronunciation

Pinyin is the official phonetic system for transcribing the Mandarin pronunciations of Chinese characters into the Latin alphabet. *Pīnyīn* 拼音 literally means "spelled-out sounds.

Letter	English approximation
a	father
b	bay / spit
p	pay / pit
m	may / mummy
f	fair / fun
d	day / stop
t	take / top
n	nay / nit
l	lay / love
g	gay / skill
k	kay / kill
h	hay
j	jeep / church
q	cheer / punch
x	she / push
zh	junk / choke
ch	church / chin
sh	shirt / shoe
r	leisure / reduce
z	reads

c	hats / cats
s	say / sun
y	yea / yes
w	way / water
o	saw
e	her
i	(no illustration)
i	see
u	rude
ü	French tu, German Fühlen
er	are
ai	eye
ei	eight
ao	now
ou	oh
an	can
en	turn
ang	German Gang
eng	sung
ong	German Lunge
ia	Asia

ie	yes
iao	yeowl
iu	yoke / yukon
ian	yen
in	in
iang	e+yang
ing	sing
iong	German Jünger
ua	guano
uo	wall
uai	wife
uan	one
un	went
uang	oo+ahng
üe	ü+eh
üan	ü+an
ün	German grün
kongr	corn
wanr	w + far
dianr	d + yar

About the Author

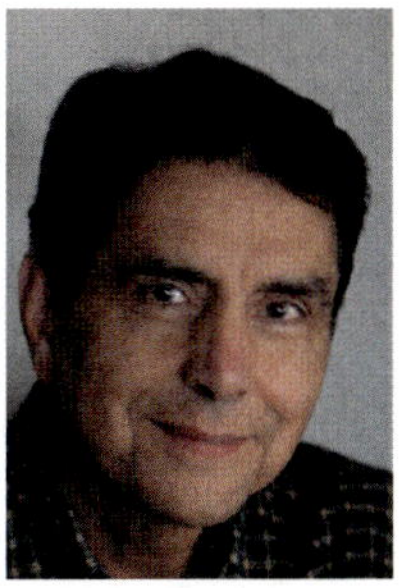

Hamid Montakab – graduated from the Medical School of Paris and further did his residency in surgery and Gynaecology. He concurrently completed a degree program in Acupuncture at the AFA School in Paris, after which he spent four months in intensive training at the Men Wa and ISA schools in Hong Kong. He then spent some time exploring the Traditional medicines in the Philippines and India, where he also practiced combining TCM with Allopathic and Ayurvedic medicines.

Between 1980-85 Hamid practiced in America, obtaining the Oregon Acupuncture Board and the National Acupuncture Board (NCCA). Later, he completed trainings in Chinese Herbal Medicine, Osteopathy and Visceral Osteopathy in Europe. Since 1985 he has been practicing and lecturing in Switzerland, France and Germany.

Dr. Montakab was commissioned by the Swiss National Science Foundation to conduct a scientific research study on Acupuncture and Insomnia. He has also done a smaller study on Acupuncture in Atopic Dermatitis at the Geneva University Hospital. Dr. Montakab was the co-founder of the Swiss Professional Organisation for TCM (SBO-TCM) and it's president from 1995 till 2000.

With his wife Solange, they founded the Academy of Chinese Healing Arts in Switzerland in 1986. With his background in Eastern and Western medical practices, and his exposure to the practice of Chinese Medicine in Europe, China and America, he brings his students the combined sum of his experiences in the field of Traditional as well as Classical Chinese Medicine. He currently practices in Savièse-Switzerland and teaches internationally.

Other related titles by Hamid Montakab:

- "Treatment of Acute ankle sprains with Acupuncture" (1977 thesis);
- “The Diagnostic chart in TCM” (1978)
- "Pulse Diagnosis in Chinese Medicine" (1980)
- "Acupuncture and Insomnia" (1990 study)
- Co-author of "Stresskrankheiten" (Elsevier 2006)
- " Acupuncture for Insomnia/ Sleep and Dreams in Chinese Medicine (Thieme 2012);
- "Acupuncture Point and Channel Energetics/ Bridging the Gap" (Kiener 2014)
- Co-author of "Behandlung von Schlafstörungen" (MS 2015)
- "Acupuncture for Headaches, Eyes and ENT Pathologies" (Singing Dragon 2019)

About the Co-authors

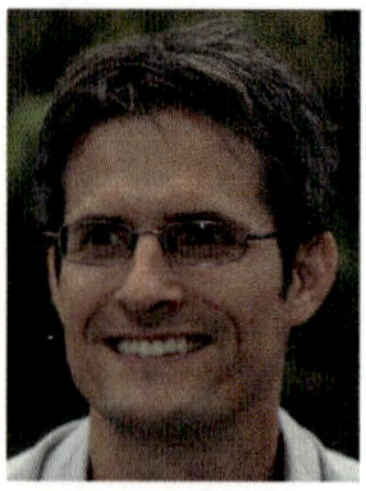

Simon Becker – studied Chinese medicine in the US and later in China. He was the President of the Swiss Professional Association (SBO-TCM) from 2003 to 2010. Currently he is the deputy head of the Department of Chinese Medicine of the Lake Hospital Horgen as well as a TCM-expert at Lian Chinaherb company. Simon Becker is the principal of Chiway Academy of Asian medicine in Winterthur. He teaches in Switzerland and abroad and is the author of "A Handbook of Chinese Hematology", "The Treatment of Cardiovascular Diseases with Chinese Medicine" and "Correcting the Errors in the Forest of Medicine". He specializes in Chinese herbal medicine and particularly in paediatrics and cancer support.

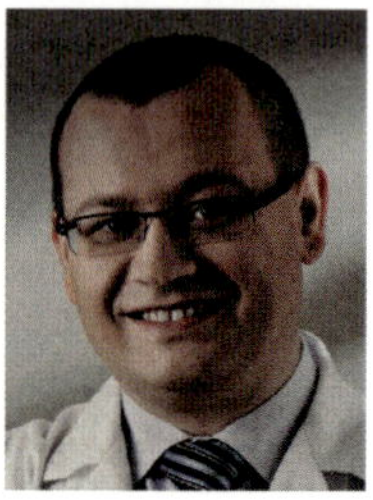

Dr. Bartosz Chmielnicki – trained as an MD and later in acupuncture in Poland. He was the co-founder of "Compleo" and Silesian Academy of Acupuncture and the president of Silesian Chapter and board member of the Polish Acupunture Association. Between 2010 and 2014 he was elected the president of Classical Acupuncture Association. He has co-authored numerous seminars on basic acupuncture and for pain management at the Colleguim Medicum of Jagiellonian University in Cracow. Dr. Chmielnicki practices currently at Compleo in Katowice as well as at the Pain Management outpatient clinic in Tychy. He is deeply involved in teaching in Poland and abroad as well as publishing various articles and is the author of a book about pulse diagnosis in Chinese Medicine.

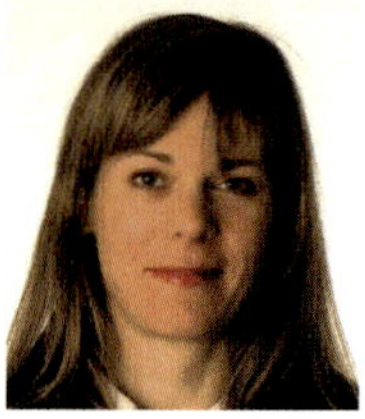

Christine Dam – after studying Chinese dietetics and Naturopathy in Germany, she completed her education in acupuncture and Chinese herbal medicine in Zurich, followed by practical trainings in China. Christine Dam has been practicing and teaching Chinese dietary therapy and acupuncture in Zürich and is currently in charge of the Chinese dietary therapy department at Chiway Academy of Asian medicine in Winterthur.

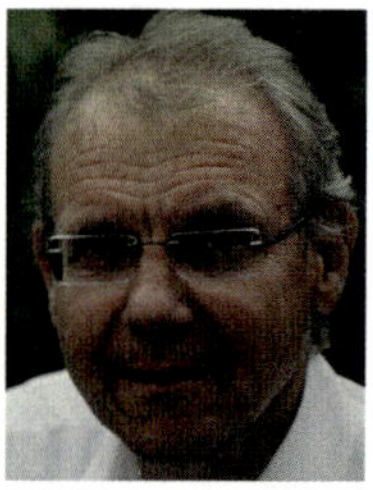

Dr. Stefan Englert – after completing his medical studies he specialised in Chinese Medicine in Ravensburg. He was the founding member of the German scientific Society of TCM (DWG TCM e.V.) and head of the medical association for TCM in reproductive medicine (DGRM). Dr. Englert is the Co-Director of the Chiway Academy of Asian medicine in Winterthur. He is the author of “Großes Handbuch der chinesischen Phytotherapie und Akupunktur”, „Behandlung von Menopause und klimakterischen Beschwerden“ and „Checkliste Chinesische Diätetik”, and co-editor of the series “Praxisreihe Traditionelle Chinesische Medizin”. He is currently the head of the department of Acupuncture and TCM scientific research and training programs at the Dresden International University and a lecturer at the University of Ulm and a member of the examination committee of the German medical association in Baden-Württemberg. Dr. Englert practices in Ravensburg with an integrative approach of TCM and Western medicine.

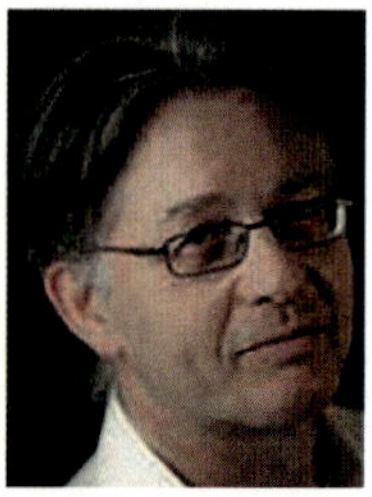

Peter Firebrace – graduated in Acupuncture from the International College of Oriental Medicine in England, then did further studies with the European School of Acupuncture in Paris and the College of Traditional Chinese Medicine in Chengdu, China. He has also studied Chinese language and philosophy with the Ricci Institute in Paris. Past Principal of ICOM, he is a co-founder of Monkey Press which produces the "Chinese Medicine from the Classics" series, co-author of "A Guide to Acupuncture", he has produced educational DVDs on the "Roots of Chinese Medicine" and "The Body Map of Chinese Medicine", a book of related poems entitled "Cloud Falls Rap" and two albums of songs and music videos on

Chinese medical and Daoist themes, "Sea Gong" and "Chinese Medicine Blues". Peter Firebrace currently practices in London and teaches internationally.

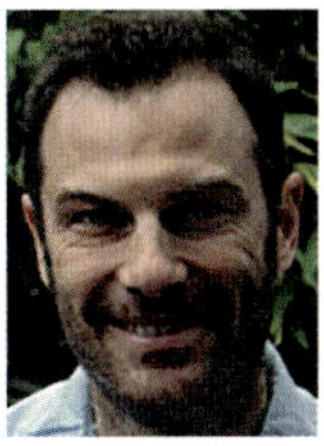

Phillip Haas – studied anthropology in particular exploring the traditional Mayan medicine. He later trained in Chinese Medicine at the Academy or Chinese Healing Arts in Switzerland as well as in Munich and Chengdu-China, further specialising in Tuina massage. Currently he practices Acupuncture and Tuina-massage as well as teaching at the Chiway Academy of Asian medicine in Winterthur in Switzerland.

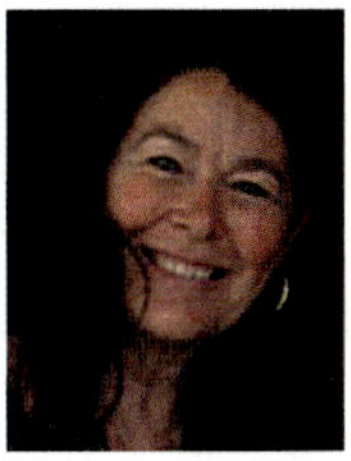

Solange Montakab-Pont – trained as a Yoga instructor and later studied Naturopathy, Auriculotherapy, Acupuncture and Chinese herbal medicine in Switzerland and in France. She did further trainings in Osteopathy and Visceral Osteopathy in France. For decades, she practiced *Qi Gong* and meditation, in particular the Daoist and Buddhist approaches. Her particular interest in human psychology led her to the study of a variety of psychotherapeutic methods such as re-birthing, de-hypnotherapy, trans-personal psychotherapy. Inspired by these Eastern and Western methods, she has created her own personal brand of working with patients that she has named "Psycho-energetics". Solange Montakab was the co-founder of the Academy of Chinese Healing Arts and co-author of "Acupuncture for Insomnia". Currently she practices TCM in her private practice in Saviese and is a senior teacher at Chiway Academy of Asian medicine in Winterthur.

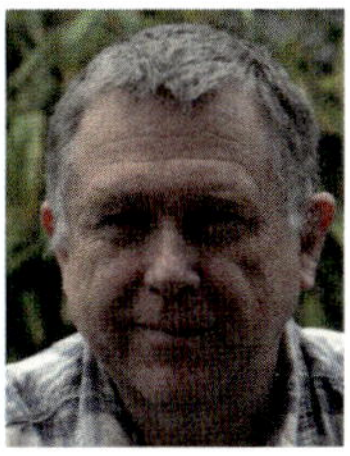

Bernhard Nessensohn – studied Natural Healing in Germany and later graduated in Acupuncture from the Academy of Chinese Healing Arts in Switzerland as well as a teacher's training in *Qi Gong* and Psychosomatics under master Li. He further completed courses in 5-Element and Stems and Branches Acupuncture in Holland with J. Duveen and P. van Kervel as well as *Taiji* with master Fei. He was a board member of the SBO-TCM, and currently is a senior teacher and lecturer at the Academy of Asian medicine in Winterthur. Bernhard Nessensohn has his own private practice in TCM in Heiden, as well as in Holland, where he also teaches Qi Gong and Taiji.

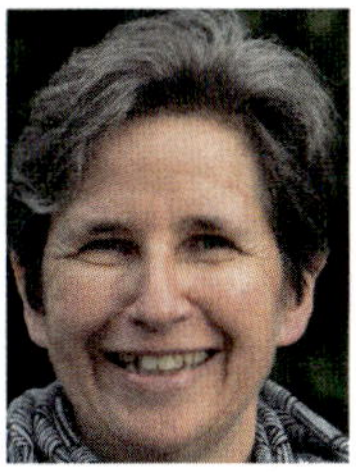

Christine Reist – graduated in Acupuncture and Chinese Herbal Medicine from the Academy of Chinese Healing Arts in Switzerland. Her studies in sinology, social sciences and antroplogy at the university of Zurich are the basis of her knowledge of the Chinese culture and language. For the past 30 years she has practiced *Qi Gong* and *Taijiquan* with various teachers in Switzerland and China, especially Hunyuan-Style *Taijiquan* with Master Feng Zhiqiang. Since 1995 she has been a disciple of Hu Yuexian, younger daughter of the famous martial artist and physician, Hu Yaozhen. With Hu Yuexian's support she practises and teaches Hu Yaozhen's method of medical *Qi Gong*, as well as the application of *Qi Gong* in acupuncture. The exploration of the common roots of these two methods is her main interest and inspires her teachings at the Chiway Academy of Asian medicine in Winterthur.

Made in the USA
Las Vegas, NV
18 May 2026

47218756R00276